Health-Promoting Components of Fruits and Vegetables in Human Health

Special Issue Editors

M. Monica Giusti
Taylor C. Wallace

MDPI • Basel • Beijing • Wuhan • Barcelona • Belgrade

MDPI

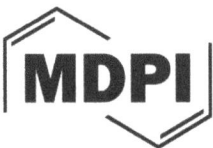

Special Issue Editors

M. Monica Giusti
The Ohio State University
USA

Taylor C. Wallace
George Mason University
USA

Editorial Office
MDPI AG
St. Alban-Anlage 66
Basel, Switzerland

This edition is a reprint of the Special Issue published online in the open access journal *Nutrients* (ISSN 2072-6643) in 2016 (available at: http://www.mdpi.com/journal/nutrients/special_issues/fruits_and_vegetables).

For citation purposes, cite each article independently as indicated on the article page online and as indicated below:

Author 1; Author 2. Article title. *Journal Name* **Year**, *Article number*, page range.

First Edition 2017

ISBN 978-3-03842-628-8 (Pbk)
ISBN 978-3-03842-629-5 (PDF)

Table of Contents

About the Special Issue Editors

M. Monica Giusti, is a Professor at the Food Science and Technology Department, The Ohio State University, and gradate faculty at the Universidad Nacional Agraria, La Molina. Her research is focused on the chemistry and functionality of flavonoids, with emphasis on anthocyanins. Her research has generated over 100 peer-reviewed publications, 2 books and 6 patents. She was named the 2011 TechColumbus Outstanding Woman in Technology, the 2013 OSU Early Career Innovator of the Year and received the 2017 Educator Award from the North American Colleges and Teachers in Agriculture. Dr. Giusti is a member of the American Chemical Society, the Institute of Food Technologists (IFT) and the AOAC. Before joining Ohio State, Dr. Giusti was a faculty member at the University of Maryland. Dr. Giusti, born in Lima, Peru, received a Food Engineer degree from the Universidad Nacional Agraria, Peru and Master's and Doctorate degrees in Food Science from Oregon State University.

Taylor C. Wallace, PhD, CFS, FACN is the Principal and CEO at the Think Healthy Group and a Professor in the Department of Nutrition and Food Studies at George Mason University. His research interests are in the area of nutritional interventions to promote health and prevent the onset of chronic disease. Dr. Wallace's background includes a PhD Food Science and Nutrition from The Ohio State University. Dr. Wallace is a regularly sourced mainstream media expert. In his free time, he manages and operates a large food and nutrition blog (www.DrTaylorWallace.com) that provides science-based nutrition, food safety, and food technology information to the general public. Dr. Wallace is a fellow of the American College of Nutrition (ACN), the 2015 recipient of the Charles A. Regus Award, given by the ACN for original research in the field of nutrition, and the Deputy Editor of the Journal of the American College of Nutrition.

Preface to "Health-Promoting Components of Fruits and Vegetables in Human Health"

It is well accepted that diets rich in colorful fruits and vegetables are linked to health longevity, and a reduced risk for the development of chronic diseases. Fruits and vegetables are major sources of dietary bioactive compounds, defined by the U.S. National Institutes of Health (NIH) as "compounds that are constituents of foods and dietary supplements, other than those needed to meet basic human nutritional needs, which are responsible for changes in health status." These compounds are generally thought to be safe in food at normal consumption levels (e.g., anthocyanins in berries). Their biological activities may be dependant of the presence of a single compound (e.g., lutein in spinach) or class of compounds (e.g., avenanthramides in oats) for which optimal effects may be achieved through consumption of mixtures where the exact identity and composition are often unknown. Classes of similar compounds are commonly found in similar types of plants; however, their ratios and relative concentrations in the food can vary significantly because of environmental influences, such as cultivation, soil, altitude, and weather conditions. Substantial scientific evidence is available for some health promoting bioactives, including dose-response relations, and statistically significant relations with improved physiologic performance and/or reduction in the risk of chronic disease. Although mixtures and/or specific bioactives may have a marked effect on human health, it should be recognized that they are not pharmaceuticals and their intended use should be in helping consumers to achieve healthier lifestyles and maintain or extend normal physiological functions during the process of aging through consumption of fruits and vegetables. Critical to the field of nutrition science will be development of dietary recommendations for bioactives. However, several limitations relating to absorption, distribution, metabolism and excretion of many dietary bioactives still exist and must be better understood in the scientific literature.

This book has the purpose of effectively and accurately communicating modern-day research to a large group of scientific audiences ranging from university classrooms to industry product developers and basic researchers in the fields of nutrition and food science. The search for an international assortment of expert scientists working on the health-promoting components of fruits and vegetables who were qualified to contribute manuscripts to this book were indeed an exciting editorial challenge. The interdisciplinary range of content that is covered by the different manuscripts made this work particularly intellectually stimulating. We would like to personally thank each contributing author for their dedication to producing a high-quality manuscript for this book (a reproduction of a Special Edition of the journal Nutrients). The unique expertise of each distinguished scientist in their particular field makes this book authoritative and cutting-edge.

It is our hope that this book will strengthen our understanding of how many dietary bioactive compounds from fruits and vegetables, influence long-term health maintenance and disease prevention.

M. Monica Giusti and Taylor C. Wallace

Special Issue Editors

nutrients

MDPI

Article

Cancer Prevention and Health Benefices of Traditionally Consumed *Borago officinalis* Plants

María-Dolores Lozano-Baena [1,*,†], Inmaculada Tasset [2,†], Andrés Muñoz-Serrano [3], Ángeles Alonso-Moraga [3] and Antonio de Haro-Bailón [1]

[1]   Department of Plant Breeding, Institute of Sustainable Agriculture, CSIC, Av. Menéndez Pidal s/n, Córdoba E-14004, Spain; adeharobailon@ias.csic.es

[2]   Department of Developmental and Molecular Biology, Institute for Aging Studies, Albert Einstein College of Medicine, 1300 Morris Park Avenue, Bronx, NY 10461, USA; inmaculada.tasset@einstein.yu.edu

[3]   Department of Genetics, Gregor Mendel Building, Faculty of Science, University of Córdoba, Campus Rabanales, Córdoba 14014, Spain; ge1ams@uco.es (A.M.-S.); ge1almoa@uco.es (Á.A.-M.)

*   Correspondence: mdlozano@ias.csic.es; Tel.: +34-957-218-674

†   These authors contributed equally to this work.

Received: 19 November 2015; Accepted: 11 January 2016; Published: 18 January 2016

Abstract: Nowadays, healthy eating is increasing the demand of functional foods by societies as sources of bioactive products with healthy qualities. For this reason, we tested the safety of the consumption of *Borago officinalis* L. and its main phenolic components as well as the possibility of its use as a nutraceutical plant to help in cancer prevention. The *in vivo Drosophila* Somatic Mutation and Recombination Test (SMART) and *in vitro* HL-60 human cell systems were performed, as well-recognized methods for testing genotoxicity/cytotoxicity of bioactive compounds and plant products. *B. officinalis* and the tested compounds possess antigenotoxic activity. Moreover, *B. officinalis* wild type cultivar exerts the most antigenotoxic values. Cytotoxic effect was probed for both cultivars with IC_{50} values of 0.49 and 0.28 mg·mL^{-1} for wild type and cultivated plants respectively, as well as their constituent rosmarinic acid and the assayed phenolic mixture (IC_{50} = 0.07 and 0.04 mM respectively). *B. officinalis* exerts DNA protection and anticarcinogenic effects as do its component rosmarinic acid and the mixture of the main phenolics presented in the plant. In conclusion, the results showed that *B. officinalis* may represent a high value plant for pleiotropic uses and support its consumption as a nutraceutical plant.

Keywords: *Borago officinalis*; health; safety; dietary bioactives; vegetables; SMART; HL-60; cancer prevention

1. Introduction

Healthy eating is one of the most pursued objectives in today's society. The increased demand for food with protection properties against diseases has made herbal products a principal target for industry requirements and government recommendations. In this sense, people usually search for plants according to their well recognized benefits for human health, and most commonly herbal components are considered commercial products [1]. However, reports that show protective effects in some species are often conflicting or present variable results.

Borage (*Borago officinalis* L., *Boraginaceae*), also known as starflower, is a native annual plant in the Mediterranean region that has been used since ancient times for culinary and medicinal purposes, for the treatment of swelling and inflammation, respiratory complaints and melancholy ("I, Borage, bring always courage," translation of the old verse "*Ego borago gaudia semper ago*") [2]. Also, health properties such as anti-obesity, diuretic, emollient, lenitive, laxative, anti-anemic, menstrual analgesic and antipyretic properties are recorded [3–5]. In this sense, borage leaves (>60%

of the plant matter) are considered by industries as a by-product, so it could be used as an economic source of healthy products [6].

Vegetable use of borage is common in Germany (as an ingredient in green sauce, made in Frankfurt), Crete and in the Italian region of Liguria (to fill traditional ravioli pasta). Vegetable borage is also very popular in the cuisine of the Spanish regions of Aragon and Navarra (*i.e.*, boiled and sautéed with garlic, served with potatoes). Borage is used by naturopathic practitioners in the regulation of metabolism and the hormonal system, being considered a good remedy for premenstrual syndrome and menopause symptoms, such as hot flashes [7,8]. In Iran, people make tea (Gol Gav Zaban tea) to relieve colds, flu, bronchitis, rheumatoid arthritis, and kidney inflammation [9]. Recently, interest in borage has been renewed because its seeds appear to be the richest known plant source of gamma linolenic (all *cis*-6,9,12 octadecatrienoic) acid (GLA), which is an intermediate of indispensable compounds in the body, such as prostaglandin E1 and its derivatives [10–14]. All these facts have generated an increasing interest in *B. officinalis* production and researchers are now establishing the best management practices in order to optimize crop performance [15,16]. Furthermore, borage is used by industries as an antioxidant due to its bioactive compound content, *i.e.*, phenolics, responsible for most plant properties [17–19]. The phenolic content of edible parts (leaves and petioles) of *B. officinalis* had been previously determined, with rosmarinic, syringic and sinapic acids being the major phenolics in all plant growth stages [20–22]. These three compounds act as bioactive molecules and exert antioxidant and anti-inflammatory properties [23–25]. Specially, rosmarinic acid is investigated and employed by the food and pharmaceutical industries [26].

The complexity of plant composition and the human digestion process requires validated models that represent this relation as closely and in a manner as valuable for research as possible. For this reason, we have selected the *in vivo Drosophila melanogaster* and *in vitro* HL-60 human cancer cell system as two complementary, sensitive, low-cost and rapid eukaryotic assays, able to detect the potential mutagenic and carcinogenic effects of tested compounds [27–30].

We present the first report proving the antigenotoxic and anticarcinogenic properties of two *B. officinalis* varieties (wild and cultivated) as well as of their major phenolics: rosmarinic, syringic and sinapic acids. Moreover, the interaction between these bioactive compounds is tested, highlighting their potential use and commercialization by industries for products with health benefits as dietary bioactives.

2. Materials and Methods

2.1. Plant Material

Two *Borago officinalis* L. varieties were selected for this work: blue-flowered (BF, wild type, accession Bo IAS 2008-07, collected in Córdoba in December 2009, Southern Spain) and white-flowered (WF type, accession Bo IAS 2008-08, traditionally cultivated in Navarra in December 2009, Northern Spain). These genotypes are part of a *B. officinalis* germplasm bank in the Institute of Sustainable Agriculture (IAS-CSIC, Córdoba, Spain). Plants were grown on an experimental farm at the IAS (N 37°8', W 4°8') wherein climate is typically Mediterranean, with an average annual rainfall of 650 mm. The soil is deep and sandy-loam, classified as a Typic Xerofluvent. Leaves and petioles from 5 plants of each variety were harvested when they reached the optimal stage to be consumed (55 days after sowing), weighed, frozen (24 h at −80 °C) and lyophilized with a freeze-drier Telstar model Cryodos-50 (Telstar, Terrasa, Spain). After lyophilisation, dry material was weighed again, grounded for about 20 s in a Janke and Kunkel Model A10 mill (IKA-Labortechnik, Staufen, Germany), mixed and kept at room temperature and in darkness to preserve their properties until use.

2.2. Chemicals

The single compounds, rosmarinic ($C_{18}H_{16}O_8$), syringic ($C_{19}H_{10}O_5$) and sinapic ($C_{11}H_{12}O_5$) acids, were purchased from Sigma-Aldrich (St. Louis, MO, USA).

2.3. Drosophila Experiments

2.3.1. Fly Stocks and Crosses

The *D. melanogaster* system was selected for the determination of the safety of *B. officinalis* consumption as a well-recognized method to analyze vegetable complex mixtures using SMART [31,32]. This test was used in order to evaluate the genotoxic and antigenotoxic activity of *B. officinalis* leaves and petioles as well as their selected bioactive compounds [33]. This activity was measured by direct visualization of the occurrence of recessive mutations in the wing hairs of two different *D. melanogaster* strains. Flies from experiments carried these visible wing genetic markers: the flare (*flr*) strain *flr³/ln (3LR) TM3, Bdˢ* [34] and the multiple wing-hair (*mwh*) strain *mwh/mwh* [35]. The marker flare (*flr³*, 3_38.3) produces individual malformed hairs and the marker multiple wing hairs (*mwh*, 3_0.3) produces multiple hairs per cell. Larvae used in treatments come from two types of crosses: the standard cross with *flr³/TM3, Bdˢ* females mated to *mwh/mwh* males and the reciprocal cross.

2.3.2. Larvae Treatments

Optimal fertile flies were anesthetized under CO_2 narcotisation for cross selection and then placed in new vials for fertilization. After that, hybrid eggs from crossing were collected over an 8 h period and emerged larvae (72 $\pm$ 4 h later) were cleaned up for a few seconds in sterile distilled water to remove feeding medium rests [33]. For genotoxicity analysis (simple treatments), groups of 100 larvae were transferred into vials containing 0.85 g of *Drosophila* Instant Medium (Formula 4–24, Carolina Biological Supply, Burlington, NC, USA) wetted with 4 mL of a mixture of distilled water and increasing concentrations of samples: *B. officinalis* BF and WF (1.25, 2.5, and 5 mg·mL^{-1}), RO (0.35, 0.7, 1.39 and 2.78 mM), SY (0.16, 0.32, 0.63 and 1.26 mM), SI (0.15, 0.29, 0.58 and 1.16 mM) and the mixture of these three bioactive compounds at each concentration assayed individually. Bioactive compound concentrations were chosen on the basis of their known content in *B. officinalis* species [11]. For antigenotoxicity analysis (combined treatments) the same number of vials were prepared but treatment media were mixed with H_2O_2 0.12 M as mutagenic agent. Vials with the medium mixed with distilled water or H_2O_2 (0.12 M) were used as negative and positive controls respectively. Larvae were fed on these media until pupation (about 48 h). After emergence, resulting adult flies were sacrificed under CO_2 narcotisation and stored in a 70% ethanol solution in sterile water. Emerged adults were counted for toxicity evaluation and transheterozygous wings (*mwh flr⁺/mwh⁺ flr³*) were mounted on microscope slides and wing hair mutations (spots) scored, using a photonic microscope (Nikon) at 400× magnification for genotoxicity and antigenotoxicity evaluation.

2.4. HL-60 Experiments

2.4.1. Cell Cultures

The human acute promyelocytic leukemia cell line HL-60 was routinely grown in suspension in RPMI medium (Invitrogen, Madrid, Spain) containing glutamine (200 mM, Sigma-Aldrich, St. Louis, MO, USA), antibiotics (100IU penicillin mL^{-1} and 100 µg streptomycin mL^{-1}, Sigma-Aldrich) and supplemented with 10% heat-inactivated foetal bovine serum (Linus, Cultek, Madrid, Spain) and placed in an incubator (Shel Lab, Cornelious, OR, USA) with a 5% CO_2 humidified atmosphere at 37 °C [36]. HL-60 cells were subcultured every 2–3 days to maintain logarithmic growth and they were allowed to grow for 48 h before use [37]. Cultures were plated at a density of 12.5×10^4 cells mL^{-1} in 40 mL culture flasks (25 cm^2).

2.4.2. Cell Treatments

Cytotoxic activity was measured as growing inhibition or decreased viability on HL-60 cells following a previous protocol modified by us [38]. For assays, cells were placed in 12-well culture plates (1×10^5 cells mL^{-1}; final volume = 2 mL per well) and treated with different filtered

(Millipore "non-pyrogenic", "sterile-R", 0.2 μm filter) RPMI solutions with the selected concentrations of *B. officinalis* BF and WF plant samples (0.125, 0.25, 0.5, 1 and 2 mg· mL^{-1}), RO (0.07, 0.14, 0.28, 0.55, 1.1 and 2.2 mM), SY (0.03, 0.06, 0.13, 0.25, 0.5 and, 1 mM), SI (0.03, 0.06, 0.12, 0.23, 0.5 and, 1 mM) and the mixture of these three bioactive compounds at each individually assayed concentration. Cells were counted after 72 h treatment. Tested concentrations were calculated according to those used for *in vivo* assays to equal the range of tested doses. Untreated cultures were used as negative control.

2.4.3. Trypan Blue Dye Exclusion Assay

Cell viability was determined by the Trypan Blue dye exclusion test. Cells were stained with an equal volume of Trypan Blue commercial solution (Sigma-Aldrich) and counted using a hemocytometer at room temperature under a light inverted microscope (AE30/31, Motic, Barcelona, Spain).

2.5. Statistical Analysis

The determination of Toxicity (T) of treatments in *D. melanogaster* was performed following this formula [39]:

$$T = (N° \text{ of emerging individuals in treatment}/N° \text{ of emerging individuals in the negative control}) \times 100 \qquad (1)$$

Differences in *D. melanogaster* survival between treatments at each concentration with respect to negative control were analyzed with a Chi-square test. This procedure was also performed for the analysis of each simple treatment with their correspondent combined treatment.

For the evaluation of genotoxic effects, the frequencies of spots per fly of each treated series were compared to the concurrent negative control for each class of mutational clone as well as between simple and combined treatments for the same concentration comparisons. Spots were grouped into three different categories: single (a small single spot corresponding to one or two cells exhibiting the *mwh* phenotype), large (a large single spot corresponding to three or more cells showing *mwh* or *flr³* phenotypes) and twin (a large spot corresponding to three or more cells showing adjacent both *mwh* and *flr³* phenotypes). A multiple-decision procedure was used to categorize results as positive, inconclusive or negative [40]. Inconclusive and positive results were evaluated by the non-parametric *U* test of Mann, Whitney and Wilcoxon [41]. The inhibition percentage (IP) of genotoxicity was calculated from the total frequencies of spots per wing, following this formula [42]:

$$IP = (\text{genotoxin alone} - \text{sample} + \text{genotoxin}) \times 100/(\text{genotoxin alone}) \qquad (2)$$

Significant differences of IP for each treatment respect to the positive control were analyzed with a Chi-square test.

Cytotoxic effect evaluation was determined after each culture incubation period, establishing a growth curve and determining IC$_{50}$ values by regression analysis of the curves. Viability estimated regressions of leukemia cells are presented as a survival percentage with respect to controls at 72 h growth and plotted as mean viability $\pm$ standard error of at least three independent replicas for each treatment and concentration.

Statistical analyses were performed using a Microsoft 2007 Excel spreadsheet. The non-parametric U test of Mann, Whitney and Wilcoxon was performed with the SPSS Statistic 17.0 software (SPSS, Inc., Chicago, IL, USA).

3. Results and Discussion

3.1. In Vivo *Assays*

Tables 1–3 show the results obtained in *D. melanogaster* experiments for edible leaves and petioles of *B. officinalis* of the selected varieties, blue flowered (BF) and white flowered (WF), and their bioactive compounds, rosmarinic (RO), syringic (SY) and sinapic (SI) acids. The negative controls produced mutation rates which fall into the normal range obtained in other laboratories, thus the data in discussion comply with the expected spots per wing with no anomalous or borderline controls [43,44]. The positive control used in this study was hydrogen peroxide (H_2O_2). This oxidative mutagen has been used in many mutation assays and it is known that an excess of H_2O_2 can influence the expression of a high number of genes [45]. As previously reported, H_2O_2 affects *D. melanogaster* survival and creates an excess of small single spots, with no significant induction of twin spot excess [29,39]. The genotoxic results for H_2O_2 validate the assay as an appropriate system for screening between mutagens (positive controls as H_2O_2) and non-mutagens (water controls or safe plants and bioactive compounds).

Table 1. Toxicity of *Borago officinalis* plant material, blue flowered (BF) and white flowered (WF), and the bioactive compounds, rosmarinic (RO), syringic (SY) and sinapic (SI) acids.

				Survival [1] % Treatments			
	Simple		Combined [2]		Simple		Combined [2]
H_2O		100		H_2O_2 (0.12 M)		37.87 *	
	BF (mg·mL^{-1})				WF (mg·mL^{-1})		
1.25		100	52.44 *,‡	1.25		97.78	33.33 *,‡
2.5		100	54 *,‡	2.5		63.11 *	27.56 *,‡
5		82 *	86.89 *	5		71.33 *	17.33 *,‡
	RO (mM)				SY (mM)		
0.35		48.44 *	49.56 *	0.16		39.78 *	31.11 *,‡
0.7		22.22 *	31.11 *,‡	0.32		42.67 *	29.33 *,‡
1.39		33.33 *	45.56 *,‡	0.63		31.11 *	20.44 *,‡
2.78		21.33 *	38.89 *,‡	1.26		58.22 *	36.89 *,‡
	SI (mM)				RO + SY + SI (mM)		
0.15		78.22 *	64 *,‡	a [3]		48.67 *	24.44 *,‡
0.29		60.22 *	58.89 *	b		55.11 *	34.67 *,‡
0.58		69.33 *	39.78 *,‡	c		74.44 *	57.78 *,‡
1.16		55.11 *	43.56 *,‡	d		44.89 *	53.78 *,‡

[1] Survival expressed in percentage as total emerged adults of each treatment with respect to H_2O control total emerged adults; [2] Combined treatments using standard medium and 0.12 M H_2O_2; [3] Letters *a–d* correspond to the lowest, two intermediate and highest concentrations respectively assayed for each single compound once their mixture is assayed; * Significance levels with respect to the negative control (untreated, H_2O) group ($p \leqslant 0.05$); ‡ Significance levels between simple and combined treatment for the same concentration comparisons ($p \leqslant 0.05$).

Table 2. Genotoxicity of *Borago officinalis* plant material: blue flowered (BF) and white flowered (WF); and the bioactive compounds: rosmarinic (RO), syringic (SY) and sinapic (SI) acids.

		Mutation Rate (Spots/Wing) Diagnosis [1]			
	N° of Wings	Small Single Spots 1–2 Cells $m = 2$	Large Single Spots >2 Cells $m = 5$	Twin Spots $m = 5$	Total Spots $m = 2$
H_2O	212	0.26 (54)	0.04 (8)	0.03 (5)	0.32 (67)
H_2O_2 (0.12 M)	168	0.60 (94) +	0.07 (11) −	0.06 (4) −	0.65 (109) +
		BF (mg·mL^{-1})			
1.25	40	0.13 (5) −	0.03 (1) −	0.05 (2) −	0.20 (8) −
2.5	54	0.22 (12) −	0.06 (3) −	0.02 (1) −	0.30 (16) −
5	66	0.29 (19) −	0.03 (2) −	0.05 (3) −	0.36 (24) −
		WF (mg·mL^{-1})			
1.25	66	0.26 (17) −	0.03 (2) −	0.05 (3) −	0.33 (22) −
2.5	50	0.26 (13) −	0.08 (4) −	0.02 (1) −	0.36 (18) −
5	90	0.36 (32) −	0.02 (2) −	0.01 (1) −	0.39 (35) −

Table 2. *Cont.*

		Mutation Rate (Spots/Wing) Diagnosis [1]			
	N° of Wings	Small Single Spots 1–2 Cells $m = 2$	Large Single Spots >2 Cells $m = 5$	Twin Spots $m = 5$	Total Spots $m = 2$
		RO (mM)			
0.35	16	0.38 (6) −	0	0	0.38 (6) −
0.7	34	0.21 (7) −	0	0.06 (2) −	0.26 (9) −
1.39	22	0.18 (4) −	0	0.05 (1) −	0.23 (5) −
2.78	38	0.16 (6) −	0.05 (2) −	0	0.21 (8) −
		SY (mM)			
0.16	40	0.30 (12) −	0.05 (2) −	0.03 (1) −	0.38 (15) −
0.32	30	0.20 (6) −	0.07 (2) −	0	0.27 (8) −
0.63	48	0.19 (9) −	0.02 (1) −	0	0.21 (10) −
1.26	32	0.22 (7) −	0.06 (2) −	0	0.28 (9) −
		SI (mM)			
0.15	24	0.38 (9) −	0.04 (1) −	0.04 (1) −	0.46 (11) −
0.29	32	0.39 (12) −	0.10 (3) −	0	0.48 (15) −
0.58	30	0.33 (10) −	0.07 (2) −	0	0.40 (12) −
1.16	40	0.23 (9) −	0.03 (1) −	0.03 (1) −	0.28 (11) −
		RO + SY + SI (mM)			
a [2]	26	0.15 (4) −	0	0.04 (1) −	0.19 (5) −
b	34	0.12 (4) −	0.03 (1) −	0	0.15 (5) −
c	32	0.22 (7) −	0.13 (4) +	0	0.34 (11) −
d	22	0.41 (9) −	0.05 (1) −	0	0.45 (10) −

[1] Statistical diagnoses: + (positive) and − (negative) [40,41]. Significance levels $\alpha = \beta = 0.05$, one-sided test without Bonferroni correction; [2] Letters *a–d* correspond to the lowest, two intermediate and highest concentrations respectively assayed for each single compound once their mixture is assayed.

Table 3. Antigenotoxicity of *Borago officinalis* plant material: blue flowered (BF) and white flowered (WF); and the bioactive compounds: rosmarinic (RO), syringic (SY) and sinapic (SI) acids.

		Mutation Rate (Spots/Wing) Diagnosis [1]			
	N° of Wings	Small Single Spots 1–2 Cells $m = 2$	Large Single Spots >2 Cells $m = 5$	Twin Spots $m = 5$	Total Spots $m = 2$
H_2O	212	0.26 (54)	0.04 (8)	0.03 (5)	0.32 (67)
H_2O_2 (0.12 M)	168	0.60 (94) +	0.07 (11) −	0.06 (4) −	0.65 (109) +
		BF $(mg \cdot mL^{-1})$			
1.25	30	0.13 (4) −	0.03 (1) −	0	0.17 (5) −
2.5	34	0.24 (8) −	0.03 (1) −	0	0.26 (9) −
5	18	0.17 (3) −	0.06 (1) −	0	0.23 (4) −
		WF $(mg \cdot mL^{-1})$			
1.25	10	0.30 (3) −	0.10 (1) −	0	0.40 (4) −
2.5	28	0.32 (9) −	0	0	0.32 (9) −
5	24	0.25 (6) −	0.04 (1) −	0	0.29 (7) −
		RO (mM)			
0.35	30	0.17 (5) −	0	0	0.17 (5) −
0.7	40	0.35 (14) −	0.08 (3) −	0.03 (1) −	0.45 (18) −
1.39	22	0.14 (3) −	0.14 (3) −	0	0.27 (6) −
2.78	52	0.21 (11) −	0	0.04 (2) −	0.25 (13) −
		SY (mM)			
0.16	22	0.23 (5) −	0	0	0.23 (5) −
0.32	10	0.30 (3) −	0	0	0.30 (3) −
0.63	32	0.28 (9) −	0	0	0.28 (9) −
1.26	22	0.32 (7) −	0	0	0.32 (7) −

Table 3. *Cont.*

| | N° of Wings | Mutation Rate (Spots/Wing) Diagnosis [1] | | | |
		Small Single Spots 1–2 Cells $m = 2$	Large Single Spots >2 Cells $m = 5$	Twin Spots $m = 5$	Total Spots $m = 2$
		SI (mM)			
0.15	12	0.42 (5) −	0	0	0.42 (5) −
0.29	8	0.25 (2) −	0	0	0.25 (2) −
0.58	22	0.27 (6) −	0.09 (2) −	0.05 (1) −	0.41 (9) −
1.16	28	0.25 (7) −	0.04 (1) −	0	0.29 (8) −
		RO + SY + SI (mM)			
a [2]	38	0.29 (11) −	0	0	0.29 (11) −
b	26	0.27 (7) −	0.15 (4) +	0	0.42 (11) −
c	17	0.18 (3) −	0	0	0.18 (3) −
d	12	0.25 (3) −	0.08 (1) −	0	0.33 (4) −

[1] Statistical diagnoses: + (positive) and − (negative) [40,41]. Significance levels $\alpha = \beta = 0.05$, one-sided test without Bonferroni correction; [2] Letters *a–d* correspond to the lowest, two intermediate and highest concentrations respectively assayed for each single compound once their mixture is assayed.

3.1.1. Toxicity Assays

Table 1 summarizes the toxicity results obtained for analyzed samples expressed as percentage of emerged adults from treatment compared with the emerged adults from the negative control (survival control corrected).

All treatments at all assayed concentrations significantly affected *D. melanogaster* survival except plant samples of *B. officinalis* BF at concentrations 1.25 and 2.5 mg·mL^{-1} and *B. officinalis* WF at 1.25 mg·mL^{-1}. The highest concentration of *B. officinalis* BF reduced the *D. melanogaster* survival to less than 20%. Intermediate and highest *B. officinalis* WF assayed concentrations decreased *D. melanogaster* survival to 63.11% and 71.33% respectively. Regarding borage toxicity, the American Herbal Products Association's Botanical Safety Handbook recommends *Borago* ssp. leaf consumption sporadically due to their pyrrolizidine alkaloid content [46,47]. However, current revisions of *Borago* ssp. properties suggest that the complex bioactive compound leaf composition of this species is more beneficial than harmful for human health because of its phenolic content [3]. This fact could explain the difference we have found between *B. officinalis* BF and WF toxicity levels. On average, the bioactive compounds reduced *D. melanogaster* larval survival by around 50% (LD$_{50}$), normal values for toxicity assays and no dose effect was observed. RO showed the largest reduction in survival, with the highest RO concentration being the most toxic treatment (21.33%). Other authors have also found RO toxicity by oral administration [48]. However, these authors recommend the use of RO in human inflammatory diseases because of its protective effect in the stomach unlike commonly used anti-inflammatory products that possess serious disadvantages for human health. The addition of H$_2$O$_2$ to the medium in combined treatments contributed to reducing *D. melanogaster* larval survival in all samples when compared to simple treatments, with the exception of the highest *B. officinalis* BF concentration as well as all RO assayed concentrations and highest mixture concentration. These treatments had a protective effect against H$_2$O$_2$ damage (detoxification), interfering with H$_2$O$_2$ oxidative action and slightly increasing *D. melanogaster* larval survival. Nevertheless, only in the case of RO treatments this effect was significant. Contrarily, the application of RO mixed with SY and SI (mixture treatment) did not present any protective additive effects with the exception of highest tested concentration. Thus, the addition of H$_2$O$_2$ to the medium in mixture treatments reduced *D. melanogaster* survival to a greater degree than applying RO alone in combined treatments. However, the mixture survival ended up quite similar to RO survival in combined treatments (survival average of 42.67 and 41.28 respectively). Previous reports showed that the *B. officinalis* beneficial effect on health depends on the composition of phenolics having synergic effects [20,49]. This fact could explain why the mixture of selected bioactive compounds did not exert the same protective effects as RO when it is added alone to a larvae feeding medium in combined treatments. *B. officinalis* WF treatments resulted in the highest survival reduction (average of 66.32%) when combining with H_2O_2. Moreover, the combined (H_2O_2) treatment at the highest *B. officinalis* WF concentration produced the highest reduction of *D. melanogaster* survival decreasing this value to 17.33%. The H_2O_2 toxic effect was enhanced also by lowest and intermediate *B. officinalis* BF concentrations with an average survival reduction of ~50%.

3.1.2. Genotoxicity Assays

Table 2 summarizes the genotoxicity results obtained in the Somatic Mutation and Recombination Test (SMART) as total mutations per wing observed in treatments with *B. officinalis* plant and bioactive compound samples.

It is remarkable that no concentration of plant samples was significantly different from the negative control, but contrarily, some of the treatments showed lower mutation rates (from 0.20 to 0.30) than the negative control (0.32). Although a healthy and non-genotoxic effect of many herbal products is generally expected, it is necessary to empirically check this assumption for parts of the plants that are usually consumed [1,50]. This result is also displayed for plant phenolic products for which pharmacological potential has been widely tested but no complete understanding of their mechanism of action has been elucidated [51].

At present, very little is known about the lack of genotoxicity of *B. officinalis* plants with no direct work reporting genotoxic effects, although a previous work determined the genotoxicity of pirrolizidine alkaloids (compounds present in *B. officinalis* plants) using SMART [52]. This work classified pirrolizidine compounds as genotoxic but this effect varied widely depending on their chemical structures. Similarly to the plant sample results, the main bioactive constituents of *B. officinalis*, RO, SY and SI phenols, were not mutagenic in the *Drosophila* wing spot test as expected from the negative results for the plant. A multitude of beneficial biological activities have been described for RO (astringent, antioxidative, anti-inflammatory, antimutagen, antibacterial and antiviral), so the non-mutagenic results obtained in the wing spot test were expected [24]. Our results also agree with those of Pereira *et al.* [53] that showed no genotoxic effect of RO (doses of 2 and 8 mg·kg^{-1}) using the comet assay in brain tissue and peripheral blood in rats. In conclusion, *B. officinalis* plants and their selected components did not exert any DNA damage on the *mwh/flr* eukaryotic system of *D. melanogaster*.

3.1.3. Antigenotoxicity Assays

In this work we present results on the antigenotoxic activity of *B. officinalis* leaves and petioles which could be considered as a health benefits index. Our results for combined treatments in the SMART, showed in Table 3, account for the desmutagenic activity of the selected substances when assayed against H_2O_2.

The inhibition percentage (IP) ranged between 30.77% and 73.85% in tested samples. The highest detoxification potential appeared in the highest *B. officinalis* BF concentration (Figure 1a) as well as RO at 0.35 mM (Figure 2a). The lowest detoxification potential corresponded to RO treatments at 0.7 mM (Figure 2a). All these samples corresponded to combined treatments (adding H_2O_2 to samples). No dose effect relationship was observed. The detoxifying ability of highest *B. officinalis* BF and lowest RO assayed concentrations against mutations produced by H_2O_2 can be explained by the direct interaction of phenols contained in the plants which act as scavengers of reactive oxygen species before the larvae uptake and H_2O_2 reaches the DNA [54]. In this respect, RO, SY and SI behaved as desmutagens with a high antioxidative capacity, which has also been shown when they are extracted from borage defatted seeds [55].

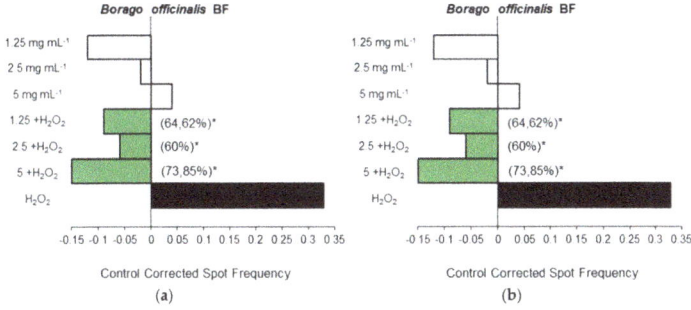

Figure 1. Antigenotoxic activity of *Borago officinalis* plant material: (**a**) blue flowered (BF) and (**b**) white flowered (WF) plant material expressed as mutation frequency corrected to control. Strength of inhibition on the capability of H_2O_2 (0.12 M) to induce mutated cells is also shown (Inhibition Percentage in brackets). White columns correspond with tested concentrations of simple treatments, green with combined treatments and black with spot frequencies induced by H_2O_2. * Significance levels with respect to the positive control (H_2O_2) group ($p \leqslant 0.05$).

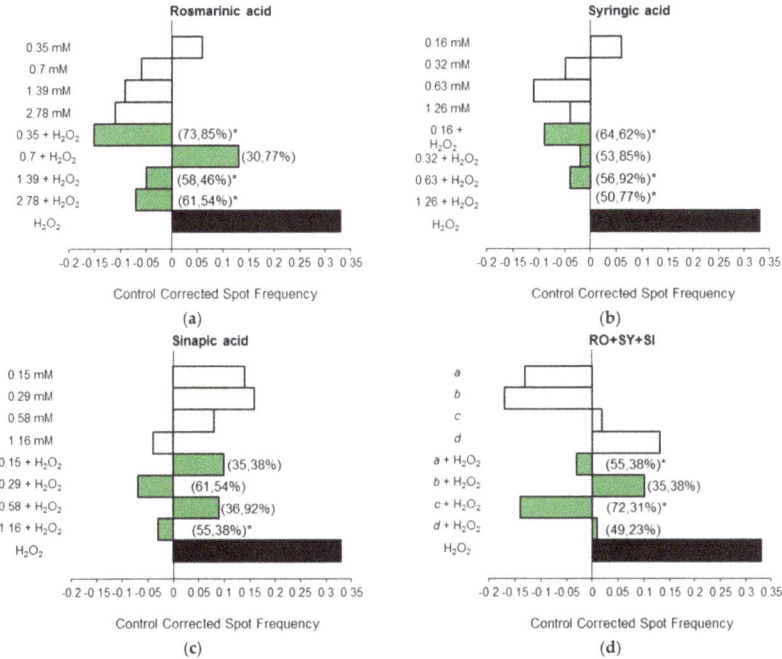

Figure 2. Antigenotoxic activity of *Borago officinalis* bioactive compounds: (**a**) RO; (**b**) SY; (**c**) SI and (**d**) mixture (RO + SY + SI) expressed as mutation frequency corrected to control. Strength of inhibition on the capability of H_2O_2 (0.12 M) to induce mutated cells is also shown (Inhibition Percentage in brackets). Light green columns correspond with tested concentrations of simple treatments, green with combined treatments and black column corresponds to spot frequencies induced by H_2O_2. Letters *a–d* in graphic (**d**) correspond to the lowest, two intermediate and highest concentrations respectively assayed for each single compound once their mixture is assayed. * Significance levels with respect to the positive control (H_2O_2) group ($p \leqslant 0.05$).

Our results for RO bioactive compound are in accordance with prior reports showing its protective effect against H_2O_2 damage in other *in vivo* systems like rats as well as *in vitro* systems [56,57]. This antigenotoxic effect has also been demonstrated against the DNA damage brought on by the mutagen ethyl methanesulfonate in males from *D. melanogaster* using the sex-linked recessive lethal (SLRL) test [58]. The other phenolics assayed, SY and SI, possess lower antigenotoxic activity with SI being the least effective in reducing mutations induced by H_2O_2 (Figure 2b,c). In accordance with these results, SI has been recently used in order to determine its genotoxic/antigenotoxic activity in the V79 cell line [59]. This phenolic was found to be antigenotoxic but in a way that depends on the dose, with the lower concentrations (below 2 mM, as our assayed concentrations) being those that significantly reduce DNA damage. As discussed for toxicity results, no additive effect in phenolic mixture was found in any assayed concentration (Figure 2d). In this sense, phenolic borage content varies depending on the plant stage, tested phenolics being the major bioactive constituents during plant growth [20,49]. This fact might suggest that the antigenotoxic effect found in our samples corresponds to a specific phenolic or the addition of each phenolic effect. However, our results showed that phenolic effects are not additives but synergic.

3.2. In Vitro Assays

Cytotoxicity Assays

The human acute promyelocytic leukemia cell line HL-60 has been used as a model on a wide variety of substances that are candidates to be used as anticarcinogens and has proved to be a robust test system for pilot screening experiments [30,39,60]. That is why we have selected this system to elucidate the inhibitory capacity of tumour growth for the different samples studied. Our results are shown in Figure 3 as the relative HL-60 growth rate with different concentrations of *B. officinalis* BF and WF plant samples and their main active components (RO, SY and SI) regarding their concurrent control cultures.

A dose-response curve was observed for *B. officinalis* BF and WF plant material (Figure 3a,b) which exhibited IC_{50} values of 0.49 and 0.28 mg·mL^{-1} respectively. This cytotoxic effect of borage was also found in the Vero line of African green monkey kidney cells with an IC_{50} value of 0.2 mg·mL^{-1} (similar to that obtained for our borage WF samples) [61].

In the case of phenolic compounds, the IC_{50} could only be determined for RO (0.07 mM) and mixture (0.04 mM of RO equivalent units) samples with a marked slope in the case of phenol mixture. Interestingly, no viable cells could be detected when RO was added to the cell medium (alone or in the mixture) at concentrations over 0.55 mM (Figure 3c,f). Other studied cancer cell lines have been shown to be more sensitive to RO exposure than HL-60 cells, a fact that enhances the disease prevention properties of RO [62,63]. Also, *in vivo* studies in mice conclude that the RO anticarcinogenic activity is related to the activity of this phenol in inhibiting inflammation and scavenging reactive oxygen species [64]. In our experiments, the phenols SY and SI did not affect HL-60 growth (Figure 3d,e). The lack of cytotoxicity in HL-60 experiments that we have found for SY is in accordance with previous determination that indicated no cytotoxic effect of SY in extracts of *Elaphomyces granulates* at concentrations up to ~31 µg·mL^{-1} using this cell line [65]. Moreover, Fabiani *et al.* [66] found that SY did not induce apoptosis in HL-60 cell when is applied to the cell medium at a concentration of 0.1 mM. It has been reported that SI biotransformation by plant peroxidases results in an anticarcinogenic effect from its derivates in HL-60 cells [67]. This fact could explain the difference that we found between its antigenotoxic effect in *D. melanogaster* individuals and the lack of SI cytotoxicity in HL-60 cells, SI derivates being responsible for healthy actions instead of the phenol. As in the case of antigenotoxicity experiments, the cytotoxic effect of the mixture did not correspond to the addition of each individually assayed phenolic. Moreover, the fact that mixture samples presented the highest anticarcinogenic effect proves that the phenolic mixture produces a synergic healthy effect.

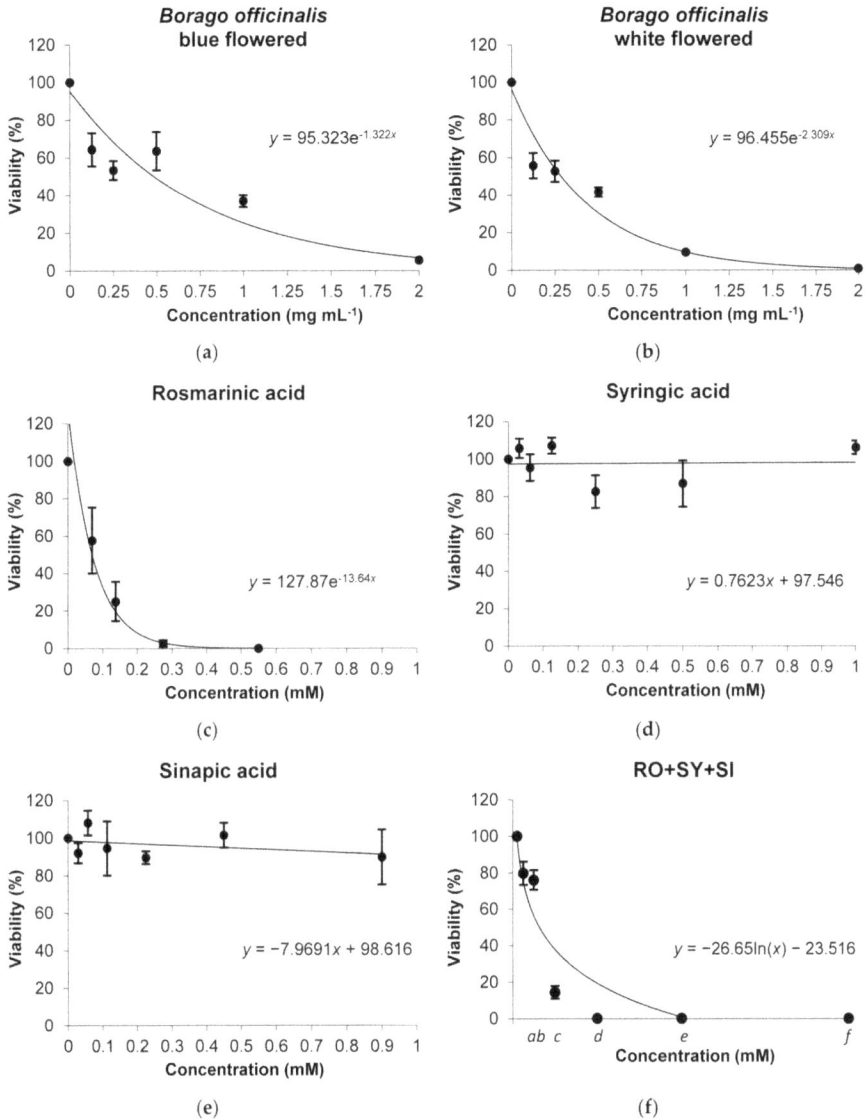

Figure 3. Survival of HL-60 cultures treated with different concentrations of: *Borago officinalis* (**a**) blue flowered (BF) and (**b**) white flowered (WF) plant material; and bioactive compounds: (**c**) RO; (**d**) SY; (**e**) SI and (**f**) mixture (RO + SY + SI; italic letters from *a–f* correspond to the concentrations respectively assayed for each single compound once their mixture is assayed.). Survival estimated regressions are plotted as percentages with respect to the control counted from at least three independent experiments (mean ± SD).

4. Conclusions

We have provided a primer on antigenotoxicity and tumoricide activities of edible parts (leaves and petioles) of two borage varieties and some of its bioactive principles. The *in vivo* assays showed their safe use for human consumption and their antigenotoxicity potency, supporting their protective DNA damage activity and consequently their health benefits. Our results in the *in vitro* assays highlight *B. officinalis* fresh plant use as a nutraceutical plant and as a potential source of dietary bioactives with an outstanding anticarcinogenic activity. In this sense, *B. officinalis* is a desirable Mediterranean plant adapted to the European climate and a good source of pharmaceutical products, which has made *B. officinalis* a fashionable topic in plant research. Borage breeders have to take this eventual insight as a unique opportunity. Exploitation of this vegetable could be focused on a dual perspective: on the one hand, these cultivars could be partially used for bioactive resources and on the other, as a part for growing a unique plant. The wide spread of *B. officinalis* cultivars for industrial purposes should be used to advise world markets about the pleiotropic uses of this vegetable, not only as a source of products but also as a nutraceutical fresh-consumed plant.

In brief, the varieties studied here show that *B. officinalis* could be put on the table not as a silent partner with other vegetables but as something more than a salad due to its protective and chemopreventive activities.

Acknowledgments: Acknowledgments: We are grateful to C. Gómez-Díaz (S.C.A.I., University of Córdoba, Spain) for supplying HL-60 cell line. This work was supported by the Andalusian Government (Research Project PAI 07-AGR-02759). We thank Eileen Brophy for the grammatical revision of the text.

Author Contributions: Author Contributions: Authors who: (1) conceived and designed the experiments: A.H.-B., Á.A.-M.; (2) performed the experiments: M.-D.L.-B., I.T.; (3) analyzed the data: M.-D.L.-B., Á.A.-M., A.M.-S.; (4) contributed reagents/materials/analysis tools: A.H.-B., Á.A.-M.; (5) wrote the paper: M.-D.L.-B., Á.A.-M., A.H.-B. All authors have read and approved the final manuscript.

Conflicts of Interest: Conflicts of Interest: The authors declare no conflict of interest. The founding sponsors had no role in the design of the study; in the collection, analyses, or interpretation of data; in the writing of the manuscript, and in the decision to publish the results.

Abbreviations

BF	*Borago officinalis* blue-flowered
CO_2	carbon dioxide
DNA	deoxyribonucleic acid
flr	flare
H_2O_2	hydrogen peroxide
HL-60	human acute promyelocytic leukemia cell line
IC_{50}	half maximal inhibitory concentration
IP	inhibition percentage
LD_{50}	median lethal dose
mwh	multiple wing-hair
RO	rosmarinic acid
SI	sinapic acid
SMART	somatic mutation and recombination test
SY	syringic acid
T	toxicity
WF	*Borago officinalis* white-flowered

References

1. Zhou, S.; Koh, H.L.; Gao, Y.; Gong, Z.Y.; Lee, E.J.D. Herbal bioactivation: The good, the bad and the ugly. *Life Sci.* **2004**, *74*, 935–968. [CrossRef] [PubMed]
2. Gerard, J. *The History of Plants*; Woodward, M., Ed.; Senate, Studio Editions Ltd.: London, UK, 1927; pp. 185–186.
3. Basar, S.N.; Rani, S.; Farah, S.A.; Zaman, R. Review on *Borago officinalis*: A Wonder Herb. *Int. J. Biol. Pharm. Res.* **2013**, *4*, 582–587.

4. Leporatti, M.L.; Ivancheva, S. Preliminary comparative analysis of medicinal plants used in the traditional medicine of Bulgaria and Italy. *J. Ethnopharmacol.* **2003**, *87*, 123–142. [CrossRef]
5. Marrelli, M.; Loizzo, M.R.; Nicoletti, M.; Menichini, F.; Conforti, F. *In vitro* investigation of the potential health benefits of wild Mediterranean dietary plants as anti-obesity agents with alpha-amylase and pancreatic lipase inhibitory activities. *J. Sci. Food Agric.* **2014**, *94*, 2217–2224. [CrossRef] [PubMed]
6. De Ciriano, M.G.I.; García-Herreros, C.; Larequi, E.; Valencia, I.; Ansorena, D.; Astiasarán, I. Use of natural antioxidants from lyophilized water extracts of *Borago officinalis* in dry fermented sausages enriched in ω-3 PUFA. *Meat Sci.* **2009**, *83*, 271–277. [CrossRef] [PubMed]
7. Barre, D. Potential of evening primrose, borage, black currant, and fungal oils in human health. *Ann. Nutr. Metab.* **2001**, *45*, 47–57. [CrossRef] [PubMed]
8. Bendich, A. The potential for dietary supplements to reduce premenstrual syndrome (PMS) symptoms. *J. Am. Coll. Nutr.* **2000**, *19*, 3–12. [CrossRef] [PubMed]
9. Simmons, S. *A Treasury of Persian Cuisine*, 2nd ed.; Stamford House Publishing: Hong Kong, China, 2007.
10. Del Río-Celestino, M.; Font, R.; de Haro-Bailón, A. Distribution of the fatty acids content in edible organs and seed fractions of borage (*Borago officinalis* L.). *J. Sci. Food Agric.* **2008**, *88*, 248–255. [CrossRef]
11. Guil-Guerrero, J.L.; García-Maroto, F.; Vilches-Ferrón, M.A.; López-Alonso, D. Gamma-linolenic acid from fourteen *Boraginaceae* species. *Ind. Crops Prod.* **2003**, *18*, 85–89. [CrossRef]
12. Gunstone, F.D. Gamma-linolenic acid—Occurrence and physical and chemical properties. *Prog. Lipid Res.* **1992**, *31*, 145–161. [CrossRef]
13. Janick, J.; Simon, J.E.; Quinn, J.; Beaubaire, N. Borage: A source of gamma-linolenic acid. In *Herbs, Spices and Medicinal Plants*; Cracker, L.E., Simon, J.E., Eds.; Oryx Press: Phoenix, Arizona, 1989; Volume 4, pp. 145–168.
14. Jaramillo, G.; Vilela, A. Critical size for reproduction and ontogenetic changes in the allocation patterns of wild and domesticated species of evening primrose (*Oenothera* L.). *Ind. Crop. Prod.* **2015**, *65*, 324–327. [CrossRef]
15. El Hafid, R.; Blade, S.F.; Hoyano, Y. Seeding date and nitrogen fertilization effects on the performance of borage (*Borago officinalis* L.). *Ind. Crop. Prod.* **2002**, *16*, 193–199. [CrossRef]
16. Gilbertson, P.K.; Berti, M.T.; Johnson, B.L. Borage cardinal germination temperatures and seed development. *Ind. Crop. Prod.* **2014**, *59*, 202–209. [CrossRef]
17. Asadi-Samani, M.; Bahmani, M.; Rafieian-Kopaei, M. The chemical composition, botanical characteristic and biological activities of *Borago officinalis*: A review. *Asian Pac. J. Trop. Med.* **2014**, *7*, S22–S28. [CrossRef]
18. Segovia, F.; Lupo, B.; Peiró, S.; Gordon, M.H.; Almajano, M.P. Extraction of antioxidants from borage (*Borago officinalis* L.) leaves—Optimization by response surface method and application in oil-in-water emulsions. *Antioxidants* **2015**, *3*, 339–357. [CrossRef]
19. Zemmouri, H.; Ammar, S.; Boumendjel, A.; Messarah, M.; el Feki, A.; Bouaziz, M. Chemical composition and antioxidant activity of *Borago officinalis* L. leaf extract growing in Algeria. *Arabian J. Chem.* **2014**. [CrossRef]
20. Mhamdi, W.; Aidi, W.W.; Chahed, T.; Ksouri, R.; Marzouk, B. Phenolic compounds and antiradical scavenging activity changes during *Borago officinalis* stalk leaf development. *Asian J. Chem.* **2010**, *22*, 6397–6402.
21. Chlopcíková, S.; Psotová, J.; Miketová, P.; Sousek, J.; Lichnovský, V.; Simánek, V. Chemoprotective effect of plant phenolics against anthracycline-induced toxicity on rat cardiomyocytes. Part II. Caffeic, chlorogenic and rosmarinic acids. *Phytother. Res.* **2004**, *18*, 408–413. [CrossRef] [PubMed]
22. Gamaniel, K.; Samuel, B.B.; Kapu, D.S.; Samson, A.; Wagner, H.; Okogun, J.I.; Wambebe, C. Anti-sickling, analgesic and anti-inflammatory properties of 3,5-dimethoxy-4-hydroxy benzoic acid and 2,3,4-trihydroxyacetophenone. *Phytomedicine* **2000**, *7*, 105–110. [CrossRef]
23. Niwa, T.; Doi, U.; Kato, Y.; Osawa, T. Inhibitory mechanism of sinapinic acid against peroxynitrite-mediated tyrosine nitration of protein *in vitro*. *FEBS Lett.* **1999**, *459*, 43–46. [CrossRef]
24. Petersen, M.; Simmonds, M.S. Rosmarinic acid. *Phytochemistry* **2003**, *62*, 121–125. [CrossRef]
25. Segovia, F.J.; Luengo, E.; Corral-Pérez, J.J.; Raso, J.; Almajano, M.P. Improvements in the aqueous extraction of polyphenols from borage (*Borago officinalis* L.) leaves by pulsed electric fields: Pulsed electric fields (PEF) applications. *Ind. Crop. Prod.* **2014**, *65*, 390–396. [CrossRef]
26. Galwey, N.W.; Shirlin, A.J. Selection of borage (*Borago officinalis*) as a seed crop for pharmaceutical uses. *Heredity* **1990**, *65*, 249–257. [CrossRef]

27. Kelber, O.; Wegener, T.; Steinhoff, B.; Staiger, C.; Wiesner, J.; Knöss, W.; Kraft, K. Assessment of genotoxicity of herbal medicinal products: Application of the "bracketing and matrixing" concept using the example of *Valerianae radix* (valerian root). *Phytomedicine* **2014**, *2*, 1124–1129. [CrossRef]

28. Prasad, B.R.; Hegde, S.N. Use of *Drosophila* as a model organism in medicine. *J. Med. Med. Sci.* **2010**, *1*, 589–593.

29. Romero-Jiménez, M.; Campos-Sánchez, J.; Analla, M.; Muñoz-Serrano, A.; Alonso-Moraga, Á. Genotoxicity and antigenotoxicity of some traditional medicinal herbs. *Mutat. Res.* **2005**, *585*, 147–155. [CrossRef] [PubMed]

30. Lozano-Baena, M.D.; Tasset, I.; Obregón-Cano, S.; de Haro-Bailon, A.; Muñoz-Serrano, A.; Alonso-Moraga, Á. Antigenotoxicity and tumor growing inhibition by leafy *Brassica carinata* and sinigrin. *Molecules* **2015**, *20*, 15748–15765. [CrossRef] [PubMed]

31. Anter, J.; Campos-Sánchez, J.; el Hamss, R.; Rojas-Molina, M.; Muñoz-Serrano, A.; Analla, M.; Alonso-Moraga, Á. Modulation of genotoxicity by extra-virgin olive oil and some of its distinctive components assessed by use of the *Drosophila* wing-spot test. *Mutat. Res. Genet. Toxicol. Environ. Mutagen.* **2010**, *703*, 137–142. [CrossRef] [PubMed]

32. Rojas-Molina, M.; Campos-Sánchez, J.; Analla, M.; Muñoz-Serrano, A.; Alonso-Moraga, Á. Genotoxicity of vegetable cooking oils in the *Drosophila* wing spot test. *Environ. Mol. Mutagen.* **2005**, *45*, 90–95. [CrossRef] [PubMed]

33. Graf, U.; Würgler, F.E.; Katz, A.J.; Frei, H.; Juon, H.; Hall, C.B.; Kale, P.G. Somatic mutation and recombination test in *Drosophila melanogaster*. *Environ. Mol. Mutagen.* **1984**, *6*, 153–188. [CrossRef]

34. Ren, N.; Charlton, J.; Adler, P.N. The flare gene, which encodes the AIP1 protein of *Drosophila*, functions to regulate F-actin disassembly in pupal epidermal cells. *Genetics* **2007**, *176*, 2223–2234. [CrossRef] [PubMed]

35. Yan, J.; Huen, D.; Morely, T.; Johnson, G.; Gubb, D.; Roote, J.; Adler, P.N. The multiple-wing-hairs gene encodes a novel GBD-FH3 domain-containing protein that functions both prior to and after wing hair initiation. *Genetics* **2008**, *180*, 219–228. [CrossRef] [PubMed]

36. Collins, S.J.; Ruscetti, F.W.; Gallagher, R.E.; Gallo, R.C. Terminal differentiation of human promyelocytic leukaemia cells induced by dimethyl sulfoxide and other polar compounds. *Proc. Natl. Acad. Sci. USA* **1978**, *75*, 2458–2462. [CrossRef] [PubMed]

37. Tai, J.; Cheung, S.; Chan, E.; Hasman, D. *In vitro* culture studies of *Sutherlandia frutescens* on human tumor cell lines. *J. Ethnopharmacol.* **2004**, *93*, 9–19. [CrossRef] [PubMed]

38. Zhu, C.Y.; Loft, S. Effect of chemopreventive compounds from *Brassica* vegetables on NAD(P)H: Quinine reductase and induction of DNA strand breaks in murine hepa1c1c7 cells. *Food Chem. Toxicol.* **2003**, *41*, 455–462. [CrossRef]

39. Tasset-Cuevas, I.; Fernández-Bedmar, Z.; Lozano-Baena, M.D.; Campos-Sánchez, J.; de Haro-Bailón, A.; Muñoz-Serrano, A.; Alonso-Moraga, Á. Protective effect of borage seed oil and gamma linolenic acid on DNA: *in vivo* and *in vitro* studies. *PLoS ONE* **2013**, *8*, e56986. [CrossRef] [PubMed]

40. Frei, H.; Würgler, F.E. Statistical methods to decide whether mutagenicity test data from *Drosophila* assays indicate a positive, negative, or inconclusive result. *Mutat. Res.* **1988**, *203*, 297–308. [CrossRef]

41. Frei, H.; Würgler, F.E. Optimal experimental design and sample size for the statistical evaluation of data from somatic mutation and recombination tests (SMART) in *Drosophila*. *Mutat. Res.* **1995**, *334*, 247–258. [CrossRef]

42. Abraham, S.K. Antigenotoxicity of coffee in the *Drosophila* assay for somatic mutation and recombination. *Mutagenesis* **1994**, *9*, 383–386. [CrossRef] [PubMed]

43. Alonso-Moraga, Á.; Graf, U. Genotoxicity testing of antiparasitic nitrofurans in the *Drosophila* wing somatic mutation and recombination test. *Mutagenesis* **1989**, *4*, 105–110. [CrossRef]

44. Graf, U.; Alonso-Moraga, Á.; Castro, R.; Díaz-Carrillo, E. Genotoxicity testing of different types of beverages in the wing somatic mutation and recombination test. *Food Chem. Toxicol.* **1994**, *32*, 423–430. [CrossRef]

45. Allen, R.G.; Tresini, M. Oxidative stress and gene regulation. *Free Radic. Biol. Med.* **2000**, *28*, 463–499. [CrossRef]

46. Larson, K.M.; Roby, M.R.; Stermitz, F.R. Unsaturated pyrrolizidines from Borage (*Borago officinalis*) a common garden herb. *J. Nat. Prod.* **1984**, *47*, 747–748. [CrossRef]

47. McGuffin, M.; Hobbs, C.; Upton, R.; Goldberg, A. *American Herbal Products Association's Botanical Safety Handbook*, 2nd ed.; Boca Raton, CRC Press: Florida, CA, USA, 1997.

48. Zenk, M.; Etschenberg, E.; Graf, E. Use of Rosmarinic Acid in the Treatment of Inflammations and Pharmaceutical Products Used Therein. U.S. Patent 4329361, 11 May 1982.
49. Mhamdi, B.; Wannes, W.A.; Sriti, J.; Jellali, I.; Ksouri, R.; Marzouk, B. Effect of harvesting time on phenolic compounds and antiradical scavenging activity of *Borago officinalis* seed extracts. *Ind. Crop. Prod.* **2010**, *31*, e1–e4. [CrossRef]
50. Bast, A.; Chandler, R.F.; Choy, P.C.; Delmulle, L.M.; Gruenwald, J.; Halkes, S.B.A.; Keller, K.; Koeman, J.H.; Peters, P.; Przyrembel, H.; *et al.* Botanical health products, positioning and requirements for effective and safe use. *Environ. Toxicol. Pharmacol.* **2002**, *12*, 195–211. [CrossRef]
51. Naczk, M.; Shahidi, F. Phenolic compounds in plant foods: Chemistry and health benefits. *J. Food Sci. Nutr.* **2003**, *8*, 200–218. [CrossRef]
52. Frei, H.; Luthy, J.; Brauchli, J.; Zweifel, U.; Wurgler, F.E.; Schlatter, C. Structure/activity relationships of the genotoxic potencies of sixteen pyrrolizidine alkaloids assayed for the induction of somatic mutation and recombination in wing cells of *Drosophila melanogaster*. *Chem. Biol. Interact.* **1992**, *83*, 1–22. [CrossRef]
53. Pereira, P.; Tysca, D.; Oliveira, P.; Brum, L.F.S.; Picada, J.N.; Ardenghi, P. Neurobehavioral and genotoxic aspects of rosmarinic acid. *Pharmacol. Res.* **2005**, *52*, 199–203. [CrossRef] [PubMed]
54. Kada, T.; Inoue, T.; Namiki, M. Environmental desmutagens and antimutagens. In *Environmental Mutagenesis, Carcinogenesis and Plant Biology*; Klekowski, E.J., Ed.; Praeger: New York, NY, USA, 1982; pp. 133–152.
55. Wettasinghe, M.; Shahidi, F. Scavenging of reactive-oxygen species and DPPH free radicals by extracts of borage and evening primrose meals. *Food Chem.* **2000**, *70*, 17–26. [CrossRef]
56. De Oliveira, N.C.; Sarmento, M.S.; Nunes, E.A.; Porto, C.M.; Rosa, D.P.; Bona, S.R.; da Silva, J. Rosmarinic acid as a protective agent against genotoxicity of ethanol in mice. *Food Chem. Toxicol.* **2012**, *50*, 1208–1214. [CrossRef] [PubMed]
57. Lee, H.J.; Cho, H.S.; Park, E.; Kim, S.; Lee, S.Y.; Kim, C.S.; Kim do, K.; Kim, S.J.; Chun, H.S. Rosmarinic acid protects human dopaminergic neuronal cells against hydrogen peroxide-induced apoptosis. *Toxicology* **2008**, *250*, 109–115. [CrossRef] [PubMed]
58. Mladenović, M.; Matić, S.; Stanić, S.; Solujić, S.; Mihailović, V.; Stanković, N.; Katanić, J. Combining molecular docking and 3-D pharmacophore generation to enclose the *in vivo* antigenotoxic activity of naturally occurring aromatic compounds: Myricetin, quercetin, rutin, and rosmarinic acid. *Biochem. Pharmacol.* **2013**, *86*, 1376–1396. [CrossRef] [PubMed]
59. Hameed, H.; Aydin, S.; Başaran, A.; Basaran, N. Effects of sinapic acid on oxidative DNA damage in V79 cell line. In Proceedings of the 11th International Comet Assay Workshop, Conference Abstract: ICAW 2015, Antwerpen, Belgium, 1–4 September 2015. [CrossRef]
60. Fernández-Bedmar, Z.; Anter, J.; de la Cruz-Ares, S.; Muñoz-Serrano, A.; Alonso-Moraga, Á.; Pérez-Guisado, J. Role of citrus juices and distinctive components in the modulation of degenerative processes: Genotoxicity, antigenotoxicity, cytotoxicity, and longevity in *Drosophila*. *J. Toxicol. Environ. Health A* **2011**, *74*, 1052–1066. [CrossRef] [PubMed]
61. Leos-Rivas, C.; Verde-Star, M.J.; Torres, L.O.; Oranday-Cardenas, A.; Rivas-Morales, C.; Barron-Gonzalez, M.P.; Morales-Vallarta, M.R.; Cruz-Veja, D.E. *In vitro* amoebicidal activity of borage (*Borago officinalis*) extract on *Entamoeba histolytica*. *J. Med. Food* **2011**, *14*, 866–869. [CrossRef] [PubMed]
62. Lin, L.; Gao, Q.; Cui, C.; Zhao, H.; Fu, L.; Chen, L.; Yang, B.; Luo, W.; Zhao, M. Isolation and identification of ent-kaurane-type diterpenoids from *Rabdosia serra* (MAXIM.) HARA leaf and their inhibitory activities against HepG-2, MCF-7, and HL-60 cell lines. *Food Chem.* **2012**, *131*, 1009–1014. [CrossRef]
63. Yesil-Celiktas, O.; Sevimli, C.; Bedir, E.; Vardar-Sukan, F. Inhibitory effects of rosemary extracts, carnosic acid and rosmarinic acid on the growth of various human cancer cell lines. *Plant Foods Hum. Nutr.* **2010**, *65*, 158–163. [CrossRef] [PubMed]
64. Osakabe, N.; Yasuda, A.; Natsume, M.; Yoshikawa, T. Rosmarinic acid inhibits epidermal inflammatory responses: Anticarcinogenic effect of *Perilla frutescens* extract in the murine two-stage skin model. *Carcinogenesis* **2004**, *25*, 549–557. [CrossRef] [PubMed]
65. Stanikunaite, R.; Khan, S.I.; Trappe, J.M.; Ross, S.A. Cyclooxygenase-2 inhibitory and antioxidant compounds from the truffle *Elaphomyces granulatus*. *Phytother. Res.* **2009**, *23*, 575–578. [CrossRef] [PubMed]

66. Fabiani, R.; Rosignoli, P.; Fuccelli, R.; Pieravanti, F.; de Bartolomeo, A.; Morozzi, G. Involvement of hydrogen peroxide formation on apoptosis induction by olive oil phenolic compounds. *Czech J. Food Sci.* **2009**, *27*, S197–S199.

67. Liu, H.L.; Wan, X.; Huang, X.F.; Kong, L.Y. Biotransformation of sinapic acid catalyzed by Momordica charantia peroxidase. *J. Agric. Food Chem.* **2007**, *55*, 1003–1008. [CrossRef] [PubMed]

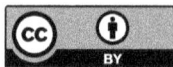

nutrients

MDPI

Review

Dietary Natural Products for Prevention and Treatment of Liver Cancer

Yue Zhou [1], Ya Li [1], Tong Zhou [1], Jie Zheng [1], Sha Li [3] and Hua-Bin Li [1,2,*]

[1]   Guangdong Provincial Key Laboratory of Food, Nutrition and Health, School of Public Health,
      Sun Yat-Sen University, Guangzhou 510080, China; zhouyuesysu@163.com (Y.Z.); saferide@126.com (Y.L.);
      zwky740359@163.com (T.Z.); zhengj37@mail2.sysu.edu.cn (J.Z.)
[2]   South China Sea Bioresource Exploitation and Utilization Collaborative Innovation Center,
      Sun Yat-Sen University, Guangzhou 510006, China
[3]   School of Chinese Medicine, The University of Hong Kong, Hong Kong, China; lishasl0308@163.com
*   Correspondence: lihuabin@mail.sysu.edu.cn; Tel.: +86-20-873-323-91

Received: 11 January 2016; Accepted: 1 March 2016; Published: 10 March 2016

Abstract: Liver cancer is the most common malignancy of the digestive system with high death rate. Accumulating evidences suggests that many dietary natural products are potential sources for prevention and treatment of liver cancer, such as grapes, black currant, plum, pomegranate, cruciferous vegetables, French beans, tomatoes, asparagus, garlic, turmeric, ginger, soy, rice bran, and some edible macro-fungi. These dietary natural products and their active components could affect the development and progression of liver cancer in various ways, such as inhibiting tumor cell growth and metastasis, protecting against liver carcinogens, immunomodulating and enhancing effects of chemotherapeutic drugs. This review summarizes the potential prevention and treatment activities of dietary natural products and their major bioactive constituents on liver cancer, and discusses possible mechanisms of action.

Keywords: liver cancer; fruit; vegetable; spice; anticancer

1. Introduction

Globally, liver cancer is the second most common cause of cancer death, accounting for more than 700,000 deaths every year [1,2]. Hepatocellular carcinoma (HCC) is the major type of liver cancer (70%–80%), followed by intrahepatic cholangiocarcinoma [3]. The main risk factors for liver cancer are hepatitis B/hepatitis C virus infection, alcohol consumption, aflatoxin B1 and metabolic disorders [4]. Liver cancer is usually an aggressive malignancy associated with poor prognosis, and the five-year survival rate is estimated to be less than 9%. Surgical interventions including liver resection, liver transplantation and percutaneous ablation are regarded as the most effective approach with curative potential for liver cancer. Unfortunately, due to numerous lesions, and extrahepatic metastasis, only about 20% of liver cancer patients are suitable for surgery. On the other hand, chemotherapeutic drugs for liver cancer are limited, and Sorafenib is the most common prescription. The large phase III trials demonstrated that Sorafenib could improve overall survival and time to progression [5,6]. However, its clinical benefits remains modest, and it was reported that Sorafenib was useful for around 30% patients, and drug resistance developed within six months [7]. Furthermore, problems such as hepatotoxicity, recurrence, drug resistance and other adverse effects exist in current therapeutics, which urge researchers to find alternative treatment.

Diet plays a pivotal role in cancers. Epidemiological studies suggested that decreased overall cancer risks might be correlated with regular intake of a high fiber, low fat diet accompanied by significant consumption of fruits and vegetables [8,9]. Therefore, dietary natural products could provide novel and fascinating preventive or therapeutic options for liver cancer. Researchers have found a variety of anticancer effects of dietary natural products, such as inhibiting tumor cell growth and metastasis, protecting against liver carcinogens, immunomodulating and enhancing effects of chemotherapeutic drugs [10–12]. Furthermore, many dietary natural products displayed selective inhibition against cancer cells [13]. This discrimination is very important for liver cancer treatment, since the majority of patients suffers from severely compromised liver function or liver cirrhosis and can not afford further losses of normal liver cells [4]. This review summarizes the prevention and treatment action of dietary natural products and their major bioactive constituents on liver cancer, and discusses the mechanism of action.

2. Fruits

The high content of polyphenols gives fruits remarkable antioxidant activity and may help lessen the risk of cancer [14–16]. Indeed, many fruits and their major bioactive constituents showed anticancer potential in various bioassay systems and animal models.

2.1. Grape

Grape products are well recognized healthy dietary components against many pathophysiologic processes. Stilbenes, anthocyanins, and procyanidins, which are abundant in grape skin, seeds and red wines, have been reported to possess strong antioxidant and anti-inflammatory properties [17]. A team isolated two fractions (TP-4 and TP-6) from grape cell culture with strong chemopreventive properties in an *in vitro* human DNA topoisomerase II assay [18]. TP-6, the procyanidin-rich fraction, selectively inhibited cell viability of HepG2 cancer cells, yet caused no toxicity to normal PK15 pig kidney cells [13]. Liver cancer is enriched with blood vessels, and angiogenesis plays a key role in cancer metastasis and relapse. The treatment of grape procyanidin in a liver cancer xenograft model exerted anti-angiogenic activity in a dose dependent manner by suppressing proliferation of vascular endothelial cells [19]. Researchers also suggested a possible anti-carcinogenic use against HCC for grape seed extracts from winery waste. The seed extract treatment in HepG2 cells induced DNA damage, enhanced NO production, p53 upregulation and significant decrease of total PARP expression, thus promoting apoptosis [20].

2.2. Black Currant

Black currant (*Ribes nigrum* L.) fruits are widely consumed, and are known to possess strong antioxidant and anti-inflammatory activities due to high content of anthocyanins (250 mg/100 g fresh fruit), which have been suggested to have potent anti-tumor properties. Utilizing HepG2 cells, an *in vitro* study found that the anthocyanin-rich fraction of black currant significantly inhibited cell proliferation [21]. Compared with other parts, black currant skin extract (BCSE) was a better source of anthocyanins with cyanidin-3-*O*-rutinoside as the predominant one. In a chemically induced rat model of liver cancer, administration of dietary BCSE (100 or 500 mg/kg for 22 weeks) dose dependently suppressed diethylnitrosamine triggered liver γ-glutamyl transpeptidase-positive preneoplastic foci. BCSE also alleviated lipid peroxidation and expression of cyclooxygenase-2, heat shock proteins (HSP70 and HSP90), inducible nitric oxide synthase and 3-nitrotyrosine as well as upregulated many hepatic antioxidant and detoxifying enzymes including glutathione *S*-transferase, quinone oxidoreductase and uridine diphosphate glucuronosyltransferase isoenzymes. The mechanistic study offered substantial evidence that the inhibition of inflammatory cascade via modulating the NF-κB signaling pathway, and suppression of oxidative stress through activating Nrf2 signaling pathway could contribute to the preventive properties of black currant bioactive components against diethylnitrosamine induced hepatocarcinogenesis [10,22]. Similarly, in a diethylnitrosamine initiated and phenobarbital promoted two stage liver cancer rat model, BCSE reduced the incidence, total number, size and multiplicity of preneoplastic hepatic nodules in a dose responsive manner. Further study revealed that the pro-apoptosis via up-regulation of Bax and simultaneously down-regulation of Bcl-2 expression are probably implicated in BCSE-mediated anticancer effects [23].

2.3. Plum

Immature plum (*Prunus salicina* Lindl.) fruits contain high contents of natural phenolic phytochemicals, which may be effective dietary natural antioxidants and preventive agents of cancer [24]. The total polyphenol content was 10 g/kg dry weight in extracts of immature plum, and (−)-epicatechin (34.7%) and (−)-gallocatechin gallate (28.6%) were major components. Extract of immature plum induced extrinsic apoptosis in HepG2 cells as evidenced by caspase-8, -10, and -3 activation as well as DNA fragmentation [25]. Another *in vitro* study found anti-metastasis property of immature plum extract in HepG2 cells. Mechanistic analysis suggested that the effects were achieved through inhibition of transcriptional expression of MMP-9 gene via suppressing the nuclear translocations of NF-κB and AP-1 [11]. In liver metabolism of exogenous compounds, phase I reactions are often associated with the metabolic activation of carcinogens, while phase II reactions mediate the detoxify process by facilitating elimination. A team found that pretreatment of immature plum extracts in rat alleviated the carcinogenicity of benzo(α)pyrene (B(α)P) through upregulating the synthesis of enzymes implicated in detoxification [26].

2.4. Other Fruits

Pomegranate is gaining increasing attention for its potent antioxidant activities due to rich polyphenol contents, such as anthocyanins, hydrolysable tannins and proanthocyanidins. It was reported that pomegranate bioactive constituents were capable of suppressing diethylnitrosamine induced hepatocarcinogenesis in rats by suppressing oxidative insult through Nrf2-mediated redox signaling pathway and inhibiting inflammatory response via NF-κB-regulated inflammatory pathway. The result provided ample support for potent tumor inhibitory activities of pomegranate at an early stage of hepatocarcinogenesis [27,28].

In China, drinking jujube tea was believed to provide synergic health effects from jujube and tea. Researchers investigated the combined effects of jujube and green tea extract and the underlying mechanisms in an *in vitro* study using HepG2 cells. The combined treatment selectively inhibited cell viability of HepG2 cells, without apparent toxic effects on the normal rat hepatocytes. Furthermore, the combination caused G_1 cell cycle arrest, which might be associated with increased level of p53 and p21$^{Waf1/Cip1}$ and decreased cyclin E levels. The treatment also enhanced anti-tumor effects via downregulating A proliferation inducing ligand (APRIL), a member of the TNF family which was reported to promote cancer cell growth [29,30].

Apples are well known healthy foods. The flavonoid-enriched fraction isolated from apple peels, at dose of 50 μg total monomeric polyphenols/mL, selectively inhibited cell proliferation of HepG2 cells, which was comparable to the currently prescribed drug Sorafenib. At the same time, the extract showed very low toxicity to normal liver cells. The induction of apoptosis, G_2/M cell cycle arrest and inhibition of DNA topoisomerase II were suggested to underlie these anti-tumor activities [31].

Sugar apple or sweetsop (*Annona squamosa* L.) is native to the tropical American. The seed extract of the fruit was traditionally used as a remedy against "malignant sores" (cancer) in China. The studies have demonstrated that annonaceous acetogenins, possessing potent anticancer activities, are the major bioactive components of *A. squamosa* seeds. In a recent study, the seed extract showed significant cytotoxicity against HepG2 cells with an IC_{50} of 0.36 μg/mL. The subsequent study in a H22 liver cancer cells transplanted rat model corroborated the findings of *in vitro* study. Oral administration of *A. squamosa* seed extract inhibited the growth of tumor cells with a maximum inhibitory rate of 69.55%. In addition, no adverse effects were observed in response to the extract [32].

Sea Buckthorn (*Hippophae rhamnoides* L.) is a thorny deciduous herb native to Europe and Asia. The fruits are tasty and contain rich nutrients and bioactive substances. The flavonoids of *H. rhamnoides* have been reported to possess antioxidant, immunomodulatory and hepatoprotective activities [33].

Isorhamnetin is an important flavonol aglycone isolated from the plant. *In vitro* study showed that isorhamnetin inhibited cell viability (IC_{50}, 74.4 ± 1.13 µg/mL) of BEL-7402 human HCC cells in a time- and dose- dependent manner. The treatment also induced the appearance of a hypodiploid peak, which might due to the promotion of apoptosis [34]. Gac fruit (*Momordica cochinchinensis*) is a delicious wild fruit widely consumed in the Southeast Asia. An *in vitro* study showed that the water extract of Gac fruit exerted antiproliferative activities in HepG2 cells. Immunoblotting found that the treatment downregulated cyclin A, Cdk2, $p27^{waf1/Kip1}$, which might explain the induced S phase arrest. Researchers suggested that a water-soluble protein with molecular weight of 35 kDa was responsible for the anticancer properties [35]. Mangosteen is a common tropical fruit. The fruit hulls contain many xanthones such as α-, β- and γ-mangostin which have diverse biological activities. The antiproliferative activity of xanthones from mangosteen has been demonstrated in several human cancer cell lines from brain, breast and colon. A recent study demonstrated that γ-mangostin had antiproliferative activity in HepG2 cells via induction of apoptosis [36]. Litchi fruit pericarp extract inhibited cancer cell growth (IC_{50}, 80 µg/mL) and colony formation *in vitro*. In murine hepatoma bearing-mice, the daily administration of the extract also suppressed tumor growth in a dose-dependent way, with 0.6 g/kg/day inhibited 44.23% ($p < 0.01$) tumor growth [37]. Auraptene is an antioxidant from citrus fruit. Post-treatment of auraptene to *N,N*-diethylnitrosamine challenged rats effectively inhibited tumor progression, presumably by negative selection for cancer cells with β-catenin mutation [38]. In an *in vivo* study using Swiss albino mice, both treatments of mango pulp extract and lupeol, a triterpene present in mango, ameliorated DMBA induced alterations in liver [39]. Another study reported that 3,5,7,3′,4′-pentahydroxy-flavonol-3-*O*-β-D-glucopyranoside, ursolic acid and quercetin, which were isolated from cranberry, demonstrated potent antiproliferative effects against HepG2 cells [40].

3. Vegetables

Epidemiological studies suggested a favorable role of high consumption vegetables, such as cruciferous vegetables, tomatoes and legumes, in cancer risks, particularly of the digestive tract. According to a recent meta-analysis, the intake of vegetables was inversely associated with risk of liver cancer (RR, 0.78; 95% CI, 0.62–0.99) [41].

3.1. Cruciferous Vegetables

Many species from the Cruciferae family are widely cultivated and consumed vegetables. Epidemiological studies pointed out consumption of cruciferous vegetables, such as cauliflower, broccoli, watercress and Brussel sprouts, with low risks of various cancers. This anticancer effect has been attributed to high contents of glucosinolates and isothiocyanates in cruciferous vegetables (Figure 1). Radishes (*Raphanus sativus* L.) contained high concentrations of glucosinolates, isothiocyanates and polyphenols [42]. For instance, 4-methylsulfanyl-3-butenyl glucosinolate, also referred to as glucoraphasatin, is a glucosinolate which is most abundant in *Raphanus sativus*. It has been well accepted that an effective way for achieving anti-tumor activities is facilitating phase II detoxification enzyme systems, such as NAD(P)H: quinone oxidoreductase 1 (NQO1), glutathione-*S*-transferase and phenolsulfotransferases, thereby promoting the detoxification of reactive metabolites of carcinogenic compounds [43]. Indeed, numerous studies have demonstrated the anti-tumor effects of glucosinolates which were associated with promotion of such enzyme activities [44]. However, it was suggested that isothiocyanate, rather than glucosinolate itself, possessed anticarcinogenic activity. For instance, in precision-cut rat liver slices, low concentrations of glucoraphasatin as well as its corresponding isothiocyanate derived from radish sprouts potently upregulated hepatic phase II detoxification enzymes involved in the metabolism of chemical carcinogens, including mycotoxins, heterocyclic amines and polycyclic aromatic hydrocarbons, while it left the cytochrome P450 enzymes such as the CYP1 family unaffected [45]. Furthermore, sulforaphane (SUL), an isothiocyanate particularly high in broccoli, was reported to transcriptionally increase the expression of CYP1A1 in a time- and dose-responsive fashion in Hepa 1c1c7 and HepG2 cells [46]. However, it was suggested that SUL was highly reactive and was further metabolized to the N-acetyl-L-cysteine (NAC) conjugate in humans. The SUL-NAC showed greater effects of inhibition against murine hepatoma cells and induction of activities of quinone reductase, a phase II detoxification enzyme [47]. Sinigrin, a main aliphatic glucosinolate present in cruciferous vegetables, is hydrolyzed to allylisothiocyanate (AITC). Both treatments of AITC and synthetic NAC-AITC dose dependently inhibited the growth of Hepa1c1c7 murine hepatoma cells. The increased activity and mRNA expression of quinine reductase might be responsible for the observed anticancer effects [48]. Besides, in SK-Hep 1 human hepatoma cells, the treatment of the two compounds dose dependently suppressed cancer cell adhesion, invasion, and migration through downregulating matrix metalloproteinase (MMP)-2/-9 at a transcriptional level [49]. Rutabaga (*Brassica napobrassica*) is a popular vegetable in North Europe and North America. Extract of rutabaga (especially eight day sprouts) exerted selective antiproliferative and pro-apoptotic effects in HepG2 cells, while it had less potent effects on the growth of normal mammalian Chinese hamster ovary cells [50].

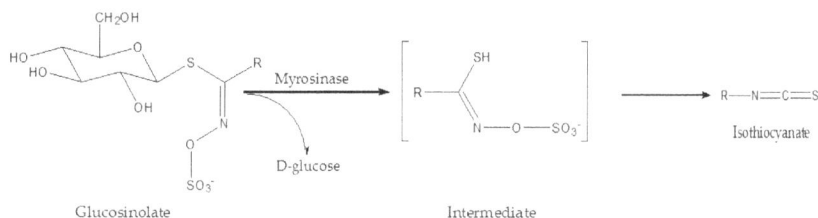

Figure 1. The general structure of glucosinolates and their enzymatic conversion to isothiocyanates by myrosinase.

3.2. French Bean

A study evaluated the antiproliferative activities of aqueous extracts from aerial parts of French bean (*Phaseolus vulgaris*). The extracts at 400 and 800 mg/mL displayed potent antioxidant activities, and also suppressed the growth of HepG2 cells by 57% and 74%, respectively [51]. Phytochemical analysis of the seed coats from *P. vulgaris* identified 24 compounds, including 12 triterpenoids and seven flavonoids. Several compounds exhibited antiproliferative activities with IC_{50} ranging from 32.1 ± 6.3 to 779.3 ± 37.4 ìM [52]. Legume lectins are usually the abundant storage proteins in legumes. In recent years, lectin has received special attention as therapeutic agents due to its diverse biological functions including anti-tumor, antibacterial and anti-HIV activities. A dimeric 64-kDa hemagglutinin was isolated from dried seeds of *P. vulgaris* with a high yield (1.1 g/100 g seeds). The compound displayed a modest inhibition against the growth of HepG2 cells (IC_{50}, 100 µM), without interfering in normal liver WRL 68 cells [53]. Later, the team purified a new legume lectin (BTKL) from seeds of *P. vulgaris*, which possessed strong selectively cytotoxicity to HepG2 cells (IC_{50}, 7.9 ± 0.5 µM). According to their study, the potential mechanisms of the anti-tumor activities of BTKL include: (1) inducing apoptosis and necrosis; (2) promoting NO production via the upregulation of iNOS; and (3) triggering the release of pro-inflammatory cytokines such as IL-1β, IL-2, TNF-α, and INF-γ [54]. In another study, a hemagglutinin isolated from *P. vulgaris* showed stronger antiproliferative properties than concanavalin A in the HepG2 cancer cell line [55].

3.3. Tomato

It was reported that tomato contains an average of 11.6–14 mg/kg lycopene. The compound is an unsaturated carotenoid with high antioxidant activity, which has been reported to modulate cell proliferation, differentiation, and apoptosis [56,57]. Therefore, lycopene might serve as a rational approach in combating HCC. The pre-treatment of lycopene from tomatoes to *N*-nitrosamines challenged mice ameliorated the carcinogenic damage, as shown by decrease of oxidative stress, chromosomal and membrane abnormalities [58]. Moreover, lycopene administration markedly suppressed the expression of anti-apoptotic gene and upregulated caspase 3, 9 and p53 expression, leading to enhanced apoptosis in response to *N*-nitrosamine insult [59]. Besides, in *N*-nitrosodiethylamine (NDEA)-challenged mice, decrease of tumor incidence (42.05%), multiplicity (3.42), and burden (1.39) as well as increase of survival rate were observed upon lycopene pretreatment to NDEA-treated animals. Histopathological analysis showed a reduction of aggressive tumor nodules formation [60]. Collectively, these results may support anti-tumor properties of lycopene during early stages of chemical induced hepatocarcinogenesis.

Beside lycopene, tomatine, a glycoalkaloid contained much higher in green tomato than the red one, may also possess anti-tumor properties. *In vivo* study indicated that anti-tumor effects of tomatine acted through a different mechanism, including induction of antigen-specific cellular immunity and direct destruction of cancer cell membranes. A commercial tomato glycoalkaloid tomatine (10:1 mixture of α-tomatine and dehydrotomatine) exerted dose-dependent inhibition against HepG2 cancer cells and was reported to be more potent than the anticancer drug doxorubicin. These findings suggested that consumers might also benefit from eating high-tomatine containing green tomatoes [61].

3.4. Asparagus

Asparagus (*Asparagus officinalis* L.) is a popular vegetable often used in soups, salads and vegetable dishes. Several studies revealed numerous pharmacological activities associated with *A. officinalis*, such as anti-inflammation, anti-mutagenicity, and cytotoxicity. Polysaccharides, steroidal saponins and flavonoids extracted from the plant were suggested to be main constituents responsible for its bioactivities.

Asparagus polysaccharide has been clinically adopted to treat various cancers including breast cancer, leukemia, and lung cancer. A recent study reported that the asparagus polysaccharide selectively inhibited cell proliferation of HepG2 (IC_{50}, 5.7 mg/mL) and Hep3B (IC_{50}, 9.39 mg/mL) cell lines with less toxicity on normal human hepatocellular 7702 cells (IC_{50}, 20.92 mg/mL). Mechanistic study revealed that the induction of G_2/M phase arrest and apoptosis by asparagus polysaccharide via modulation of Bax, Bcl-2 and capase-3 contributed to the effects [62]. In addition, asparagus polysaccharide was a good embolic candidate in transcatheter arterial chemoembolization (TACE), a minimally invasive treatment for unresectable HCC. The combined treatment of asparagus polysaccharide with TACE markedly suppressed liver tumor growth as well as prolonged survival time in rat model with little toxicity [63].

Asparanin A, a steroidal saponin isolated from *A. officinalis*, has displayed antiproliferative activities against many cancers, such as esophageal cancer, gastric cancer, lung cancer and leukemia [64]. Asparanin A also exerted dose- and time-dependent inhibition against HepG2 cells with IC_{50} at 6.20 ± 0.56 μmol/L. The treatment induced G_2/M cell cycle arrest through downregulating Cdk1, Cdk4, and cyclin A and simultaneously upregulating p21$^{WAF1/Cip1}$. Besides, the promotion of apoptosis via both the intrinsic and extrinsic pathway was observed upon asparanin A treatment to HepG2 cells [65].

3.5. Other Vegetables

The treatment of mung bean sprouts (MBS) extract showed different cytotoxicity against HepG2 cells (IC_{50}, 14.04 ± 1.5 mg/mL) and normal human cells (IC_{50}, 163.97 ± 5.73 mg/mL). The selectivity index for HepG2 cells was 11.94 ± 1.2. Mechanisms underlying the anti-tumor properties of MBS included induction of apoptosis (Bax and capase-8), increase of anti-tumor cytokines (TNF-α and IFN-β), promotion of IFN-γ production, and upregulation of cell-mediated immunity through immunopolarization [66].

Momordica charantia lectin (MCL) is a type II ribosome inactivating protein derived from bitter gourd, a vegetable and traditional herbal medicine in China. The treatment of MCL significantly suppressed HCC cell growth *in vitro* and *in vivo* through inducing G_2/M phase arrest, apoptosis and autophagy [67]. Besides, MAP30, a type I ribosome inactivating protein purified from bitter gourd, demonstrated both cytostatic and cytotoxic effects in cultured Hep G2 cells. The activities were attributed to activation of extrinsic and intrinsic caspase apoptosis and induction of S phase cell cycle arrest. The anti-tumor role of MAP30 was also demonstrated *in vivo* [68]. RNase MC2 is a ribonuclease from *M. charantia*, and could enhance apoptotic death both *in vitro* and in HepG2-bearing mice [69].

Perilla frutescens L. is widely used for its pleasant aroma and the leaves are eaten as a delicious vegetable. Ingredients extracted from the plant, including rosmarinic acid, caffeic acid and apigenin were reported to exert antiproliferative activities against a wide range of cancers. A study reported that isoegomaketone, a compound isolated from *P. frutescens*, significantly inhibited cell growth and xenograft tumor formation probably through blocking the PI3K/Akt signaling pathway of HCC cells [70]. A study evaluated the antioxidant activity, contents of total phenolics, anthocyanin and chlorogenic acid, and *in vitro* anticancer capacity of potato. Among the tested samples, *Solanum pinnatisectum*, which possessed the highest antioxidant activity, also showed the strongest antiproliferative effects against liver cancer cells [71]. It was suggested that the glycoalkaloids from potatoes possessed anti-tumor abilities. The treatment of potato glycoalkaloids, especially α-chaconine dose dependently inhibited HepG2 cell growth in the range of 0.1–10 µg/mL, with lower cytotoxicity to normal liver cells [72]. Celery (*Apium graveolens* L.) is frequently used as vegetable worldwide. Its seeds, possessing potent antioxidant and anti-inflammatory abilities, are traditionally used to treat liver indurations. Phytochemical analysis reported that main bioactive constituents in celery seeds were apigenin, linamarose, and vitamins A and C. Pretreatment of rats with celery seed extracts dose dependently suppressed chemically induced hepatocarcinogenesis as evidenced by reduction of γ-GT positive foci [73].

4. Spices

4.1. Garlic

Epidemiologic evidence suggested that high consumption of garlic protected against various cancers. Organo-sulphur compounds (OSC), such as alliin, allicin, diallyl disulfide, diallyl sulfide, allyl mercaptan, and S-allylcysteine, were reported to be major ingredients with anti-tumor properties in garlic (Figure 2) [74,75]. For instance, administration of garlic powders to rat inhibited DNA damage by 35%–60% induced by N-nitrosodimethylamine in liver as assessed by the comet assay. The effect was attributed to the high alliin concentration in samples [76]. Subsequently, researchers investigated the anticancer effects of selected OSC from garlic against chemical induced DNA damage using HepG2 cells. The study showed that all the OSC tested except allyl mercaptan markedly inhibited aflatoxin B1 induced DNA damage, while allyl mercaptan administration significantly reduced DNA breaks induced by dimethylnitrosamine. Benzo(α)pyrene genotoxicity was effectively suppressed by diallyl disulfide. Besides, all the tested OSC inhibited DNA damage of direct-acting agents, H_2O_2 and methyl methanesulfonate [77]. In another study using rat hepatoma cells, sodium 2-propenyl thiosulfate was found to be a potent inducer of quinone reductase [78]. In Hep3B HCC cells, hexane extracts of garlic promoted ROS production and subsequent dysregulation of mitochondrial membrane potential, leading to enhanced apoptotic cell death [79]. Similarly, allicin was also able to induce apoptotic cell death through overproduction of ROS in Hep3B human HCC cell line [80]. The propensity to metastasis of HCC leads to recurrence and poor prognosis. S-allylcysteine was observed to suppress proliferation and metastasis of HCC in a metastatic HCC cell line MHCC97L and *in vivo* xenograft liver cancer model. The potential mechanisms included (1) to inhibit cancer cell migration and invasion by suppressing VEGF and increasing E-cadherin; (2) to promote cell apoptotic death via downregulating Bcl-2,-xl and upregulating caspase-3, -9 activities; and (3) to induce S cell cycle arrest [79]. On the other hand, an *in vitro* study reported that the water-soluble garlic extracts were more potent inhibitor of HepG2 cells than the oil-soluble compound diallyl disulfide by inducing a p53/p21-mediated G_2/M phase arrest and apoptosis [81]. A team evaluated the anti-tumor activities of a unique garlic preparation, namely aged garlic extract in rats. The preparation inhibited diethylnitrosamine induced preneoplastic lesions in liver, presumably through slowing the proliferation rate of liver cells [82]. It is known that immune functions are usually deficient in advanced-cancer patients. A clinical trial of patients with advanced cancer in digestive system (84% were liver cancer) reported that the aged garlic extract had a positive effect on natural-killer cell activities [83].

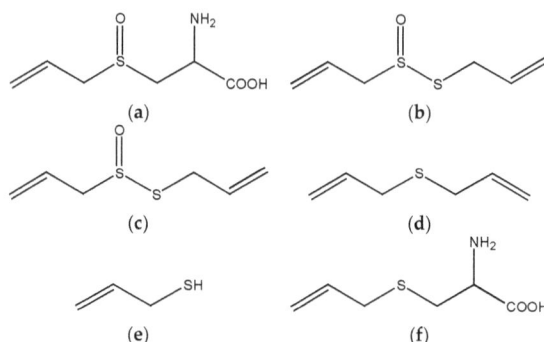

Figure 2. The chemical structures of several organo-sulphur compounds in garlic: (**a**) alliin; (**b**) allicin; (**c**) diallyl disulfide; (**d**) diallyl sulfide; (**e**) allyl mercaptan; and (**f**) *S*-allylcysteine.

4.2. Turmeric

Turmeric (*Curcuma longa* L.) is a popular spice in Asia, especially in India. In HBV X protein transgenic mice, *Curcuma longa* extracts led to less visceral fat, lower ratio of liver to body weight and delayed pathogenesis. Since HBV infection plays a key role in the development and progression of liver cirrhosis and HCC, the spice may be a good candidate against HBV-related liver cancer [84]. Curcumin is a yellow pigment from *Curcuma longa* with numerous bioactivities including antioxidant, anti-inflammatory and anticancer activities. In an *in vivo* study, curcumin demonstrated anticancer activity against chemical induced hepatocarcinogenesis. The administration of curcumin reduced hyper plastic nodule, liver damage markers, body weight loss and hypoproteinemia in the liver of diethylnitrosamine/phenobarbital challenged Wistar rats [85]. The protective effects of curcumin against liver cancer also involved the enhanced degradation of hypoxia-inducible factor, and curcumin could promote apoptosis of Hep 3B cells [86]. It was suggested that curcumin glucuronide was the main form of curcumin in plasma following oral administration in rats, because most curcumin was conjugated after absorption. This conjugated compound showed weaker anticancer activities against HepG2 cancer cells [87]. Beside curcumin, curcuma oil possessed hepatoprotective properties, and sesquiterpenoids might be its main bioactive ingredients. Treatment of curcuma oil alleviated concanavalin A induced oxidative stress and inflammation in mice. The oil also induced apoptosis of Hepa1-6 cancer cells in a time-/dose-dependent manner *in vitro* and inhibited inoculated tumor cell growth *in vivo* [88]. Aromatic tumerone (ar-tumerone) is another volatile oil from *C. longa*. The IC_{50} of ar-tumerone were 64.8 ± 7.1 µg/mL for HepG2, 102.5 ± 11.5 µg/mL for Huh-7, and 122.2 ± 7.6 µg/mL for Hep3B liver cancer cell line. Further analysis showed that the ar-turmerone-induced apoptotic cell death of HepG2 was a result of ROS-mediated ERK and JNK kinases activation [89].

4.3. Pepper

An *in vitro* study showed that pepper extracts reduced cell viability of rat hepatoma McA-RH7777, while displaying no cytotoxicity, even protected against basal death of normal rat hepatocytes in the case of *Piper putumayoense*. The selective cytotoxicity was attributed to the intracellular accumulation of ROS [90].

The glycoprotein (24 kD) isolated from *Zanthoxylum piperitum* could prevent chemical-induced liver carcinogenesis by immunomodulation and promotion of apoptosis. In diethylnitrosamine treated Balb/c mice, the glycoprotein (20 mg/kg) enhanced expression of perforin, granzyme B and NK cell activities, as well as pro-apoptotic factors (bid, capase-3 and cytochrome c) in liver [91]. The metastasis of tumor required degradation of extracellular matrix. MMP-2/-9 promoted this process, while TIMP-1/-2, the endogenous inhibitors of MMPs, was negatively related to tumor metastasis. *In vitro* studies using HA22T cancer cell line, treatment of *Zanthoxylum avicennae* extract not only suppressed cell proliferation through induction of G_2/M cell cycle arrest and apoptosis, but also inhibited cell metastasis, invasion via downregulating MMP-2/-9 and upregulating TIMP-1/-2 [92–94]. Subsequent mechanistic analysis revealed that the activation of phosphatase 2A was behind those anti-tumor effects. An essential oil was extracted from dried pericarp of *Zanthoxylum schinifolium*, which mainly consisted of 29.9% geranyl acetate, 15.8% citronella and 15.4% sabinene. This volatile extract dose dependently promoted ROS production in HepG2 cells, leading to increased apoptotic cell death. The extract also exerted anti-tumor activities in Huh-7 human liver cancer cell transplanted nude mice [95].

4.4. Ginger

It was reported that ginger could be a promising candidate for cancer prevention [96–98]. In a chemical induced liver cancer rat model, 50 mg/kg daily treatment of ginger significantly reduced serum liver cancer markers (α-fetoprotein, CEA), as well as liver tissue growth factors [99]. The inhibition of inflammation and promotion of apoptosis were implicated in the protection of ginger against liver cancer. For instance, the suppression of inflammatory responses as evidenced by decreased NF-κB and TNF-α was found in ginger (100 mg/kg) treated rat hepatoma model [100]. Besides, ginger extracts dose dependently inhibited cell proliferation of the HEp-2 cell line (IC_{50}, 900 μg/mL), which was mediated though ROS induced apoptotic death. Further analysis of active ingredients by GC-MS revealed the existence of geraniol, pinostrobin and clavatol [101]. In addition, the studies suggested that 6-shogaol and 6-gingerol, two compounds isolated from ginger, exhibited anti-metastasis effects against liver cancer cells via downregulation of MMP-9, urokinase-type plasminogen (6-shogaol) and upregulation of TIMP-1 [102]. Moreover, 6-shogaol could also effectively induce ROS-mediated caspase-dependent apoptosis in a multidrug resistance hepatoma cell line [103].

4.5. Other Spices

Star anise (*Illicium verum*) is widely consumed as a condiment in Asian countries. In an NDEA/phenobarbital induced liver cancer model, the administration of star anise during the promotion stage exhibited anti-carcinogenic potential in the liver tissue of rat. The treatment ameliorated tumor burden (decrease of liver weight, nodule incidence, size, volume and multiplicity), decreased oxidative stress (restoration of superoxide dismutase activity) and upregulated phase II detoxifying enzymes (glutathione-*S*-transferase) [104].

Saffron is the dried stigmas of *Crocus sativus* L., which are commonly consumed as spice and food colorant. Saffron has been proposed as a potential treatment for cancer. The IC_{50} of saffron against HepG2 cells was 950 μg/mL. The inhibition of cancer cell viability by saffron involved apoptosis, but was not associated with ROS production [105]. The induction of apoptosis was also observed in saffron treated rats after diethylnitrosamine administration. Besides, saffron reduced tumor burden and oxidative damage as well as suppressed inflammatory responses in the liver tissue [106].

Galangal (*Alpinia officinarum* H.) is a spice in southern China. Galagin, a flavonol from *A. Officinarum*, could promote apoptotic death of HCC cells in the intrinsic mitochondrial pathway via activation of capase-8 and Bid [107]. The diarylheptanoids isolated from the roots also possessed modest cytotoxicity against HepG2 liver cancer cells [108]. Isoobtusilactone A is isolated from *Cinnamomum kotoense* leave. The compound could induce apoptotic cell death (IC_{50}, 37.5 μmol/L) through overproduction of ROS in HepG2 cells [109]. In addition, *in vitro* studies showed that the

ROS-mediated anticancer effect was also involved in the promotion of TRAIL-related apoptosis by isoobtusilactone A [110]. A study showed that basil extract could inhibit the sulfotransferase induced procarcinogenesis by suppressing DNA adducts formation in HepG2 cells and in rat hepatoma model [111]. In addition, carnosic acid from rosemary exerted anti-tumor activities against aflatoxin B1 through reduced oxidative stress in HepG2 cells [112].

5. Soy

The decreased cancer risks of Asian population traditionally eating a soy-based diet have been associated with the abundant soy isoflavones with antioxidant activities, especially daidzein and genistein [113]. For instance, the treatment of daidzein at a non-toxic dose enhanced the activity and transcriptionally upregulated the expression of catalase in Huh-7 and HepG2 human liver cancer cells [114]. In another study, a trypsin inhibitor isolated from Hokkaido large black soybeans exerted antiproliferative (IC_{50}, 140 μmol/L) activities against HepG2 cells [115]. Similarly, a trypsin inhibitor (19 kD) from Chinese black soybean *Glycine max* inhibited growth of HepG2 cells with an IC_{50} of about 25 μmol/L [116]. However, it is of note that the role of soy isoflavones as food supplements in cancer prevention is controversial. It was reported that genistein possessed abilities to promote proliferation of estrogen-dependent breast cancer *in vivo*, which could be ameliorated by other components in soy foods [117]. Thus, the consumption of soy-based foods rather than purified soy isoflavones might be safer for women at high risk of breast cancer.

6. Cereals

Rice bran is a byproduct of rice milling. In a study, gastrointestinal-resistant peptide hydrolysates prepared from rice bran were fractionated into different size. Trypan blue dye exclusion assay showed that the <5, 5–10 kD fractions significantly suppressed ($p < 0.05$) growth of HegG2 cells *in vitro* [118]. The byproduct is also a source of phytic acid [119], which has been reported to possess anticancer abilities. Phytic acid from rice bran could dose-dependently suppress HepG2 cancer cell proliferation with an IC_{50} of 2.49 mmol/L. The growth inhibition was correlated to enhanced apoptosis as shown by upregulated capase-3/-9, Bax and p53 [120]. Pigmented rice usually contained more bioactive compounds, such as flavones, phenolics, tannin, tocopherols and sterols [121]. For example, Payao, a pigmented rice cultivar from Thailand, was reported to be a rich source of anthocyanin (5.80 mg/g). The extract of Payao could significantly inhibit HepG2 cell growth [122].

Corn is a widely cultivated economic crop. Polysaccharides from corn silk exerted anti-tumor effects and extended survival time of H22 hepatoma-bearing mice. The enhanced immune function, as evidenced by increase of IL-2/-6, and TNF-α, peripheral white blood cells counts, thymus and spleen index following the polysaccharides treatment, might delineate these anti-tumor activities [123]. *Coix lacryma*, also called semen coicis, is a grass-like relative of corn in China. Extract from the seed of *Coix lacryma* time- and dose-dependently promoted apoptotic death of HepG2 cancer cells through upregulation of capase-8 [124]. According to an *in vitro* study, the ethyl acetate and hexane extracts of buckwheat hull selectively inhibited cell growth by 75.3% and 83.6% of Hep3B liver cancer cells, while the inhibition rates against normal control cells were lower than 35% [125].

7. Edible Macro-Fungi

Edible macro-fungi have a long history of use for its nutrition value and flavors. It is also a rich source of bioactive compounds, especially polysaccharide [126]. Recently, the exploration of edible macro-fungi for tumor prevention and treatment has been carried out in various model systems.

Agaricus blazei M. has been suggested to have anticancer activities. There was evidence that the mushroom could improve immune function and life quality of gynecological cancer patients taking chemotherapy [127]. Besides, the extract from *A. blazei* meycelial could decrease formation of abnormal collagen fiber in HCC cells [128], which might be very helpful since liver cirrhosis is highly implicated in the development of liver cancer. The anti-tumor property of *A. blazei* was also proved in Smmu 7721 hepatoma-bearing mice [129]. Further studies isolated several compounds with anti-tumor activities against liver cancer. For instance, the β-glucan from *A. blazei* protected against benzo(á)pyrene induced DNA damage in HepG2 cells by binding to the carcinogen, scavenging free radicals and probably modulating cell metabolism [130]. Two compounds, namely blazeispirols A and C from *A. blazei* displayed potent antiproliferative activities against Hep3B cells (IC$_{50}$, 2.8 and 4.5 μg/mL) and HepG2 cells (IC$_{50}$, 1.4 and 2.0 μg/mL) [131]. Mechanistic study reported that bazeispirol A inhibited Hep3B cancer cell growth in a dose- and time-dependent manner through promoting apoptotic death [132].

Pleurotus pulmonarius had potent antioxidant activities. Pretreatment of *P. pulmonarius* to Huh7 hepatoma bearing-nude mice significantly reduced the incidence and size of tumors without obvious adverse effects [133]. Furthermore, *P. Pulmonarius* could inhibit invasion and drug-resistance of hepatoma cells. The inhibition of the PI3K/AKT signaling pathway was suggested to be the underlying mechanism [134]. In another study, protein isolated from the dried fruiting bodies of *Pleurotus eryngii* dose dependently suppressed HepG2 cell proliferation through apoptosis without apparent toxicity to normal liver Chang cells [135]. A polysaccharide (120 kDa) from *Pleurotus abalones* also possessed antiproliferative properties in HepG2 cells [136]. In addition, the polysaccharide-rich fraction of *Lentinula edodes* mycelia effectively killed HepG2 cells through the capase-3/-8 mediated extrinsic apoptosis pathway, but showed minor cytotoxicity on normal control cells [137].

AAL-2 is a novel lectin (43.175 kDa) from *Agrocybe aegerita*. *In vitro* study reported that the lectin could bind to the surface of liver cancer cells, resulting in apoptotic cell death. Furthermore, AAL-2 administration inhibited tumor growth and extended survival time in hepatoma-bearing mice [138]. The study reported a glycoprotein (FVE) with immunomodulatory properties from *Flammulina velutipes* [139]. In hepatoma-bearing mice, the oral treatment of FVE (10 mg/kg) significantly prolonged survival time and reduced tumor size, through inducing cytotoxic immune response by enhancing innate and adaptive immunity. Besides, IFN-γ was suggested to participate in this process [140]. Iso-suillin, isolated from *Suillus luteus*, selectively suppressed proliferation, induced G$_1$ cell cycle arrest and promoted apoptotic death of SMMC-7721 human liver cancer cells, without obvious cytotoxicity against normal human lymphocytes [141]. *O*-orsellinaldehyde was isolated from *Grifola frondosa*. The compound exhibited selective potent cytotoxicity against Hep3B cells (IC$_{50}$, 3.6 μg/mL) through apoptosis [142]. In addition, *p*-terphenyl derivatives from *Thelephora aurantiotincta* induced G$_1$ phase arrest in human hepatoma cells probably through iron chelation [143].

8. Effects of Combination of Dietary Natural Products with Anticancer Treatments

Chemotherapy and radiotherapy are commonly used cancer therapies. However, the toxic adverse effects and drug resistance restrict their clinical effectiveness. Dietary natural products and their bioactive components could improve efficacy, decrease dose, and ameliorate toxic effects of anticancer drugs, and the combination of natural products with anticancer treatments could offer an attractive strategy for liver cancer treatment. Resistance to apoptosis is a common trait of many cancer cells, which has become a hurdle in traditional anticancer therapies. Asparagus polysaccharide could potentiate the tumoricidal activities of mitomycin *in vitro* and *in vivo*, reducing the amount of drug used without causing deleterious effects. The promotion of apoptosis was suggested to contribute to the activities [62]. In another study, *Momordica charantia* lectin enhanced Sorafenib induced apoptosis by 3.37 folds in HepG2 cells. Consistently with the *in vitro* finding, the combined treatment at a physiologically safe dose completely arrested HepG2 xenograft tumor growth [67]. Extracts of Payao (pigment rice) also sensitized HepG2 cells to cytotoxicity of vinblastine, which was suggested to be achieved through a mitochondrial apoptosis pathway [122]. In addition, enhancing anticancer activities through promotion of intracellular drug accumulation was observed in several studies. For instance, compared with doxorubicin alone, the combination of grape proanthocyanidin and doxorubicin markedly inhibited H22 tumor growth. The promotion of doxorubicin-induced apoptosis via intracellular doxorubicin accumulation is likely to be the underlying mechanism [144]. Epigallocatechin gallate also induced intracellular accumulation of doxorubicin in a human chemoresistant liver cancer cell line through suppressing the activity of a P-glycoprotein efflux pump [145]. NF-κB regulates cell survival and its activation contributes to drug resistance via inhibiting the pro-apoptotic effects of chemotherapy. The studies demonstrated that *Agaricus blazei* and *Hericium erinaceus* could sensitize doxorubicin-mediated apoptosis through inhibiting NF-κB activation [146,147]. It was reported that the PI3K/AKT pathway contributed to drug resistance of cancer cells, and inactivation of the pathway by *Pleurotus pulmonarius* significantly enhanced the sensitivity of HCC cells to cisplatin [134]. In addition, the destruction of lymphocytes and immunosuppression were problems associated with anticancer therapies. A study showed that combined treatment of polysaccharides from *Lentinus edodes* and *Tricholoma matsutake* enhanced anticancer activities of 5-fluorouracil against H22 cells. Besides, compared with 5-fluorouracil alone, the combination performed better in reducing tumor weight and volume in mice model. It was suggested that the enhanced activities of NK cells and cytotoxic T lymphocytes, the increased secretion of cytokines (TNF-α and IFN-γ) and frequency of CD4[+] and CD8[+] T cells in the spleen as well as maintenence of the relative weight of the thymus and spleen all contributed to chemo-sensitizing activities of *Lentinus edodes* and *Tricholoma matsutake* [12]. On the other hand, liver is considered to be sensitive to radiation, and radiotherapy itself could induce liver damage. Compared with radiotherapy alone, the combination of apricot supplementation and radiotherapy exerted synergistically protective effects against DMBA (7,12-dimethylbenz(a)anthracene) induced liver damage and carcinogenesis in rats through alleviating apoptosis and oxidative stress [148].

Finally, some dietary natural products for the prevention and treatment of liver cancer are summarized in Table 1. In addition, some effects of dietary natural products against liver cancer are shown in Figure 3.

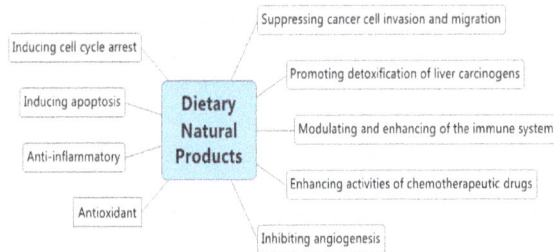

Figure 3. Some effects of dietary natural products against liver cancer.

Table 1. Effects of dietary natural products against liver cancer.

Natural Products	Bioactive Components	Study Type	Bioactivities and Potential Mechanisms	References
Fruits				
Grape	procyanidins	*in vitro*	selective cytotoxicity to cancer cells	[13]
		in vivo	inhibiting tumor angiogenesis; promoting doxorubicin induced apoptosis	[19,144]
	Flavan-3-ol	*in vitro*	inducing apoptosis, DNA damage and Suppressing expression of oncoprotein Her-2	[20]
Black currant	anthocyanins	*in vivo*	protecting against diethylnitrosamine induced hepatocarcinogenesis by inducting apoptosis and suppressing oxidative stress and inflammation	[10]
Plum	polyphenols	*in vitro*	inducing extrinsic apoptosis and inhibiting migration	[11,25]
		in vivo	protecting against B(α)P liver damage through regulating enzymes involved detoxification	[26]
Pomegranate	polyphenols	*in vivo*	protecting against diethylnitrosamine induced hepatocarcinogenesis by suppressing oxidative stress and inflammatory responses	[27,28]
Apple	polyphenols	*in vitro*	inducing apoptosis, G2/M cell cycle arrest and inhibiting DNA topoisomerase II in cancer cells	[31]

Table 1. *Cont.*

Natural Products	Bioactive Components	Study Type	Bioactivities and Potential Mechanisms	References
Sweetsop	annonaceous acetogenins	*in vitro* and *in vivo*	exerting cytotoxicity against HepG2 cells and inhibiting tumor growth in hepatoma bearing mice	[32]
Sea buckthorn	isorhamnetin	*in vitro*	promoting apoptosis of human hepatoma cells	[34]
Gac fruit	a water soluble protein	*in vitro*	inducing S phase arrest in cancer cells	[35]
Mangosteen	γ-mangostin	*in vitro*	inducing apoptosis in cancer cells	[36]
Citrus fruit	auraptene	*in vivo*	suppressing tumor progression in *N,N*-diethylnitrosamine challenged rats by negative selection for cancer cells with β-catenin mutation	[38]
Mango	lupeol	*in vivo*	ameliorating DMBA insult induced alterations in liver	[39]
Vegetables				
Radish	Glucoraphasa-tin, isothiocyanate	*in vitro*	upregulating hepatic phase II detoxification enzymes involved in the metabolism of chemical carcinogens	[45]
Broccoli	sulforaphane	*in vitro*	upregulating CYP1A1 and quinone reductase	[46,47]
Rutabaga	NA	*in vitro*	exerting selective antiproliferative and pro-apoptotic effects in cancer cells	[50]
French bean	triterpenoids, flavonoids	*in vitro*	exhibiting antiproliferative activities against cancer cells	[52]
	lectins	*in vitro*	exerting selectively cytotoxicity to cancer cells via promoting apoptosis, necrosis, NO production and release of proinflammatory cytokines	[54]
Tomato	lycopene	*in vivo*	protecting against chemical induced liver carcinogenesis through inducing apoptosis	[59,60]
	tomatine	*in vivo*	inducing antigen-specific cellular immunity and direct destructing cancer cell membranes	[61]
Asparagus	polysaccharides	*in vitro* and *in vivo*	selectively inhibiting cancer cell proliferation and enhancing the tumoricidal activities of mitomycin	[62]
		in vivo	serving as a good embolic candidate in transcatheter arterial chemoembolization	[63]
	asparanin A	*in vitro*	inducing G2/M cell cycle arrest and apoptosis	[65]
Mung bean sprouts	NA	*in vitro*	increasing apoptosis, anti-tumor cytokines (TNF-α and IFN-β), IFN-γ production and upregulating cell-mediated immunity	[66]
Bitter gourd	lectin	*in vitro*	inducing G2/M phase arrest, apoptosis, autophagy and enhancing the anti-tumor effects of Sorafenib	[67]
	MAP30	*in vitro* and *in vivo*	inducing apoptosis and S phase cell cycle arrest	[68]
Purple perilla	Isoegomake-tone	*in vitro* and *in vivo*	inhibiting cell growth and xenograft tumor formation probably through blocking the PI3K/Akt signaling pathway	[70]
Potato	glycoalkaloids	*in vitro*	selectively inhibiting cancer cell growth	[72]
Celery	pigenin, linamarose, Vitamins A/C	*in vivo*	dose dependently suppressing chemically induced hepatocarcinogenesis	[73]
Spices				
Garlic	Organo-sulphur compounds	*in vitro*	inhibiting chemical induced DNA damage	[77]
	sodium 2-propenyl thiosulfate	*in vitro*	upregulating quinone reductase	[78]
	allicin	*in vitro*	inducing apoptosis through overproduction of ROS	[80]
	S-allylcysteine	*in vitro* and *in vivo*	inducing apoptosis and S phase arrest, inhibiting cancer cell migration and invasion	[78]
	aged garlic extract	*in vivo*	inhibiting diethylnitrosamine induced preneoplastic lesions in liver	[81]
		clinical trial	enhancing natural-killer cell activities	[83]

Table 1. *Cont.*

Natural Products	Bioactive Components	Study Type	Bioactivities and Potential Mechanisms	References
Turmeric	NA	*in vivo*	protecting against HBV-related liver cancer	[84]
	curcumin	*in vitro* and *in vivo*	demonstrating anti-tumor activity against chemical induced hepatocarcinogenesis	[85]
	Sesquiterpe-noids	*in vitro* and *in vivo*	alleviating concanavalin A induced oxidative stress and inflammation, inhibiting cancer cell growth	[88]
	aromatic tumerone	*in vitro*	inducing apoptotic cell death via ROS-mediated ERK and JNK kinases activation	[89]
Pepper	NA	*in vitro*	selective cytotoxicity against rat hepatoma cells through intracellular accumulation of ROS	[90]
	glycoprotein	*in vivo*	preventing chemical induced liver carcinogenesis by immunomodulation and promotion of apoptosis	[91]
	NA	*in vitro*	inducing G2/M cell cycle arrest and apoptosis, inhibiting cell metastasis, invasion via down-regulating MMP-2/-9 and up-regulating TIMP-1/-2	[92–94]
	geranyl acetate, citronella, sabinene	*in vitro* and *in vivo*	increasing apoptotic cell death through ROS production	[95]
Ginger	NA	*in vivo*	inhibiting inflammation and promoting apoptosis	[100]
	geraniol, pinostrobin, clavatol	*in vitro*	inhibiting cancer cell proliferation though ROS-mediated apoptotic death	[101]
	6-shogaol, 6-gingerol	*in vitro*	suppressing metastasis via down-regulation of MMP-9, urokinase-type plasminogen and up-regulation of TIMP-1	[102]
Star anise	NA	*in vivo*	ameliorating tumor burden, oxidative stress and upregulating phase II detoxifying enzymes	[104]
Saffron	NA	*in vitro* and *in vivo*	inducing apoptosis and decreasing tumor burden, oxidative damage and inflammatory responses	[105,106]
Galangal	galagin	*in vitro*	promoting mitochondrial apoptotic death	[107]
Cinnamon	Isoobtusilac-tone A	*in vitro*	inducing apoptotic cancer cell death through overproduction of ROS	[109,110]
Basil	NA	*in vitro* and *in vivo*	inhibiting sulfotransferase induced procarcinogenesis by suppressing DNA adducts formation	[111]
Rosemary	carnosic acid	*in vitro*	protecting against aflatoxin B1 through reduced oxidative stress	[112]
Soy	trypsin inhibitor	*in vitro*	inhibiting cancer cell growth	[115,116]
Cereals				
Rice bran	peptide hydrolysates, phytic acid	*in vitro*	inhibiting cancer cell growth	[118,120]
Pigmented rice	anthocyanin	*in vitro*	synergistically promoting the cytotoxicity of vinblastine through a mitochondrial apoptosis pathway	[122]
Corn silk	polysaccharides	*in vivo*	enhancing immune function and extending survival time	[123]
Semen coicis	NA	*in vitro*	dose-dependently promoting apoptotic death of cancer cells through upregulation of capase-8	[124]
Edible macro-fungi				
Agaricus blazei	NA	*in vitro*	sensitizing doxorubicin induced apoptotic death of cancer cells; decreasing formation of abnormal collagen fiber	[128,146]
	β-glucan	*in vitro*	protecting against B(α)P induced DNA damage by binding to the carcinogen, scavenging free radicals and probably modulating cell metabolism	[130]
	blazeispirols A and C	*in vitro*	displaying potent antiproliferative activities against Hep3B cells and HepG2 cells	[131]

Table 1. *Cont.*

Natural Products	Bioactive Components	Study Type	Bioactivities and Potential Mechanisms	References
Pleurotus pulmonarius	NA	*in vitro* and *in vivo*	reducing the incidence and size of tumor; inhibiting invasion and drug-resistance of hepatoma cells; enhancing cytotoxicity of cisplatin	[133,134]
Lentinula edodes	polysaccharide	*in vitro*	selectively killing HepG2 cells through the capase-3/-8 mediated extrinsic apoptosis pathway	[137]
Agrocybe aegerita	lectin	*in vitro*	binding to the surface of liver cancer cells, resulting apoptotic cell death	[138]
Flammulina velutipes	FVE (glycoprotein)	*in vivo*	prolonging survival time and reduced tumor size through inducing cytotoxic immune response	[140]
Suillus luteus	iso-suillin	*in vitro*	selectively inducing G1 cell cycle arrest and apoptotic death in cancer cells	[141]
Grifola frondosa	O-orsellinaldehyde	*in vitro*	exhibiting selective potent cytotoxicity against Hep3B cells	[142]

NA stands for not available.

9. Conclusions

Accumulating evidence suggested that many dietary natural products could be potential sources for prevention and treatment of liver cancer, and the following are notable for their potential anti-hepatoma properties, including (1) grapes, black currant, plum, pomegranate, and the isolated flavonoids, tannins, proanthocyanidins; (2) cruciferous vegetables (isothiocyanates), French beans (lectins), tomatoes (lycopene and tomatine), asparagus (polysaccharides and saponins); (3) garlic (organo-sulphur compounds), turmeric (curcumin), ginger (6-shogaol and 6-gingerol); and (4) soy, rice bran, and polysaccharides from edible macro-fungi. These dietary natural products and their active components could affect the development and progression of liver cancer in various ways, such as inhibiting tumor cell growth and metastasis, protecting against liver carcinogens, immunomodulating and enhancing effects of chemotherapeutic drugs. In the future, attention should be paid to the isolation of active compounds, the illustration of action mechanisms, bioavailability, potential toxicity and adverse effects, and more studies are required concerning the clinical efficacy of dietary natural products and their bioactive components.

Acknowledgments: This work was supported by the National Natural Science Foundation of China (No. 81372976), Key Project of Guangdong Provincial Science and Technology Program (No. 2014B020205002), and the Hundred-Talents Scheme of Sun Yat-Sen University.

Author Contributions: Y.Z. and H.B.L. conceived and designed the review. Y.Z., Y.L., T.Z. and J.Z. wrote the review. S.L. and H.B.L. revised the review. All authors discussed and approved the final version.

Conflicts of Interest: The authors declare no conflict of interest.

References

1. Marquardt, J.U.; Andersen, J.B.; Thorgeirsson, S.S. Functional and genetic deconstruction of the cellular origin in liver cancer. *Nat. Rev. Cancer* **2015**, *15*, 653–667. [CrossRef] [PubMed]
2. Torre, L.A.; Bray, F.; Siegel, R.L.; Ferlay, J.; Lortet-Tieulent, J.; Jemal, A. Global cancer statistics, 2012. *CA Cancer J. Clin.* **2015**, *65*, 87–108. [CrossRef] [PubMed]
3. De Jong, M.C.; Nathan, H.; Sotiropoulos, G.C.; Paul, A.; Alexandrescu, S.; Marques, H.; Pulitano, C.; Barroso, E.; Clary, B.M.; Aldrighetti, L.; *et al.* Intrahepatic cholangiocarcinoma: An international multi-institutional analysis of prognostic factors and lymph node assessment. *J. Clin. Oncol.* **2011**, *29*, 3140–3145. [CrossRef] [PubMed]
4. Chatterjee, R.; Mitra, A. An overview of effective therapies and recent advances in biomarkers for chronic liver diseases and associated liver cancer. *Int. Immunopharmacol.* **2015**, *24*, 335–345. [CrossRef] [PubMed]
5. Bruix, J.; Raoul, J.L.; Sherman, M.; Mazzaferro, V.; Bolondi, L.; Craxi, A.; Galle, P.R.; Santoro, A.; Beaugrand, M.; Sangiovanni, A.; *et al.* Efficacy and safety of sorafenib in patients with advanced hepatocellular carcinoma: Subanalyses of a phase III trial. *J. Hepatol.* **2012**, *57*, 821–829. [CrossRef] [PubMed]

6. Peng, S.l.; Zhao, Y.; Xu, F.; Jia, C.J.; Xu, Y.Q.; Dai, C.L. An updated meta-analysis of randomized controlled trials assessing the effect of sorafenib in advanced hepatocellular carcinoma. *PLoS ONE* **2014**, *9*, e112530. [CrossRef] [PubMed]
7. Chen, J; Jin, R.A.; Zhao, J.; Liu, J.H.; Ying, H.N.; Yan, H.; Zhou, S.J.; Liang, Y.L.; Huang, D.Y.; Liang, X.; *et al.* Potential molecular, cellular and microenvironmental mechanism of Sorafenib resistance in hepatocellular carcinoma. *Cancer Lett.* **2015**, *367*, 1–11.
8. Soerjomataram, I.; Oomen, D.; Lemmens, V.; Oenema, A.; Benetou, V.; Trichopoulou, A.; Coebergh, J.W.; Barendregt, J.; de Vries, E. Increased consumption of fruit and vegetable and future cancer incidence in selected European countries. *Eur. J. Cancer* **2010**, *46*, 2563–2580. [CrossRef] [PubMed]
9. Turati, F.; Rossi, M.; Pelucchi, C.; Levi, F.; La Vecchia, C. Fruit and vegetables and cancer risk: A review of southern European studies. *Br. J. Nutr.* **2015**, *113*, 102–110. [CrossRef] [PubMed]
10. Thoppil, R.J.; Bhatia, D.; Barnes, K.F.; Haznagy-Radnai, E.; Hohmann, J.; Darvesh, A.S.; Bishayee, A. Black currant anthocyanins abrogate oxidative stress through Nrf2-mediated antioxidant mechanisms in a rat model of hepatocellular carcinoma. *Curr. Cancer Drug Targets* **2012**, *12*, 1244–1257. [CrossRef] [PubMed]
11. Yu, M.H.; Gwon, I.H.; Gyu, L.S.; Kim, D.I.; Jeong, S.H.; Lee, I.S. Inhibitory effect of immature plum on PMA-induced MMP-9 expression in human hepatocellular carcinoma. *Nat. Prod. Res.* **2009**, *23*, 704–718. [CrossRef] [PubMed]
12. Ren, M.; Ye, L.; Hao, X.; Ren, Z.; Ren, S.; Xu, K.; Li, J. Polysaccharides from *Tricholoma matsutake* and *Lentinus edodes* enhance 5-fluorouracil-mediated H22 cell growth inhibition. *J. Tradit. Chin. Med.* **2014**, *34*, 309–316. [CrossRef]
13. Jo, J.Y.; de Mejia, E.G.; Lila, M.A. Cytotoxicity of bioactive polymeric fractions from grape cell culture on human hepatocellular carcinoma, murine leukemia and non-cancerous PK15 kidney cells. *Food Chem. Toxicol.* **2006**, *44*, 1758–1767. [CrossRef] [PubMed]
14. Fu, L.; Xu, B.T.; Xu, X.R.; Gan, R.Y.; Zhang, Y.; Xia, E.Q.; Li, H.B. Antioxidant capacities and total phenolic contents of 62 fruits. *Food Chem.* **2011**, *129*, 345–350. [CrossRef]
15. Li, F.; Li, S.; Li, H.B.; Deng, G.F.; Ling, W.H.; Wu, S.; Xu, X.R.; Chen, F. Antiproliferative activity of peels, pulps and seeds of 61 fruits. *J. Funct. Foods* **2013**, *5*, 1298–1309. [CrossRef]
16. Deng, G.F.; Shen, C.; Xu, X.R.; Kuang, R.D.; Guo, Y.J.; Zeng, L.S.; Gao, L.L.; Lin, X.; Xie, J.F.; Xia, E.Q.; *et al.* Potential of fruit wastes as natural resources of bioactive compounds. *Int. J. Mol. Sci.* **2012**, *13*, 8308–8323. [CrossRef] [PubMed]
17. Xia, E.Q.; Deng, G.F.; Guo, Y.J.; Li, H.B. Biological activities of polyphenols from grapes. *Int. J. Mol. Sci.* **2010**, *11*, 622–646. [CrossRef] [PubMed]
18. Jo, J.; Gonzalez De Mejia, E.; Lila, M.A. Effects of grape cell culture extracts on human topoisomerase II catalytic activity and characterization of active fractions. *J. Agric. Food Chem.* **2005**, *53*, 2489–2498. [CrossRef] [PubMed]
19. Feng, L.L.; Liu, B.X.; Zhong, J.Y.; Sun, L.B.; Yu, H.S. Effect of grape procyanidins on tumor angiogenesis in liver cancer xenograft models. *Asian Pac. J. Cancer Prev.* **2014**, *15*, 737–741. [CrossRef] [PubMed]
20. Scola, G.; Fernandes, C.L.C.; Menin, E.; Salvador, M. Suppression of oncoprotein Her-2 and DNA damage after treatment with Flavan-3-ol *Vitis labrusca* extract. *Anticancer Agents Med. Chem.* **2013**, *13*, 1088–1095. [CrossRef] [PubMed]
21. Bishayee, A.; Haznagy-Radnai, E.; Mbimba, T.; Sipos, P.; Morazzoni, P.; Darvesh, A.S.; Bhatia, D.; Hohmann, J. Anthocyanin-rich black currant extract suppresses the growth of human hepatocellular carcinoma cells. *Nat. Prod. Commun.* **2010**, *5*, 1613–1618. [PubMed]
22. Bishayee, A.; Thoppil, R.J.; Mandal, A.; Darvesh, A.S.; Ohanyan, V.; Meszaros, J.G.; Haznagy-Radnai, E.; Hohmann, J.; Bhatia, D. Black currant phytoconstituents exert chemoprevention of diethylnitrosamine-initiated hepatocarcinogenesis by suppression of the inflammatory response. *Mol. Carcinog.* **2013**, *52*, 304–317. [CrossRef] [PubMed]
23. Bishayee, A.; Mbimba, T.; Thoppil, R.J.; Haznagy-Radnai, E.; Sipos, P.; Darvesh, A.S.; Folkesson, H.G.; Hohmann, J. Anthocyanin-rich black currant (*Ribes nigrum* L.) extract affords chemoprevention against diethylnitrosamine-induced hepatocellular carcinogenesis in rats. *J. Nutr. Biochem.* **2011**, *22*, 1035–1046. [CrossRef] [PubMed]

24. Ramos, S.; Alia, M.; Bravo, L.; Goya, L. Comparative effects of food-derived polyphenols on the viability and apoptosis of a human hepatoma cell line (HepG2). *J. Agric. Food Chem.* **2005**, *53*, 1271–1280. [CrossRef] [PubMed]

25. Yu, M.H.; Im, H.G.; Kim, H.I.; Lee, I.S. Induction of apoptosis by immature plum in human hepatocellular carcinoma. *J. Med. Food* **2009**, *12*, 518–527. [CrossRef] [PubMed]

26. Kim, H.J.; Yu, M.H.; Lee, I.S. Inhibitory effects of methanol extract of plum (*Prunus salicina* L., cv. "Soldam") fruits against benzo(α)pyrene-induced toxicity in mice. *Food Chem. Toxicol.* **2008**, *46*, 3407–3413. [CrossRef] [PubMed]

27. Bishayee, A.; Thoppil, R.J.; Darvesh, A.S.; Ohanyan, V.; Meszaros, J.G.; Bhatia, D. Pomegranate phytoconstituents blunt the inflammatory cascade in a chemically induced rodent model of hepatocellular carcinogenesis. *J. Nutr. Biochem.* **2013**, *24*, 178–187. [CrossRef] [PubMed]

28. Bishayee, A.; Bhatia, D.; Thoppil, R.J.; Darvesh, A.S.; Nevo, E.; Lansky, E.P. Pomegranate-mediated chemoprevention of experimental hepatocarcinogenesis involves Nrf2-regulated antioxidant mechanisms. *Carcinogenesis* **2011**, *32*, 888–896. [CrossRef] [PubMed]

29. Huang, X.; Kojima-Yuasa, A.; Xu, S.; Kennedy, D.O.; Hasuma, T.; Matsui-Yuasa, I. Combination of *Zizyphus jujuba* and green tea extracts exerts excellent cytotoxic activity in HepG2 cells via reducing the expression of APRIL. *Am. J. Chin. Med.* **2009**, *37*, 169–179. [CrossRef] [PubMed]

30. Huang, X.; Kojima-Yuasa, A.; Xu, S.; Norikura, T.; Kennedy, D.O.; Hasuma, T.; Matsui-Yuasa, I. Green tea extract enhances the selective cytotoxic activity of *Zizyphus jujuba* extracts in HepG2 cells. *Am. J. Chin. Med.* **2008**, *36*, 729–744. [CrossRef] [PubMed]

31. Sudan, S.; Rupasinghe, H.P. Flavonoid-enriched apple fraction AF4 induces cell cycle arrest, DNA topoisomerase II inhibition, and apoptosis in human liver cancer HepG2 cells. *Nutr. Cancer* **2014**, *66*, 1237–1246. [CrossRef] [PubMed]

32. Chen, Y.; Xu, S.S.; Chen, J.W.; Wang, Y.; Xu, H.Q.; Fan, N.B.; Li, X. Anti-tumor activity of *Annona squamosa* seeds extract containing annonaceous acetogenin compounds. *J. Ethnopharmacol.* **2012**, *142*, 462–466. [CrossRef] [PubMed]

33. Gao, X.; Ohlander, M.; Jeppsson, N.; Björk, L.; Trajkovski, V. Changes in antioxidant effects and their relationship to phytonutrients in fruits of sea buckthorn (*Hippophae rhamnoides* L.) during maturation. *J. Agr. Food Chem.* **2000**, *48*, 1485–1490. [CrossRef]

34. Teng, B.S.; Lu, Y.H.; Wang, Z.T.; Tao, X.Y.; Wei, D.Z. *In vitro* anti-tumor activity of isorhamnetin isolated from *Hippophae rhamnoides* L. against BEL-7402 cells. *Pharmacol. Res.* **2006**, *54*, 186–194. [CrossRef] [PubMed]

35. Tien, P.G.; Kayama, F.; Konishi, F.; Tamemoto, H.; Kasono, K.; Hung, N.T.; Kuroki, M.; Ishikawa, S.E.; Van, C.N.; Kawakami, M. Inhibition of tumor growth and angiogenesis by water extract of Gac fruit (*Momordica cochinchinensis* Spreng). *Int. J. Oncol.* **2005**, *26*, 881–889. [CrossRef] [PubMed]

36. Chang, H.F.; Wu, C.H.; Yang, L.L. Antitumour and free radical scavenging effects of γ-mangostin isolated from *Garcinia mangostana* pericarps against hepatocellular carcinoma cell. *J. Pharm. Pharmacol.* **2013**, *65*, 1419–1428. [CrossRef] [PubMed]

37. Wang, X.; Wei, Y.; Yuan, S.; Liu, G.; Zhang, Y.L.; Wang, W. Potential anticancer activity of litchi fruit pericarp extract against hepatocellular carcinoma *in vitro* and *in vivo*. *Cancer Lett.* **2006**, *239*, 144–150. [CrossRef] [PubMed]

38. Hara, A.; Sakata, K.; Yamada, Y.; Kuno, T.; Kitaori, N.; Oyama, T.; Hirose, Y.; Murakami, A.; Tanaka, T.; Mori, H. Suppression of β-catenin mutation by dietary exposure of auraptene, a citrus antioxidant, in *N,N*-diethylnitrosamine-induced hepatocellular carcinomas in rats. *Oncol. Rep.* **2005**, *14*, 345–351. [CrossRef] [PubMed]

39. Prasad, S.; Kalra, N.; Shukla, Y. Hepatoprotective effects of lupeol and mango pulp extract of carcinogen induced alteration in Swiss albino mice. *Mol. Nutr. Food Res.* **2007**, *51*, 352–359. [CrossRef] [PubMed]

40. He, X.; Liu, R.H. Cranberry phytochemicals: Isolation, structure elucidation, and their antiproliferative and antioxidant activities. *J. Agric. Food Chem.* **2006**, *54*, 7069–7074. [CrossRef] [PubMed]

41. Luo, A.; Wang, F.; Luo, D.; Hu, D.; Mao, P.; Xie, W.; He, X.; Kan, W.; Wang, Y. Consumption of vegetables may reduce the risk of liver cancer: Results from a meta-analysis of case-control and cohort studies. *Clin. Res. Hepatol. Gas.* **2015**, *39*, 45–51. [CrossRef] [PubMed]

42. Hanlon, P.R.; Barnes, D.M. Phytochemical composition and biological activity of 8 varieties of radish (*Raphanus sativus* L.) sprouts and mature taproots. *J. Food Sci.* **2011**, *76*, C185–C192. [CrossRef] [PubMed]

43. Yeh, C.T.; Yen, G.C. Effect of vegetables on human phenolsulfotransferases in relation to their antioxidant activity and total phenolics. *Free Radic. Res.* **2005**, *39*, 893–904. [CrossRef] [PubMed]
44. Hanlon, P.R.; Webber, D.M.; Barnes, D.M. Aqueous extract from Spanish black radish (*Raphanus sativus* L. Var. niger) induces detoxification enzymes in the HepG2 human hepatoma cell line. *J. Agric. Food Chem.* **2007**, *55*, 6439–6446. [CrossRef] [PubMed]
45. Abdull, R.A.; De Nicola, G.R.; Pagnotta, E.; Iori, R.; Ioannides, C. 4-Methylsulfanyl-3-butenyl isothiocyanate derived from glucoraphasatin is a potent inducer of rat hepatic phase II enzymes and a potential chemopreventive agent. *Arch. Toxicol.* **2012**, *86*, 183–194. [CrossRef] [PubMed]
46. Anwar-Mohamed, A.; El-Kadi, A.O. Sulforaphane induces CYP1A1 mRNA, protein, and catalytic activity levels via an AhR-dependent pathway in murine hepatoma Hepa 1c1c7 and human HepG2 cells. *Cancer Lett.* **2009**, *275*, 93–101. [CrossRef] [PubMed]
47. Hwang, E.S.; Jeffery, E.H. Induction of quinone reductase by sulforaphane and sulforaphane *N*-acetylcysteine conjugate in murine hepatoma cells. *J. Med. Food* **2005**, *8*, 198–203. [CrossRef] [PubMed]
48. Hwang, E.S.; Lee, H.J. Induction of quinone reductase by allylisothiocyanate (AITC) and the *N*-acetylcysteine conjugate of AITC in Hepa1c1c7 mouse hepatoma cells. *Biofactors* **2006**, *26*, 7–15. [CrossRef] [PubMed]
49. Hwang, E.S.; Lee, H.J. Allyl isothiocyanate and its *N*-acetylcysteine conjugate suppress metastasis via inhibition of invasion, migration, and matrix metalloproteinase-2/-9 activities in SK-Hep 1 human hepatoma cells. *Exp. Biol. Med. (Maywood)* **2006**, *231*, 421–430. [PubMed]
50. Pasko, P.; Bukowska-Strakova, K.; Gdula-Argasinska, J.; Tyszka-Czochara, M. Rutabaga (*Brassica napus* L. var. napobrassica) seeds, roots, and sprouts: A novel kind of food with antioxidant properties and proapoptotic potential in HepG2 hepatoma cell line. *J. Med. Food* **2013**, *16*, 749–759. [CrossRef] [PubMed]
51. Spanou, C.; Stagos, D.; Aligiannis, N.; Kouretas, D. Influence of potent antioxidant leguminosae family plant extracts on growth and antioxidant defense system of Hep2 cancer cell line. *J. Med. Food* **2010**, *13*, 149–155. [CrossRef] [PubMed]
52. Dong, M.; He, X.; Liu, R.H. Phytochemicals of black bean seed coats: Isolation, structure elucidation, and their antiproliferative and antioxidative activities. *J. Agric. Food Chem.* **2007**, *55*, 6044–6051. [CrossRef] [PubMed]
53. Lam, S.K.; Ng, T.B. Isolation and characterization of a French bean hemagglutinin with antitumor, antifungal, and anti-HIV-1 reverse transcriptase activities and an exceptionally high yield. *Phytomedicine* **2010**, *17*, 457–462. [CrossRef] [PubMed]
54. Fang, E.F.; Pan, W.L.; Wong, J.H.; Chan, Y.S.; Ye, X.J.; Ng, T.B. A new *Phaseolus vulgaris* lectin induces selective toxicity on human liver carcinoma Hep G2 cells. *Arch. Toxicol.* **2011**, *85*, 1551–1563. [CrossRef] [PubMed]
55. Wong, J.H.; Wan, C.T.; Ng, T.B. Characterisation of a haemagglutinin from Hokkaido red bean (*Phaseolus vulgaris* cv. Hokkaido red bean). *J. Sci. Food Agric.* **2010**, *90*, 70–77. [CrossRef] [PubMed]
56. Wang, Y.; Ausman, L.M.; Greenberg, A.S.; Russell, R.M.; Wang, X.D. Dietary lycopene and tomato extract supplementations inhibit nonalcoholic steatohepatitis-promoted hepatocarcinogenesis in rats. *Int. J. Cancer* **2010**, *126*, 1788–1796. [CrossRef] [PubMed]
57. Koul, A.; Arora, N.; Tanwar, L. Lycopene mediated modulation of 7,12-Dimethlybenz(α) anthracene induced hepatic clastogenicity in male Balb/c mice. *Nutr. Hosp.* **2010**, *25*, 304–310. [PubMed]
58. Gupta, P.; Bansal, M.P.; Koul, A. Lycopene modulates initiation of *N*-nitrosodiethylamine induced hepatocarcinogenesis: Studies on chromosomal abnormalities, membrane fluidity and antioxidant defense system. *Chem. Biol. Interact.* **2013**, *206*, 364–374. [CrossRef] [PubMed]
59. Gupta, P.; Bansal, M.P.; Koul, A. Evaluating the effect of lycopene from *Lycopersicum esculentum* on apoptosis during NDEA induced hepatocarcinogenesis. *Biochem. Biophys. Res. Commun.* **2013**, *434*, 479–485. [CrossRef] [PubMed]
60. Gupta, P.; Bansal, M.P.; Koul, A. Spectroscopic characterization of lycopene extract from *Lycopersicum esculentum* (Tomato) and its evaluation as a chemopreventive agent against experimental hepatocarcinogenesis in mice. *Phytother. Res.* **2013**, *27*, 448–456. [CrossRef] [PubMed]
61. Friedman, M.; Levin, C.E.; Lee, S.U.; Kim, H.J.; Lee, I.S.; Byun, J.O.; Kozukue, N. Tomatine-containing green tomato extracts inhibit growth of human breast, colon, liver, and stomach cancer cells. *J. Agric. Food Chem.* **2009**, *57*, 5727–5733. [CrossRef] [PubMed]

62. Xiang, J.; Xiang, Y.; Lin, S.; Xin, D.; Liu, X.; Weng, L.; Chen, T.; Zhang, M. Anticancer effects of deproteinized asparagus polysaccharide on hepatocellular carcinoma *in vitro* and *in vivo*. *Tumour Biol.* **2014**, *35*, 3517–3524. [CrossRef] [PubMed]

63. Weng, L.L.; Xiang, J.F.; Lin, J.B.; Yi, S.H.; Yang, L.T.; Li, Y.S.; Zeng, H.T.; Lin, S.M.; Xin, D.W.; Zhao, H.L.; *et al.* Asparagus polysaccharide and gum with hepatic artery embolization induces tumor growth and inhibits angiogenesis in an orthotopic hepatocellular carcinoma model. *Asian Pac. J Cancer. Prev.* **2014**, *15*, 10949–10955. [CrossRef] [PubMed]

64. Huang, X.; Lin, Y.; Kong, L. Steroids from the roots of *Asparagus officinalis* and their cytotoxic activity. *J. Integr. Plant Biol.* **2008**, *50*, 717–722. [CrossRef] [PubMed]

65. Liu, W.; Huang, X.F.; Qi, Q.; Dai, Q.S.; Yang, L.; Nie, F.F.; Lu, N.; Gong, D.D.; Kong, L.Y.; Guo, Q.L. Asparanin A induces G_2/M cell cycle arrest and apoptosis in human hepatocellular carcinoma HepG2 cells. *Biochem. Biophys. Res. Commun.* **2009**, *381*, 700–705. [CrossRef] [PubMed]

66. Hafidh, R.R.; Abdulamir, A.S.; Bakar, F.A.; Jalilian, F.A.; Abas, F.; Sekawi, Z. Novel molecular, cytotoxical, and immunological study on promising and selective anticancer activity of mung bean sprouts. *BMC Complement. Altern. Med.* **2012**, *12*, 208. [CrossRef] [PubMed]

67. Zhang, C.Z.; Fang, E.F.; Zhang, H.T.; Liu, L.L.; Yun, J.P. *Momordica charantia* lectin exhibits antitumor activity towards hepatocellular carcinoma. *Investig. New Drugs* **2015**, *33*, 1–11. [CrossRef] [PubMed]

68. Fang, E.F.; Zhang, C.Z.; Wong, J.H.; Shen, J.Y.; Li, C.H.; Ng, T.B. The MAP30 protein from bitter gourd (*Momordica charantia*) seeds promotes apoptosis in liver cancer cells *in vitro* and *in vivo*. *Cancer Lett.* **2012**, *324*, 66–74. [CrossRef] [PubMed]

69. Fang, E.F.; Zhang, C.Z.; Zhang, L.; Fong, W.P.; Ng, T.B. *In vitro* and *in vivo* anticarcinogenic effects of RNase MC2, a ribonuclease isolated from dietary bitter gourd, toward human liver cancer cells. *Int. J. Biochem. Cell Biol.* **2012**, *44*, 1351–1360. [CrossRef] [PubMed]

70. Wang, Y.; Huang, X.; Han, J.; Zheng, W.; Ma, W. Extract of *Perilla frutescens* inhibits tumor proliferation of HCC via PI3K/AKT signal pathway. *Afr. J. Tradit. Complement. Alt. Med.* **2013**, *10*, 251–257. [CrossRef]

71. Wang, Q.; Chen, Q.; He, M.; Mir, P.; Su, J.; Yang, Q. Inhibitory effect of antioxidant extracts from various potatoes on the proliferation of human colon and liver cancer cells. *Nutr. Cancer* **2011**, *63*, 1044–1052. [CrossRef] [PubMed]

72. Friedman, M.; Lee, K.R.; Kim, H.J.; Lee, I.S.; Kozukue, N. Anticarcinogenic effects of glycoalkaloids from potatoes against human cervical, liver, lymphoma, and stomach cancer cells. *J. Agric. Food Chem.* **2005**, *53*, 6162–6169. [CrossRef] [PubMed]

73. Sultana, S.; Ahmed, S.; Jahangir, T.; Sharma, S. Inhibitory effect of celery seeds extract on chemically induced hepatocarcinogenesis: Modulation of cell proliferation, metabolism and altered hepatic foci development. *Cancer Lett.* **2005**, *221*, 11–20. [CrossRef] [PubMed]

74. Arnault, I.; Haffner, T.; Siess, M.H.; Vollmar, A.; Kahane, R.; Auger, J. Analytical method for appreciation of garlic therapeutic potential and for validation of a new formulation. *J. Pharm. Biomed. Anal.* **2005**, *37*, 963–970. [CrossRef] [PubMed]

75. Iciek, M.; Kwiecien, I.; Chwatko, G.; Sokolowska-Jezewicz, M.; Kowalczyk-Pachel, D.; Rokita, H. The effects of garlic-derived sulfur compounds on cell proliferation, caspase 3 activity, thiol levels and anaerobic sulfur metabolism in human hepatoblastoma HepG2 cells. *Cell Biochem. Funct.* **2012**, *30*, 198–204. [CrossRef] [PubMed]

76. Singh, V.; Belloir, C.; Siess, M.H.; Le Bon, A.M. Inhibition of carcinogen-induced DNA damage in rat liver and colon by garlic powders with varying alliin content. *Nutr. Cancer* **2006**, *55*, 178–184. [CrossRef] [PubMed]

77. Belloir, C.; Singh, V.; Daurat, C.; Siess, M.H.; Le Bon, A.M. Protective effects of garlic sulfur compounds against DNA damage induced by direct- and indirect-acting genotoxic agents in HepG2 cells. *Food Chem. Toxicol.* **2006**, *44*, 827–834. [CrossRef] [PubMed]

78. Chang, H.S.; Ko, M.; Ishizuka, M.; Fujita, S.; Yabuki, A.; Hossain, M.A.; Yamato, O. Sodium 2-propenyl thiosulfate derived from garlic induces phase II detoxification enzymes in rat hepatoma H4IIE cells. *Nutr. Res.* **2010**, *30*, 435–440. [CrossRef] [PubMed]

79. Ng, K.T.; Guo, D.Y.; Cheng, Q.; Geng, W.; Ling, C.C.; Li, C.X.; Liu, X.B.; Ma, Y.Y.; Lo, C.M.; Poon, R.T.; *et al.* A garlic derivative, *S*-allylcysteine (SAC), suppresses proliferation and metastasis of hepatocellular carcinoma. *PLoS ONE* **2012**, *7*, e31655. [CrossRef] [PubMed]

80. Chu, Y.L.; Ho, C.T.; Chung, J.G.; Raghu, R.; Lo, Y.C.; Sheen, L.Y. Allicin induces anti-human liver cancer cells through the p53 gene modulating apoptosis and autophagy. *J. Agric. Food Chem.* **2013**, *61*, 9839–9848. [CrossRef] [PubMed]

81. De Martino, A.; Filomeni, G.; Aquilano, K.; Ciriolo, M.R.; Rotilio, G. Effects of water garlic extracts on cell cycle and viability of HepG2 hepatoma cells. *J. Nutr. Biochem.* **2006**, *17*, 742–749. [CrossRef] [PubMed]

82. Uda, N.; Kashimoto, N.; Sumioka, I.; Kyo, E.; Sumi, S.; Fukushima, S. Aged garlic extract inhibits development of putative preneoplastic lesions in rat hepatocarcinogenesis. *J. Nutr.* **2006**, *136*, 855S–860S. [PubMed]

83. Ishikawa, H.; Saeki, T.; Otani, T.; Suzuki, T.; Shimozuma, K.; Nishino, H.; Fukuda, S.; Morimoto, K. Aged garlic extract prevents a decline of NK cell number and activity in patients with advanced cancer. *J. Nutr.* **2006**, *136*, 816S–820S. [PubMed]

84. Kim, J.; Ha, H.L.; Moon, H.B.; Lee, Y.W.; Cho, C.K.; Yoo, H.S.; Yu, D.Y. Chemopreventive effect of *Curcuma longa* Linn on liver pathology in HBx transgenic mice. *Integr. Cancer Ther.* **2011**, *10*, 168–177. [CrossRef] [PubMed]

85. Sreepriya, M.; Bali, G. Chemopreventive effects of embelin and curcumin against *N*-nitrosodiethylamine/phenobarbital-induced hepatocarcinogenesis in Wistar rats. *Fitoterapia* **2005**, *76*, 549–555. [CrossRef] [PubMed]

86. Strofer, M.; Jelkmann, W.; Depping, R. Curcumin decreases survival of Hep3B liver and MCF-7 breast cancer cells: The role of HIF. *Strahlenther. Onkol.* **2011**, *187*, 393–400. [CrossRef] [PubMed]

87. Shoji, M.; Nakagawa, K.; Watanabe, A.; Tsuduki, T.; Yamada, T.; Kuwahara, S.; Kimura, F.; Miyazawa, T. Comparison of the effects of curcumin and curcumin glucuronide in human hepatocellular carcinoma HepG2 cells. *Food Chem.* **2014**, *151*, 126–132. [CrossRef] [PubMed]

88. Li, Y.; Shi, X.; Zhang, J.; Zhang, X.; Martin, R.C. Hepatic protection and anticancer activity of curcuma: A potential chemopreventive strategy against hepatocellular carcinoma. *Int. J. Oncol.* **2014**, *44*, 505–513. [CrossRef] [PubMed]

89. Cheng, S.B.; Wu, L.C.; Hsieh, Y.C.; Wu, C.H.; Chan, Y.J.; Chang, L.H.; Chang, C.M.; Hsu, S.L.; Teng, C.L.; Wu, C.C. Supercritical carbon dioxide extraction of aromatic turmerone from *Curcuma longa* L. inn. induces apoptosis through reactive oxygen species-triggered intrinsic and extrinsic pathways in human hepatocellular carcinoma HepG2 cells. *J. Agric. Food Chem.* **2012**, *60*, 9620–9630. [CrossRef] [PubMed]

90. Lizcano, L.J.; Siles, M.; Trepiana, J.; Hernandez, M.L.; Navarro, R.; Ruiz-Larrea, M.B.; Ruiz-Sanz, J.I. Piper and vismia species from Colombian Amazonia differentially affect cell proliferation of hepatocarcinoma cells. *Nutrients* **2015**, *7*, 179–195. [CrossRef] [PubMed]

91. Lee, J.; Lee, S.J.; Lim, K.T. ZPDC glycoprotein (24 kDa) induces apoptosis and enhances activity of NK cells in *N*-nitrosodiethylamine-injected Balb/c. *Cell Immunol.* **2014**, *289*, 1–6. [CrossRef] [PubMed]

92. Dung, T.D.; Feng, C.C.; Kuo, W.W.; Pai, P.; Chung, L.C.; Chang, S.H.; Hsu, H.H.; Tsai, F.J.; Lin, Y.M.; Huang, C.Y. Suppression of plasminogen activators and the MMP-2/-9 pathway by a *Zanthoxylum avicennae* extract to inhibit the HA22T human hepatocellular carcinoma cell migration and invasion effects *in vitro* and *in vivo* via phosphatase 2A activation. *Biosci. Biotechnol. Biochem.* **2013**, *77*, 1814–1821. [CrossRef] [PubMed]

93. Dung, T.D.; Chang, H.C.; Binh, T.V.; Lee, M.R.; Tsai, C.H.; Tsai, F.J.; Kuo, W.W.; Chen, L.M.; Huang, C.Y. *Zanthoxylum avicennae* extracts inhibit cell proliferation through protein phosphatase 2A activation in HA22T human hepatocellular carcinoma cells *in vitro* and *in vivo*. *Int. J. Mol. Med.* **2012**, *29*, 1045–1052. [PubMed]

94. Dung, T.D.; Chang, H.C.; Chen, C.Y.; Peng, W.H.; Tsai, C.H.; Tsai, F.J.; Kuo, W.W.; Chen, L.M.; Huang, C.Y. *Zanthoxylum avicennae* extracts induce cell apoptosis through protein phosphatase 2A activation in HA22T human hepatocellular carcinoma cells and block tumor growth in xenografted nude mice. *Int. J. Mol. Med.* **2011**, *28*, 927–936. [PubMed]

95. Paik, S.Y.; Koh, K.H.; Beak, S.M.; Paek, S.H.; Kim, J.A. The essential oils from *Zanthoxylum schinifolium* pericarp induce apoptosis of HepG2 human hepatoma cells through increased production of reactive oxygen species. *Biol. Pharm. Bull.* **2005**, *28*, 802–807. [CrossRef] [PubMed]

96. Choudhury, D.; Das, A.; Bhattacharya, A.; Chakrabarti, G. Aqueous extract of ginger shows antiproliferative activity through disruption of microtubule network of cancer cells. *Food Chem. Toxicol.* **2010**, *48*, 2872–2880. [CrossRef] [PubMed]

97. Manju, V.; Nalini, N. Chemopreventive efficacy of ginger, a naturally occurring anticarcinogen during the initiation, post-initiation stages of 1,2 dimethylhydrazine-induced colon cancer. *Clin. Chim. Acta* **2005**, *358*, 60–67. [CrossRef] [PubMed]

98. Park, K.K.; Chun, K.S.; Lee, J.M.; Lee, S.S.; Surh, Y.J. Inhibitory effects of 6-gingerol, a major pungent principle of ginger, on phorbol ester-induced inflammation, epidermal ornithine decarboxylase activity and skin tumor promotion in ICR mice. *Cancer Lett.* **1998**, *129*, 139–144. [CrossRef]

99. Mansour, M.A.; Bekheet, S.A.; Al-Rejaie, S.S.; Al-Shabanah, O.A.; Al-Howiriny, T.A.; Al-Rikabi, A.C.; Abdo, A.A. Ginger ingredients inhibit the development of diethylnitrosoamine induced premalignant phenotype in rat chemical hepatocarcinogenesis model. *Biofactors* **2010**, *36*, 483–490. [CrossRef] [PubMed]

100. Habib, S.H.; Makpol, S.; Abdul, H.N.; Das, S.; Ngah, W.Z.; Yusof, Y.A. Ginger extract (*Zingiber officinale*) has anti-cancer and anti-inflammatory effects on ethionine-induced hepatoma rats. *Clinics* **2008**, *63*, 807–813. [CrossRef] [PubMed]

101. Vijaya, P.V.; Arul, D.C.S.; Ramkuma, K.M. Induction of apoptosis by ginger in HEp-2 cell line is mediated by reactive oxygen species. *Basic Clin. Pharmacol. Toxicol.* **2007**, *100*, 302–307. [CrossRef] [PubMed]

102. Weng, C.J.; Wu, C.F.; Huang, H.W.; Ho, C.T.; Yen, G.C. Anti-invasion effects of 6-shogaol and 6-gingerol, two active components in ginger, on human hepatocarcinoma cells. *Mol. Nutr. Food Res.* **2010**, *54*, 1618–1627. [CrossRef] [PubMed]

103. Chen, C.Y.; Liu, T.Z.; Liu, Y.W.; Tseng, W.C.; Liu, R.H.; Lu, F.J.; Lin, Y.S.; Kuo, S.H.; Chen, C.H. 6-shogaol (alkanone from ginger) induces apoptotic cell death of human hepatoma p53 mutant Mahlavu subline via an oxidative stress-mediated caspase-dependent mechanism. *J. Agric. Food Chem.* **2007**, *55*, 948–954. [CrossRef] [PubMed]

104. Yadav, A.S.; Bhatnagar, D. Chemo-preventive effect of Star anise in *N*-nitrosodiethylamine initiated and phenobarbital promoted hepato-carcinogenesis. *Chem. Biol. Interact.* **2007**, *169*, 207–214. [CrossRef] [PubMed]

105. Tavakkol-Afshari, J.; Brook, A.; Mousavi, S.H. Study of cytotoxic and apoptogenic properties of saffron extract in human cancer cell lines. *Food Chem. Toxicol.* **2008**, *46*, 3443–3447. [CrossRef] [PubMed]

106. Amin, A.; Hamza, A.A.; Bajbouj, K.; Ashraf, S.S.; Daoud, S. Saffron: A potential candidate for a novel anticancer drug against hepatocellular carcinoma. *Hepatology* **2011**, *54*, 857–867. [CrossRef] [PubMed]

107. Zhang, H.T.; Wu, J.; Wen, M.; Su, L.J.; Luo, H. Galangin induces apoptosis in hepatocellular carcinoma cells through the caspase 8/t-Bid mitochondrial pathway. *J. Asian Nat. Prod. Res.* **2012**, *14*, 626–633. [CrossRef] [PubMed]

108. An, N.; Zou, Z.M.; Tian, Z.; Luo, X.Z.; Yang, S.L.; Xu, L.Z. Diarylheptanoids from the rhizomes of *Alpinia officinarum* and their anticancer activity. *Fitoterapia* **2008**, *79*, 27–31. [CrossRef] [PubMed]

109. Chen, C.Y.; Liu, T.Z.; Chen, C.H.; Wu, C.C.; Cheng, J.T.; Yiin, S.J.; Shih, M.K.; Wu, M.J.; Chern, C.L. Isoobtusilactone A-induced apoptosis in human hepatoma HepG2 cells is mediated via increased NADPH oxidase-derived reactive oxygen species (ROS) production and the mitochondria-associated apoptotic mechanisms. *Food Chem. Toxicol.* **2007**, *45*, 1268–1276. [CrossRef] [PubMed]

110. Chen, C.Y.; Yiin, S.J.; Hsu, J.L.; Wang, W.C.; Lin, S.C.; Chern, C.L. Isoobtusilactone A sensitizes human hepatoma HepG2 cells to TRAIL-induced apoptosis via ROS and CHOP-mediated up-regulation of DR5. *J. Agric. Food Chem.* **2012**, *60*, 3533–3539. [CrossRef] [PubMed]

111. Jeurissen, S.M.; Punt, A.; Delatour, T.; Rietjens, I.M. Basil extract inhibits the sulfotransferase mediated formation of DNA adducts of the procarcinogen 1'-hydroxyestragole by rat and human liver S9 homogenates and in HepG2 human hepatoma cells. *Food Chem. Toxicol.* **2008**, *46*, 2296–2302. [CrossRef] [PubMed]

112. Costa, S.; Utan, A.; Speroni, E.; Cervellati, R.; Piva, G.; Prandini, A.; Guerra, M.C. Carnosic acid from rosemary extracts: A potential chemoprotective agent against aflatoxin B1. An *in vitro* study. *J. Appl. Toxicol.* **2007**, *27*, 152–159. [CrossRef] [PubMed]

113. Limer, J.L.; Speirs, V. Phyto-oestrogens and breast cancer chemoprevention. *Breast Cancer Res.* **2004**, *6*, 119–127. [CrossRef] [PubMed]

114. Kampkotter, A.; Wiegand, C.; Timpel, C.; Rohrdanz, E.; Chovolou, Y.; Kahl, R.; Watjen, W. Increased expression of catalase in human hepatoma cells by the soy isoflavone, daidzein. *Basic Clin. Pharmacol. Toxicol.* **2008**, *102*, 437–442. [CrossRef] [PubMed]

115. Ho, V.S.; Ng, T.B. A Bowman-Birk trypsin inhibitor with antiproliferative activity from Hokkaido large black soybeans. *J. Pept. Sci.* **2008**, *14*, 278–282. [CrossRef] [PubMed]

116. Ye, X.; Ng, T.B. A trypsin-chymotrypsin inhibitor with antiproliferative activity from small glossy black soybeans. *Planta Med.* **2009**, *75*, 550–556. [CrossRef] [PubMed]
117. Helferich, W.G.; Andrade, J.E.; Hoagland, M.S. Phytoestrogens and breast cancer: A complex story. *Inflammopharmacology* **2008**, *16*, 219–226. [CrossRef] [PubMed]
118. Kannan, A.; Hettiarachchy, N.; Johnson, M.G.; Nannapaneni, R. Human colon and liver cancer cell proliferation inhibition by peptide hydrolysates derived from heat-stabilized defatted rice bran. *J. Agric. Food Chem.* **2008**, *56*, 11643–11647. [CrossRef] [PubMed]
119. LIU, Z. Grain phytic acid content in japonica rice as affected by cultivar and environment and its relation to protein content. *Food Chem.* **2005**, *89*, 49–52. [CrossRef]
120. Al-Fatlawi, A.A.; Al-Fatlawi, A.A.; Irshad, M.; Zafaryab, M.; Rizvi, M.M.; Ahmad, A. Rice bran phytic acid induced apoptosis through regulation of Bcl-2/Bax and p53 genes in HepG2 human hepatocellular carcinoma cells. *Asian Pac. J. Cancer Prev.* **2014**, *15*, 3731–3736. [CrossRef] [PubMed]
121. Deng, G.F.; Xu, X.R.; Zhang, Y.; Li, D.; Gan, R.Y.; Li, H.B. Phenolic compounds and bioactivities of pigmented rice. *Crit. Rev. Food Sci.* **2013**, *53*, 296–306. [CrossRef] [PubMed]
122. Banjerdpongchai, R.; Wudtiwai, B.; Sringarm, K. Cytotoxic and apoptotic-inducing effects of purple rice extracts and chemotherapeutic drugs on human cancer cell lines. *Asian Pac. J. Cancer Prev.* **2014**, *14*, 6541–6548. [CrossRef] [PubMed]
123. Yang, J.; Li, X.; Xue, Y.; Wang, N.; Liu, W. Anti-hepatoma activity and mechanism of corn silk polysaccharides in H22 tumor-bearing mice. *Int. J. Biol. Macromol.* **2014**, *64*, 276–280. [CrossRef] [PubMed]
124. Lu, Y.; Zhang, B.Y.; Jia, Z.X.; Wu, W.J.; Lu, Z.Q. Hepatocellular carcinoma HepG2 cell apoptosis and caspase-8 and Bcl-2 expression induced by injectable seed extract of *Coix lacryma*-jobi. *Hepatob. Pancreatic. Dis. Int.* **2011**, *10*, 303–307. [CrossRef]
125. Kim, S.H.; Cui, C.B.; Kang, I.J.; Kim, S.Y.; Ham, S.S. Cytotoxic effect of buckwheat (*Fagopyrum esculentum* Moench) hull against cancer cells. *J. Med. Food.* **2007**, *10*, 232–238. [CrossRef] [PubMed]
126. Guo, Y.J.; Deng, G.F.; Xu, X.R.; Wu, S.; Li, S.; Xia, E.Q.; Li, F.; Chen, F.; Ling, W.H.; Li, H.B. Antioxidant capacities, phenolic compounds and polysaccharide contents of 49 edible macro-fungi. *Food Funct.* **2012**, *3*, 1195–1205. [CrossRef] [PubMed]
127. Ahn, W.S.; Kim, D.J.; Chae, G.T.; Lee, J.M.; Bae, S.M.; Sin, J.I.; Kim, Y.W.; Namkoong, S.E.; Lee, I.P. Natural killer cell activity and quality of life were improved by consumption of a mushroom extract, *Agaricus blazei* Murill Kyowa, in gynecological cancer patients undergoing chemotherapy. *Int. J. Gynecol. Cancer* **2004**, *14*, 589–594. [CrossRef] [PubMed]
128. Sorimachi, K.; Akimoto, K.; Koge, T. Inhibitory effect of *Agaricu blazei* Murill components on abnormal collagen fiber formation in human hepatocarcinoma cells. *Biosci. Biotechnol. Biochem.* **2008**, *72*, 621–623. [CrossRef]
129. Wu, M.F.; Lu, H.F.; Hsu, Y.M.; Tang, M.C.; Chen, H.C.; Lee, C.S.; Yang, Y.Y.; Yeh, M.Y.; Chung, H.K.; Huang, Y.P.; et al. Possible reduction of hepatoma formation by Smmu 7721 cells in SCID mice and metastasis formation by B16F10 melanoma cells in C57BL/6 mice by *Agaricus blazei* Murill extract. *Vivo* **2011**, *25*, 399–404.
130. Angeli, J.P.; Ribeiro, L.R.; Bellini, M.F.; Mantovani, M.S. β-glucan extracted from the medicinal mushroom *Agaricus blazei* prevents the genotoxic effects of benzo(α)pyrene in the human hepatoma cell line HepG2. *Arch. Toxicol.* **2009**, *83*, 81–86. [CrossRef] [PubMed]
131. Su, Z.Y.; Hwang, L.S.; Kuo, Y.H.; Shu, C.H.; Sheen, L.Y. Black soybean promotes the formation of active components with antihepatoma activity in the fermentation product of *Agaricus blazei*. *J. Agric. Food Chem.* **2008**, *56*, 9447–9454. [CrossRef] [PubMed]
132. Su, Z.Y.; Tung, Y.C.; Hwang, L.S.; Sheen, L.Y. Blazeispirol A from *Agaricus blazei* fermentation product induces cell death in human hepatoma Hep3B cells through caspase-dependent and caspase-independent pathways. *J. Agric. Food Chem.* **2011**, *59*, 5109–5116. [CrossRef] [PubMed]
133. Xu, W.W.; Li, B.; Lai, E.T.; Chen, L.; Huang, J.J.; Cheung, A.L.; Cheung, P.C. Water extract from *Pleurotus pulmonarius* with antioxidant activity exerts *in vivo* chemoprophylaxis and chemosensitization for liver cancer. *Nutr. Cancer* **2014**, *66*, 989–998. [CrossRef] [PubMed]
134. Xu, W.; Huang, J.J.; Cheung, P.C. Extract of *Pleurotus pulmonarius* suppresses liver cancer development and progression through inhibition of VEGF-induced PI3K/AKT signaling pathway. *PLoS ONE* **2012**, *7*, e34406. [CrossRef] [PubMed]

135. Mariga, A.M.; Yang, W.J.; Mugambi, D.K.; Pei, F.; Zhao, L.Y.; Shao, Y.N.; Hu, Q. Antiproliferative and immunostimulatory activity of a protein from *Pleurotus eryngii*. *J. Sci. Food Agric.* **2014**, *94*, 3152–3162. [CrossRef] [PubMed]

136. Wang, C.R.; Ng, T.B.; Li, L.; Fang, J.C.; Jiang, Y.; Wen, T.Y.; Qiao, W.T.; Li, N.; Liu, F. Isolation of a polysaccharide with antiproliferative, hypoglycemic, antioxidant and HIV-1 reverse transcriptase inhibitory activities from the fruiting bodies of the abalone mushroom *Pleurotus abalonus*. *J. Pharm. Pharmacol.* **2011**, *63*, 825–832. [CrossRef] [PubMed]

137. Yukawa, H.; Ishikawa, S.; Kawanishi, T.; Tamesada, M.; Tomi, H. Direct cytotoxicity of *Lentinula edodes* mycelia extract on human hepatocellular carcinoma cell line. *Biol. Pharm. Bull.* **2012**, *35*, 1014–1021. [CrossRef] [PubMed]

138. Jiang, S.; Chen, Y.; Wang, M.; Yin, Y.; Pan, Y.; Gu, B.; Yu, G.; Li, Y.; Wong, B.H.; Liang, Y.; *et al.* A novel lectin from *Agrocybe aegerita* shows high binding selectivity for terminal N-acetylglucosamine. *Biochem. J.* **2012**, *443*, 369–378. [CrossRef] [PubMed]

139. Hsieh, C.W.; Lan, J.L.; Meng, Q.; Cheng, Y.W.; Huang, H.M.; Tsai, J.J. Eosinophil apoptosis induced by fungal immunomodulatory peptide-fve via reducing IL-5α receptor. *J. Formos. Med. Assoc.* **2007**, *106*, 36–43. [CrossRef]

140. Chang, H.H.; Hsieh, K.Y.; Yeh, C.H.; Tu, Y.P.; Sheu, F. Oral administration of an Enoki mushroom protein FVE activates innate and adaptive immunity and induces anti-tumor activity against murine hepatocellular carcinoma. *Int. Immunopharmacol.* **2010**, *10*, 239–246. [CrossRef] [PubMed]

141. Jia, Z.Q.; Chen, Y.; Yan, Y.X.; Zhao, J.X. Iso-suillin isolated from *Suillus luteus*, induces G_1 phase arrest and apoptosis in human hepatoma SMMC-7721 cells. *Asian Pac. J. Cancer Prev.* **2014**, *15*, 1423–1428. [CrossRef] [PubMed]

142. Lin, J.T.; Liu, W.H. o-Orsellinaldehyde from the submerged culture of the edible mushroom *Grifola frondosa* exhibits selective cytotoxic effect against Hep 3B cells through apoptosis. *J. Agric. Food Chem.* **2006**, *54*, 7564–7569. [CrossRef] [PubMed]

143. Norikura, T.; Fujiwara, K.; Yanai, T.; Sano, Y.; Sato, T.; Tsunoda, T.; Kushibe, K.; Todate, A.; Morinaga, Y.; Iwai, K.; Matsue, H. p-terphenyl derivatives from the mushroom *Thelephora aurantiotincta* suppress the proliferation of human hepatocellular carcinoma cells via iron chelation. *J. Agric. Food Chem.* **2013**, *61*, 1258–1264. [CrossRef] [PubMed]

144. Zhang, X.Y.; Bai, D.C.; Wu, Y.J.; Li, W.G.; Liu, N.F. Proanthocyanidin from grape seeds enhances anti-tumor effect of doxorubicin both *in vitro* and *in vivo*. *Pharmazie* **2005**, *60*, 533–538. [PubMed]

145. Liang, G.; Tang, A.; Lin, X.; Li, L.; Zhang, S.; Huang, Z.; Tang, H.; Li, Q.Q. Green tea catechins augment the antitumor activity of doxorubicin in an *in vivo* mouse model for chemoresistant liver cancer. *Int. J. Oncol.* **2010**, *37*, 111–123. [PubMed]

146. Lee, J.S.; Hong, E.K. *Agaricus blazei* Murill enhances doxorubicin-induced apoptosis in human hepatocellular carcinoma cells by NFκB-mediated increase of intracellular doxorubicin accumulation. *Int. J. Oncol.* **2011**, *38*, 401–408. [PubMed]

147. Lee, J.S.; Hong, E.K. *Hericium erinaceus* enhances doxorubicin-induced apoptosis in human hepatocellular carcinoma cells. *Cancer Lett.* **2010**, *297*, 144–154. [CrossRef] [PubMed]

148. Karabulut, A.B.; Karadag, N.; Gurocak, S.; Kiran, T.; Tuzcu, M.; Sahin, K. Apricot attenuates oxidative stress and modulates of Bax, Bcl-2, caspases, NFκ-B, AP-1, CREB expression of rats bearing DMBA-induced liver damage and treated with a combination of radiotherapy. *Food Chem. Toxicol.* **2014**, *70*, 128–133. [CrossRef] [PubMed]

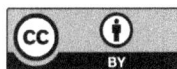

nutrients

MDPI

Article

Antiproliferative Activity of Triterpene Glycoside Nutrient from Monk Fruit in Colorectal Cancer and Throat Cancer

Can Liu [1,2,3], Longhai Dai [2], Yueping Liu [1,3,]*, Long Rong [4], Dequan Dou [1,]*, Yuanxia Sun [2] and Lanqing Ma [1,3,]*

[1]   Key Laboratory of Urban Agriculture (North) of Ministry of Agriculture, Beijing University of Agriculture, Beijing 102206, China; liucan808@163.com
[2]   National Engineering Laboratory for Industrial Enzymes, Tianjin Institute of Industrial Biotechnology, Chinese Academy of Sciences, Tianjin 300308, China; dai_lh@tib.cas.cn (L.D.); sun_yx@tib.cas.cn (Y.S.)
[3]   Beijing Collaborative Innovation Center for Eco-Environmental Improvement with Forestry and Fruit Trees, Beijing 102206, China
[4]   School of Biological Science and Medical Engineering, Beihang University, Beijing 100191, China; ronglong64@163.com
*   Correspondence: liuyueping@bua.edu.cn (Y.L.); Doudequan@126.com (D.D.); lqma@bac.edu.cn (L.M.); Tel.: +86-10-8079-9163 (D.D.); +86-10-8079-7305 (L.M.)

Received: 27 April 2016; Accepted: 3 June 2016; Published: 13 June 2016

Abstract: Colorectal cancer and throat cancer are the world's most prevalent neoplastic diseases, and a serious threat to human health. Plant triterpene glycosides have demonstrated antitumor activity. In this study, we investigated potential anticancer effects of mogroside IVe, a triterpenoid glycoside from monk fruit, using *in vitro* and *in vivo* models of colorectal and laryngeal cancer. The effects of mogroside IVe on the proliferation of colorectal cancer HT29 cells and throat cancer Hep-2 cells were determined by 3-(4,5-dimethylthiazol-2-yl)-2,5-diphenyltetrazolium bromide (MTT) assay, and the expression levels of p53, phosphorylated ERK1/2, and MMP-9 were analyzed by western blotting and immunohistochemistry. The results indicated that mogroside IVe inhibited, in a dose-dependent manner, the proliferation of HT29 and Hep-2 cells in culture and in xenografted mice, which was accompanied by the upregulation of tumor suppressor p53, and downregulation of matrix metallopeptidase 9 (MMP-9) and phosphorylated extracellular signal-regulated kinases (ERK)1/2. This study revealed the suppressive activity of mogroside IVe towards colorectal and throat cancers and identified the underlying mechanisms, suggesting that mogroside IVe may be potentially used as a biologically-active phytochemical supplement for treating colorectal and throat cancers.

Keywords: mogroside IVe; monk fruit; colorectal cancer; throat cancer

1. Introduction

Natural products play an important role in contemporary cancer therapy [1,2], and a substantial number of clinically-used chemicals are derived from plants [3–5]. Monk fruit (*Siraitia grosvenorii*) is a cucurbitaceous herb widely planted in the Guangxi province of China, which produces high-potency sweeteners increasingly popular in the food industry as additives in low-calorie drinks or foods [6]. A study on adverse effect of monk fruit has shown that its extracts and individual compounds are essentially non-toxic [7]. Mogroside IVe, a triterpenoid glycoside from monk fruit, consists of an aglycone (mogrol) and four glucose groups [8]. However, despite the presence of glucose residues, mogroside IVe exerts an antihyperglycemic effect and could regulate blood sugar levels in diabetic patients [9]. Mogroside IVe is responsible, in part, for the intense sweetness of the fruit and is estimated to be about 392 times sweeter than sucrose [10].

Colorectal cancer and throat cancer are the world's most prevalent neoplastic diseases and a serious threat to human health [11,12]. Diet and exercise have been established as important factors in cancer prevention, and many triterpene glycosides have demonstrated antitumor activity [13–15]. However, the pharmacological properties of mogroside IVe in preventing colorectal and laryngeal cancers remain unknown. As no negative side effects associated with the ingestion of monk fruit extracts have been reported, in 2014, Food and Drug Administration (FDA) acknowledged mogrosides as Generally Recognized as Safe (GRAS) and approved their use as general-purpose food sweeteners, indicating their safety as pharmacological agents. In this study, we investigated potential anticancer effects of mogroside IVe, including the ability to induce cancer cell apoptosis and inhibit proliferation using *in vitro* and *in vivo* models.

2. Materials and Methods

2.1. Cells and Compounds

Colorectal cancer HT29 and throat cancer Hep-2 cell lines were obtained from the Typical Culture Preservation Commission Cell Bank, Chinese Academy of Sciences (Shanghai, China). HT29 and Hep-2 cells were cultured in Dulbecco's Modified Eagle medium (DMEM) (Gibco Invitrogen) supplemented with penicillin (100 U/mL), streptomycin (100 μg/mL), and 10% fetal bovine serum (FBS), at 37 °C in a 5% CO_2 incubator. Mogroside IVe was purchased from Must Bio-Technology Co., Ltd. (Chengdu, China).

2.2. Identification of Mogroside IVe

The chemical structure of mogroside IVe was confirmed by liquid chromatography electrospray ionization mass spectrometry (LC-ESI-MS) analysis as previously described, with slight modifications [16]. LC-ESI-MS was performed in positive ion mode at the scan range of 100–1500 m/z; 0.1% formic acid was used as a mobile phase additive.

2.3. Measurement of Cell Proliferation

HT29 and Hep-2 cells were seeded into 96-well plates (1×10^4 cells/well) and treated with vehicle (PBS) or increasing concentrations (0–250 μmol/L) of mogroside IVe for 48 h. Cell viability was assessed by MTT assay; the absorbance was read at a wavelength of 570 nm using a spectrophotometer as previously described [14].

2.4. Mouse Studies

All animal experiments were performed in accordance with institutional guidelines approved by the Beijing University of Agriculture. Xenograft tumor models were established by implanting 1×10^7 HT29 or Hep-2 cells subcutaneously into male BALB/c nude mice (eight weeks old, 25–30 g) purchased from Charles River Ltd. (Beijing, China). Then, mice were randomly assigned into four groups (*n* = 8 per group): three treatment groups received intravenous injections of mogroside IVe (2 mg/kg, 10 mg/kg, and 30 mg/kg) three times per week for five weeks, while the control group received saline. Tumor size was measured with a vernier caliper and monitored twice weekly, andtumor volume was calculated as V = (L $\times$ W^2)/2, where L is the length and W is the width of the tumor. At day 35 post-implantation, mice were euthanized by intraperitoneal injection of sodium pentobarbital (150–200 mg/kg), and tumors were harvested for further analysis.

2.5. Immunoblotting and Immunohistochemistry

The level of protein expression in cultured cells was determined by immunoblotting as previously described [17,18] using primary antibodies against MMP-9 (Santa Cruz Biotechnology Inc., Santa Cruz, CA, USA), p53, phospho-ERK1/2, total ERK, and β-actin (all Sigma-Aldrich, St. Louis, MO, USA). Protein expression in xenografted tumors was analyzed by immunohistochemistry. Tumor tissues were fixed immediately after harvesting in 10% phosphate-buffered formalin, embedded in paraffin, and tissue sections were stained with the antibodies indicated above.

2.6. Apoptosis Assessment

Tumor sections prepared as above were analyzed for cell apoptosis by the TUNEL assay using the *In Situ* Cell Death Detection Kit, POD (Roche Diagnostics, Mannheim, Germany) as described previously [19,20]. After TUNEL staining, tumor sections were mounted using Vectashield supplemented with 4′-6-diamidino-2-phenylindole (DAPI; H-1200, Vector Laboratories, Burlingame, CA, USA) for nuclei detection and the images were acquired under a confocal laser scanning microscope.

2.7. Statistical Analysis

All *in vitro* experiments were repeated at least three times. Statistical analysis was performed using GraphPad Prism 5 (GraphPad Software, Inc., La Jolla, CA, USA). Statistical significance was determined by Student's *t*-test, and *p* values < 0.05 were considered statistically significant.

3. Results

3.1. Identification of Mogroside IVe

The structure of mogroside IVe was confirmed by mass spectrometry. Fragment patterns of mogroside IVe included m/z ratios of 1125.6124 $[M + H]^+$, 963.5564 $[M + H-Glc]^+$, 801.4997 $[M + H-2Glc]^+$, and 639.4541 $[M + H-3Glc]^+$ (Figure 1).

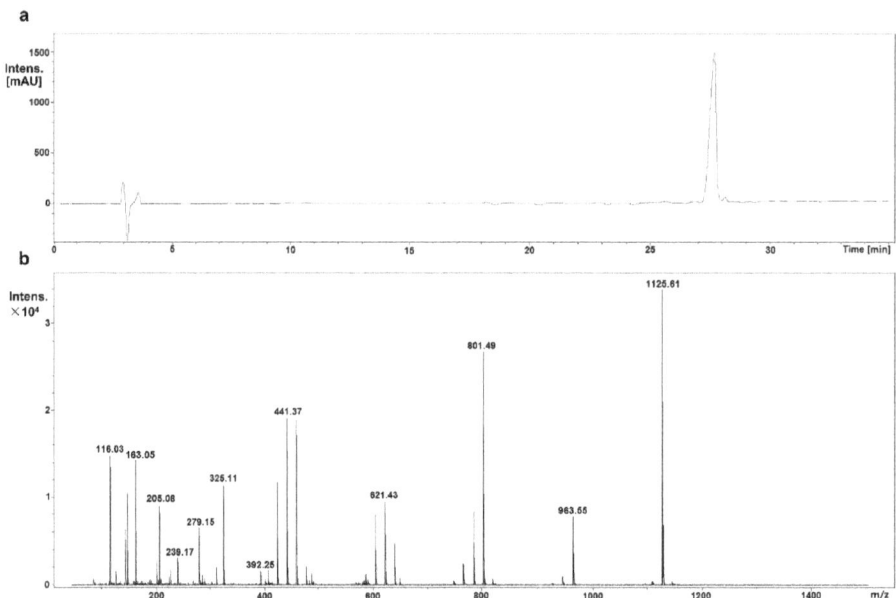

Figure 1. HPLC and mass spectra of mogroside IVe. (**a**) LC chromatogram of mogroside IVe standard; (**b**) Mass spectrum of mogroside IVe standard.

3.2. Mogroside IVe Inhibits the Proliferation of HT29 and Hep-2 Cells

The effect of mogroside IVe on cell proliferation was measured by MTT assay. HT29 and Hep-2 cells were cultured in the presence of different concentrations (0–250 µmol/L) of mogroside IVe for

48 h. The results demonstrated that mogroside IVe inhibited the proliferation of both HT29 and Hep-2 cells in a dose-dependent manner (Figure 2b,c). Figure 2d shows significant morphological changes induced by mogroside IVe in both cell lines. While control (PBS-treated) cells were similar in size and regularly shaped, some of mogroside IVe-treated cells were detached from the surface and lysed, as evidenced by the presence of cell debris, or formed apoptotic bodies.

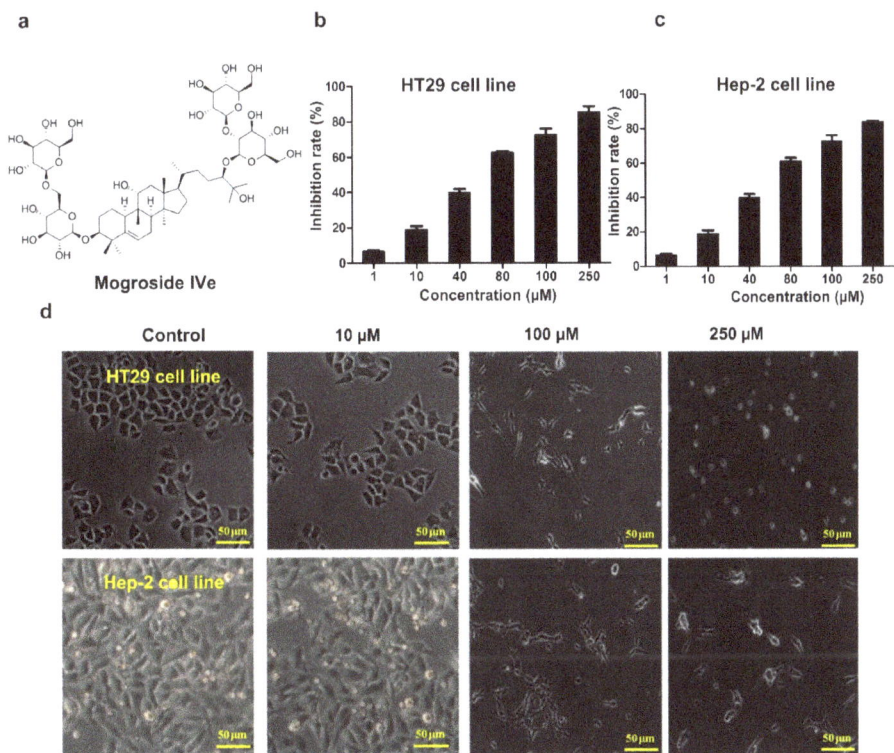

Figure 2. Mogroside IVe inhibits the proliferation of cultured cancer cells. (**a**) Chemical structure of mogroside IVe; (**b,c**) Mogroside IVe suppressed the proliferation of HT29 (**b**) and Hep-2 (**c**) cells in a dose-dependent manner. The results represent the mean ± SD of three independent experiments performed in triplicate; (**d**) Significant morphological changes were induced in cancer cells by mogroside IVe.

3.3. Effect of Mogroside IVe on the Phosphorylation of ERK1/2, and the Expression of p53 and MMP-9

Next, we examined the mechanism underlying mogroside IVe inhibition of cancer cell proliferation. As tumor suppressor protein p53, extracellular signal-regulated kinasesERK1/2, and matrix metallopeptidase 9 (MMP-9) are implicated in cancer cell proliferation and metastasis, we examined their expression in HT29 and Hep-2 cells. The results indicated that mogroside IVe, in a dose-dependent manner, significantly suppressed the phosphorylation of ERK1/2 (Figure 3a,b), while upregulating the expression of p53 (Figure 3c,d) and downregulating that of MMP-9 (Figure 3e,f). These findings strongly suggested that phospho-ERK1/2, p53, and MMP-9 may be molecular targets of mogroside IVe.

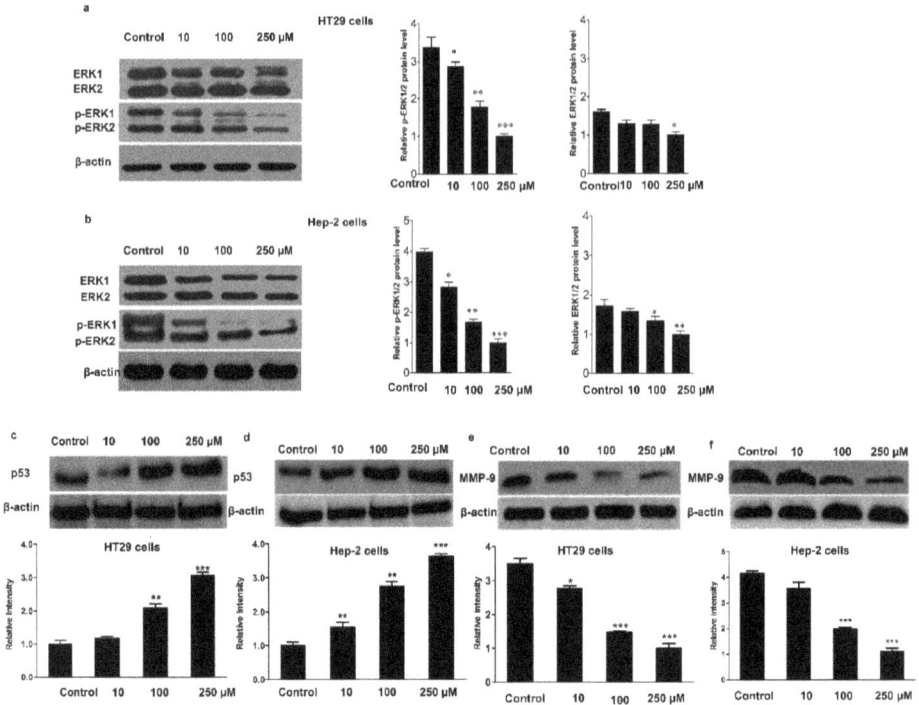

Figure 3. Mogroside IVe regulates ERK1/2 phosphorylation, and p53 and MMP-9 expression. HT29 and Hep-2 cells were treated with the indicated concentrations of mogroside IVe and analyzed for protein expression by Western blotting. (**a,b**) Mogroside IVe inhibited ERK1/2 phosphorylation in HT29 (**a**) and Hep-2 (**b**) cells; (**c,d**) Mogroside IVe enhanced p53 expression in HT29 (**c**) and Hep-2 (**d**) cells; (**e,f**) Mogroside IVe inhibited MMP-9 expression in HT29 (**e**) and Hep-2 (**f**) cells. The data represent the mean $\pm$ SD of three independent experiments performed in triplicate. * $p < 0.05$, ** $p < 0.01$, *** $p < 0.001$ compared to control.

3.4. Anticancer Effect of Mogroside IVe in Mice

To investigate the effect of mogroside IVe on tumor growth *in vivo*, we developed an animal xenograft model of HT29- and Hep-2 cell-derived tumors. In HT29 and Hep-2 xenografted mice, mogroside IVe showed statistically significant inhibition of tumor growth (Figure 4a,b). After five weeks of treatment with mogroside IVe, all mice were euthanized, and the tumors were weighed. Consistent with the tumor volumes estimated by external measurements, tumor weight in mogroside IVe-treated mice was significantly less than that in control mice by day 35. The results presented in Figure 4, confirmed that the treatment with mogroside IVe significantly inhibited the growth of HT29- and Hep-2-derived tumors.

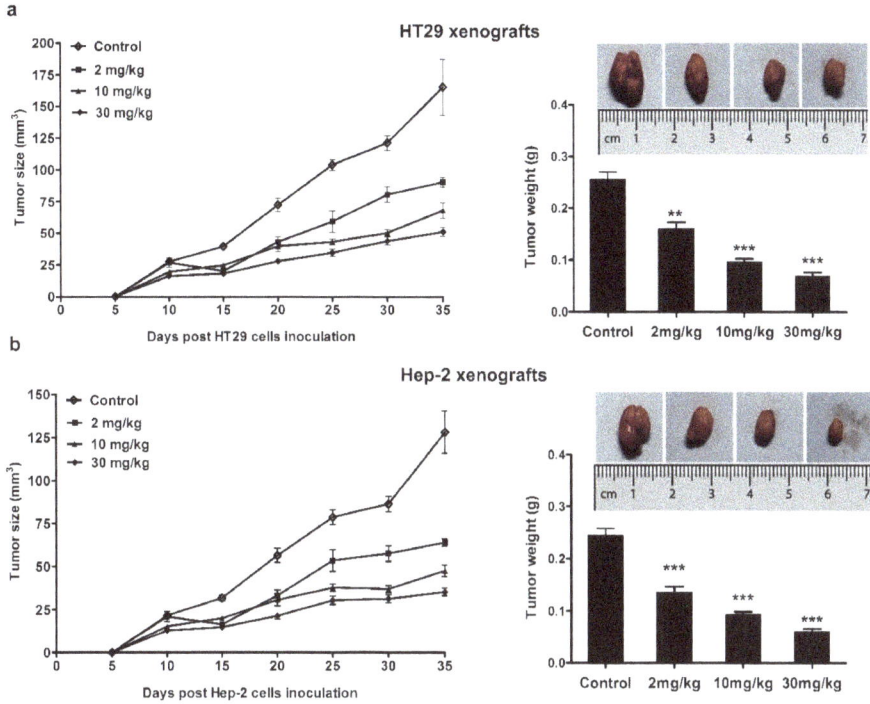

Figure 4. Mogroside IVe inhibits the growth of HT29- and Hep-2-derived tumors. Mice were implanted 1×10^7 HT29 or Hep-2 cells subcutaneously and injected 2 mg/kg, 10 mg/kg, and 30 mg/kg of mogroside IVe three times a week for five weeks; the control group was injected saline. (**a**) Mogroside IVe reduced the size (left panel) and weight (right panel) of HT29-derived tumors; (**b**) Mogroside IVe reduced the size (left panel) and weight (right panel) of Hep-2-derived tumors. Statistical significance between control and treated animals were evaluated by Student's *t*-test (*n* = 8). ** $p < 0.01$; *** $p < 0.001$ compared to control.

3.5. Mogroside IVe Induces Apoptosis of Tumor Cells in Mice

The induction of apoptosis in cancer cells is an important aspect of tumor-suppressing activity exerted by anticancer agents. As revealed by the TUNEL assay, mogroside IVe-treated mice demonstrated a significant increase in the number of apoptotic bodies (stained red) in cancer cell xenografts compared with control (Figure 5a,b), suggesting that the suppression of tumor growth in mice injected with mogroside IVe was due to increased apoptosis of tumor cells.

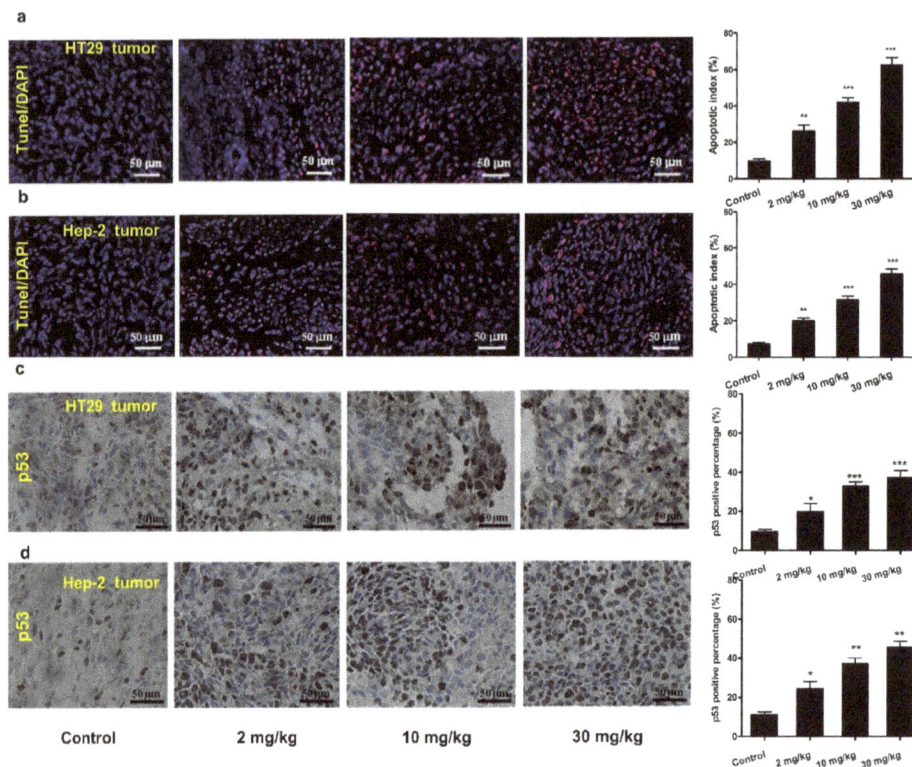

Figure 5. Mogroside IVe induced apoptosis in HT29 and Hep-2 cell-derived tumors by upregulating p53 levels. (**a**,**b**) Detection of apoptotic cells (stained red) in tumors using the TUNEL assay. Mogroside IVe induced apoptosis in HT29 (**a**) and Hep-2 (**b**) tumors in a dose-dependent manner; (**c**,**d**) Mogroside IVe increased p53 expression in HT29 (**c**) and Hep-2 (**d**) tumors. * $p < 0.05$, ** $p < 0.01$, *** $p < 0.001$ compared to control.

To investigate the mechanism by which mogroside IVe induced apoptosis in HT29- and Hep-2-derived tumors, they were evaluated by immunohistochemistry, which revealed significantly increased p53 expression in the tumors from mogroside IVe-treated mice compared with those from the control group (Figure 5c,d). This observation indicated that mogroside IVe induced tumor cell apoptosis by promoting p53 expression.

3.6. Effect of Mogroside IVe on ERK1/2 Phosphorylation and MMP-9 Expression in Vivo

ERK1/2 phosphorylation-dependent signaling is required to support the invasion of HT29 and Hep-2 cells through activation of the downstream pathways [21,22]. MMP-9 is a zinc-dependent protease implicated in cancer cell invasion and metastasis [23]. Immunohistochemistry analysis indicated that mogroside IVe markedly decreased the levels of phospho-ERK1/2 and downregulated MMP-9 expression in the tumors of treated mice in a dose-dependent manner (Figure 6).

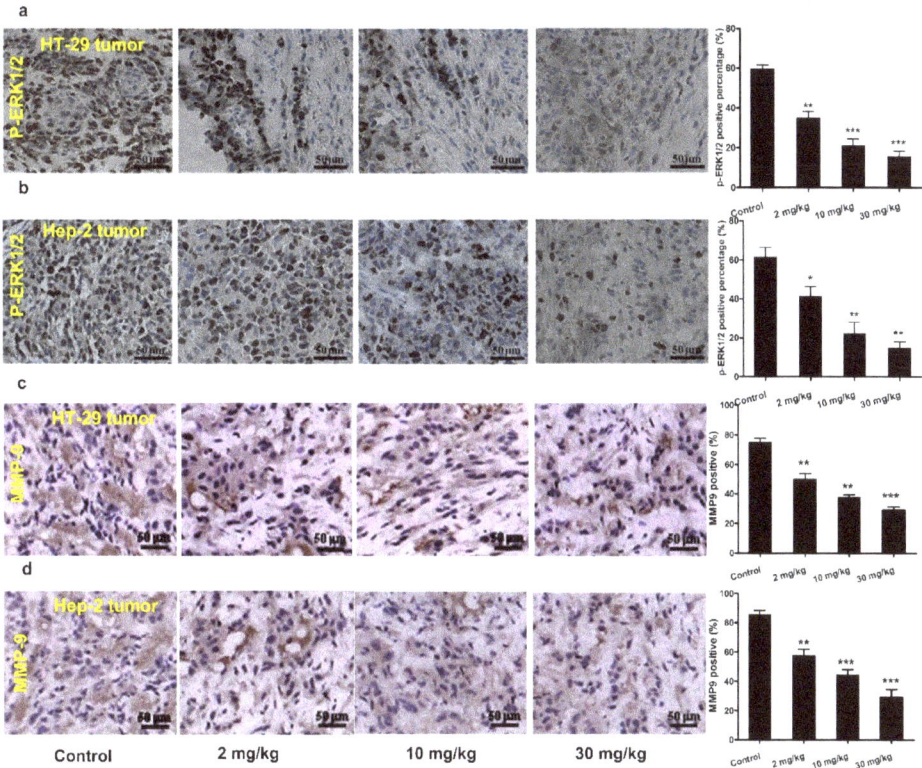

Figure 6. Immunohistochemical analysis of p-ERK1/2 and MMP-9 expression in HT29 and Hep-2 cell-derived tumors. (**a,b**) Mogroside IVe inhibited Erk1/2 phosphorylation in HT29 (**a**) and Hep-2 (**b**) tumors in a dose-dependent manner; (**c,d**) The number of MMP-9–positive cells was reduced after mogroside IVe treatment in HT29 (**c**) and Hep-2 (**d**) tumors compared with the control group. * $p < 0.05$, ** $p < 0.01$, and *** $p < 0.001$ compared to control.

4. Discussion

Our results indicate that mogroside IVe, a triterpenoid glycoside from monk fruit used as a strong sweetener, has a potential to prevent the development of colorectal and laryngeal cancers because it significantly inhibited the proliferation of HT29 and Hep-2 cells *in vitro* (Figure 2b–d), and, consistently, demonstrated an anticancer effect in mice with HT29- and Hep-2-derived xenografted tumors (Figure 4).

The TUNEL assay showed that the ability of mogroside IVe to suppress tumor growth may be based, at least in part, on the induction of apoptosis in cancer cells (Figure 5a,b). Previous studies have indicated that many apoptotic signals associated with cell death in HT29 and Hep-2 cells are mediated by p53 because enhanced p53 expression induces tumor cell apoptosis [24–27]. In agreement with these findings, in our xenograft model mogroside IVe significantly increased the expression level of p53 in tumors (Figure 5c,d), which was corroborated by the *in vitro* results (Figure 3c,d). Overall, these data suggest that mogroside IVe induced p53-mediated apoptosis in HT29 and Hep-2 cancer cells.

Cell invasion is a critical step in cancer progression as it facilitates metastasis [28–30], which is a critical factor in determining the survival of cancer patients [31–33]. MMP-9 is thought to play an important role in HT29 and Hep-2 cancer cell migration and invasion [34,35], and our findings indicated that mogroside IVe treatment downregulatedMMP-9 expression in HT29 and Hep-2 cells both *in vitro* (Figure 3e,f) and *in vivo* (Figure 6c,d). These results were supported by the observation that mogroside IVe inhibited the phosphorylation of ERK1/2 (Figure 3a,b and Figure 6a,b), which acts as an upstream regulator of MMP-9 expression [36–39]. Together, these findings suggest that mogroside IVe may suppress MMP-9 expression via inhibition of ERK1/2 phosphorylation-dependent activation. As MMP-9 is considered to play a critical role in the migration and invasion of HT29 and Hep-2 cancer cells, we can speculate that mogroside IVe may also inhibit cancer invasion and metastasis. However, future *in vitro* and *in vivo* studies are required to test this hypothesis and confirm that mogroside IVe can prevent or reduce cancer cell migration and invasion.

In conclusion, we demonstrated that mogroside IVe has the ability to suppress the proliferation of colorectal cancer and throat cancer cells by inducing apoptosis through upregulation of p53, and downregulation of p-ERK1/2 and MMP-9 levels, strongly indicating anticancer activity. Thus, we highlighted, for the first time, the role and mechanism of mogroside IVe as a phytochemical with anti-colorectal cancer and anti-throat cancer activity. As mogroside IVe does not have side effects and is used as a sweetener in many low-calorie foods and drinks, its application as a dietary supplement may have benefits over conventional drugs in terms of cancer prevention effects and user compliance.

Acknowledgments: This work was supported by the Foundation of Beijing Talent Training Scheme (No. 2015000020124G243), the Foundation of Beijing University of Agriculture (No. GZL2015010, 2017516005), and the "863" Program (No. 2012AA021403).

Author Contributions: Dequan Dou and Lanqing Ma designed the project, Can Liu and Longhai Dai carried out the assays and statistical analysis, Long Rong and Yuanxia Sun wrote the manuscript, and Yueping Liu edited the manuscript. All authors have read and approved the final version.

Conflicts of Interest: The authors declare no conflict of interest.

Abbreviations

The following abbreviations are used in this manuscript:

MMP-9	matrix metallopeptidase 9
ERK	extracellular signal-regulated kinase
p53	tumor suppressor p53
HPLC	high performance liquid chromatography

References

1. Newman, D.J.; Cragg, G.M.; Snader, K.M. Natural products as sources of new drugs over the period 1981–2002. *J. Nat. Prod.* **2003**, *66*, 1022–1037. [CrossRef] [PubMed]
2. Agbarya, A.; Ruimi, N.; Epelbaum, R.; Ben-Arye, E.; Mahajna, J. Natural products as potential cancer therapy enhancers: A preclinical update. *SAGE Open Med.* **2014**, *2*. [CrossRef] [PubMed]
3. Nobili, S.; Lippi, D.; Witort, E.; Donnini, M.; Bausi, L.; Mini, E.; Capaccioli, S. Natural compounds for cancer treatment and prevention. *Pharmacol. Res.* **2009**, *59*, 365–378. [CrossRef] [PubMed]
4. Mukherjee, A.K.; Basu, S.; Sarkar, N.; Ghosh, A.C. Advances in cancer therapy with plant based natural products. *Curr. Med. Chem.* **2001**, *8*, 1467–1486. [CrossRef] [PubMed]
5. Butler, M.S. The role of natural product chemistry in drug discovery. *J. Nat. Prod.* **2004**, *67*, 2141–2153. [CrossRef] [PubMed]
6. Li, X.; Lopetcharat, K.; Drake, M. Parents' and children's acceptance of skim chocolate milks sweetened by monk fruit and stevia leaf extracts. *J. Food Sci.* **2015**, *80*, S1083–S1092. [CrossRef] [PubMed]
7. Chun, L.I.; Lin, L.M.; Feng, S.; Wang, Z.M.; Huo, H.R.; Li, D.; Jiang, T.L. Chemistry and pharmacology of *Siraitia grosvenorii*: A review. *Chin. J. Nat. Med.* **2014**, *12*, 89–102.
8. Kasai, R.; Nie, R.L.; Nashi, K.; Ohtani, K.; Zhou, J.; Tao, G.D.; Tanaka, O. Sweet cucurbitane glycosides from fruits of *Siraitia siamensis* (chi-zi luo-han-guo), a Chinese folk medicine. *Agric. Biol. Chem.* **1989**, *53*, 3347–3349. [CrossRef]

9. Suzuki, Y.A.; Tomoda, M.; Murata, Y.; Inui, H.; Sugiura, M.; Nakano, Y. Antidiabetic effect of long-term supplementation with *Siraitia grosvenori* on the spontaneously diabetic Goto–Kakizaki rat. *Br. J. Nutr.* **2007**, *97*, 770–775. [CrossRef] [PubMed]

10. Matsumoto, K.; Kasai, R.; Ohtani, K.; Tanaka, O. Minor cucurbitane-glycosides from fruits of *Siraitia grosvenori* (Cucurbitaceae). *Chem. Pharm. Bull.* **1990**, *38*, 2030–2032. [CrossRef]

11. Center, M.M.; Jemal, A.; Ward, E. International trends in colorectal cancer incidence rates. *Cancer Epidemiol. Biomark. Prev.* **2009**, *18*, 1688–1694. [CrossRef] [PubMed]

12. Meijer van Putten, J.B. Mouth and throat cancer; new developments. *Ned. Tijdschr. Tandheelkd.* **1996**, *103*, 31–32. [PubMed]

13. Careaga, V.; Bueno, C.C.; Alche, L.; Maier, M. Antiproliferative, cytotoxic and hemolytic activities of a triterpene glycoside from *Psolus patagonicus* and its desulfated analog. *Chemotherapy* **2009**, *55*, 60–68. [CrossRef] [PubMed]

14. Dyshlovoy, S.A.; Menchinskaya, E.S.; Venz, S.; Rast, S.; Amann, K.; Hauschild, J.; Otte, K.; Kalinin, V.I.; Silchenko, A.S.; Avilov, S.A.; *et al.* The marine triterpene glycoside frondoside A exhibits activity *in vitro* and *in vivo* in prostate cancer. *Int. J. Cancer* **2015**, *32*, 1601–1618.

15. Qin, Z.; Yong, X.; Wang, J.F.; Li, H.; Long, T.T.; Li, Z.; Wang, Y.M.; Dong, P.; Xue, C.H. *In vitro* and *in vivo* anti-tumour activities of echinoside A and ds-echinoside A from *Pearsonothuria graeffei*. *J. Sci. Food Agric.* **2012**, *92*, 965–974.

16. Dai, L.; Liu, C.; Zhu, Y.; Zhang, J.; Men, Y.; Zeng, Y.; Sun, Y. Functional characterization of cucurbitadienol synthase and triterpene glycosyltransferase involved in biosynthesis of mogrosides from *Siraitia grosvenorii*. *Plant Cell Physiol.* **2015**, *56*, 1172–1182. [CrossRef] [PubMed]

17. Hohmann, A.W.; Faulkner, P. Monoclonal antibodies to baculovirus structural proteins: determination of specificities by Western blot analysis. *Virology* **1983**, *125*, 432–444. [CrossRef]

18. Shacter, E.; Williams, J.A.; Lim, M.; Levine, R.L. Differential susceptibility of plasma proteins to oxidative modification: examination by western blot immunoassay. *Free Radic. Biol. Med.* **1994**, *17*, 429–437. [CrossRef]

19. Park, H.Y.; Kim, J.H.; Park, C.K. Activation of autophagy induces retinal ganglion cell death in a chronic hypertensive glaucoma model. *Cell Death Dis.* **2012**, *3*. [CrossRef] [PubMed]

20. Susini, L.; Besse, S.; Duflaut, D.; Lespagnol, A.; Beekman, C.; Fiucci, G.; Atkinson, A.R.; Busso, D.; Poussin, P.; Marine, J.C.; *et al.* TCTP protects from apoptotic cell death by antagonizing bax function. *Cell Death Differ.* **2008**, *15*, 1211–1220. [CrossRef] [PubMed]

21. Popovic, V.; Zivkovic, J.; Davidovic, S.; Stevanovic, M.; Stojkovic, D. Mycotherapy of Cancer: An update on cytotoxic and antitumor activities of mushrooms, bioactive principles and molecular mechanisms of their action. *Curr. Top Med. Chem.* **2013**, *13*, 2791–2806. [CrossRef] [PubMed]

22. Zhou, Y.; Feng, X.; Liu, Y.L.; Ye, S.C.; Wang, H.; Tan, W.K.; Tian, T.; Qiu, Y.M.; Luo, H.S. Down-regulation of miR-126 is associated with colorectal cancer cells proliferation, migration and invasion by targeting IRS-1 via the AKT and ERK1/2 signaling pathways. *PLoS ONE* **2013**, *8*. [CrossRef] [PubMed]

23. Moulik, S.; Sen, T.; Dutta, A.; Banerji, A. Phosphatidylinositol 3-Kinase and NF-kappaB Involved in Epidermal Growth Factor-Induced Matrix Metalloproteinase-9 Expression. *J. Cancer Mol.* **2008**, *4*, 55–60.

24. Giono, L.E.; Manfredi, J.J. The p53 tumor suppressor participates in multiple cell cycle checkpoints. *J. Cell Physiol.* **2006**, *209*, 13–20. [CrossRef] [PubMed]

25. Merchant, A.K.; Loney, T.L.; Maybaum, J. Expression of wild-type p53 stimulates an increase in both Bax and Bcl-xL protein content in HT29 cells. *Oncogene* **1996**, *13*, 2631–2637. [PubMed]

26. Reyes-Zurita, F.J.; Pachón-Peña, G.; Lizárraga, D.; Rufino-Palomares, E.E.; Cascante, M.; Lupiáñez, J.A. The natural triterpenemaslinic acid induces apoptosis in HT29 colon cancer cells by a JNK-p53-dependent mechanism. *BMC Cancer* **2011**, *11*. [CrossRef] [PubMed]

27. Corbiere, C.; Liagre, B.; Terro, F.; Beneytout, J.-L. Induction of antiproliferative effect by diosgenin through activation of p53, release of apoptosis-inducing factor (AIF) and modulation of caspase-3 activity in different human cancer cells. *Cell Res.* **2004**, *14*, 188–196. [CrossRef] [PubMed]

28. Kenny, H.A.; Swayamjot, K.; Coussens, L.M.; Ernst, L. The initial steps of ovarian cancer cell metastasis are mediated by MMP-2 cleavage of vitronectin and fibronectin. *J. Clin. Invest.* **2008**, *118*, 1367–1379. [CrossRef] [PubMed]

29. Van Zijl, F.V.; Krupitza, G.; Mikulits, W. Initial steps of metastasis: cell invasion and endothelial transmigration. *Mutat. Res. Rev. Mutat.* **2011**, *728*, 23–34. [CrossRef] [PubMed]

30. Bogenrieder, T.; Herlyn, M. Axis of evil: Molecular mechanism of cancer metastasis. *Oncogene* **2003**, *22*, 6524–6536. [CrossRef] [PubMed]

31. Leung, S.Y.; Chen, X.; Chu, K.M.; Yuen, S.T.; Mathy, J.; Ji, J.; Chan, A.S.Y.; Li, R.; Law, S.; Troyanskaya, O.G.; *et al.* Phospholipase A2 group IIA expression in gastric adenocarcinoma is associated with prolonged survival and less frequent metastasis. *Proc. Natl. Acad. Sci. USA* **2003**, *99*, 16203–16208. [CrossRef] [PubMed]

32. Maheswaran, S.; Haber, D.A. Circulating tumor cells: A window into cancer biology and metastasis. *Curr. Opin. Genet. Dev.* **2010**, *20*, 96–99. [CrossRef] [PubMed]

33. Scott, V.; Weinberg, R.A. Tumor metastasis: molecular insights and evolving paradigms. *Cell* **2011**, *147*, 275–292.

34. Abrassart, S.; Peter, R.; Hoffmeyer, P. Thymoquinone as an anticancer agent: evidence from inhibition of cancer cells viability and invasion *in vitro* and tumor growth *in vivo*. *Fundam. Clin. Pharmacol.* **2013**, *27*, 557–569.

35. Li, R.; Pan, Y.; He, B.; Xu, Y.; Gao, T.; Song, G.; Sun, H.; Deng, Q.; Wang, S. Downregulation of CD147 expression by RNA interference inhibits HT29 cell proliferation, invasion and tumorigenicity *in vitro* and *in vivo*. *Int. J. Oncol.* **2013**, *43*, 1885–1894. [PubMed]

36. Xie, Z.; Singh, M.; Singh, K. Differential regulation of matrix metalloproteinase-2 and -9 expression and activity in adult rat cardiac fibroblasts in response to interleukin-1β. *J. Biol. Chem.* **2004**, *279*, 39513–39519. [CrossRef] [PubMed]

37. Padmaja, K.; Kasyapa, C.S.; Lesleyann, H.; Cowell, J.K. LGI1, a putative tumor metastasis suppressor gene, controls *in vitro* invasiveness and expression of matrix metalloproteinases in glioma cells through the ERK1/2 pathway. *J. Biol. Chem.* **2004**, *279*, 23151–23157.

38. Moshal, K.; Sen, U.N.; Henderson, B.; Steed, M.; Ovechkin, A.; Tyagi, S. Regulation of homocysteine-induced MMP-9 by ERK1/2 pathway. *Am. J. Physiol. Cell Physiol.* **2006**, *290*, C883–C891. [CrossRef] [PubMed]

39. Sun, D.K.; Yang, S.I.; Kim, H.C.; Chan, Y.S.; Ko, K.H. Inhibition of GSK-3β mediates expression of MMP-9 through ERK1/2 activation and translocation of NF-κB in rat primary astrocyte. *Brain Res.* **2007**, *1186*, 12–20. [CrossRef] [PubMed]

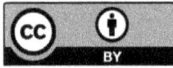

nutrients

MDPI

Article

Concord and Niagara Grape Juice and Their Phenolics Modify Intestinal Glucose Transport in a Coupled in Vitro Digestion/Caco-2 Human Intestinal Model

Sydney Moser [1], Jongbin Lim [1], Mohammad Chegeni [1], JoLynne D. Wightman [2],
Bruce R. Hamaker [1,3,*] and Mario G. Ferruzzi [1,3]

[1] Department of Food Science, Purdue University, West Lafayette, IN 47907, USA; moser6@purdue.edu (S.M.);
     lim175@purdue.edu (J.L.); mchegeni@purdue.edu (M.C.); mferruzz@purdue.edu (M.G.F.)
[2] Welch Foods Inc., Concord, MA 01742, USA; jwightman@welchs.com
[3] Whistler Center for Carbohydrate Research, Purdue University, West Lafayette, IN 47907, USA
*   Correspondence: mferruzz@purdue.edu; Tel.: +1-765-494-0625

Received: 22 April 2016; Accepted: 30 June 2016; Published: 5 July 2016

Abstract: While the potential of dietary phenolics to mitigate glycemic response has been proposed, the translation of these effects to phenolic rich foods such as 100% grape juice (GJ) remains unclear. Initial in vitro screening of GJ phenolic extracts from American grape varieties (V. labrusca; Niagara and Concord) suggested limited inhibitory capacity for amylase and α-glucosidase (6.2%–11.5% inhibition; $p < 0.05$). Separately, all GJ extracts (10–100 μM total phenolics) did reduce intestinal trans-epithelial transport of deuterated glucose (d7-glu) and fructose (d7-fru) by Caco-2 monolayers in a dose-dependent fashion, with 60 min d7-glu/d7-fru transport reduced 10%–38% by GJ extracts compared to control. To expand on these findings by assessing the ability of 100% GJ to modify starch digestion and glucose transport from a model starch-rich meal, 100% Niagara and Concord GJ samples were combined with a starch rich model meal (1:1 and 1:2 wt:wt) and glucose release and transport were assessed in a coupled in vitro digestion/Caco-2 cell model. Digestive release of glucose from the starch model meal was decreased when digested in the presence of GJs (5.9%–15% relative to sugar matched control). Furthermore, transport of d7-glu was reduced 10%–38% by digesta containing bioaccessible phenolics from Concord and Niagara GJ compared to control. These data suggest that phenolics present in 100% GJ may alter absorption of monosaccharides naturally present in 100% GJ and may potentially alter glycemic response if consumed with a starch rich meal.

Keywords: grape juice; anthocyanins; carbohydrate digestion; glucose transport

1. Introduction

On average, Americans consume 0.43 gallons per capita of grape juice (GJ) annually, making GJ the third most commonly consumed juice in the US [1]. Native American Concord and Niagara grape cultivars are sources for production of purple and white juice, respectively. Both grapes and their corresponding juices are well established sources of nutrients and bioactive phenolic compounds, including flavan-3-ols, flavonols, stilbenes, phenolic acids and, for Concord grapes, anthocyanins [2–5]. With total phenolic and anthocyanin levels reported as high as 2900 mg/L and 880 mg/L, respectively, for 100% Concord GJ and similarly high levels of phenolics in 100% Niagara GJ, these products can be significant contributors to health promoting phytochemicals [4].

Phenolic rich 100% Concord GJ consumption has been reported to have health promoting activities including improved cardiovascular and cognitive function [6–8]. Primary outcomes mediated by Concord GJ include increased flow mediated dilation, decreased platelet aggregation, modulation of low density lipoprotein (LDL) oxidation lag time, and improved memory function and brain signaling (reviewed by Blumberg et al. [6]; Krikorian et al. [7,8]). While promising, these benefits have been observed with consumption of between ~12 and 20 oz of 100% juice and 100% GJ contains ~36 g sugar per 240 mL serving [9]. While fruit juices have been reported to have similar glycemic response to whole fruits when matched by sugar load [10], realization of these benefits remains challenged by consumer concern related to the higher sugar content and risk for obesity and diabetes. Therefore, while evidence for the benefits of GJ and GJ phenolics continues to expand, there remains a hesitation in recommending 100% GJ consumption to certain populations due to its natural high sugar content.

Over the past decade, the potential of phenolics to modulate glucose homeostasis has emerged (reviewed by Hanhineva et al. [11] and Williamson et al. [12]). Specifically, phenolics derived from foods including berries, juices, tea and coffee have demonstrated the ability to modulate intestinal digestion of starch by inhibition of amylase and glucosidase enzymes as well as intestinal glucose absorption through inhibition of glucose transporters such as GLUT 2 [13–20]. While primarily based on experiments with purified phenolics and phenolic extracts, these data would suggest that sugar in the context of a phenolic rich food or beverage may be processed differently in the intestine resulting in a modified glycemic response. Interestingly, while similar glycemic responses have been observed between grape juice and fruit, juice resulted in lower insulin response [21]. Johnston et al. [22] previously reported that 3 h glycemic response from both clear and cloudy 100% apple juice was in fact lower in healthy volunteers compared to a phenolic-free, sugar-matched placebo beverage. While no mechanistic test were performed, the authors postulated that phenolics in apple juices, including phloridzin or other polyphenols, may be responsible, in part, for the observed delay in intestinal absorption of glucose. In a related fashion, chronic consumption of 100% Concord GJ (8 weeks) decreased fasting blood glucose levels compared to placebo beverage [23]. These results do in fact suggest that specific 100% juice components might modify glucose absorption and/or homeostasis in humans.

While these data are promising, additional insight into the ability and mechanisms by which GJ phenolics may modulate glucose absorption is required. Also, considering the potential mechanism of phenolic inhibition of starch digestive enzyme and glucose transport, it is important to consider the potential impact of a complex meal on these effects. Although clinical studies remain the gold standard for investigating health-related outcomes, in vitro models provide an effective screening tool to investigate mechanistic steps and screen a broader set of food matrix factors that impact nutrient and phytonutrient bioavailability prior to refining designs for clinical evaluation [24–28]. Leveraging a similar approach, the specific objectives of this study were to (1) examine the potential for 100% GJ phenolics to modulate carbohydrate digestion and intestinal glucose transport in vitro; and (2) determine if bioaccessible phenolics from 100% GJ can alter carbohydrate digestion and intestinal glucose transport in the presence of a starch rich meal using a coupled in vitro digestion/Caco-2 model.

2. Materials and Methods

2.1. Chemicals, Solutions and Standards

Chromatography solvents, acids and salts including acetonitrile, methanol and water, formic acid and ammonium formate in addition to phenolic standards (gallic acid, caffeic acid, epicatechin, quercetin-3-*O*-glucoside, quercetin-3-glucuronide, quercetin, resveratrol, and cyanidin-3-*O*-glucoside) were purchased from Sigma-Aldrich, (St. Louis, MO, USA). Material for test meal including nonfat dry milk (NFDM; Maple Island, North St. Paul, MN, USA) and corn starch (Tate and Lyle) were purchased at a local market. Materials for in vitro digestion including urea (U5378), uric acid (U2625), porcine mucin (M2378), α-amylase (A3176), pepsin (P7125), lipase (L3126), pancreatin (P1750) bile salt (B8631) extract, KH_2PO_4 (VWR), K_2SO_4 (Riedel-de Haën), potassium citrate, sodium citrate, KCl,

CaCO$_3$, MgCO$_3$ (Sigma-Aldrich) and Tris-HCl were also purchased from Sigma-Aldrich. NaCl, HCl, and NaHCO$_3$ were purchased from Mallinckrodt (Phillipsburg, NJ, USA). Reagents for enzyme inhibition assays including dimethylsulfoxide (DMSO), acarbose, phosphoric acid, α-amylase (A3176), rat intestinal α-glucosidase, NaCl, glucose oxidase-peroxidase, maltose, maltotriose, maltotetrose and maltopentose, were obtained from Sigma-Aldrich. Cell culture reagents including Dulbecco's Modified Eagles Medium (DMEM), non-essential amino acids (NEAA), penicillin/streptomycin (pen/strep), and phosphate buffered saline (PBS) were purchased from Lonza (Walkersville, MD, USA). Cell culture reagents including 4-(2-hydroxylethyl)-1-piperazineethanes (HEPES), bovine serum albumin (free fatty acid free) (FFA) and glucose-free DMEM were purchased from Sigma-Aldrich. NaHCO$_3$, monosodium phosphate, and disodium phosphate were obtained from J.T. Baker (Center Valley, PA, USA). Fetal bovine serum (FBS) (Atlanta Biologicals, Lawrenceville, GA, USA), gentamycin (J.R. Scientific, Woodland, CA, USA), trypsin (Thermo Scientific, Waltham, MA, USA), glucose and fructose (Research Products International Corps, Mt. Prospect, IL, USA), and D-glucose-1,2,3,4,5,6,6-d7 (d7-glu) and D-Fructose-1,1,3,4,5,6,6-d7 (d7-fru) (Sigma-Aldrich) were used in glucose transport experiments.

2.2. Grape Juice Samples

One hundred percent Niagara and Concord GJ were provided by Welch Foods Inc. (Concord, MA, USA) (Table 1). One hundred percent juices were produced from two harvest years (2013 and 2014) and were pasteurized and maintained refrigerated at 4 °C until used in experiments. The Niagara GJs were processed with and without the addition of sulfur dioxide.

Table 1. Description of 100% grape juice samples assessed [1].

Grape Juice Description	Form of Juice	Sugar Content
Niagara, 2013 harvest	Reconstituted from concentrate	16.0° Brix
SO$_2$ Niagara, 2013 harvest	Reconstituted from concentrate	16.0° Brix
Concord, 2013 harvest	Not from concentrate	16.5° Brix
Niagara, 2014 harvest	Reconstituted from concentrate	16.0° Brix
SO$_2$ Niagara, 2014 harvest	Not from concentrate	13.3° Brix
Concord, 2014 harvest	Not from concentrate	15.9° Brix

[1] All samples received from Welch's Foods Inc.

2.3. Phenolic Extraction

Phenolics were extracted from aliquots (5 mL) of GJ by solid phase extraction (Oasis® HLB 6cc (150 mg) extraction cartridges) using the method of Song et al. [29]. Briefly, 5 mL of juice were loaded onto the SPE cartridges (Milford, MA, USA) and rinsed with 2% formic acid in water. Elution of phenolics was completed with 2% formic acid in methanol. Eluates were dried down under nitrogen and kept frozen (−80 °C) until analysis. Total phenolic content of extracts was measured using a modified Folin-Ciocalteau assay as described by Waterhouse et al. [30].

2.4. Analysis of Polyphenol and Anthocyanin-Rich Fractions by LC-MS

Dried GJ extracts were resolubilized in 2.0% formic acid in water and characterized by LC-MS using methods of Song et al. [29] with minor modification. Single ion responses (SIRs) were used to quantify individual GJ phenolics. Phenolic acids, flavonoids and stilbenoids were quantified using multi-level response curves constructed with authentic standards of each phenolic species identified by co-chromatography with limited exception. Piceid concentration (a resveratrol glucoside) was estimated using a resveratrol calibration curve. Concentration of all quercetin-*O*-glucosides was estimated using quercetin-3-*O*-glucoside. Finally, concentrations of anthocyanins were determined using a calibration curve constructed from cyanidin-3-*O*-glucoside.

2.5. Impact of GJ Phenolic Extracts on Starch Digestive Enzymes in Vitro

Impact of GJ phenolic extracts on starch digestion by α-amylase and α-glucosidase was determined as described by Lee et al. [31]. Briefly, GJ phenolic extracts were dissolved in DMSO (5 mM).

A waxy maize starch solution (1 g/50 mL) was prepared in 20 mM sodium phosphate buffer and boiled to achieve gelatinization (20 min). Starch solutions (50 µL) were then combined with GJ phenolic extract (15 µL, delivering 10–500 µM of total phenols), pancreatic α-amylase (37 °C, 10 U/37.5 µL) and phosphate buffer (20 mM, pH 6.8). Samples were incubated for 10 min after which the reaction was terminated by boiling. Samples were diluted 10× in water prior to quantification of maltose and maltotriose by HPAEC-ECD. Percent inhibition of α-amylase by GJ phenolics was calculated relative to vehicle control (DMSO with no GJ extract) and compared to positive control acarbose.

Inhibition of α-glucosidase by GJ phenolics was assessed using a Megazyme glucose assay kit (Megazyme Inc., Chicago, IL, USA). Briefly, rat intestinal α-glucosidase solution (1 g/10 mL, 10 µL) was mixed with inhibitor (10 µL, 100–5000 µM total polyphenols). Sodium phosphate (0.1 M, pH 6.8, 70 µL) was added to the enzyme-inhibitor solution and the mixture was vortexed well. Maltose solution (10 µL, 100 mg/mL) was then added. The reaction mixture was incubated at 37 °C for 90 min. Enzymes were inactivated by placing the samples in boiling water. Samples were then centrifuged. The supernatant was collected and diluted 10×. Glucose content was determined by addition of glucose oxidase-peroxidase reagent and measuring absorbance at 510 nm. Percent inhibition of α-glucosidase by phenolic extracts and acarbose was determined by comparing the difference in absorbance between control and extract relative to absorbance of the control.

2.6. Inhibition of Glucose/Fructose Transport through Caco-2 Human Intestinal Cell Monolayers by GJ Phenolic Extracts

Potential for inhibition of glucose and fructose intestinal transport by GJ phenolic extract was assessed using a three-compartment Caco-2 human intestinal cell culture model. Caco-2 (TC7 clone) cells were maintained in DMEM supplemented with 10% v/v FBS, 1% v/v NEAA, 1% v/v HEPES, 1% v/v pen/strep and 0.1% v/v gentamicin. Cells were seeded (2.12×10^5 cells/cm^2), grown and differentiated in 6 well insert plates (Corning® Transwell® polyester membrane, Corning Inc., Oneonta, AL, USA, 24 mm diameter, pore size 0.4 µm) under a humidified atmosphere of air/CO$_2$ (95:5) at 37 °C. All experiments used differentiated monolayers (electrical resistance >250 Ω) at passages 90–95, with transport studies conducted 21–24 days post-confluency. Cells were incubated in glucose-free DMEM for 2 h preceding treatment. Test media for initial experiments was prepared by solubilizing glucose and fructose (9 mM each), d7-glu and d7-fru (3 mM each), and GJ phenolic extracts in PBS pH 5.5 (delivering 10–100 µM total phenolics, respectively). Cellular viability was assessed using the MTT assay (Biotium, Hayward, CA, USA). Highly differentiated cell monolayers treated with phenolic extracts and digesta (at concentrations >100 µM) for 4 h were found to have >95% viability. Test media was applied to the apical surface of cell monolayers. After 60 min incubation, basolateral and apical media were collected and cells were washed twice with 0.1% fatty acid free PBS. Membranes were then washed with ice cold PBS to terminate glucose transport, and cells were collected by scraping and frozen until analysis. All treatments were performed in quadruplicate.

2.7. Analysis of d7-Glucose and d7-Fructose Concentration in Basolateral Media by LC-MS

Basolateral media (100 µL) was extracted using acetone (0.5 mL), dried down under nitrogen, resolubilized in mobile phase (0.6 mL), and centrifuged (14,000 rpm, 5 min) prior to analysis for the chlorine adduct of d7-glu and d7-fru by LC-TOF-MS [32]. 10 µL of sample was injected on a Waters ACQUITY UPLC H-Class system equipped with an ACQUITY QDa mass detector. Separation was achieved according to a method by Liu et al. [33] with minor modification. A Waters BEH-amide column (2.1 mm id × 150 mm, 2.5 µM particle size) was heated to 30 °C under isocratic conditions with flow rate of 0.65 mL/min for 6 min and mobile phase 87:13 acetonitrile:water with 8 mM ammonium formate, pH 9.8. Conditions were as follows: ionization mode: ESI (−); mass: 222 m/z; capillary voltage: 0.8 kV; cone voltage: 20 V; probe temp: 350 °C; desolvation temp: 600 °C. Glucose, fructose, d7-glu and d7-fru concentrations were calculated using calibration curves made from authentic standards.

2.8. Impact of 100% GJ on Glucose Release/Transport in a Coupled in Vitro Digestion/Caco-2 Model

To extend beyond GJ extracts, a coupled three-stage in vitro digestion/Caco-2 model was used to determine if bioaccessible GJ phenolics could inhibit starch digestion and/or glucose transport with or without a co-consumed starch rich meal. Initially 100% GJ or sugar matched phenolic free control (~10 mL) was introduced to a three-stage in vitro digestion with oral, gastric and small intestinal phase as described by Moser et al. [34] and modified according to conditions described by Vermeirssen et al. [35] to include rat intestinal powder (0.15 g/reaction) as a source of α-glucosidase. Aliquots of undigested beverage starting material (SM), and centrifuged aqueous intestinal digesta (AQ) containing bioaccessible GJ phenolics were collected and acidified with aqueous acetic acid (1% total in sample) and stored frozen at $-80\,^{\circ}C$ until phenolic analysis by HPLC-MS (outlined above). A separate aliquot of AQ digesta was then diluted 2:7 with PBS (pH 5.5) (delivering ~21–56 μM total bioaccessible GJ phenolics, ~24 mM monosaccharides), spiked with d7-glu (6 mM), and applied to the apical surface of Caco-2 monolayers. A matching phenolic-free control was prepared by solubilizing glucose and fructose (24 mM total) with d7-glu (6 mM each) in blank AQ digesta diluted 2:7 with PBS. Treatments were replicated in quadruplicate. Transport of d7-glu was followed as described previously.

In a second experiment, 100% GJ was co-digested with a test meal consisting of a starch/nonfat dry milk model meal. The model meal was prepared by mixing corn starch and non-fat dry milk (NFDM) in double-distilled water (10% v/v each). The mixture was then heated (95 $^{\circ}C$, 30 min) and cooled slowly to 4 $^{\circ}C$. The resulting product was blended and an aliquot (5 g) was combined with 2.5 or 5 g of 100% GJ (Concord or SO_2 Niagara, 2013 harvest) or sugar-matched control beverage (50:50 Glucose:Fructose; 16° Brix) prior to introduction to the oral phase of digestion. Starting materials (GJ plus model meal) and final AQ digesta were collected and stored ($-80\,^{\circ}C$). Bioaccessibility of phenolics was determined by comparing individual phenolic content of AQ digesta relative to starting material. The extent of starch digestion was determined by comparison of initial glucose content in starting material to that in final AQ digesta. Percentage inhibition of starch digestion by GJ was determined by comparing release of glucose from starch during digestion of model meal with grape juice relative to phenolic-free control. Following digestion, the ability of co-digested GJ to further inhibit glucose transport was determined by diluting AQ digesta 2:7 with PBS (pH 5.5) containing 6 mM d7-glu (delivering ~5–16 μM total bioaccessible phenolics, determined using Folin-Ciocalteu assay [30]) and applying to the apical surface of Caco-2 monolayers. Feeding material containing AQ from high and low level GJ samples contained ~12 mM and 6 mM glucose and fructose. Matching phenolic-free controls were prepared. Treatments were replicated in quadruplicate. Transport of d7-glu (6 mM) was tracked and compared to control matched for sugar content.

2.9. Data Analysis

Data for polyphenol, anthocyanin, and (d7)-glu and (d7)-fru content of GJ samples, AQ digesta and basolateral material are expressed as mean $\pm$ SEM. Relative (%) bioaccessibility is defined as the percentage of polyphenol recovered in final digesta from that in starting material. Absolute bioaccessibility (μM) is the amount of phenolic available in digesta relative to that present in starting material, calculated by multiplying % bioaccessibility by concentration (μM) of phenolic in starting material. Percent (%) glucose release from corn starch by α-amylase was calculated as the fraction of glucose released compared to negative control. Glucose transport is expressed as concentration (μM) of d7-gluc appearing in the basolateral compartment over time. Percent (%) glucose transport was calculated on the basis of initial d7-glu content in the apical compartment at time 0. In order to facilitate comparison between treatments and control for variability between individual replicates, percentage (%) glucose transport was normalized using the d7-glu transport from control. Differences in phenolic profile, bioaccessibility data, enzyme inhibitory activity and glucose transport for each GJ or GJ extract were performed using JMP (Version 12, SAS Institute, Cary, NC, USA), and evaluated using Tukey's test or *t*-test. All significant differences testing used $\alpha < 0.05$.

3. Results

3.1. Phenolic and Anthocyanin Profiles of 100% Grape Juice

Phenolic content including anthocyanins and non anthocyaninin phenolics (Table 2) in Niagara and Concord GJ were comparable to that reported previously [5,36]. Several phenolic species previously reported in these native American grape varieties were observed including phenolic acids, flavonoids, stilbenes and anthocyanins. Concord GJ had higher levels of total phenolics compared to Niagara GJ for both 2013 and 2014 harvest juices. Further, GJ produced from 2013 harvest grapes had higher ($p < 0.05$) levels of caftaric acid, epicatechin, quercetin, quercetin-3-*O*-glucoside and specific anthocyanins compared to that from 2013 harvest grapes. Overall, phenolic acids, quercetin, and resveratrol were the most prominent phenolics observed in all samples, with levels up to 1134 μM. Use of SO_2 during Niagara GJ processing did result in higher phenolics levels in finished juice compared to untreated juice ($p < 0.05$).

Anthocyanins were present in GJ at lower levels compared to other phenolics (Table 2). Consistent with a report by Wang et al. [37], cyanidin and delphinidin derivatives were primary contributors to total anthocyanin content in Concord GJs. Concord GJ contained 2427.5–3092.0 ng/100 mL total anthocyanins compared to 111.1–131.9 mg/100 mL non-anthocyanin phenolics. Specifically, cyanidin-3,5-*O*-diglucoside and delphinidin-3-*O*-glucoside were the most abundant anthocyanins in Concord GJ, present up to 710.0 and 877.4 ng/100 mL, respectively. Further, cyanidin-3-*O*-p-coumaroyl-5-*O*-diglucoside and delphinidin-3-*O*-p-coumaroylglucoside were the only anthocyanins detected and tentatively identified in Niagara GJ and only at low levels (25.8–55.0 and 111.0–124.4 nmol/100 mL, respectively).

3.2. Modulation of α-Amylase and α-Glucosidase Activity by Grape Juice Phenolic Extracts

The ability of GJ phenolic extracts (50–500 μM) to inhibit α-amylase and α-glucosidase was determined in vitro. Only results from higher level phenolics experiments (300 and 500 μM) are shown (Table 3) as no activity was observed at less than 300 μM (data not shown). For both assays, the positive control (acarbose) decreased α-amylase and α-glucosidase activity significantly ($p < 0.05$) with complete inhibition of α-amylase activity observed at 300 μM. α-Glucosidase inhibition was observed by 300 μM and 500 μM acarbose at 88.9% and 92.4%, respectively.

GJ phenolic extracts demonstrated only modest inhibitory capacity for α-amylase and α-glucosidase (Table 3). At 500 μM, GJ phenolic extracts only modestly decreased α-amylase activity compared to phenolic-free control, with 2013 extracts (7.9%–9.4% inhibition) generally having greater ($p < 0.05$) impact compared to 2014 extracts (0.7%–9.2% inhibition). α-Amylase inhibition at lower GJ phenolic levels was not observed. Conversely, all GJ extracts exhibited modest α-glucosidase inhibitory capacity at both 300 and 500 μM. The 2013 harvest GJ extracts had similar inhibitory capacity for α-glucosidase (5.4%–11.5% inhibition) compared to 2014 extracts (3.8%–9.3% inhibition).

3.3. Modulation of Glucose Transport across Caco-2 Intestinal Cells by Grape Juice Phenolic Extracts

Previous studies have shown that various plant-derived phenolic extracts have ability to decrease basolateral glucose transport [18–20]. To determine if GJ phenolics exhibit similar activity, their ability to modulate intestinal glucose and fructose transport was assessed using a three-compartment Caco-2 human intestinal cell model. GJ extracts between 10 and 100 μM of total phenolics were able to reduce transport of d7-fru and d7-glu compared to control, with effect generally being increased with increased concentration (Figure 1; Table S1). Inhibition was similar across all GJ extracts and was greater for d7-fru compared to d7-glu transport, ranging from 10.9% to 41.3% and from 4.7% to 35.7% inhibition for d7-fru and d7-glu transport, respectively. Overall, extracts from Niagara GJ with and without SO_2 had similar effect on transport of d7-glu and d7-fru and generally exhibited a greater ability to inhibit transport relative to Concord GJ extracts.

Table 2. Content (μM) of individual non-anthocyanin phenolics and anthocyanins in three types of grape juices over two harvest years [1,2,3,4].

Phenolic Content (mg/100 mL)

100% Juice: Grape, Harvest Year	Gallic Acid	Caffeic Acid	Caftaric Acid	Epicatechin	Quercetin-3-O-glucoside	Quercetin 3,4-O-diglucoside	Quercetin-3-O-glucuronide	Quercetin	Isorhamnetin	Piceid	Resveratrol	Sum
Niagara, 2013	5.0 ± 0.4 [b]	3.4 ± 0.1 [c]	4.2 ± 0.1 [e]	NC	NC	2.2 ± 0.2 [c]	NC	16.8 ± 0.2 [d]	4.9 ± 0.1 [b]	0.8 ± 0.01 [f]	7.1 ± 0.2 [d]	44.5 ± 1.2 [e]
SO_2 Niagara, 2013	1.9 ± 0.04 [d]	5.2 ± 0.5 [b,c]	9.6 ± 0.2 [d]	1.5 ± 0.1 [c]	NC	2.0 ± 0.2 [c]	NC	19.8 ± 1.1 [c]	6.2 ± 0.4 [b]	5.3 ± 0.3 [a]	13.3 ± 0.7 [a]	64.8 ± 3.2 [d]
Concord, 2013	8.1 ± 0.4 [a]	11.1 ± 0.2 [a]	20.8 ± 0.7 [b]	7.9 ± 0.7 [b]	5.9 ± 0.4 [b]	4.2 ± 0.2 [a]	4.9 ± 0.3 [a]	30.0 ± 0.5 [b]	12.6 ± 0.4 [a]	2.2 ± 0.02 [d]	3.5 ± 0.1 [f]	111.1 ± 3.8 [b]
Niagara, 2014	4.0 ± 0.2 [b,c]	4.2 ± 0.2 [c]	2.9 ± 0.1 [e]	2.4 ± 0.3 [c]	NC	2.5 ± 0.2 [c]	NC	20.6 ± 0.1 [c]	5.0 ± 0.1 [b]	1.4 ± 0.03 [e]	10.3 ± 0.1 [c]	53.4 ± 1.3 [e]
SO_2 Niagara, 2014	2.9 ± 0.6 [c,d]	7.6 ± 1.7 [b]	16.9 ± 0.9 [c]	11.6 ± 0.9 [a]	NC	3.3 ± 0.4 [b]	NC	31.1 ± 0.6 [b]	10.3 ± 1.3 [a]	4.9 ± 0.06 [b]	11.7 ± 0.01 [b]	100.4 ± 6.7 [c]
Concord, 2014	8.9 ± 0.4 [a]	12.8 ± 0.6 [a]	25.1 ± 0.7 [a]	12.6 ± 1.2 [a]	7.8 ± 0.5 [a]	4.3 ± 0.3 [a]	3.8 ± 0.2 [b]	34.3 ± 0.3 [a]	13.1 ± 0.5 [a]	4.3 ± 0.2 [c]	5.1 ± 0.2 [e]	131.9 ± 4.9 [a]

Anthocyanin Content (mg/100 mL)

100% Juice: Grape, Harvest Year	Cyanidin-3,5-O-diglucoside	Cyanidin-3-O-acetyl glucoside	Cyanidin-3-O-glucoside	Delphinidin-3,5-O-diglucoside	Peonidin-3,5-O-diglucoside	Peonidin-3-O-glucoside	Peonidin-3-O-acetyl glucoside	Delphinidin-3-O-glucoside	Delphinidin-3-O-acetyl glucoside
Concord, 2013	623.5 ± 38.7 [a]	87.5 ± 15.8 [a]	74.8 ± 7.9 [b]		144.7 ± 13.5 [a]	13.6 ± 2.6 [b]	10.7 ± 2.4 [a]	620.5 ± 45.0 [b]	113.2 ± 13.0 [b]
Concord, 2014	710.0 ± 60.5 [a]	40.8 ± 17.4 [a]	106.9 ± 13.4 [a]		150.4 ± 11.5 [a]	19.2 ± 2.0 [a]	15.9 ± 3.3 [a]	877.4 ± 66.0 [a]	210.3 ± 27.7 [a]

Anthocyanin Content (mg/100 mL)

100% Juice: Grape, Harvest Year	Delphinidin-3-O-p-coumaroyl-5-O-diglucoside	Delphinidin-3-O-p-coumaroyl glucoside	Petunidin-3-O-glucoside	Petunidin-3-O-acetyl glucoside	Petunidin-3-O-p-coumaroyl-5-O-diglucoside	Malvidin-3-O-glucoside	Malvidin-3-O-acetyl glucoside	Sum
Concord, 2013	122.3 ± 20.6 [b]	199.8 ± 6.0 [a]	191.1 ± 17.2 [a]	35.0 ± 3.5 [b]	35.3 ± 7.4 [a]	133.4 ± 8.0 [b]	22.3 ± 3.3 [b]	2427.5 ± 205.0 [b]
Concord, 2014	212.1 ± 40.8 [a]	211.7 ± 9.1 [a]	210.1 ± 20.2 [a]	61.9 ± 10.1 [a]	58.2 ± 11.7 [a]	168.4 ± 14.5 [a]	38.8 ± 6.4 [a]	3092.0 ± 314.6 [a]

[1] Values represent mean ± standard error of mean from a triplicate analysis; [2] NC = Non Detected; [3] Presence of different letter (a, b) between values indicates significant differences in concentration of phenolic class between grape juices ($p < 0.05$); [4] Cyanidin-3-O-p-coumaroyl-5-O-diglucoside and delphinidin-3-O-p-coumaroyl glucoside were present in Niagara juices at 0.9 ± 0.01 to 1.9 ± 0.1 and 3.7 ± 0.1 to 4.1 ± 0.1 μM, respectively.

Table 3. Inhibition (%) of α-amylase and glucosidase activity by grape juice phenolic extracts.

Inhibitor	Inhibitor Concentration (µM GAE) [1]	Percent (%) Inhibition	
		α-Amylase	α-Glucosidase
Negative Control	0	0	0
Acarbose (Positive Control)	500	103.2 ± 5.1	92.4 ± 1.2
	300	102.0 ± 6.1	88.9 ± 0.9
	5	30.5 ± 2.9	6.2 ± 0.8
	3	17.6 ± 5.1	2.3 ± 0.5
Niagara, 2013	500	7.9 ± 4.5 [a,b,*]	10.0 ± 4.2 [a,b,*]
	300	4.5 ± 2.2 [b,c,*]	6.6 ± 2.9 [a,b,*]
SO$_2$ Niagara, 2013	500	9.4 ± 3.3 [a,*]	11.5 ± 3.1 [a,*]
	300	−3.9 ± 2.0 [f]	7.1 ± 2.6 [a,b,*]
Concord 2013	500	8.7 ± 4.3 [a,*]	9.2 ± 0.8 [a,b,*]
	300	−3.4 ± 2.0 [f]	5.4 ± 2.1 [b,*]
Niagara, 2014	500	0.7 ± 1.7 [d,e]	6.2 ± 3.4 [a,b,*]
	300	−1.9 ± 2.6 [e,f]	3.8 ± 2.0 [b]
SO$_2$ Niagara, 2014	500	9.2 ± 3.9 [a,*]	7.1 ± 2.7 [a,b,*]
	300	0.5 ± 1.0 [d,e]	4.2 ± 2.1 [b]
Concord 2014	500	3.4 ± 1.4 [c,d,*]	9.3 ± 3.2 [a,b,*]
	300	−1.2 ± 2.1 [e,f]	4.9 ± 1.2 [b]

Experiments represent average of *n* = 3 replicates; Preliminary dose finding experiments conducted with range of 10–1000 µM of phenolic extracts; Presence of different letter between values indicates significant differences in percentage inhibition between GJ extracts ($p < 0.05$); * indicates significant differences in percent inhibition by inhibitor compared to negative control ($p < 0.05$); [1] Total phenolics in digesta determined using Folin-Ciocalteu Assay and expressed as gallic acid equivalents (GAE); HPAEC-ECD and inhibition of α-glucosidase by glucose oxidase-peroxidase assay.

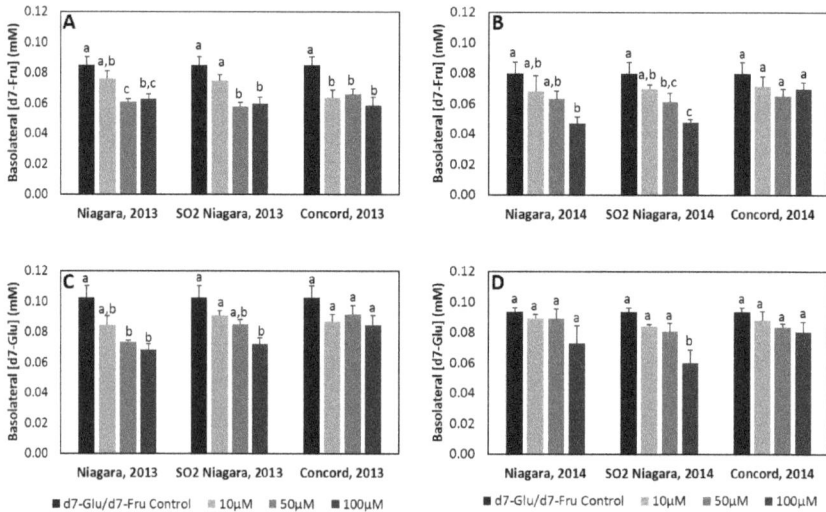

Figure 1. Impact of 2013 and 2014 harvest grape juice extracts on d7-fructose (**A,B**) or d7-glucose (**C,D**) transport across Caco-2 human intestinal cell monolayer. Data is represented as concentration of deuterated sugar in basolateral compartment at 60 min. Data represent mean ± SEM for *n* = 4 replicate wells at each time point. Presence of different letters between values indicates significant differences in glucose transport between treatments within each concentration ($p < 0.05$).

3.4. Influence of Bioaccessible Phenolics from 100% Grape Juice Phenolics on Carbohydrate Digestion and Glucose Transport When Co-Digested with Starch Rich Model Test Meal

In order to better understand the extent to which inhibition of starch digestion and glucose transport from GJ extracts translates to 100% GJ and whole food systems, Niagara and Concord GJs were subjected to an in vitro gastrointestinal digestion model with and without a starch based model meal. Bioaccessibility of GJ phenolics from each juice was determined to evaluate differences in delivery of phenolics in the upper GI tract from AQ digesta based on grape variety (Concord, Niagara), harvest year (2013, 2014), and SO_2 treatment (Table 4). The impact of bioaccessible phenolics on intestinal transport of glucose was also assessed (Figure 2). Additionally, the impact of co-digestion of GJ with a starch rich model meal on bioaccessibility of phenolics from GJ, starch digestion, and intestinal transport of glucose was assessed (Tables 5 and 6; Figure 3 and Table S2).

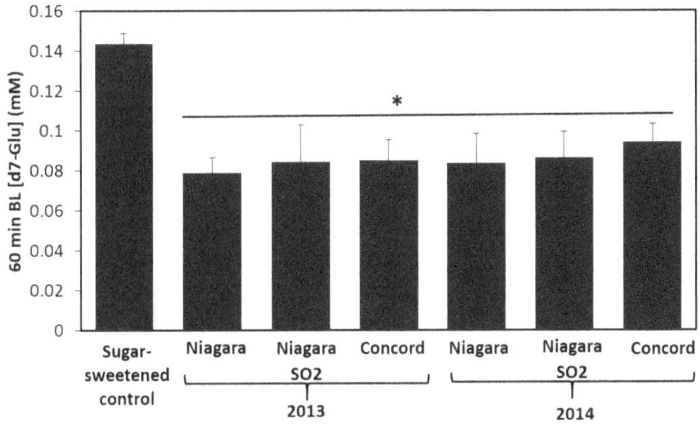

Figure 2. Impact of 2013 and 2014 100% grape juice aqueous digesta (AQ) on d7-glucose transport across Caco-2 human intestinal cell monolayers over 60 min. Data represent mean $\pm$ SEM for $n = 4$ replicate wells. * indicates significant difference in basolateral glucose concentration (mM) compared to control ($p < 0.05$).

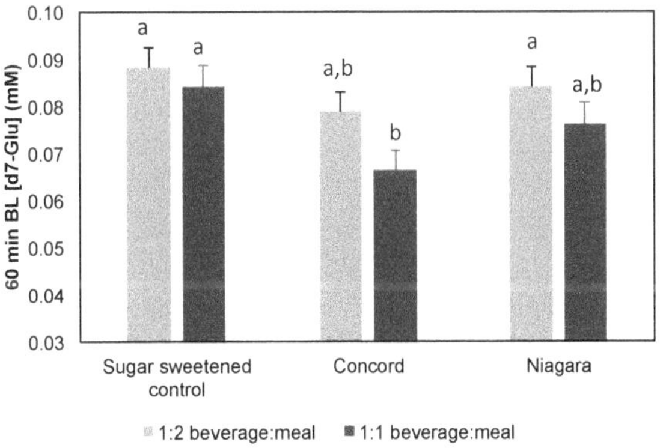

Figure 3. d7-Glucose transport across Caco-2 human intestinal cell monolayers from AQ digesta of co-digested GJ and starch rich test meal. Data is represented as a concentration of deuterated glucose in basolateral compartment at 60 min by treatment compared to control over 60 min. Data represent mean $\pm$ SEM for $n = 4$ replicate wells at each time point. Presence of different letter between values indicates significant differences in d7-glucose transport between treatments within the same ratio of beverage to meal.

Table 4. Relative (%) and absolute (μM or nM) bioaccessibility of non-anthocyanin phenolics and anthocyanins for three types of grape juices over two harvest years [1,2,3,4,5].

Non-Anthocyanin Phenolic Relative Bioaccessibility (%)

100% Juice: Grape, Harvest Year	Gallic Acid	Caffeic Acid	Caftaric Acid	Epicatechin	Quercetin 3,4-diglucoside	Quercetin	Isorhamnetin	Piceid	Resveratrol
Niagara, 2013	32.0 ± 9.2 [a,b]	24.8 ± 2.6 [b]	39.5 ± 0.6 [a,b]	NC [e]	16.9 ± 6.8 [a]	8.4 ± 0.8 [a]	20.9 ± 0.8 [a]	22.1 ± 1.2 [a]	18.7 ± 1.9 [b]
SO₂ Niagara, 2013	31.7 ± 4.4 [a]	36.1 ± 4.2 [a,b]	32.7 ± 1.7 [b]	27.4 ± 3.0 [a]	21.7 ± 8.5 [a]	7.6 ± 0.5 [a]	18.5 ± 1.9 [a]	10.3 ± 0.3 [c,d]	17.5 ± 1.6 [b]
Concord, 2013	29.6 ± 6.6 [a]	29.1 ± 3.6 [b]	32.2 ± 1.6 [b]	18.5 ± 1.4 [c]	15.7 ± 7.4 [a]	2.6 ± 0.5 [b]	7.6 ± 0.4 [b]	14.8 ± 2.0 [b]	26.6 ± 1.7 [a]
Niagara, 2014	29.7 ± 5.8 [a]	27.5 ± 2.0 [b]	56.0 ± 15.0 [a]	11.8 ± 2.0 [d]	13.8 ± 4.6 [a]	2.1 ± 0.2 [b]	7.6 ± 0.2 [b]	12.6 ± 0.1 [b,c]	14.6 ± 1.4 [b]
SO₂ Niagara, 2014	22.0 ± 1.5 [a]	44.7 ± 8.0 [a]	31.6 ± 3.2 [b]	24.3 ± 2.1 [a,b]	16.7 ± 8.8 [a]	1.7 ± 0.3 [b]	4.1 ± 0.4 [c]	8.9 ± 1.3 [c,d]	16.8 ± 2.3 [b]
Concord, 2014	29.2 ± 2.5 [a]	28.7 ± 5.7 [b]	30.3 ± 5.2 [b]	21.3 ± 1.3 [b,c]	12.2 ± 5.0 [a]	1.8 ± 0.5 [b]	3.3 ± 0.3 [c]	8.1 ± 1.2 [d]	17.6 ± 3.8 [b]

Anthocyanin Relative Bioaccessibility (%)

100% Juice: Grape, Harvest Year	Cyanidin-3,5-O-diglucoside	Peonidin-3,5-O-diglucoside	Delphinidin-3-O-glucoside	Delphinidin-3-O-acetyl glucoside	Delphinidin-3-O-p-coumaroyl-glucoside	Petunidin-3-O-glucoside	Malvidin-3-O-glucoside
Concord, 2013	18.0 ± 0.9 [a]	25.7 ± 1.5 [a]	12.0 ± 1.1 [a]	6.3 ± 1.8 [a]	10.1 ± 0.8 [a]	23.0 ± 1.9 [a]	37.2 ± 1.7 [a]
Concord, 2014	13.1 ± 1.2 [b]	18.7 ± 1.1 [b]	8.1 ± 1.3 [b]	3.7 ± 0.9 [b]	6.3 ± 0.6 [b]	19.9 ± 2.9 [a]	30.0 ± 4.8 [b]

Non-Anthocyanin Phenolic Absolute Bioaccessibility (μM)

100% Juice: Grape, Harvest Year	Gallic Acid	Caffeic Acid	Caftaric Acid	Epicatechin	Quercetin 3,4-diglucoside	Quercetin	Isorhamnetin	Piceid	Resveratrol
Niagara, 2013	91.0 ± 20.0 [b]	47.5 ± 6.2 [b]	53.4 ± 0.6 [e]	NC	8.2 ± 3.4 [a]	46.5 ± 3.7 [a]	21.2 ± 0.7 [b]	8.2 ± 0.4 [c]	57.8 ± 4.6 [c,d]
SO₂ Niagara, 2013	36.3 ± 5.6 [c]	103.6 ± 8.8 [b]	100.9 ± 5.2 [d]	13.7 ± 1.3 [c]	9.2 ± 3.7 [a]	50.3 ± 5.6 [a]	23.7 ± 1.1 [a]	24.2 ± 1.6 [a]	102.7 ± 14.0 [a]
Concord, 2013	139.0 ± 25.9 [a]	179.1 ± 22.3 [a]	214.3 ± 8.8 [b]	50.7 ± 7.1 [b]	14.3 ± 6.9 [a]	25.9 ± 4.7 [b]	19.9 ± 0.7 [b]	14.1 ± 1.9 [b]	40.4 ± 1.8 [c,d]
Niagara, 2014	68.7 ± 10.6 [b,c]	64.8 ± 6.3 [b]	53.3 ± 15.2 [e]	9.5 ± 0.9 [c]	7.8 ± 3.4 [a]	14.0 ± 1.2 [b]	8.0 ± 0.1 [c]	7.8 ± 0.2 [c]	66.1 ± 6.9 [b,c]
SO₂ Niagara, 2014	37.0 ± 6.2 [c]	177.6 ± 37.1 [a]	169.2 ± 7.2 [c]	96.8 ± 10.5 [a]	10.5 ± 4.4 [a]	17.8 ± 2.6 [b]	8.7 ± 0.2 [c]	19.2 ± 2.6 [a,b]	86.1 ± 11.6 [a,b]
Concord, 2014	152.4 ± 14.2 [a]	202.5 ± 37.4 [a]	241.1 ± 35.8 [a]	91.5 ± 3.7 [a]	11.5 ± 4.6 [a]	20.3 ± 5.1 [b]	8.9 ± 0.5 [c]	15.3 ± 2.2 [b]	38.6 ± 7.7 [d]

Anthocyanin Absolute Bioaccessibility (nM)

100% Juice: Grape, Harvest Year	Cyanidin-3,5-O-diglucoside	Peonidin-3,5-O-diglucoside	Delphinidin-3-O-glucoside	Delphinidin-3-O-acetyl glucoside	Delphinidin-3-O-p-coumaroyl-glucoside	Petunidin-3-O-glucoside	Malvidin-3-O-glucoside
Concord, 2013	16.2 ± 1.0 [a]	5.1 ± 0.4 [a]	10.1 ± 0.4 [a]	0.9 ± 0.2 [a]	2.8 ± 0.2 [a]	5.7 ± 0.2 [a]	6.2 ± 0.3 [a]
Concord, 2014	13.4 ± 1.5 [b]	3.9 ± 0.2 [b]	9.8 ± 1.7 [a]	1.0 ± 0.2 [a]	1.8 ± 0.3 [b]	5.6 ± 1.4 [a]	6.4 ± 1.4 [a]

[1] Values represent mean ± standard error of mean from a triplicate analysis; [2] NC = Non Detected; [3] Presence of different letter between values indicates significant differences in concentration of phenolic class between grape juices ($p < 0.05$); [4] Quercetin-3-O-glucoside bioaccessibility from Concord grape juices was between 7.2% ± 2.7% to 8.1% ± 3.5%. Delphinidin-3-O-p-coumaroyl glucoside bioaccessibility from Niagara juices and Concord juices was between 8.4% ± 0.5% to 24.3% ± 1.0% and 6.3% ± 0.6% to 10.1% ± 0.8%, respectively; [5] Phenolics in GJs and digesta determined using LC-MS.

Table 5. Glucose transport by Caco-2 small intestinal epithelial cells co-treated with d7-Glu (6 mM) and aqueous digesta (AQ) or matched phenolic-free control [1,2,3,4].

Treatment	Phenolic Concentration (µM) [5]	Percent d7-Glu Transport [6]	Percent (%) d7-Glu Transported over 60 min Relative to Control [7]
Without Model Test Meal			
Control (24 mM glucose/fructose)	0	2.4 ± 0.1 [a]	100 [a]
Niagara, 2013 AQ	27.1	1.3 ± 0.1 [b]	54.8 ± 5.4 [b]
SO$_2$ Niagara, 2013 AQ	37.8	1.4 ± 0.3 [b]	58.6 ± 13.0 [b]
Concord, 2013 AQ	56.3	1.4 ± 0.2 [b]	59.2 ± 7.3 [b]
Niagara, 2014 AQ	20.8	1.4 ± 0.3 [b]	58.2 ± 10.4 [b]
SO$_2$ Niagara, 2014 AQ	39.4	1.4 ± 0.2 [b]	60.1 ± 9.0 [b]
Concord 2014 AQ	53.7	1.6 ± 0.2 [b]	65.7 ± 6.5 [b]
With Model Test Meal			
1:1 Control (12 mM glu/fru)	0	1.5 ± 0.1 [a]	100 [a]
1:2 Control (6 mM glu/fru)	0	1.3 ± 0.1 [a]	100 [a]
1:1 Concord 2013	16.4	1.1 ± 0.2 [b]	78.6 ± 7.7 [b]
1:1 SO$_2$ Niagara 2013	7.1	1.3 ± 0.2 [a,b]	90.6 ± 7.6 [a,b]
1:2 Concord, 2013	10.1	1.3 ± 0.1 [a]	89.5 ± 9.5 [a,b]
1:2 SO$_2$ Niagara 2013	4.6	1.4 ± 0.1 [a]	95.2 ± 10.2 [a]

[1] Treatments included aqueous digesta (AQ) diluted 2:7 prior to introduction to apical compartment of three-compartment Caco-2 cell model; [2] d7-Glucose (6 mM) was used as a marker for glucose transport; Diluted Concord, Niagara, and blank digesta AQ contained 15, 12, and 12 mM glucose, respectively and 12, 17, and 12 mM fructose, respectively; [3] Data represent an average of $n = 4$ wells per experiment; [4] Presence of different letter between values indicates significant differences in glucose transport between treatment and control, within experiment comparing AQ digesta from different juices or experiment comparing AQ digesta with and without model test meal ($p < 0.05$); [5] Total phenolics and sugars in digesta determined using LC-MS; [6] Percent of d7-glucose transported from apical media to basolateral compartment; [7] Amount of d7-glucose transported basolaterally over 60 min relative to daily control matched for glucose/fructose and d7-glucose.

Table 6. Percentage decrease in release of glucose from starch-rich model meal co-digested with grape juice compared with a sugar-matched control [1].

Formulation [2]	Concentration of Phenolics in Aqueous Digesta (AQ) Fraction Following Digestion (µM) [3]	Percent Decrease in Glucose Release from Corn Starch by GJ Phenolics Compared to Phenolic-Free Control [4]
1:1 Concord:Model meal	73.7	15.0
1:2 Concord: Model meal	35.4	5.9
1:1 SO$_2$ Niagara: Model meal	25.9	12.1
1:2 SO$_2$ Niagara: Model meal	17.2	6.6

[1] Experiments represent average of $n = 3$ replicates; [2] High and low 100% Concord 2013 GJ contained 473 and 236 µmol/240 mL serving total phenolics, respectively; High and low Niagara 2013 GJ contained 289 and 144 µmol/240 mL serving total phenolics, respectively; Concord and Niagara 2013 juices contained 447 and 596 mM fructose, respectively, and 531 and 427 mM glucose, respectively (determined using LC-MS); [3] Total phenolics and sugars in SM and AQ digesta determined using LC-MS; [4] Phenolic-free control was distilled water with matching glucose and fructose content.

Overall, relative bioaccessibility (Table 4) of non-anthocyanin phenolics was similar between Concord and Niagara GJ varieties and generally consistent with previous reports of phenolic bioaccessibility from fruit juices [38–40]. SO$_2$ treatment generally did not significantly alter bioaccessibility of non-anthocyanin phenolics from Niagara GJ. Phenolic acids were the most bioaccessible forms in GJ ranging from 22.0% to 56.0% relative bioaccessibility. Overall, caftaric acid was the most bioaccessible non-anthocyanin phenolic from GJ, with bioaccessibility ranging from 30.3% to 56.0%. Remaining phenolic acids as well as epicatechin and resveratrol were less bioaccessible (~11.8% to 44.7%). Quercetin, isorhamnetin, and piceid generally had higher ($p < 0.05$) relative bioaccessibility from 2013 harvest Niagara GJ compared to 2014 harvest. Although there were few trends for differences in relative bioaccessibility of phenolic acids between GJs, absolute bioaccessibility (µM) of most non-anthocyanin phenolics were significantly ($p < 0.05$) higher from SO$_2$ Niagara compared to non SO$_2$ treated Niagara GJ and phenolic acids and epicatechin were significantly higher ($p < 0.05$) from Concord GJ compared to Niagara GJs (Table 4).

Relative bioaccessibilities of individual anthocyanins from GJ were generally lower compared to other phenolics, ranging from 3.7% to 37.2% (Table 4). Notably, malvidin-3-*O*-glucoside had the highest bioaccessibility among anthocyanins (37.2% ± 1.7%) from Concord 2013 harvest GJ. Similar to the trend for phenolics, relative bioaccessibility for anthocyanins were higher ($p < 0.05$) from 2013 harvest compared to 2014 harvest Concord GJs. For Niagara GJs, delphinidin-3-O-p-coumaroylglucoside bioaccessibility was significantly higher from 2013 compared to 2014 harvest GJ (24.3% ± 1.0% compared 9.5% ± 0.1%). Unlike non-anthocyanin phenolics, anthocyanin absolute bioaccessibility from each GJ were reflective of the trends observed in relative bioaccessibility. Notably, cyanidin-3,5-O-diglucoside had highest absolute bioaccessibility (13.4–16.2 nM). Absolute bioaccessibility was low for remaining anthocyanins ranging from 0.9 to 10.1 nM.

Following assessment of bioaccessibility, AQ fractions from final digesta of juices and sugar-matched controls were diluted with PBS (pH 5.5) containing 6 mM d7-glu and applied to the apical side of Caco-2 monolayers to determine intestinal glucose transport from phenolic rich GJ. Apical to basolateral transport of d7-glu was assessed over 60 min. Compared to digesta from phenolic-free sugar matched control beverages, all media containing GJ AQ digesta reduced d7-glu transport efficiency by 34.3% to 45.2% over 60 min (Table 5, Figure 2). These results were similar to those observed from GJ extracts described earlier (Figure 1) and suggest that activities observed in extract screen are preserved through digestion.

To better understand the potential influence of macronutrients from a complex meal on the ability of GJ to influence carbohydrate digestion and glucose transport, Concord and SO_2 Niagara GJ (2013 harvest) were co-formulated with a model test meal (1:1 and 1:2 (wt:wt) in starting material) consisting of a corn starch and milk protein rich model meal and digested in vitro. Co-digestion of starch-rich model meal with Concord and SO_2 Niagara GJ at both high (1:1 GJ:model meal) and low (1:2 GJ:model meal) juice levels resulted in decreased glucose release (5.9% to 15.0% reduction) from starch digestion relative to phenolic-free sugar matched control (Table 6), suggesting bioaccessible phenolics from 100% GJ have ability to modulate glucose availability by decreasing the digestive release of glucose from starch in the small intestine.

To confirm that bioaccessible GJ phenolics resulting from co-digestion of GJ with test meal maintain the ability to modulate d7-glu intestinal transport, AQ digesta fractions from co-digestion experiments were diluted with PBS containing a final concentration of 6 mM of d7-glu. Despite lower phenolic concentration in test media, distinct inhibition of glucose transport was observed (Table 5; Figure 3). Specifically, d7-glu transport was decreased by 4.8%–21.4%, with a significant ($p < 0.05$) decline in glucose transport observed for treatment with 50% Concord GJ inclusion in the model meal.

4. Discussion

Clinical evidence exists to support the notion that certain phenolic-rich foods and beverages may modify glycemic parameters [22,23,41–46]. One hundred percent GJ is a particularly rich source of dietary phenolics but also naturally high in sugar (~36 g sugar per 240 mL serving) [9]. While it has been reported that fruit juices have similar glycemic responses to their corresponding whole fruits [10]), grape juice has also been shown to have a lower insulinemic response than corresponding grapes [21]. This may be related to the differential profile of grape juice compared to grapes and, thus, a better understanding of the interaction between GJ phenolics and the intrinsic sugar in these products is required. This study was designed to develop insight into the ability and mechanisms by which GJ phenolics may modulate starch digestion and absorption of glucose in the context of a juice matrix with and without a starch rich meal.

One mechanism that has been proposed for these effects is related to phenolic inhibition of starch digestion [47–50]. In the present study, GJ phenolic extracts (300 and 500 μM) demonstrated only modest inhibitory capacity for α-amylase and α-glucosidase (Table 3). Harvest year impacted α-amylase, but not α-glucosidase activity, with 2013 extracts generally having greater impact compared to 2014 extracts. This may be related to subtle differences in qualitative phenolic profiles from 2013 to 2014 harvest GJs as total levels appeared similar between harvest years. Phenolic rich GJ extracts had greater inhibitory activity toward α-glucosidase compared to α-amylase. Similar results were previously reported for wine grape tannins, pomace and skin extracts for inhibition of α-glucosidase (~20% to 85%), with little to no detectable impact on α-amylase activity [48,49]. Levels of phenolics required to achieve even modest inhibition were observed to be high (>300 μM). However, it is important to note that concentrations of phenolics in the gut lumen from a serving of phenolic rich food or beverage may in in fact be quite high and approach high μM to even mM levels as previously postulated [7,51]. Therefore, results here suggesting a modest ability of GJ phenolics to inhibit α-glucosidase at a 300 μM dose does support the hypothesis that consumption of GJ with starch rich foods may have relevance to starch digestion and liberation of glucose in the gut lumen.

A second mechanism by which phenolics may modulate glycemic response is through alteration of glucose intestinal transport [18–20]. In the present study, GJ extracts (10–100 μM total phenolics) reduced intestinal glucose and fructose transport by Caco-2 human intestinal cell monolayers compared to control. These findings are similar to those previously reported with plant-derived phenolic extracts [18–20] (Figure 1; Table S1). Overall, inhibition by GJ extracts was greater for d7-fru compared to d7-glu transport, with extracts from Niagara GJ generally exhibiting greater inhibitory activity relative to Concord GJ extracts. Since extracts were standardized for total phenolics, these results suggest that the qualitative phenolic profile of Niagara GJ, which is primarily composed of non-anthocyanin flavonoids and phenolic acids and minimal amounts of anthocyanins (Table 2), may be most critical to consider in selection of juices and therefore merits additional investigation as targeted modifiers of intestinal glucose transport. The mechanism behind this reduction of glucose transport may be related, in part, to the ability of GJ phenolics to inhibit expression of hexose transporters (GLUT2 and SGLT1) or through direct inhibition of these transporters. Alzaid et al. [20] demonstrated that GLUT2 and SGLT1 mRNA were significantly decreased compared to baseline by up to 85% and 70%, respectively, following treatment of cells with berry extract for over 12 h. However, although GLUT2 protein was significantly reduced compared to control by treatment of blueberry extract for 16 h, SGLT1 protein levels were not affected. In a preliminary experiment, expression of GLUT2 and SGLT1 mRNA was measured in Caco-2 monolayers exposed to 100% GJ phenolic extracts (SO$_2$ Niagara and Concord 2013) for 4 and 24 h. Interestingly, GLUT2 mRNA was significantly ($p < 0.05$) decreased two-fold following treatment by Concord GJ phenolic extract, but no significant change in SGLT1 expression was observed (Figure S1). While these preliminary results are consistent with previous observations [18–20], they cannot fully explain the observed effects in the present study. Previous reports have also demonstrated that bioavailability of select polyphenols may be increased in the presence of carbohydrates [52–54] suggesting the potential for additional interrelated mechanism impacting the transport of both phenolics and carbohydrate. Transepithelial flux of grape juice phenolics was not simultaneously monitored in this study, and, as such, it is not possible to speculate to these mechanisms. Further investigations are therefore warranted to better delineate the extent to which phenolic inhibit of natural juice sugars may be related to changes in transporter expression or function, or alternative mechanisms.

Finally, in order to better understand the extent to which these effects would be extendable to 100% GJ, Niagara and Concord GJ or matching phenolic free control were formulated with and without a starch rich model meal and digested in vitro. Differences observed in phenolic relative bioaccessibility from juice alone are suggestive of variations in grape phenolic components between harvest years (Tables 2 and 4). On the other hand, SO$_2$ treatment did not impact relative bioaccessibility of phenolics from Niagara GJ. These results logically suggest that starting concentration of phenolics in 100% GJ have a direct impact on concentration of phenolics available for interactions in the gut and ultimate stability and accessibility of phenolics in the small intestine. Following assessment of phenolic bioaccessibility, transport of glucose from AQ digesta of 100% GJ and sugar match controls by Caco-2 intestinal cells was assessed. All GJ AQ digesta reduced d7-glu transport efficiency compared to phenolic-free sugar matched control up to 45% over 60 min (Figure 2; Table 5). These results were similar to those observed from extract screening and suggest that reduced efficiency of intestinal glucose transport may be a factor to consider in assessing glycemic response from GJ relative to a phenolic free sugar sweetened beverage. Interestingly, this observation is consistent with the glycemic response of phenolic rich apple juice that has previously been shown to cause a modest reduction in glycemic response relative to sugar matched controls in healthy humans [22,41].

To build on these findings with the awareness that GJ is commonly consumed with meals, it is important to consider the consequences of co-consumed food on ability of GJ phenolics to modulate carbohydrate digestion and glucose transport. It is well known that phenolics interact non-covalently with protein and carbohydrate (reviewed by Bordenave et al. [55] and Jakobek et al. [56]). These interactions in the context of a co-consumed meal may result in changes to the activity of phenolics relative to endpoints critical to glycemic response, namely carbohydrate digestion and glucose transport. Therefore, digestion of carbohydrate from a starch and protein-rich test meal co-formulated with GJ compared to phenolic-free control was determined. Although the level of GJ phenolics in AQ digesta resulting from co-digestion of GJ with test meal was lower compared to level of phenolics from GJ extracts used in enzyme inhibition assays (Tables 3 and 5), results for inhibition of starch digestion were in fact similar. Therefore, it appears bioaccessible phenolics in the context of a complex meal still have the ability to impact digestion of carbohydrates derived from the meal. The extent to which this may be due to the proximity of phenolics and macronutrients in the meal and specific interactions that may develop through preparation and/or digestion remains to be explored.

Modifying glucose transport by GJ in the context of a digested meal was also determined. The effect of AQ digesta from GJ containing meals demonstrated only modest inhibitory effects (Figure 3) which reach significance only for 100% Concord GJ. While in contrast with extract screening that found Niagara phenolics to be more effective, this observation was not totally unexpected as the phenolic concentrations resulting from digestion of mixed meals were lower than extract and juice experiments, especially for Niagara (Table 5). Considering that in humans concentrations in the gut lumen may reach high μM to mM levels [12] from typical food doses and gut dilution, responses within a meal such as those observed with berries by Törrönen et al. [57] may be expected. While requiring additional clinical insights as to the direction and extent of this effect in vivo are required, current results, while in vitro, do reflect the modest but important changes in glycemic response observed in recent clinical trials involving phenolic-rich foods and beverages [22,23,41–46]. This is relevant considering that moderate post-prandial hyperglycemia blood glucose levels (148–199 mg/dL) have been shown to be indicative of the development of negative health effects including atherosclerosis and endothelial damage [58]. This range represents a ~6% increase compared to the recommended <140 mg/dL post-prandial (2 h) blood glucose target [59], suggesting that even subtle improvements to post-prandial blood glucose level may prevent development of negative health outcomes. Therefore, while subtle, the current observations that 100% GJ may impact both carbohydrate digestion and glucose transport both from juice and in the context of a model meal suggest that the benefits of 100% GJ may be extendable beyond the glucose derived from the juice and to the response of a full meal and, thus, have positive impacts on health.

5. Conclusions

Although high in natural sugar, 100% Concord or Niagara GJ remains a rich source of dietary phenolics that have been reported to modify glycemic parameters through alteration of carbohydrate digestion and glucose transport. Results of the current study are in general agreement with previous studies reporting the ability of phenolics to decrease α-glucosidase activity [48,49] and also indicate that 100% GJ phenolics have the ability to decrease glucose transport even following simulated oral gastric and small intestinal digestions. Further, results suggest that 100% GJ, when placed in the context of a meal, maintains the ability to decrease intestinal starch digestion and subsequent glucose transport, in a fashion consistent with promotion of healthy glucose homeostasis. Further clinical assessments of 100% GJ in the context of glycemic response are warranted to clarify the impact of both intrinsic fruit sugar in juice and the potential impact of fruit phenolics on glycemic response from a meal.

Supplementary Materials: The following are available online at http://www.mdpi.com/2072-6643/8/7/414/s1, Table S1: Glucose transport by Caco-2 small intestinal epithelial cells co-treated with sugar solution (Glu and Fru (9 mM each) and d7-Glu and d7-Fru (3 mM each) and phenolic extract from grape juice or phenolic-free control matched for sugar content, Table S2: Relative (%) bioaccessibility of marker phenolics and anthocyanins in Concord, 2013 grape juice co-digested with a protein containing corn starch gel (model meal), Table S3: Forward and reverse PCR primer sequences utilized for gene expression analysis by PCR, Figure S1: Impact grape juice phenolic extract (50 µM) treatment (4 or 24 h) has on Caco-2 expression of SGLT1 or GLUT2 compared to phenolic-free control. Data is represented as protein expression compared to control β-actin. Data represent mean ± SEM for $n = 4$ replicate wells. Presence of different letter between values indicates significant differences in protein expression between treatments within each time point ($p < 0.05$).

Acknowledgments: Funded by a grant from Welch Foods Inc. and by the USDA National Needs Fellowship. The views expressed in this manuscript are those of the author(s) and do not necessarily reflect the position or policy of Welch Foods Inc.

Author Contributions: M.G.F., B.R.H., J.D.W. and S.M. conceived and designed the experiments; S.M., J.L. and M.C. performed the experiments; S.M. and M.G.F. analyzed the data; S.M. and M.G.F. wrote the paper with B.R.H., J.D.W. and M.C. providing editorial input. M.G.F. is currently a member of the Welch's Nutrition and Health Advisory Board.

Conflicts of Interest: The authors declare no conflict of interest.

Abbreviations

The following abbreviations are used in this manuscript:

GJ	Grape juice
d7-Glu	Deuterated glucose
d7-Glu	Deuterated fructose
LDL	low density lipoprotein
GLUT2	glucose transporter 2
SGLT1	sodium-dependent glucose transporter 1
DMEM	Dulbecco's Modified Eagles Medium
NEAA	non-essential amino acids
Pen/strep	penicillin/streptomycin
HEPES	4-(2-hydroxylethyl)-1-piperazineethanes
FBS	fetal bovine serum
FFA	bovine serum albumin (free fatty acid free)
SPE	solid phase extraction
LC-MS	liquid chromatography-mass spectrometry
DMSO	dimethylsulfoxide
PBS	phosphate buffered saline
SM	starting material
AQ	aqueous (intestinal digesta)
NFDM	non-fat dry milk
HPAEC-ECD	high pressure anion exchange chromatography-electrochemical detector
PCR	polymerase chain reaction

Appendix A

Appendix A.1 Modulation of Caco-2 Glucose/Fructose Transporter Gene Expression by GJ Phenolic Extracts

Cells and experimental conditions for gene expression experiment were maintained and executed according to glucose transport experiments, with minor modifications. Test media was prepared by solubilizing glucose and fructose (12 mM each) and GJ phenolic extracts in PBS pH 5.5 (delivering 50 µM total phenolics). Test media was applied to the apical surface of cell monolayers and cells were incubated for 4 or 24 h. Cells were collected with RNAlater (Sigma-Aldrich) and frozen until analysis. Treatments were replicated in quadruplicate.

Appendix A.2 Characterization of mRNA Expression and Anthocyanin-Rich Fractions by LC-MS

Total RNA was isolated from the cultured cells using TRIzol® (Invitrogen™ Life Technologies, Paisley, UK) according to the manufacturer's instructions. RNA concentration was measured using wavelength of 260 and 280 using a NanoDrop 2000 UV-Vis Spectrophotometer (Thermo Scientific., Wilmington, DC, USA) Following first strand cDNA synthesis, expression levels of glucose transporter mRNA and GAPDH mRNA (used as a housekeeping gene) were analysed by real-time quantitative PCR using an ABI Prism 7700HT Sequence Detection System and a Power SYBR® Green PCR master mix kit (Applied Biosystems™, Cheshire, UK). The primer sequences used for each gene are given in Table S3. cDNA was then synthesized from 150 ng RNA using M-MuLV reverse transcriptase (BioLabs, Ipswich, MA, USA). Real-time q-RT-PCR was performed using a CFX Connect Real-Time PCR Detection System (BioRad, Hercules, CA, USA). The expressions of SGLT1 and GLUT2 were evaluated and the expression of housekeeping gene β-actin was assessed. The primer sequences used for each gene are given in Table S3.

References

1. United States of Department of Agriculture (USDA). *Fruit Yearbook Supply and Utilization*; USDA: Washington, DC, USA, 2015.
2. Dani, C.; Oliboni, L.S.; Vanderlinde, R.; Bonatto, D.; Salvador, M.; Henriques, J.A.P. Phenolic content and antioxidant activities of white and purple juices manufactured with organically- or conventionally-produced grapes. *Food Chem. Toxicol.* **2007**, *45*, 2574–2580. [PubMed]
3. Fuleki, T.; Ricardo-Da-Silva, J.M. Effects of cultivar and processing method on the contents of catechins and procyanidins in grape juice. *J. Agric. Food Chem.* **2003**, *51*, 640–646. [CrossRef] [PubMed]
4. Iyer, M.M.; Sacks, G.L.; Padilla-Zakour, O.I. Impact of harvesting and processing conditions on green leaf volatile development and phenolics in Concord grape juice. *J. Food Sci.* **2010**, *75*, 297–304. [CrossRef] [PubMed]
5. Stalmach, A.; Edwards, C.A.; Wightman, J.D.; Crozier, A. Identification of (poly) phenolic compounds in concord grape juice and their metabolites in human plasma and urine after juice consumption. *J. Agric. Food Chem.* **2011**, *59*, 9512–9522. [CrossRef] [PubMed]
6. Blumberg, J.B.; Vita, J.A.; Chen, C.-Y.O. Concord grape juice polyphenols and cardiovascular risk factors: Dose-response relationships. *Nutrients* **2015**, *7*, 10032–10052. [CrossRef] [PubMed]
7. Krikorian, R.; Nash, T.A.; Shidler, M.D.; Shukitt-Hale, B.; Joseph, J.A. Concord grape juice supplementation improves memory function in older adults with mild cognitive impairment. *Br. J. Nutr.* **2010**, *103*, 730–734. [CrossRef] [PubMed]
8. Krikorian, R.; Boespflug, E.L.; Fleck, D.E.; Stein, A.L.; Wightman, J.D.; Shidler, M.D.; Sadat-Hossieny, S. Concord grape juice supplementation and neurocognitive function in human aging. *J. Agric. Food Chem.* **2012**, *60*, 5736–5742. [CrossRef] [PubMed]
9. United States of Department of Agriculture (USDA). *USDA National Nutrient Database for Standard Reference Release 27*; USDA: Washington, DC, USA, 2016.
10. Wolever, T.M.S.; Vuksan, V.; Relle, L.K.; Jenkins, A.L.; Josse, R.G.; Wong, G.S.; Jenkins, D.J. Glycaemic index of fruits and fruit products in patients with diabetes. *Int. J. Food Sci. Nutr.* **1993**, *43*, 205–212. [CrossRef]
11. Hanhineva, K.; Törrönen, R.; Bondia-Pons, I.; Pekkinen, J.; Kolehmainen, M.; Mykkänen, H.; Poutanen, K. Impact of dietary polyphenols on carbohydrate metabolism. *Int. J. Mol. Sci.* **2010**, *11*, 1365–1402. [CrossRef] [PubMed]
12. Williamson, G. Possible effects of dietary polyphenols on sugar absorption and digestion. *Mol. Nutr. Food Res.* **2013**, *57*, 48–57. [CrossRef] [PubMed]
13. Jeng, T.L.; Chiang, Y.C.; Lai, C.C.; Liao, T.C.; Lin, S.Y.; Lin, T.C.; Sung, J.M. Sweet potato leaf extract inhibits the simulated in vitro gastrointestinal digestion of native starch. *J. Food Drug Anal.* **2015**, *23*, 399–406. [CrossRef]
14. Coe, S.A.; Clegg, M.; Armengol, M.; Ryan, L. The polyphenol-rich baobab fruit (*Adansonia digitata* L.) reduces starch digestion and glycemic response in humans. *Nutr. Res.* **2013**, *33*, 888–896. [CrossRef] [PubMed]

15. He, Q.; Lv, Y.; Yao, K. Effects of tea polyphenols on the activities of α-amylase, pepsin, trypsin and lipase. *Food Chem.* **2007**, *101*, 1178–1182. [CrossRef]

16. Nakai, M.; Fukui, Y.; Asami, S.; Toyoda-Ono, Y.; Iwashita, T.; Shibata, H.; Mitsunaga, T.; Hashimoto, F.; Kiso, Y. Inhibitory effects of oolong tea polyphenols on pancreatic lipase in vitro. *J. Agric. Food Chem.* **2005**, *53*, 4593–4598. [CrossRef] [PubMed]

17. Naz, S.; Siddiqi, R.; Dew, T.P.; Williamson, G. Epigallocatechin-3-gallate inhibits lactase but is alleviated by salivary proline-rich proteins. *J. Agric. Food Chem.* **2011**, *59*, 2734–2738. [CrossRef] [PubMed]

18. Manzano, S.; Williamson, G. Polyphenols and phenolic acids from strawberry and apple decrease glucose uptake and transport by human intestinal Caco-2 cells. *Mol. Nutr. Food Res.* **2010**, *54*, 1773–1780. [CrossRef] [PubMed]

19. Farrell, T.L.; Ellam, S.L.; Forrelli, T.; Williamson, G. Attenuation of glucose transport across Caco-2 cell monolayers by a polyphenol-rich herbal extract: Interactions with SGLT1 and GLUT2 transporters. *Biofactors* **2013**, *39*, 448–456. [CrossRef] [PubMed]

20. Alzaid, F.; Cheung, H.-M.; Preedy, V.R.; Sharp, P.A. Regulation of glucose transporter expression in human intestinal Caco-2 cells following exposure to an anthocyanin-rich berry extract. *PLoS ONE* **2013**, *8*, e78932. [CrossRef] [PubMed]

21. Bolton, R.P.; Heaton, K.W.; Burroughs, L.F. The role of dietary fiber in satiety, glucose, and insulin: Studies with fruit and fruit juice. *Am. J. Clin. Nutr.* **1981**, *34*, 211–217. [PubMed]

22. Johnston, K.L.; Clifford, M.N.; Morgan, L.M. Possible role for apple juice phenolic compounds in the acute modification of glucose tolerance and gastrointestinal hormone secretion in humans. *J. Sci. Food Agric.* **2002**, *82*, 1800–1805. [CrossRef]

23. Dohadwala, M.M.; Hamburg, N.M.; Holbrook, M.; Kim, B.H.; Duess, M.-A.; Levit, A.; Titas, M.; Chung, W.B.; Vincent, F.B.; et al. Effects of Concord grape juice on ambulatory blood pressure in prehypertension and stage 1 hypertension. *Am. J. Clin. Nutr.* **2010**, *92*, 1052–1059. [CrossRef] [PubMed]

24. Lipkie, T.E.; Banavara, D.; Shah, B.; Morrow, A.L.; McMahon, R.J.; Jouni, Z.E.; Ferruzzi, M.G. Caco-2 accumulation of lutein is greater from human milk than from infant formula despite similar bioaccessibility. *Mol. Nutr. Food Res.* **2014**, *58*, 2014–2022. [CrossRef] [PubMed]

25. Liu, C.-S.; Glahn, R.P.; Liu, R.H. Assessment of carotenoid bioavailability of whole foods using a Caco-2 cell culture model coupled with an in vitro digestion. *J. Agric. Food Chem.* **2004**, *52*, 4330–4337. [CrossRef] [PubMed]

26. Yun, S.; Habicht, J.-P.; Miller, D.D.; Glahn, R.P. An in vitro digestion/Caco-2 cell culture system accurately predicts the effects of ascorbic acid and polyphenolic compounds on iron bioavailability in humans. *J. Nutr.* **2004**, *134*, 2717–2721. [PubMed]

27. Thakkar, S.K.; Maziya-Dixon, B.; Dixon, A.G.O.; Failla, M.L. β-carotene micellarization during in vitro digestion and uptake by Caco-2 cells is directly proportional to β-carotene content in different genotypes of cassava. *J. Nutr.* **2007**, *137*, 2229–2233. [PubMed]

28. Mahler, G.J.; Shuler, M.L.; Glahn, R.P. Characterization of Caco-2 and HT29-MTX cocultures in an in vitro digestion/cell culture model used to predict iron bioavailability. *J. Nutr. Biochem.* **2009**, *20*, 494–502. [CrossRef] [PubMed]

29. Song, B.J.; Sapper, T.N.; Burtch, C.E.; Brimmer, K.; Goldschmidt, M.; Ferruzzi, M.G. Photo- and thermodegradation of anthocyanins from grape and purple sweet potato in model beverage systems. *J. Agric. Food Chem.* **2013**, *61*, 1364–1372. [CrossRef] [PubMed]

30. Waterhouse, A.L. Determination of total phenolics. *Curr. Protoc. Food Anal. Chem.* **2002**. [CrossRef]

31. Lee, B.-H.; Eskandari, R.; Jones, K.; Reddy, K.R.; Quezada-Calvillo, R.; Nichols, B.L.; Rose, D.R.; Hamaker, B.R.; Pinto, B.M. Modulation of starch digestion for slow glucose release through "toggling" of activities of mucosal α-glucosidases. *J. Biol. Chem.* **2012**, *287*, 31929–31938. [CrossRef] [PubMed]

32. McIntosh, T.S.; Davis, H.M.; Matthews, D.E. A liquid chromatography-mass spectrometry method to measure stable isotopic tracer enrichments of glycerol and glucose in human serum. *Anal. Biochem.* **2002**, *300*, 163–169. [CrossRef] [PubMed]

33. Liu, Z.; Lou, Z.; Ding, X.; Li, X.; Qi, Y.; Zhu, Z.; Chai, Y. Global characterization of neutral saccharides in crude and processed Radix Rehmanniae by hydrophilic interaction liquid chromatography tandem electrospray ionization time-of-flight mass spectrometry. *Food Chem.* **2013**, *141*, 2833–2840. [CrossRef] [PubMed]

34. Moser, S.; Chegeni, M.; Jones, O.G.; Liceaga, A.; Ferruzzi, M.G. The effect of milk proteins on the bioaccessibility of green tea flavan-3-ols. *Food Res. Int.* **2014**, *66*, 297–305. [CrossRef]

35. Vermeirssen, V.; Augustijns, P.; Morel, N.; Camp, J.V.; Opsomer, A.; Verstraete, W. In vitro intestinal transport and antihypertensive activity of ACE inhibitory pea and whey digests. *Int. J. Food Sci. Nutr.* **2005**, *56*, 415–430. [CrossRef] [PubMed]

36. Xu, Y.; Simon, J.E.; Ferruzzi, M.G.; Ho, L.; Pasinetti, G.M.; Wu, Q. Quantification of anthocyanidins in the grapes and grape juice products with acid assisted hydrolysis using LC/MS. *J. Funct. Foods* **2012**, *4*, 710–717. [CrossRef]

37. Wang, H.; Race, E.J.; Shrikhande, A.J. Characterization of anthocyanins in grape juices by ion trap liquid chromatography-mass spectrometry. *J. Agric. Food Chem.* **2003**, *51*, 1839–1844. [CrossRef] [PubMed]

38. Rodríguez-Roque, M.J.; Rojas-Graü, M.A.; Elez-Martínez, P.; Martín-Belloso, O. In vitro bioaccessibility of health-related compounds as affected by the formulation of fruit juice- and milk-based beverages. *Food Res. Int.* **2014**, *62*, 771–778. [CrossRef]

39. Rodríguez-Roque, M.J.; de Ancos, B.; Sánchez-Moreno, C.; Cano, M.P.; Elez-Martínez, P.; Martín-Belloso, O. Impact of food matrix and processing on the in vitro bioaccessibility of vitamin C, phenolic compounds, and hydrophilic antioxidant activity from fruit juice-based beverages. *J. Funct. Foods* **2015**, *14*, 33–43. [CrossRef]

40. Pérez-Vicente, A.; Gil-Izquierdo, A.; García-Viguera, C. In vitro gastrointestinal digestion study of pomegranate juice phenolic compounds, anthocyanins, and vitamin C. *J. Agric. Food Chem.* **2002**, *50*, 2308–2312. [CrossRef] [PubMed]

41. Törrönen, R.; Sarkkinen, E.; Niskanen, T.; Tapola, N.; Kilpi, K.; Niskanen, L. Postprandial glucose, insulin and glucagon-like peptide 1 responses to sucrose ingested with berries in healthy subjects. *Br. J. Nutr.* **2012**, *107*, 1445–1451. [CrossRef] [PubMed]

42. Ramdath, D.D.; Padhi, E.; Hawke, A.; Sivaramalingam, T.; Tsao, R. The glycemic index of pigmented potatoes is related to their polyphenol content. *Food Funct.* **2014**, *5*, 909–915. [CrossRef] [PubMed]

43. Wilson, T.; Singh, A.P.; Vorsa, N.; Goettl, C.D.; Kittleson, K.M.; Roe, C.M.; Kastello, G.M.; Ragsdale, F.R. Human glycemic response and phenolic content of unsweetened cranberry juice. *J. Med Food.* **2008**, *11*, 46–54. [CrossRef] [PubMed]

44. Hlebowicz, J.; Hlebowicz, A.; Lindstedt, S.; Björgell, O.; Höglund, P.; Holst, J.J.; Darwiche, G.; Almér, L.O. Effects of 1 and 3 g cinnamon on gastric emptying, satiety, and postprandial blood glucose, insulin, glucose-dependent insulinotropic polypeptide, glucagon-like peptide 1, and ghrelin concentrations in healthy subjects. *Am. J. Clin. Nutr.* **2009**, *89*, 815–821. [CrossRef] [PubMed]

45. Hlebowicz, J.; Darwiche, G.; Björgell, O.; Almér, L.-O. Effect of cinnamon on postprandial blood glucose, gastric emptying, and satiety in healthy subjects. *Am. J. Clin. Nutr.* **2007**, *85*, 1552–1556. [PubMed]

46. Almoosawi, S.; Tsang, C.; Ostertag, L.M.; Fyfe, L.; Al-Dujaili, E.A.S. Differential effect of polyphenol-rich dark chocolate on biomarkers of glucose metabolism and cardiovascular risk factors in healthy, overweight and obese subjects: A randomized clinical trial. *Food Funct.* **2012**, *3*. [CrossRef] [PubMed]

47. Barrett, A.; Ndou, T.; Hughey, C.A.; Straut, C.; Howell, A.; Dai, Z.; Kaletunc, G. Inhibition of α-amylase and glucoamylase by tannins extracted from cocoa, pomegranates, cranberries, and grapes. *J. Agric. Food Chem.* **2013**, *61*, 1477–1486. [CrossRef] [PubMed]

48. Zhang, L.; Hogan, S.; Li, J.; Sun, S.; Canning, C.; Zheng, S.J.; Zhou, K. Grape skin extract inhibits mammalian intestinal α-glucosidase activity and suppresses postprandial glycemic response in streptozocin-treated mice. *Food Chem.* **2011**, *126*, 466–471. [CrossRef]

49. Hogan, S.; Zhang, L.; Li, J.; Sun, S.; Canning, C.; Zhou, K. Antioxidant rich grape pomace extract suppresses postprandial hyperglycemia in diabetic mice by specifically inhibiting alpha-glucosidase. *Nutr. Metab.* **2010**, *7*. [CrossRef] [PubMed]

50. McDougall, G.J.; Shpiro, F.; Dobson, P.; Smith, P.; Blake, A.; Stewart, D. Different polyphenolic components of soft fruits inhibit α-amylase and α-glucosidase. *J. Agric. Food Chem.* **2005**, *53*, 2760–2766. [CrossRef] [PubMed]

51. Scalbert, A.; Williamson, G. Dietary intake and bioavailability of polyphenols. *J. Nutr.* **2000**, *130*, 2073–2085.

52. Schramm, D.D.; Karim, M.; Schrader, H.R.; Holt, R.R.; Kirkpatrick, N.J.; Polagruto, J.A.; Ensunsa, J.L.; Schmitz, H.H.; Keen, C.L. Food effects on the absorption and pharmacokinetics of cocoa flavanols. *Life Sci.* **2003**, *73*, 857–869. [CrossRef]

53. Peters, C.M.; Green, R.J.; Janle, E.M.; Ferruzzi, M.G. Formulation with ascorbic acid and sucrose modulates catechin bioavailability from green tea. *Food Res. Int.* **2010**, *43*, 95–102. [CrossRef] [PubMed]

54. Neilson, A.P.; George, J.C.; Janle, E.M.; Mattes, R.D.; Rudolph, R.; Matusheski, N.V.; Ferruzzi, M.G. Influence of chocolate matrix composition on cocoa flavan-3-ol bioaccessibility in vitro and bioavailability in humans. *J. Agric. Food Chem.* **2009**, *57*, 9418–9426. [CrossRef] [PubMed]

55. Bordenave, N.; Hamaker, B.R.; Ferruzzi, M.G. Nature and consequences of non-covalent interactions between flavonoids and macronutrients in foods. *Food Funct.* **2013**, *5*, 18–34. [CrossRef] [PubMed]

56. Jakobek, L. Interactions of polyphenols with carbohydrates, lipids and proteins. *Food Chem.* **2015**, *175*, 556–567. [CrossRef] [PubMed]

57. Törrönen, R.; Sarkkinen, E.; Tapola, N.; Hautaniemi, E.; Kilpi, K.; Niskanen, L. Berries modify the postprandial plasma glucose response to sucrose in healthy subjects. *Br. J. Nutr.* **2010**, *103*, 1094–1097. [CrossRef] [PubMed]

58. Hanefeld, M.; Koehler, C.; Schaper, F.; Fuecker, K.; Henkel, E.; Temelkova-Kurktschiev, T. Postprandial plasma glucose is an independent risk factor for increased carotid intima-media thickness in non-diabetic individuals. *Atherosclerosis* **1999**, *144*, 229–235. [CrossRef]

59. American College of Endocrinology Consensus Statement on Guidelines for Glycemic Control. Available online: https://www.aace.com/files/dccwhitepaper.pdf (accessed on 1 July 2016).

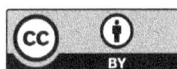

nutrients

MDPI

Review

Systematic Review of Anthocyanins and Markers of Cardiovascular Disease

Taylor C. Wallace [1,*], Margaret Slavin [1] and Cara L. Frankenfeld [2]

[1]   Department of Nutrition and Food Studies, George Mason University, Fairfax, VA 22030, USA
[2]   Department of Global and Community Health, George Mason University, Fairfax, VA 22030, USA
*   Correspondance: twallac9@gmu.edu; Tel.: +270-839-1776

Received: 7 December 2015; Accepted: 29 December 2015; Published: 9 January 2016

Abstract: Anthocyanins are dietary flavonoids commonly consumed in the diet, which have been suggested to have a preventative effect on cardiovascular disease (CVD) development among epidemiological studies. We systematically reviewed randomized controlled trials (RCTs) testing the effects of purified anthocyanins and anthocyanin-rich extracts on markers of CVD (triglycerides, total cholesterol, low-density lipoprotein (LDL) cholesterol, high-density lipoprotein (HDL) cholesterol, and blood pressure) in both healthy and diseased populations. Eligible studies included RCTs of adults published in English. We searched PubMed, Web of Science Core Collection, and BIOSIS Previews for relevant articles from inception until 1 July 2014. Twelve RCTs representing 10 studies were included in this review. Supplementation with anthocyanins significantly improved LDL cholesterol among diseased individuals or those with elevated biomarkers. Supplementation did not significantly affect other markers of CVD in either healthy individuals or those with elevated markers. No adverse effects of anthocyanins were reported across studies at levels up to 640 mg/day. Limitations of trials in the qualitative analyses include short trial duration and large variability in the dose administered within the trials. Longer-duration trials assessing dose response are needed to adequately determine whether an effect of supplementation exists.

Keywords: anthocyanins; cardiovascular disease; LDL cholesterol

1. Introduction

Cardiovascular disease (CVD) is the number one cause of death worldwide, according to the World Health Organization (WHO). The WHO predicts that by 2030, over 28 million individuals will die from CVD annually [1]. Over the past decade, there has been increased interest in lifestyle and dietary interventions to reduce CVD risk. Research has shown that individuals who adhere to US national guidelines for a healthful diet [2] and physical activity [3] have lower cardiovascular morbidity and mortality than those who do not adhere to these guidelines. Higher fruit and vegetable consumption has been suggested to be inversely associated with a decreased risk of CVD [2]. Berry consumption has recently been reviewed and has shown to be an essential fruit group in a heart-healthy diet [4]. This may be due in part to the abundance and variety of dietary bioactive components present in plant foods.

Anthocyanins are the red-orange to blue-violet pigments present in many fruits, vegetables, flowers, grains, and other plant-derived foods. Interest in the biological effects of anthocyanins has grown because of their noted presence in the human diet, as well as their potential use as a value-added alternative to synthetic colorants in many food products. Evidence from epidemiological studies supports potential preventative effects of these compounds toward the onset of CVD [5–8] in a dose-response manner in both men and women [6]. Animal and *in vitro* cell studies support biological plausibility for these compounds to favorably improve validated and surrogate biomarkers of CVD [9].

In humans, several small to medium-sized randomized controlled trials (RCTs) have assessed the effects of purified anthocyanins and anthocyanin-rich extracts on validated biomarkers of CVD in populations of both healthy and diseased adults (*i.e.*, those with elevated markers). A plethora of clinical evidence and expert reviews support increased consumption of anthocyanin-rich whole foods and CVD prevention [4]; however, to our knowledge, there is no systematic review that assesses the effect of purified anthocyanins and/or anthocyanin-rich extracts on markers of cardiovascular health among RCTs. The objective of this study was to systematically review these RCTs and to identify research gaps where additional scientific evidence is warranted. For this systematic review, we chose to evaluate validated and/or common markers used clinically as biomarkers of cardiovascular health and to diagnose cardiovascular diseases (*i.e.*, lipids, triglycerides and blood pressure). Many types of inflammatory markers have also been measured across clinical studies; however, we chose not to review these markers because of their limited clinical use and high inter- and intra-assay variability.

2. Materials and Methods

We conducted this systematic review according to the Cochrane and Preferred Reporting Items for Systematic Reviews and Meta-Analyses (PRISMA) guidelines [10,11]. This systematic review also takes into account the recommendations of Lichtenstein *et al.* [12] and Moher and Tricco [13], which highlight areas unique to the field of nutrition, that are important to consider throughout the systematic review process.

2.1. Literature Search

We searched three databases (PubMed, Web of Science Core Collection, and BIOSIS Previews) for relevant articles from inception until 1 July 2014 using the following search algorithm: (anthocyanins AND ("cholesterol, hdl" OR "cholesterol, ldl" OR "cholesterol, vldl" OR triglycerides OR lipoproteins OR hypertension)). Supplementary literature searches included examining the reference lists of all relevant studies, pertinent review articles, and the Cochrane Library Database to identify articles not identified in our initial electronic search.

2.2. Study Selection

Studies were eligible for inclusion if the following applied: (1) they were RCTs that compared purified anthocyanins or anthocyanin-rich extracts against a placebo control; (2) they involved adult participants aged ⩾18 years old; (3) they assessed the effect of purified anthocyanins or anthocyanin-rich extracts on markers of CVD (triglycerides, total cholesterol, high-density lipoprotein (HDL) cholesterol, low-density lipoprotein (LDL) cholesterol, or blood pressure); (4) the treatment group(s) reported a quantitative or quantifiable anthocyanin content; and (5) they were published in English. Three investigators (T.C.W., C.L.F., and M.S.) independently screened the titles and abstracts of articles for eligibility for inclusion in the systematic review. If consensus was reached, ineligible articles were excluded and eligible articles were moved to the next stage (full-text review) in the process. If consensus was not reached, the article was moved to the next stage, in which the full text of the selected articles was evaluated to determine the eligibility for inclusion in the systematic review. Disagreements were resolved by discussion among the reviewers until a consensus was reached.

Based on the title and abstract review, 55 eligible articles were included in the full-text review. In addition to the studies identified in the literature search, four other articles were identified from the reference lists of full-text reviewed studies and were retrieved for full-text screening (59 total studies). Based on the full-text review, 47 articles were excluded, including two studies that did not assess validated markers of CVD, 15 studies that did not assess the effect of purified anthocyanins or anthocyanin-rich extracts and/or did not report the amount of anthocyanins in the treatment, 15 non-human studies, four review or conference proceedings manuscripts, two trials that were not randomized, two trials that did not use a placebo control, four conference abstracts, one duplicated study (data published twice in separate journals), and two studies not in English (Figure 1).

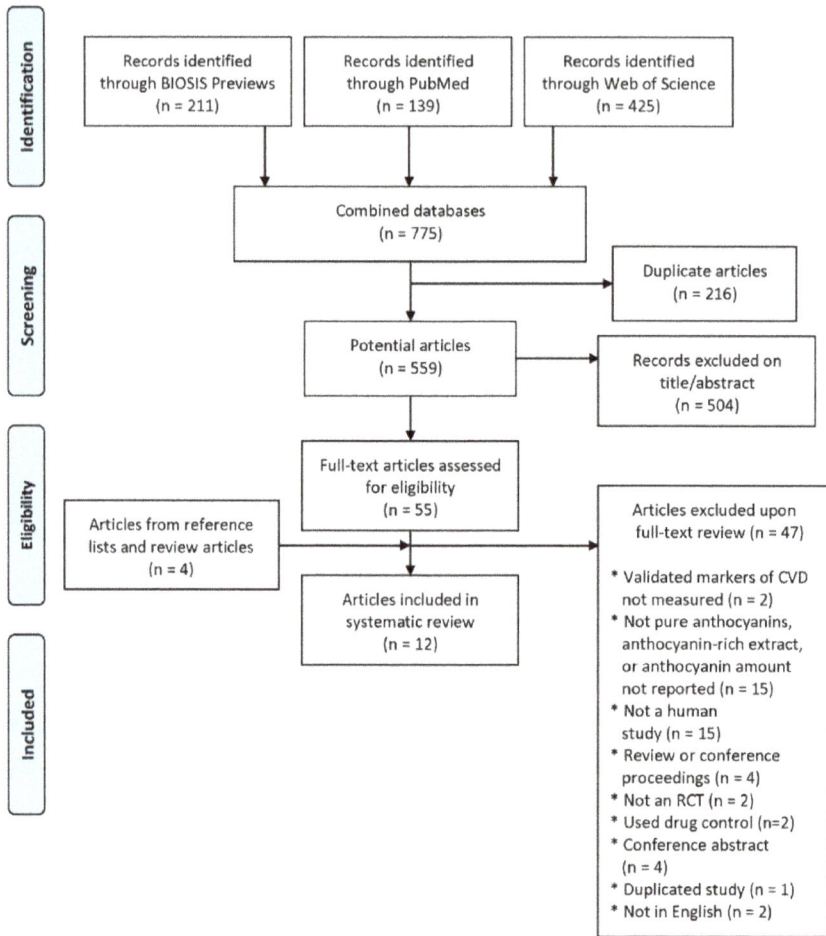

Figure 1. Flow diagram of article selection.

2.3. Data Synthesis

One investigator (C.L.F.) extracted key information from selected studies (Table 1) and two investigators (M.S. and T.C.W.) independently verified the extracted data for completeness and accuracy. The investigators resolved disagreements by consensus. Data extracted included country, sample size, participant characteristics (e.g., age, gender, and health status), dosage and duration of the treatment or intervention, follow-up period, primary end point(s), and main findings for CVD outcomes. Meta-analysis and/or meta-regression were not performed because the qualitative assessment of heterogeneity of the RCTs indicated that it would be inappropriate to statistically combine the studies. Assessment of heterogeneity included the duration of the trials (3–24 weeks), dose of anthocyanins administered (7.35–640 mg/day), raw material source of anthocyanins and therefore composition of individual anthocyanins, and the age, gender, health status, and body mass index of the studied populations.

Table 1. Study characteristics [1].

Reference	Country	Design	No. Randomized	No. Completed	Gender	Age (Year)	BMI or Weight Status	CVD-Related Disease Status	Intervention	Extract Dose	Anthocyanin Dose	Control	Intervention Length	End Point(s)
Curtis *et al.*, 2009 [14]	United Kingdom	Parallel	57	52	Postmenopausal women	<70	20–32	Healthy	Elderberry extract capsule	NR	500 mg/day	Placebo capsule	12 weeks	Triglycerides, TC, LDL, HDL, SBP, and DBP
Gurrola-Díaz *et al.*, 2010 [15]	Mexico	Parallel	152	124	Women and men	30–71	NR	Healthy and MetS	*Hibiscus sabdariffa* extract powder + preventative diet	100 mg/day	19.24 mg/day	Preventive diet	1 month	Triglycerides, TC, LDL, HDL, SBP, and DBP
Hansen *et al.*, 2005 [16]	Denmark	Parallel	70	69	Women and men	38–75	Mean 25	Healthy	Red grape extract	Full or half dose (unclear)	71 mg/day for men, 48 mg/day for women; 36 mg/day for men, 24 mg/day for women	Placebo capsule (microcrystalline cellulose)	4 weeks	TC, LDL, HDL, SBP, and DBP
Hassellund *et al.*, 2012 [17]	Norway	Crossover	31	27	Men	35–51	Mean 27	Prehypertensive	Purified anthocyanins from bilberry and black currant	NA	640 mg/day	Placebo capsule (maltodextrin)	4 weeks	SBP and DBP
Hasselund *et al.*, 2013 [18]	Norway	Crossover	31	27	Men	35–51	NR	Prehypertensive	Purified anthocyanins from bilberry and black currant	NA	640 mg/day	Placebo capsule (maltodextrin + blue color)	4 weeks	Triglycerides, TC, LDL, and HDL
Karlsen *et al.*, 2007 [19]	Norway	Parallel	120	118	Women and men	40–74	Mean 25	Healthy	Purified anthocyanins from bilberry and black currant	NA	300 mg/day	Placebo capsule (maltodextrin + blue color)	3 weeks	TC and HDL

Table 1. *Cont.*

Reference	Country	Design	No. Randomized	No. Completed	Gender	Age (Year)	BMI or Weight Status	CVD-Related Disease Status	Intervention	Extract Dose	Anthocyanin Dose	Control	Intervention Length	End Point(s)
Kianbakht *et al.*, 2014 [20]	Iran	Parallel	105	80	Women and men	20–60	Mean 30	Primary hyperlipidemia	Whortleberry extract	1050 mg/day	7.35 mg/day	Placebo capsule (toast powder)	2 months	Triglycerides, TC, LDL, and HDL
Naruszewicz *et al.*, 2007 [14]	Poland	Parallel	NR	44	Postmenopausal women, and men	Mean 66	Mean 26	Post-MI	Chokeberry extract	255 mg/day	63.75 mg/day	Placebo capsule (maltodextrin)	6 weeks	Triglycerides, TC, LDL, HDL, SBP, and DBP
Qin *et al.* 2009 [21]	China	Parallel	NR	120	Women and men	40–65	Mean 27	Dyslipidemic	Purified anthocyanins from bilberry and black currant	NA	320 mg/day	Placebo capsule (maltodextrin and pullalan)	12 weeks	Triglycerides, TC, LDL, HDL, SBP, and DBP
Soltani *et al.*, 2014 [22]	Iran	Parallel	54	50	Women and men	≥18	Mean 25	Hyperlipidemic	*Vaccinium arctostaphylos* extract	1000 mg/day	90 mg/day	Placebo capsule (calcium phosphate)	4 weeks	Triglycerides, TC, LDL, and HDL
Zhu *et al.*, 2011 [23]	China	Crossover	150	146	Women and men	40–65	Mean 26	Hypercholesterolemia	Purified anthocyanins from bilberry and black currant	NA	320 mg/day	Placebo capsule	12 weeks	SBP and DBP
Zhu *et al.* 2013 [24]	China	Parallel	150	146	Women and men	40–65	Mean 26	Hypercholesterolemia	Purified anthocyanins from bilberry and black currant	NA	320 mg/day	Placebo capsule	24 weeks	Triglycerides, TC, LDL, and HDL

[1] BMI, body mass index; CVD, cardiovascular disease; DBP, diastolic blood pressure; HDL, high-density lipoprotein; LDL, low-density lipoprotein; MetS, metabolic syndrome; MI, myocardial infarction; NA, applicable; NR, not reported; SBP, systolic blood pressure; TC, total cholesterol.

2.4. Study Quality Assessment

The 3-category Scottish Intercollegiate Guidelines Network (SIGN) grading system [25] was used to evaluate the overall methodological quality of each article that met the inclusion criteria (Table 1). Each selected article was classified as high quality, acceptable, or unacceptable. An article was graded as high quality if the majority of the outlined criteria were met, there was little or no risk of bias, and the results were unlikely to be changed by further research. An article was graded as acceptable if most of the criteria were met, there were some flaws in the study with an associated risk of bias, and/or the conclusions may change in light of further studies. An article was graded as unacceptable if most of the criteria were not met, there were significant flaws relating to key aspects of the study design, and/or the conclusions were likely to change in light of further studies.

3. Results

3.1. Study Characteristics

We identified 12 articles [14–24,26] describing 10 studies that assessed the effect of purified anthocyanins or anthocyanin-rich extracts on LDL, HDL, total cholesterol, triglycerides, or blood pressure (Figure 1). One article reported two studies in separate populations in the same publication, one in a healthy population and the other diseased [15]. Others published lipid and blood pressure results from a single trial in separate articles [17,18,23,24]. Finally, another study reported results of high-dose and low-dose anthocyanin administration [16]. Results of these two doses are presented separately in the tables, but they are considered as one study in the tallies in the ensuing discussion. Study characteristics are presented in Table 1.

The overall assessment of risk of bias in each article according to the SIGN criteria was conducted and reported as unacceptable, acceptable, or high quality. Three articles had an overall assessment of high quality [21,22,26], nine articles were of acceptable quality [14–20,23,24], and no articles were found to have an unacceptable quality rating. Tables 2–4 report the overall assessment of risk of bias of each article in proximity to study outcomes, and the full SIGN reviews by criteria are available in Supplementary Table S1.

Of the 10 separate studies, half (*n* = 5) were conducted in Europe [14,16–19,26]. Two studies were carried out in China [21,23,24], two in Iran [20,22], and one in Mexico [15]. All studies except the study published by Zhu *et al.* [23,24] were single-site trials. All studies except three [15,16,19] reported that they were double-blind in their design.

3.2. Lipoproteins

Table 2 shows the results of 10 lipoprotein studies that reported a LDL, HDL, and/or total cholesterol response to anthocyanin supplement interventions. Nine of the 10 studies included LDL as an outcome evaluated for statistical significance in the intervention group compared with the control. Four of these nine studies reported a significant decrease in LDL by the anthocyanin intervention [20–22,24]. Notably, only the studies conducted in hyperlipidemic populations demonstrated a decrease in LDL [20–22,24]. None of the studies conducted with healthy individuals or other cardiovascular-related disease statuses experienced a significant change in LDL [15,16,19,26].

Table 2. Lipoproteins [1].

Reference	SIGN Quality	Anthocyanin Dose (mg/Day)	CVD-Related Disease Status	LDL (mg/dL)				HDL (mg/dL)				Total Cholesterol (mg/dL)			
				Percent Change in Intervention	Percent Change in Control	Percent Difference Compared with Control	p	Percent Change in Intervention	Percent Change in Control	Percent Difference Compared with Control	p	Percent Change in Intervention	Percent Change in Control	Percent Difference Compared with Control	p
Curtis et al., 2009 [26]	H	500	Healthy	0.00	-5.71	5.71	NS	0.00	0.00	0.00	NS	1.85	-3.64	5.49	NS
Gurrola-Diaz et al., 2010 [15]	A	19.24	Healthy	-4.12	###	10.73	NR	3.88	0.86	3.03	NR	-4.58	-10.45	5.87	NR
Hansen et al., 2005, full [16]	A	71 or 48	Healthy	0.93	-1.26	2.19	0.643	-6.11	-9.70	3.59	<0.001	-1.48	-5.59	4.10	0.405
Hansen et al., 2005, half [16]	A	36 or 24	Healthy	3.42	-1.26	4.68	0.643	-6.11	-9.70	3.59	<0.001	-1.36	-5.59	4.22	0.405
Karlsen et al., 2007 [19]	A	300	Healthy	—	—	—	—	-1.67	-2.63	0.96	NS	-0.16	-2.38	2.22	NS
Gurrola-Diaz et al., 2010 [15]	A	19.24	MetS	-1.81	2.17	-3.98	NS	30.06	23.47	6.59	0.002	1.10	6.96	-5.86	0.019
Hasselund et al., 2013 [18]	A	640	Prehypertensive	ND	ND	ND	0.341	ND	ND	ND	0.043	ND	ND	ND	0.432
Kianbakht et al., 2014 [20]	A	7.35	Hyperlipidemic	-32.04	-9.12	-22.92	0.002	36.63	2.52	34.11	<0.001	-28.29	-2.76	-25.53	<0.001
Naruszewicz et al., 2007 [14]	A	~64	Post-MI	-0.34	-5.82	5.48	NS	2.84	1.75	1.09	NS	0.91	-3.07	3.98	NS
Qin et al., 2009 [21]	H	320	Dyslipidemic	-12.12	-0.76	-11.37	<0.001	11.55	1.74	9.81	<0.001	-2.52	-0.85	-1.67	0.435
Soltani et al., 2014 [22]	H	90	Hyperlipidemic	-8.61	2.71	-11.32	0.004	-0.35	-1.89	1.54	0.631	-15.21	1.51	-16.71	<0.001
Zhu et al., 2013 [24]	A	320	Hyperlipidemic	-10.42	0.30	-10.72	0.030	12.30	-0.81	13.10	0.036	-4.19	-3.55	-0.64	0.556

[1] Percent change is calculated as follows: (end of study value − baseline value)/(baseline value) × 100. A, acceptable; CVD, cardiovascular disease; H, high quality; HDL, high-density lipoprotein; LDL, low-density lipoprotein; MetS, metabolic syndrome; MI, myocardial infarction; ND, not determined; NR, not reported; NS, not significant; SIGN, Scottish Intercollegiate Guidelines Network.

Of the 10 lipoprotein studies, all reported the impact of intervention on HDL through statistical comparison against the control. Six studies reported a significant increase in HDL with the anthocyanin intervention [15,16,18,20,21,24]. Three of the six studies showing statistically significant increases in HDL were in subjects with hyperlipidemia [20,21,24]. One study among healthy individuals [16], one study assessing those with metabolic syndrome [19], and one study assessing those with prehypertension [18] also found statistically significant increases in HDL.

Finally, all 10 of the lipoprotein studies reported the impact of intervention on total cholesterol versus the control. Three of the 10 studies reported a significant improvement in the intervention compared with the control [15,20,22]. This includes one study in subjects with metabolic syndrome, in which both the control and intervention groups experienced increases in total cholesterol, but the magnitude of the increase was smaller in the intervention group [15]. By contrast, subjects with hyperlipidemia in the other two studies experienced dramatic lowering of LDL by 16.7% and 25.5%, respectively, in the intervention group compared with the control [20,22].

3.3. Triglycerides

Table 3 presents the nine studies that assessed triglyceride response to anthocyanin supplement interventions. Of the eight studies that reported a statistical comparison between intervention and control groups, two witnessed a significant reduction in triglycerides [20,22]. Both were conducted in subjects with hyperlipidemia.

Table 3. Triglycerides [1].

Reference	SIGN Quality	CVD-Related Disease Status	Anthocyanin Dose (mg/Day)	Percent Change in Intervention	Percent Change in Control	Percent Difference Compared with Control	P
						Triglycerides (mg/dL)	
Curtis *et al.*, 2009 [26]	H	Healthy	500	11.11	11.11	0.00	NS
Gurrola-Díaz *et al.*, 2010 [15]	A	Healthy	19.24	−8.24	−19.73	11.50	NR
Gurrola-Díaz *et al.*, 2010 [15]	A	MetS	19.24	−37.94	−17.04	−20.91	NS
Hassellund *et al.*, 2013 [18]	A	Prehypertension	640	ND	ND	ND	0.127
Kianbakht *et al.*, 2014 [20]	A	Hyperlipidemic	7.35	−18.67	−9.68	−8.99	0.002
Naruszewicz *et al.*, 2007 [14]	A	Post-MI	64	−6.15	−3.49	−2.66	NS
Qin *et al.*, 2009 [21]	H	Dyslipidemic	320	−4.24	−2.62	−1.62	0.576
Soltani *et al.*, 2014 [22]	H	Hyperlipidemic	90	−30.79	3.76	−34.55	<0.001
Zhu *et al.*, 2013 [24]	A	Hyperlipidemic	320	−4.08	−2.90	−1.18	0.462

[1] Percent change is calculated as follows: (end of study value − baseline value)/(baseline value) × 100. A, acceptable; H, high quality; CVD, cardiovascular disease; MetS, metabolic syndrome; MI, myocardial infarction; ND, not determined; NR, not reported; NS, not significant; SIGN, Scottish Intercollegiate Guidelines Network.

3.4. Blood Pressure

Table 4 shows the results of the seven studies that reported blood pressure response to anthocyanin supplement interventions. Six of the seven studies conducted a statistical test for systolic and diastolic blood outcomes in response to the intervention versus the control. Only one study that assessed individuals after myocardial infarction showed a significant decrease in systolic and diastolic blood pressure compared with the control [14].

Table 4. Blood pressure [1].

Reference	SIGN Quality	CVD-Related Disease Status	Anthocyanin Dose (mg/Day)	Systolic Blood Pressure (mmHg)				Diastolic Blood Pressure (mmHg)			
				Percent Change in Intervention	Percent Change in Control	Percent Difference Compared with Control	*p*	Percent Change in Intervention	Percent Change in Control	Percent Difference Compared with Control	*p*
Curtis *et al.*, 2009 [26]	H	Healthy	500	0.81	−4.62	5.43	NR	−1.28	−2.44	1.16	NR
Curroda-Díaz *et al.*, 2010 [15]	A	Healthy	19.2	ND	−2.09	ND	NS	ND	−2.62	ND	NS
Hansen *et al.*, 2005, full [16]	A	Healthy	71 or 48	−4.48	−3.13	−1.35	0.605	−3.66	−5.00	1.34	0.261
Hansen *et al.*, 2005, half [16]	A	Healthy	36 or 24	−1.61	−3.13	1.51	0.605	−1.27	−5.00	3.73	0.261
Curroda-Díaz *et al.*, 2010 [15]	A	MetS	19.2	−5.57	−9.04	3.47	NS	−11.25	−2.96	−8.29	NS
Hassellund *et al.*, 2012 [17]	A	Prehypertension	640	−5.59	−6.99	1.40	0.254	−13.54	−14.58	1.04	0.324
Naruszewicz *et al.*, 2007 [14]	A	Post-MI	64	−8.32	4.36	−12.68	<0.001	−8.34	1.70	−10.04	<0.001
Qin *et al.*, 2009 [21]	H	Dyslipidemic	320	−0.95	−3.33	2.38	0.888	0.00	−0.97	0.97	0.343
Zhu *et al.*, 2011 [23]	A	Hyperlipidemic	320	−5.31	−0.40	−4.91	0.245	−2.24	−1.93	−0.31	0.290

[1] Percent change is calculated as follows: (end of study value − baseline value)/(baseline value) × 100. A, acceptable; H, high quality; CVD, cardiovascular disease; MetS, metabolic syndrome; MI, myocardial infarction; ND, not determined; NR, not reported; NS, not significant; SIGN, Scottish Intercollegiate Guidelines Network.

4. Discussion

An inverse relationship between anthocyanins and anthocyanin-rich foods and CVD outcomes (e.g., mortality) has been observed among epidemiological studies. McCullough *et al.* recently observed a significant inverse dose-response relationship among 38,180 men and 60,289 women in regard to anthocyanin intake (3.8–22.2 mg/day) and age-adjusted CVD mortality [6]. This systematic review of RCTs suggests that anthocyanins may have potential to influence CVD development and progression among individuals with elevated risk biomarkers. Although most of the potential effects seen in this review were nonsignificant, improvement of biomarkers were consistent across studies, particularly in those with elevated risk biomarkers at baseline.

CVD development and progression is slow and may span decades. Nutritional interventions often show small changes in the short term but clear effects over the lifespan. Interestingly, trials that used high doses of purified anthocyanins did not observe much more of an effect compared with those studies of anthocyanin-rich extracts containing more physiologically achievable intake. No dose-response relationships were identified among the RCTs included in this review. It is possible that other dietary bioactive components present in the anthocyanin-rich extracts may exert synergistic effects or contribute to a threshold effect.

Results from animal studies suggest that anthocyanins and other polyphenols may slow or inhibit the absorption of lipids and glucose in the intestine. It has been reported that tea catechins may improve lipid profiles by inhibiting the micelle formation by bile acid [27]. Another possible mechanism for cholesterol-lowering effects of anthocyanins could be the inhibition of cholesterol synthesis. It has been shown that anthocyanins can activate AMP-activated protein kinase (AMPK) [28,29], which is involved in the regulation of energy homeostasis and influences the activity of many enzymes. One enzyme that is inhibited by AMPK is 3-hydroxy-3-methylglutaryl-coenzyme A (HMG-CoA) reductase [30]. Because HMG-CoA reductase is the limiting enzyme of cholesterol synthesis, increased AMPK activity would inhibit cholesterol synthesis and consequently lead to lower cholesterol levels. Furthermore, AMPK inhibits the activity of acetyl-CoA carboxylases ACC1 and ACC2, which leads to increased fatty acid oxidation and decreased fatty acid synthesis [30], and, accordingly, lower triglyceride concentrations. It is possible that anthocyanins may have the ability to modulate low-grade inflammation, as consumption of anthocyanin-rich foods such as berries have been suggested to affect many inflammatory markers of CVD *in vivo* [4]. Berry consumption has been suggested to be an effective strategy to counteract postprandial metabolic and oxidative stress associated with CVD, especially lipid oxidation [31]. Specific berries such as freeze-dried strawberries [32], bilberries and lingonberries [33], blueberries [34] and cranberry extracts [35], among others have shown similar favorable effects on lipid profiles those with elevated markers as suggested in our review.

In regard to blood pressure, anthocyanins have been shown to lower direct measures of arterial stiffness in a cross-sectional study of 1898 women [5]. Across the studies, most did not observe and affect of purified anthocyanins or anthocyanin-rich extracts on blood pressure.

This systematic review identified several gaps in the literature. The age range of participants in most studies was large and may contribute to the null findings of many studies, because it is likely that interventions may have a greater effect among older populations and/or those with an elevated risk of developing CVD. Compliance was also not reported in many of the included studies.

In studies that were not so heterogeneous, a meta-analysis would be carried out to assess the magnitude of effect of purified anthocyanins and anthocyanin-rich extracts on CVD biomarkers. However, we concluded from qualitative review that a meaningful summary estimate could not be obtained by meta-analysis due to high heterogeneity. The control groups included a range of different treatments (e.g., preventative diet). The duration of the studies (3–24 weeks), anthocyanin dose administered (7.35–640 mg/day), composition of the anthocyanin-rich extracts, variation in baseline status of the biomarkers, and difference in the reporting of outcome measures (e.g., mean absolute difference, or percent change) also varied.

For the purpose of developing recommended intakes, future intervention studies should be designed to assess whether a dose-response relationship of anthocyanins on markers of CVD exists. From this review, we identified gaps in the research literature that could be addressed in further studies. Data in "healthy" individuals (*i.e.*, those with risk biomarkers in the normal range) are important in developing dietary guidance for the general population; however, these data are hard to obtain in short-term clinical studies with a small population. Because larger clinical studies spanning a decade or more are expensive and difficult to control, reliance on well-designed epidemiological studies may be useful in complementing smaller clinical trial data. It may be helpful for future trials to focus on a particular anthocyanin (e.g., Cy-3-glu the most common anthocyanin present in nature), because the type of aglycon and amount of glycosylation and/or acylation of the compounds may significantly alter their biological activity as well as their transportation across the basolateral membrane. By contrast, anthocyanins are currently solely consumed as mixtures in plant-derived foods and extracts. Thus, continued research in this area is equally important. Data on study compliance and evaluation of baseline status of flavonoid and/or polyphenol intakes may improve the consistency between small clinical interventions.

5. Conclusions

Anthocyanins are abundant among plant-derived foods that are currently recommended among national and international dietary guidelines. This systematic review of RCTs adds to existing scientific evidence from observational, animal, and mechanistic studies suggesting that anthocyanins and anthocyanin-rich extracts may have the potential to affect markers of CVD. However, more carefully controlled longer-duration trials assessing dose response across various populations are needed to adequately determine whether an effect of supplementation exists. Current trials suggest that these compounds may decrease LDL cholesterol among individuals with elevated markers, with little to no safety concerns.

Supplementary Materials: Supplementary Materials: Supplementary materials can be accessed at: http://www.mdpi.com/2072-6643/8/ 1/32/s1, Table S1: SIGN checklist for controlled trials.

Author Contributions: Author Contributions: T.C.W., C.L.F., and M.S. designed the research; T.C.W., C.L.F., and M.S. conducted the research; T.C.W., C.L.F., and M.S. analyzed the data or performed statistical analysis; T.C.W., C.L.F., and M.S. wrote the paper; T.C.W. had primary responsibility for final content.

Conflicts of Interest: Conflicts of Interest: The authors declare no conflict of interest.

References

1. World Health Organization. Cardiovascular Diseases (CVDs). Fact Sheet No. 317. 2011. Available online: http://www.who.int/cardiovascular_diseases/en/ (accessed on 23 December 2014).
2. US Department of Health and Human Services, US Department of Agriculture. *Dietary Guidelines for Americans, 2010*, 7th ed.; US Government Printing Office: Washington, DC, USA, 2010.
3. US Department of Health and Human Services. *2008 Physical Activity Guidelines for Americans. ODPHP Publication No. U0036*; US Department of Health and Human Services: Washington, DC, USA, 2008.
4. Basu, A.; Rhone, M.; Lyons, T.J. Berries: Emerging impact on cardiovascular health. *Nutr. Rev.* **2010**, *66*, 168–177. [CrossRef] [PubMed]
5. Jennings, A.; Welch, A.A.; Fairweather-Tait, S.J.; Kay, C.; Minihane, A.M.; Chowienczyk, P.; Jiang, B.; Cecelja, M.; Spector, T.; Macgregor, A.; *et al.* Higher anthocyanin intake is associated with lower arterial stiffness and central blood pressure in women. *Am. J. Clin. Nutr.* **2012**, *96*, 781–788. [CrossRef] [PubMed]
6. McCullough, M.L.; Peterson, J.J.; Patel, R.; Jacques, P.F.; Shah, R.; Dwyer, J.T. Flavonoid intake and cardiovascular disease mortality in a prospective cohort of US adults. *Am. J. Clin. Nutr.* **2012**, *95*, 454–464. [CrossRef] [PubMed]
7. Mink, P.J.; Scrafford, C.G.; Barraj, L.M.; Harnack, L.; Hong, C.P.; Nettleton, J.A.; Jacobs, D.R., Jr. Flavonoid intake and cardiovascular disease mortality: A prospective study in postmenopausal women. *Am. J. Clin. Nutr.* **2007**, *85*, 895–909. [PubMed]

8. Cassidy, A.; O'Reilly, É.J.; Kay, C.; Sampson, L.; Franz, M.; Forman, J.P.; Curhan, G.; Rimm, E.B. Habitual intake of flavonoid subclasses and incident hypertension in adults. *Am. J. Clin. Nutr.* **2011**, *93*, 338–347. [CrossRef] [PubMed]

9. Wallace, T.C. Anthocyanins in cardiovascular disease. *Adv. Nutr.* **2011**, *2*, 1–7. [CrossRef] [PubMed]

10. Higgins, J.P.T.; Green, S. Cochrane Handbook for Systematic Reviews of Interventions, Version 5.1.0. Available online: http://www.cochrane-handbook.org (accessed on 24 November 2014).

11. Liberati, A.; Altman, D.G.; Tetzlaff, J.; Mulrow, C.; Gotzsche, P.C.; Ioannidis, J.P.; Clarke, M.; Devereaux, P.J.; Kleijnen, J.; Moher, D. The PRISMA statement for reporting systematic reviews and meta-analyses of studies that evaluate healthcare interventions: explanation and elaboration. *BMJ* **2009**, *339*, b2700. [CrossRef] [PubMed]

12. Lichtenstein, A.H.; Yetley, E.A.; Lau, J. Application of systematic review methodology to the field of nutrition. *J. Nutr.* **2008**, *138*, 2297–2306. [CrossRef] [PubMed]

13. Moher, D.; Tricco, A.C. Issues related to the conduct of systematic reviews: a focus on the nutrition field. *Am. J. Clin. Nutr.* **2008**, *88*, 1191–1199. [PubMed]

14. Naruszewicz, M.; Łaniewska, I.; Millo, B.; Dłużniewski, M. Combination therapy of statin with flavonoids rich extract from chokeberry fruits enhanced reduction in cardiovascular risk markers in patients after myocardial infarction (MI). *Atherosclerosis* **2007**, *194*, e179–e184. [CrossRef] [PubMed]

15. Gurrola-Díaz, C.M.; García-López, P.M.; Sánchez-Enríquez, S.; Troyo-Sanromán, R.; Andrade-González, I.; Gómez-Leyva, J.F. Effects of Hibiscus sabdariffa extract powder and preventive treatment (diet) on the lipid profiles of patients with metabolic syndrome (MeSy). *Phytomedicine* **2010**, *17*, 500–505. [CrossRef] [PubMed]

16. Hansen, A.S.; Marckmann, P.; Dragsted, L.O.; Finné Nielsen, I.L.; Neilsen, S.E.; Grønbæk, M. Effect of red wine and red grape extract on blood lipids, haemostatic factors, and other risk factors for cardiovascular disease. *Eur. J. Clin. Nutr.* **2005**, *59*, 449–455. [CrossRef] [PubMed]

17. Hassellund, S.S.; Flaa, A.; Sandvik, L.; Kjeldsen, S.E.; Rostrup, M. Effects of anthocyanins on blood pressure and stress reactivity: A double-blind randomized placebo-controlled crossover study. *J. Hum. Hypertens* **2012**, *26*, 396–404. [CrossRef] [PubMed]

18. Hassellund, S.S.; Flaa, A.; Kjeldsen, S.E.; Seljeflot, I.; Karlsen, A.; Erlund, I.; Rostrup, M. Effects of anthocyanins on cardiovascular risk factors and inflammation in pre-hypertensive men: A double-blind randomized placebo-controlled crossover study. *J. Hum. Hypertens* **2013**, *27*, 100–106. [CrossRef] [PubMed]

19. Karlsen, A.; Retterstøl, L.; Lakke, P.; Paur, I.; Kjølsrud-Bøhn, S.; Sandvik, L.; Blomhoff, R. Anthocyanins inhibit nuclear factor-κB activation in monocytes and reduce plasma concentrations of pro-inflammatory mediators in healthy adults. *J. Nutr.* **2007**, *137*, 1951–1954. [PubMed]

20. Kianbakht, S.; Abasi, B.; Dabaghian, F.H. Improved lipid profile in hyperlipidemic patients taking Vaccinium arctostaphylos fruit hydroalcoholic extract: A randomized double-blind placebo-controlled clinical trial. *Phytother. Res.* **2014**, *28*, 432–436. [CrossRef] [PubMed]

21. Qin, Y.; Xia, M.; Ma, J.; Hao, Y.T.; Liu, J.; Mou, H.Y.; Cao, L.; Ling, W. Anthocyanin supplementation improves serum LDL- and HDL-cholesterol concentrations associated with the inhibition of cholesteryl ester transfer protein in dyslipidemic subjects. *Am. J. Clin. Nutr.* **2009**, *90*, 485–492. [CrossRef] [PubMed]

22. Soltani, R.; Hakimi, M.; Asgary, S.; Ghanadian, S.M.; Keshvari, M.; Sarrafzadegan, N. Evaluation of the effects of Vaccinium arctostaphylos L. fruit extract on serum lipids and hs-CRP levels and oxidative stress in adult patients with hyperlipidemia: A randomized, double-blind, placebo-controlled clinical trial. *Evid. Based Complement. Altern. Med.* **2014**, *2014*, 217451. [CrossRef] [PubMed]

23. Zhu, Y.; Xia, M.; Yang, Y.; Liu, F.; Li, Z.; Hao, Y.; Mi, M.; Jin, T.; Ling, W. Purified anthocyanin supplementation improves endothelial function via NO-cGMP activation in hypercholesterolemic individuals. *Clin. Chem.* **2011**, *57*, 1524–1533. [CrossRef] [PubMed]

24. Zhu, Y.; Ling, W.; Guo, H.; Song, F.; Ye, Q.; Zou, T.; Li, D.; Zhang, Y.; Li, G.; Xiao, Y.; *et al.* Anti-inflammatory effect of purified dietary anthocyanin in adults with hypercholesterolemia: A randomized controlled trial. *Nutr. Metab. Cardiovasc. Dis.* **2013**, *23*, 843–849. [CrossRef] [PubMed]

25. Scottish Intercollegiate Guidelines Network (SIGN). Methodology Checklist 2: Randomized Controlled Trials. Available online: http://www.sign.ac.uk/methodology/checklists.html (accessed on 6 March 2015).

26. Curtis, P.J.; Kroon, P.A.; Hollands, W.J.; Walls, R.; Jenkins, G.; Kay, C.D.; Cassidy, A. Cardiovascular disease risk biomarkers and liver and kidney function are not altered in postmenopausal women after ingesting an elderberry extract rich in anthocyanins for 12 weeks. *J. Nutr.* **2009**, *139*, 2266–2271. [CrossRef] [PubMed]

27. Ikeda, I.; Kobayashi, M.; Hamada, T.; Tsuda, K.; Goto, H.; Imaizumi, K.; Nozawa, A.; Sugimoto, A.; Kakuda, T. Heat-epimerized tea catechins rich in gallocatechin gallate and catechin gallate are more effective to inhibit cholesterol absorption than tea catechins rich in epigallocatechin gallate and epicatechin gallate. *J. Agric. Food Chem.* **2003**, *51*, 7303–7307. [CrossRef] [PubMed]

28. Takikawa, M.; Inoue, S.; Horio, F.; Tsuda, T. Dietary anthocyanin-rich bilberry extract ameliorates hyperglycemia and insulin sensitivity via activation of AMP-activated protein kinase in diabetic mice. *J. Nutr.* **2010**, *140*, 527–533. [CrossRef] [PubMed]

29. Guo, H.; Liu, G.; Zhong, R.; Wang, Y.; Wang, D.; Xia, M. Cyanidin-3-*O*-β-glucoside regulates fatty acid metabolism via an AMP-activated protein kinase-dependent signaling pathway in human HepG2 cells. *Lipids Health Dis.* **2012**, *11*, 10. [CrossRef] [PubMed]

30. Towler, M.C.; Hardie, D.G. AMP-activated protein kinase in metabolic control and insulin signaling. *Circ. Res.* **2007**, *100*, 328–341. [CrossRef] [PubMed]

31. O'Keefe, J.H.; Gheewala, N.M.; O'Keefe, J.O. Dietary strategies for improving post-prandial and lipid profile in patients suffering from coronary artery disease. *Expert. Opin. Ther. Targets* **2008**, *51*, 249–255.

32. Basu, A.; Wilkinson, M.; Penugonda, K.; Simmons, B.; Betts, N.M.; Lyons, T.J. Freeze-dried strawberry powder improves lipid profile and lipid peroxidation in women with metabolic syndrome: Baseline and post intervention effects. *Nutr. J.* **2009**, *8*, 43. [CrossRef] [PubMed]

33. Erlund, I.; Koli, R.; Alfthan, G. Favorable effects of berry consumption on platelet function, blood pressure, and HDL cholestrol. *Am. J. Clin. Nutr.* **2008**, *87*, 323–331. [PubMed]

34. McAnulty, S.R.; McAnulty, L.S.; Morrow, J.D. Effect of daily fruit ingestion on angiotensin converting enzyme activity, blood pressure, and oxidative stress in chronic smokers. *Free Radic. Res.* **2005**, *39*, 1241–1248. [CrossRef] [PubMed]

35. Lee, I.T.; Chan, Y.C.; Lin, C.W.; Lee, W.J.; Sheu, W.H. Effect of cranberry extracts on lipid profiles in subjects with type-2 diabetes. *Diabet. Med.* **2008**, *25*, 1473–1477. [CrossRef] [PubMed]

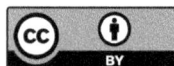

nutrients

MDPI

Article

Post-Stroke Depression Modulation and *in Vivo* Antioxidant Activity of Gallic Acid and Its Synthetic Derivatives in a Murine Model System

Seyed Fazel Nabavi [1], Solomon Habtemariam [2], Arianna Di Lorenzo [3], Antoni Sureda [4], Sedigheh Khanjani [5], Seyed Mohammad Nabavi [1,†] and Maria Daglia [3,*,†]

[1] Applied Biotechnology Research Center, Baqiyatallah University of Medical Sciences, P.O. Box 19395-5487, Tehran 19395-5487, Iran; Nabavisf@gmail.com (S.F.N.); Nabavi208@gmail.com (S.M.N.)

[2] Pharmacognosy Research Laboratories, Medway School of Science, University of Greenwich, Chatham-Maritime, Kent ME4 4TB, UK; s.habtemariam@herbalanalysis.co.uk

[3] Department of Drug Sciences, Medicinal Chemistry and Pharmaceutical Technology Section, Pavia University, Viale Taramelli 12, Pavia 27100, Italy; arianna.dilorenzo01@universitadipavia.it

[4] Grup de Nutrició Comunitària i Estrès Oxidatiu (IUNICS) and CIBEROBN (Physiopathology of Obesity and Nutrition), Universitat de les Illes Balears, Palma de Mallorca E-07122, Spain; tosugo@hotmail.com

[5] Department of Physiology, Faculty of Biological Sciences, Shahid Behshti University, P.O. Box 19615-1178, Tehran 19615-1178, Iran; s.khanjani66@yahoo.com

* Correspondence: maria.daglia@unipv.it; Tel.: +39-0382987388

† These authors contributed equally to this work.

Received: 3 March 2016; Accepted: 22 April 2016; Published: 28 April 2016

Abstract: Gallic acid (3,4,5-trihydroxybenzoic acid, GA) is a plant secondary metabolite, which shows antioxidant activity and is commonly found in many plant-based foods and beverages. Recent evidence suggests that oxidative stress contributes to the development of many human chronic diseases, including cardiovascular and neurodegenerative pathologies, metabolic syndrome, type 2 diabetes and cancer. GA and its derivative, methyl-3-*O*-methyl gallate (M3OMG), possess physiological and pharmacological activities closely related to their antioxidant properties. This paper describes the antidepressive-like effects of intraperitoneal administration of GA and two synthetic analogues, M3OMG and P3OMG (propyl-3-*O*-methylgallate), in balb/c mice with post-stroke depression, a secondary form of depression that could be due to oxidative stress occurring during cerebral ischemia and the following reperfusion. Moreover, this study determined the *in vivo* antioxidant activity of these compounds through the evaluation of superoxide dismutase (SOD) and catalase (Cat) activity, thiobarbituric acid-reactive substances (TBARS) and reduced glutathione (GSH) levels in mouse brain. GA and its synthetic analogues were found to be active (at doses of 25 and 50 mg/kg) in the modulation of depressive symptoms and the reduction of oxidative stress, restoring normal behavior and, at least in part, antioxidant endogenous defenses, with M3OMG being the most active of these compounds. SOD, TBARS, and GSH all showed strong correlation with behavioral parameters, suggesting that oxidative stress is tightly linked to the pathological processes involved in stroke and PSD. As a whole, the obtained results show that the administration of GA, M3OMG and P3OMG induce a reduction in depressive symptoms and oxidative stress.

Keywords: depression; gallic acid; ischemia; stroke

1. Introduction

Gallic acid (3,4,5-trihydroxybenzoic acid, GA, Figure 1A) is a secondary metabolite of plants, mainly formed from 3-dehydroshikimic acid through the shikimic acid pathway occurring in all plants. Thus, it is found in a wide array of foods in varying amounts according to plant species and environmental factors [1]. The main dietary sources of GA are red fruits (*i.e.*, raspberries, blueberries, and strawberries), grapes (*Vitis vinifera* L. and *Vitis aestivalis* Michx.), wine, oak bark, and gallnuts. Many plant-based foods and beverages contain GA in its esterified form and/or as GA derivatives, such as hydrolysable tannins, in addition to its free form. Green and semi-fermented or fermented teas are the most important sources of GA in the esterified forms of catechin and epicatechin, while gallotannins are not widespread in nature but have been identified in mango (*Mangifera indica* L.) and the Leguminosae and Anacardiaceae families [2].

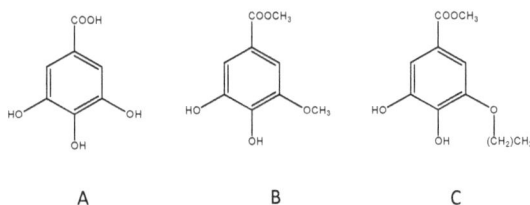

Figure 1. Chemical structure of gallic acid (**A**); methyl-3-*O*-methylgallate (**B**); and propyl-3-*O*-methylgallate (**C**).

The positive effects on human health of GA and its derivatives have been under investigation since the 1990s and many properties have been ascribed to these compounds. In addition to its well-known antioxidant activity, GA exerts anti-inflammatory, neuroprotective, cardioprotective, nephroprotective, and anticarcinogenic activities [3–6]. Moreover, it possesses antibacterial activity against different bacteria including *Escherichia coli*, *Staphylococcus aureus*, *Pseudonomas aeruginosa* and *Klebsiella pneumonia* [7]. A recent investigation has isolated a GA n-alkyl ester, methyl-3-*O*-methyl gallate (M3OMG, Figure 1B), from the leaves of *Peltiphyllum peltatum* (Torr.) Engl. (Saxifragaceae), a rhizomatous perennial herb used as a food and as a remedy in traditional medicine. A comparative *in vitro* study of the antioxidant/prooxidant activities of GA and M3OMG has revealed that M3OMG shows antioxidant activity when compared with GA, without showing prooxidant activity [8]. Further investigations on the *in vivo* antioxidant properties of M3OMG have shown that this compound is able to exert neuroprotective and cardioprotective effects against NaF-induced oxidative stress in rat brains and in erythrocyte hemolysates, respectively [9,10]. At the molecular level, GA and M3OMG exert their protective activities through different mechanisms of action. In peripheral blood mononuclear cells and EVC-304 cells, M3OMG acts through the epigenetic regulation of the expression levels of miR-17-3p, a microRNA linked to the regulation of cellular redox status [11]. Furthermore, in different prostate cancer cell subpopulations GA and M3OMG inhibit NF-kB transcriptional factor, a protein complex that controls transcription of DNA, cytokine production and cell survival [12].

Stroke is an acute cerebrovascular event caused by a reduction in the blood supplied to the brain, resulting in brain cells death. Two main types of stroke are recognized: ischemic and hemorrhagic ones. In an ischemic stroke the reduction of blood supplied to the brain is caused mainly by thrombosis due to the formation of a local blood clot causing vessels occlusion, or by embolisms due to the presence of an embolus elsewhere in the body, or by systemic hypoperfusion. The main consequences are local hypoxia, ATP decrease, and intracellular calcium increase, leading to irreversible cells damage. On the other hand, hemorrhagic stroke occurs when a weakened blood vessel ruptures. Two main types of weakened blood vessels are at the basis of hemorrhagic stroke: aneurysm and arteriovenous abnormalities, both causing bleeding into the brain after rupture. Stroke represents the second leading cause of disability in Europe and the sixth leading cause worldwide [13]. Five minutes after the onset of ischemic stroke, neurons begin to die due to oxygen and glucose deprivation, which leads to a series of negative mechanisms resulting in damage to the brain tissue. These mechanisms include oxidative stress, mitochondrial dysfunction, neuroinflammation, activation of glutamate receptors, and reduction of circulating levels of nitric oxide [14,15].

Among the complications of ischemic stroke, post-stroke depression (PSD) has high clinical relevance. One third of patients experience depression within the first year after the onset of stroke, which persists for over 20 months in 34% of elderly patients with acute stroke [16]. PSD is linked to worsened cognitive and physical outcomes, since it delays the recovery process and reduces the effect of therapy and rehabilitation. Morbidity and mortality are highly increased as a consequence. The common therapeutic approach for PSD consists of antidepressant pharmacotherapy, which is effective in increasing the number of patients reaching partial or full independence. Nevertheless, antidepressant drugs can cause side and adverse effects serious enough to make patients stop taking the medication, thus aggravating morbidity [16].

The World Health Organization reports that low fruit and vegetable intake is among the six main risk factors for cardiovascular diseases (with high blood pressure, high blood glucose, physical inactivity, overweight and obesity). Moreover, an insufficient intake of fruit and vegetables is estimated to contribute to around 9% of stroke deaths worldwide [17]. In addition, there is substantial evidence regarding the role of oxidative stress in the pathogenesis of both ischemic stroke and depression. Thus, our research group postulated the hypothesis that polyphenols and vegetable foods could have a potential therapeutic role in PSD due to their antioxidant activity [18]. Our previous research highlights the *in vivo* cardio- and neuroprotective effects of GA and its derivatives against oxidative stress [9,10,19,20]. Moreover, the benefits of GA on the brain and cognitive functions are well documented. In fact, GA reduces chronic cerebral hypoperfusion in rats and has a significant protective effect on brain cell viability [21]. In addition, GA shows antidepressive-like activity in a mouse model of unpredictable chronic mild stress [22]. A further study confirms this property by treating mice with GA brain targeted nanoparticles, which are able to improve both its antioxidant and antidepressant-like activity [23]. The antidepressive-like activity of GA has not been explored in a mouse model of PSD to date, and in view of this, the first aim of the present paper is to study the antidepressive-like effects exerted by intraperitoneal administration of GA in balb/c mice with post-stroke depression. Recent investigations into the protective effects of polyphenols have been accompanied by an increasing evaluation of their synthetic and semisynthetic analogues, which can ameliorate the bioavailability and the metabolic conversion of the original natural product, whilst maintaining both efficacy and low toxicity levels [24]. In view of this, the second aim of the present research is to evaluate the antidepressive-like activity and the *in vivo* antioxidant activity of two GA synthetic derivatives, to verify if some structural changes (*i.e.*, increase of lipophilicity) can alter the activities of these GA derivatives. The synthetic analogues, never tested on any animal model of depression, are M3OMG, previously studied by our research group regarding its *in vivo* antioxidant effect and *in vitro* epigenetic potential, and propyl-3-*O*-methylgallate, P3OMG, whose biological activities have not yet been investigated (Figure 1C).

2. Materials and Methods

2.1. Reagents and Materials

Methyl gallate, borax, dimethyl sulphate, dipropyl sulphate, sodium hydroxide, sulphuric acid, chloroform, sodium chloride and sodium sulphate were purchased from Sigma-Aldrich (St Louis, MO, USA) for the synthesis of M3OMG and P3OMG. Bovine serum albumin and a kit for protein measurement were purchased from ZiestChem Company (Tehran, Iran). 5,5-dithiobis(2-nitrobenzoic acid), ethylenediaminetetraacetic acid, nitro blue tetrazolium chloride, potassium dihydrogen phosphate, reduced glutathione, sodium dihydrogen phosphate, trichloroacetic acid, thiobarbituric acid, hydrogen peroxide, sodium carbonate, hydroxylamine chloride, ketamine, lidocaine, xylazine were purchased from Sigma-Aldrich Chemical Company, (St. Louis, MO, USA).

Other chemical reagents and solvents were of analytical grade or pure and were purchased from Merck Chemical Company (Darmstadt, Germany).

2.2. M3OMG and P3OMG Syntheses

The synthesis of M3OMG and P3OMG was performed as reported by Nabavi *et al.* [9,10]. In brief, an aliquot of 10 g of methyl gallate was added to a mixture of borax (80 g) and water (800 mL) undergoing stirring for 30 min. Using a dropping funnel, dimethyl sulphate (30 mL) and dipropyl sulphate (30 mL) and NaOH (13 g in 50 mL water) were added dropwise from two sides of the reaction flask over 2.5 h, to synthetize M3OMG and P3OMG, respectively. After leaving the reaction mixtures to be stirred overnight, concentrated sulphuric acid (50 mL) was added. The mixtures were further stirred for 1 h and submitted to liquid extraction five times with CHCl3 (1 L). The combined chloroform extracts were washed with 500 mL of brine (26% NaCl) and dried over anhydrous sodium sulphate. Removal of the solvent under reduced pressure gave pure M3OMG and P3OMG, which were used for the *in vivo* pharmacological tests.

2.3. Animals

Five-week old male balb/c mice weighing 20–25 g, purchased from the Pasteur Institute of Iran, were used in the study. All mice were kept in the animal room at $24 \pm 2\,^{\circ}\mathrm{C}$ under a 12/12 h light/dark cycle and $60\% \pm 5\%$ humidity. Food and water were provided *ad libitum*. All mice were allowed to acclimatize with the testing room for 24 h prior to behavioral examinations. In this study, behavioral examination was performed between 10:00 a.m. and 2:00 p.m. The animal experiments were processed following internationally accepted ethical guidelines for the care of laboratory animals in accordance with Principles of Laboratory Animals Care (NIH Publication No. 85-23, revised 1996). The ethical approval number is "81/021, 10 July 2002".

2.4. Stroke Inducing

For the induction of ischemic stroke, mice were anaesthetized through the intraperitoneal administration of a mixture of ketamine (60 mg/kg) and xylazine (5 mg/kg). Bilateral common carotid artery occlusion (BCCAO) was performed as per the standard experimental animal model of ischemic stroke. In brief, both right and left carotid arteries were selected and clamped for 5 min by vascular clamps (time of ischemia). Thereafter, the vascular clamps were removed for the next 10 min (time of reperfusion), and both carotid arteries were subsequently clamped again for 5 min. Finally, the vascular clamps were removed and blood circulation was allowed to return in both carotid arteries. The surgical incisions were sutured and anaesthetized with lidocaine solution as a local anesthetic drug and the area was washed with an antiseptic solution. All mice were transported to an individual cage, kept at the standard temperature and allowed to recover normal body temperature. Rectal temperature was checked every day and animals at $37 \pm 1\,^{\circ}\mathrm{C}$ were used in the study. In addition, we eliminated animals with abnormal behavior, diarrhea or seizures [25].

2.5. GA, M3OMG and P3OMG Administration

Animals were randomly divided into 8 groups of 10 animals each. GA, M3OMG and P3OMG were intraperitoneally administered in two doses (25 and 50 mg/kg body weight) for a week. After the last application, depressive-like behaviors of all animals were tested using despair swimming and tail suspension tests.

2.6. Examination of Stroke-Induced Anhedonia

For the examination of stroke-induced anhedonia, water bottles were removed from animal cages for a period of 6 h. Thereafter, two bottles were provided to each animal cage. The first bottle was filled with sucrose solution (2%, % *w/v*) and the second bottle was filled with water. This test is based on the evaluation of the volumes of consumed sucrose and water. Total volumes of sucrose solution and water were recorded over a period of 6 h [26].

2.7. Despair Swimming Test (DST)

The despair swimming test is one of the most common animal models for the examination of depressive-like behaviors. In brief, mice were individually placed in an open cylinder (25 cm height and 10 cm diameter) containing fresh water at $24 \pm 2\,^\circ C$ (19 cm of height). The animals were forced to swim for a period of 6 min, with times recorded for periods of immobility (the period during which animals have no horizontal movement, merely keeping their head above the water surface), climbing (the period of active vertical movement, in which animals try to keep their forelegs above the water surface) and swimming (the period of horizontal movement in which animals cross the water surface) [27].

2.8. Tail Suspension Test (TST)

The tail suspension test is another common model for the examination of depressive-like behaviors in experimental animals. In brief, mice were suspended at a height of 58 cm for a period of 5 min through the use of adhesive tape attached 1 cm from the tail tip of each animal. The time of immobility, defined as the amount of time spent motionless during the 5 min test, was recorded [25].

2.9. Anesthesia and Tissue Collection

At the end of the experimental period, the mice were anesthetized by the intraperitoneal administration of ketamine (60 mg/kg) and xylazine (5 mg/kg) after withholding food for 12 h. The brain was removed and kept at $-60\,^\circ C$ prior to biochemical assessment.

2.10. Preparation of Tissue Homogenate

The whole brain tissue of each animal was homogenized in 100 mM phosphate buffer saline (1:10, % *w/v*) containing ethylenediaminetetraacetic acid (1 mM, pH 7.4) and centrifuged (12,000 g, 30 min, 4 °C). The supernatant was separated and used for biochemical analysis.

2.11. Measurement of Protein Content

The protein content of the homogenates of brain was determined using the Bradford method with bovine serum albumin as the standard [28].

2.12. Estimation of Lipid Peroxidation

Lipid peroxidation, expressed as thiobarbituric acid-reactive substance (TBARS) formation, was determined with the method used by Di Lorenzo *et al.* [26]. Brain tissue homogenates containing 1 mg protein were mixed with trichloroacetic acid (1 mL, 20%) and thiobarbituric acid (2 mL, 0.67%) and then incubated for 1 h at 100 °C. After cooling, the precipitate was removed by centrifugation. The absorbance of the reaction mixtures was measured at $\lambda = 532$ nm using a blank containing all the reagents with the exception of tissue homogenates.

2.13. Determination of Superoxide Dismutase Activity

Superoxide dismutase (SOD) activity was examined according to the method used by Misra and Fridovich [29]. The reaction mixtures consisted of sodium carbonate (1 mL, 50 mM), nitroblue tetrazolium (0.4 mL, 25 µM), and freshly prepared hydroxylamine hydrochloride (0.2 mL, 0.1 mM). The reaction mixtures were mixed by inversion followed by the addition of clear supernatant of homogenates of brain tissue (0.1 mL, 1:10, % *w/v*). The change in absorbance of the reaction mixture was recorded at $\lambda = 560$ nm.

2.14. Determination of Catalase Activity

The enzyme catalase converts hydrogen peroxide into oxygen and water. Catalase activity was measured using the method described by Nabavi *et al.* [30]. The tissue homogenates (containing 5 μg of protein) were mixed with hydrogen peroxide (2.1 mL, 7.5 mM) and a time scan was performed for 10 min at $\lambda = 240$ nm and 25 °C. The disappearance of peroxide due to catalase activity was observed. One unit of catalase activity is defined as the amount of enzyme that reduces 1 μmol of hydrogen peroxide in a minute.

2.15. Determination of Reduced Glutathione Level

Reduced glutathione (GSH) level was determined with Ellman's method [31]. Brain tissue homogenates (720 μL) were double diluted and trichloroacetic acid (5%) was added to precipitate their protein content. After centrifugation ($12,000 \times g$, 5 min) the supernatant was taken, 5,5-dithiobis 2-nitrobenzoic acid solution (Ellman's reagent) was added and the absorbance of the reaction mixture was measured at $\lambda = 417$ nm. A standard curve was drawn using known levels of reduced glutathione solution. Using this standard calibration curve, reduced glutathione levels were calculated for the homogenates.

2.16. Statistical Analysis

Statistical analysis was carried out with the SPSS statistical software package version 21.0 (SPSS Inc., Chicago, IL, USA).Results were expressed as means $\pm$ SD, and $p < 0.01$ was considered statistically significant. A Shapiro-Wilk W-test was applied to assess the normal distribution of the data. The statistical significance of the data was assessed by one-way variance analysis. When significant differences were found, Bonferroni *post hoc* testing was used to determine the differences between the groups involved. Possible bivariate correlations between different parameters were analyzed. Variables were also adjusted for multiple linear regression models in order to evaluate the association between enzyme activities (SOD and Cat), the marker of lipid peroxidation (TBARS), and the content of GSH, with each of the registered behavioral parameters.

3. Results and Discussion

In the initial phase of the investigation, M3OMG and P3OMG were synthesized as reported in the Materials and Methods section [11]. Their purity was estimated at over 95% (See Supplementary Materials). Then, GA, M3OMG, and P3OMG were studied for their *in vivo* antidepressant-like and antioxidant activities. Experimental animals were divided into three major groups: (a) a control group of healthy mice; (b) a BCCAO group of animals, which underwent bilateral common carotid artery occlusion (BCCAO); (c) 6 groups treated with GA, M3OMG and P3OMG at two different doses (25 mg/kg and 50 mg/kg). As previously demonstrated [25], bilateral common carotid artery occlusion caused anhedonia, a representative symptom of acute ischemic stroke. In fact, the results reported in Figure 2 show that the BCCAO group was characterized by a significant ($p < 0.01$) increase in water consumption and a significant ($p < 0.01$) drop in sucrose solution consumption compared to the normal group, demonstrating the validity of this animal model in the study of ischemic stroke.

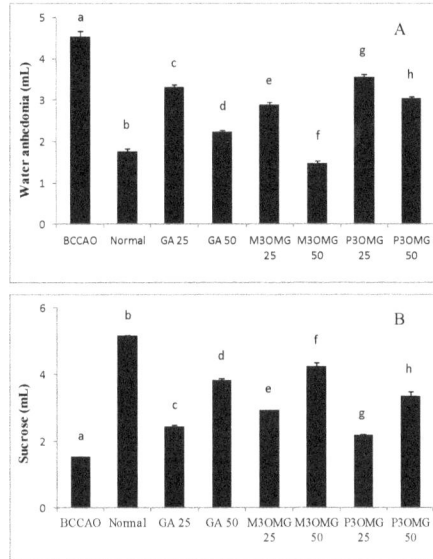

Figure 2. Volume of water (**A**) and sucrose solution (**B**) consumption in the stroke-induced anhedonia model. Data are shown as a mean (mL) $\pm$ SD (n = 3); different letters indicate statistically significant differences ($p < 0.01$) between the two groups.

Intraperitoneal administration of GA, M3OMG and P3OMG significantly ($p < 0.01$) modified water and sucrose solution consumption in a dose-dependent manner at both dosages tested, producing an improvement in the anhedonia state when compared with the BCCAO group (Figure 2A,B, respectively). The largest improvement in anhedonia was provided by M3OMG at both doses, which was able to restore normal water consumption at the 50 mg/kg dose. The least active compound was found to be P3OMG: at the highest dose (50 mg/kg) it showed the same activity ($p = 0.033$) on water consumption as M3OMG administered at the lowest dose (25 mg/kg).

The BCCAO animal model is also a suitable system to study depressive-like behavior through the use of two validated and commonly used tests, the despair swimming test (DST) and the tail suspension test (TST). DST is an important model of depressive-like behavior in which animals are forced to swim in a cylindrical container filled with water. Climbing, swimming and immobility periods are registered for the 6 min duration of the test [25]. At both concentrations and in a dose-dependent manner, the tested compounds showed antidepressive-like activity, significantly ($p < 0.01$) increasing the climbing and swimming times and decreasing the immobility time with respect to the BCCAO group (Figures 3–5 respectively).

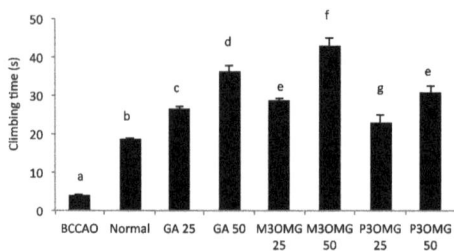

Figure 3. Effects of intraperitoneal administration of GA, M3OMG and P3OMG on climbing time in the despair swimming test. Data are a mean (s) $\pm$ SD ($n = 7$); different letters indicate statistically significant differences ($p < 0.01$) between the two groups.

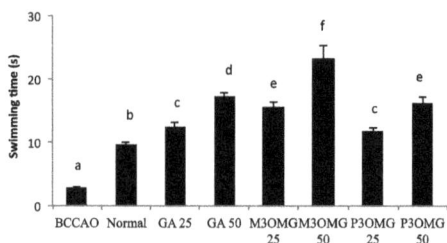

Figure 4. Effects of intraperitoneal administration of GA, M3OMG and P3OMG on swimming time in the despair swimming test. Data are a mean (s) $\pm$ SD ($n = 7$); different letters indicate statistically significant differences ($p < 0.01$) between the two groups.

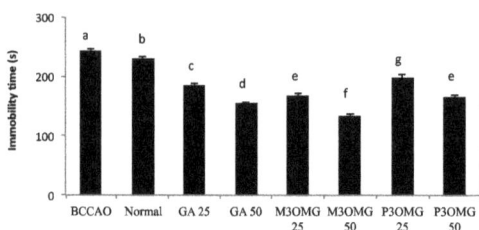

Figure 5. Effects of intraperitoneal administration of GA, M3OMG and P3OMG on immobility time in the despair swimming test. Data are a mean (s) $\pm$ SD ($n = 7$); different letters indicate statistically significant differences ($p < 0.01$) between the two groups.

For all the parameters registered and at both doses, the most active compound was found to be M3OMG, whilst the least active was P3OMG, which here too shows the same activity ($p \geqslant 0.01$) at the highest dosage (50 mg/kg) as M3OMG administered at the lowest dosage (25 mg/kg).

TST describes the depressive behavior of experimental animals through the determination of immobility time in unavoidable and inescapable stress conditions. An antidepressant agent reduces the immobility times for unsuccessful attempts to escape [32]. For both concentrations and in a dose-dependent manner, GA, M3OMG and P3OMG showed high antidepressive-like activity, significantly ($p < 0.01$) decreasing the immobility time of the treated mice compared with that of the BCCAO group (Figure 6). Here too, M3OMG results as the most active compound at both doses.

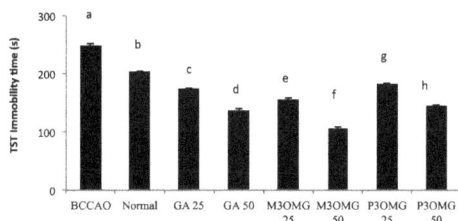

Figure 6. Effects of the intraperitoneal administration of GA, M3OMG and P3OMG on the tail suspension model. Data are a mean (s) $\pm$ SD ($n = 7$); different letters indicate statistically significant differences ($p < 0.01$) between the two groups.

In our previous review, we reported that there is a growing body of evidence that supports oxidative stress as playing a fundamental role in the pathogenesis of both ischemic stroke and major depression. Thus, we formulated the hypothesis that oxidative stress is also involved in the pathogenesis of post-stroke depression, and antioxidant substances could thus be useful in the treatment of this pathology [18]. Considering the *in vitro* and *in vivo* antioxidant and neuroprotective effects of GA and its related compounds, which are well documented in the literature [19,33–36], the present study was extended to the evaluation of the *in vivo* protective effect of GA, M3OMG and P3OMG against oxidative stress. The antioxidant activities of SOD and Cat, the degree of lipid peroxidation, (expressed in TBARS levels), and GSH levels were determined for mouse brains. As expected, stroke induced a significant ($p < 0.01$) increase in TBARS levels, revealing high oxidative stress in the BCCAO group. The treatment with GA, M3OMG and P3OMG significantly ($p < 0.01$) decreased TBARS levels at both tested concentrations, even though the compounds were not able to completely restore normal conditions (Figure 7A). Among the tested compounds, M3OMG was found to be the most active at both dosages (25 and 50 mg/kg), whilst P3OMG was less active. In fact, at the highest dose P3OMG showed the same activity ($p = 0.196$) as M3OMG administered at the lowest concentration. As far as endogenous antioxidant defenses are concerned, the induction of stroke was found to cause a significant ($p < 0.01$) decrease in SOD and Cat activities and GSH levels in comparison with the control group, confirming a relevant oxidative stress condition in the BCCAO group. Although the administration of GA, M3OMG and P3OMG improved endogenous antioxidant defenses, increasing SOD and Cat activities and GSH levels compared to the BCCAO group, the registered values did not attain those determined in the normal group (Figure 7B–D, respectively). M3OMG again exerted the highest antioxidant activity at both dosages, compared to GA and P3OMG, resulting as the most promising antioxidant compound with potential uses in the treatment of post-stroke depression.

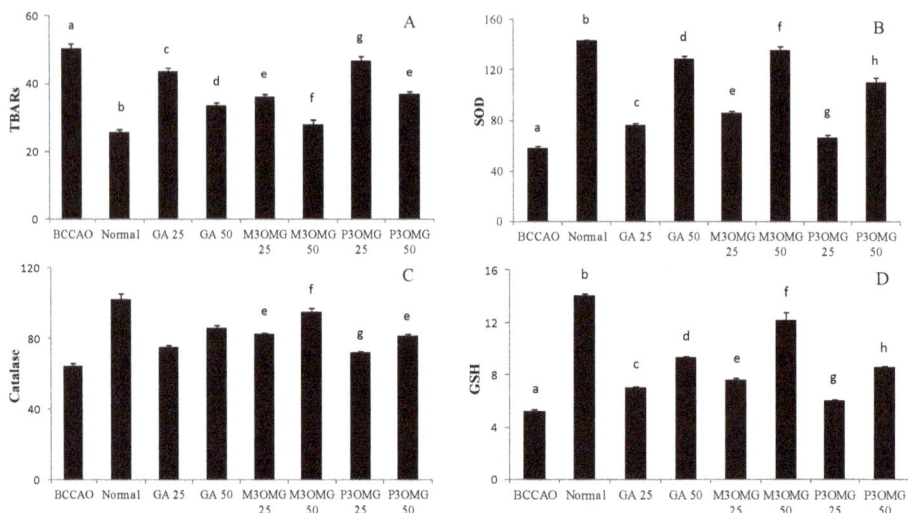

Figure 7. Effects of intraperitoneal administration of GA, M3OMG and P3OMG on oxidative stress levels in mouse brain tissue: TBARS levels, expressed as nmol MDA eq/g tissues (**A**); SOD activity, expressed as U/mg per protein (**B**); Cat activity, expressed as µg/mg per protein (**C**); and GSH levels, expressed as µg/mg per protein (**D**). Data are a mean ± SD (*n* = 7); different letters indicate statistically significant differences (*p* < 0.01) between the two groups.

To explore the relationship between the results obtained from behavioral tests and antioxidant assays in more depth, we evaluated possible bivariate correlations between the independent variables, consisting of enzyme activities (SOD and Cat), the marker of lipid peroxidation (TBARS), and the content of GSH, with the registered behavioral parameters taken as dependent variables (Table 1). Statistical significance was found for the associations of GSH, SOD and TBARS, with all the dependent variables. The highest significant associations were found between SOD and the dependent climbing and swimming variables, and for GSH and TBARS with immobility and immobility registered in TST. There were no significant associations between Cat activity and any of the studied behavioral parameters. These results support the hypothesis that oxidative stress is closely related and tightly linked to post-stroke depression.

Table 1. Multiple linear regression analysis on the dependent variables of climbing, swimming, immobility, and immobility in tail-suspension test (TST). *p* < 0.05 was considered statistically significant.

Antioxidant Enzymes/Marker of Lipid Peroxidation		Climbing	Swimming	Immobility	Immobility (TST)
Cat	β	0.586	0.256	−1.961	−1.730
	p	0.190	0.285	0.178	0.292
GSH	β	−7.125	−3.241	28.265	27.411
	p	0.000	0.000	0.000	0.000
SOD	β	0.340	0.135	−1.149	−1.220
	p	0.004	0.029	0.003	0.005
TBARS	β	−1.098	−0.646	4.210	5.045
	p	0.037	0.023	0.015	0.010

4. Conclusions

In this study we have demonstrated that the intraperitoneal administration of GA, M3OMG and P3OMG restores behavioral parameters indicative of depression to healthy levels in experimental animals in which PSD has been induced by bilateral common carotid artery occlusion. M3OMG was found to be more active than GA and P3OMG, decreasing anhedonia and improving depressive-like behavior. In all behavioral tests, GA was found to be less effective than M3OMG at both doses, and P3OMG administered at the highest dose (50 mg/kg) showed the same activity as M3OMG administered at the lowest dose (25 mg/kg). These data suggest that increasing lipophilicity, moving from GA to M3OMG, increases the antidepressive-like activity while a further increase of lipophilicity, moving from M3OMG to the propyl derivative, does not correspond to an increase in activity.

The *in vivo* antioxidant activity exerted by GA, M3OMG and P3OMG supports the hypothesis that oxidative stress, which occurs during cerebral ischemia and the following reperfusion, is implicated in the pathogenesis of PSD. M3OMG shows the highest capacity to improve SOD and Cat activities, GSH levels and decrease TBARS levels, which confirms that this compound shows higher activity than GA and P3OMG. The relationship found between the results obtained from behavioral tests and antioxidant assays corroborates our hypothesis that oxidative stress is closely related and tightly linked to stroke and post-stroke depression. It is very interesting to highlight that bivariate correlations were shown for associations between GSH, SOD and TBARS, and all behavioral parameters, while no significant associations between Cat activity and any behavioral parameters were found. These last results seems to suggest that the capacity of these exogenous antioxidant compounds to modulate depressive symptoms is probably exerted primarily through SOD activity, GSH levels and a decrease in lipid peroxidation instead of through Cat activity.

Though GA and its derivatives were administered through intraperitoneal injection rather than oral ingestion, the obtained results are interesting because they show a new biological function of these hydroxy-benzoic compounds. Future studies will be performed using the oral route of administration in view of a future use for these compounds in food supplements or drugs, and to mimic the ingestion of these polyphenols as part of plant based foods and beverages. In conclusion, this work represents the first attempt to demonstrate the positive effect of GA and its synthetic derivatives on post-stroke depression and to correlate this protective activity with their antioxidant activity.

Supplementary Materials: The following are available online at http://www.mdpi.com/2072-6643/8/5/248/s1.

Acknowledgments: Antoni Sureda was supported by Spanish Ministry of Health and Consumer Affairs (CIBEROBN CB12/03/30038). We thank the EPSRC National Mass Spectrometry Facility (Singleton Park, Swansea, UK) for acquiring the MS data.

Author Contributions: Seyed Mohammad Nabavi, Solomon Habtemariam and Maria Daglia designed the paper, Maria Daglia collected and selected the literature data, Antoni Sureda and Seyed Fazel Nabavi analyzed the data, Arianna Di Lorenzo, Sedigheh Khanjani, Maria Daglia and Seyed Mohammad Nabavi wrote the paper. All authors participated in the analysis and interpretation of literature data, revised the paper and approved the final manuscript.

Conflicts of Interest: The authors declare no conflict of interest.

References

1. Herrmann, K.M.; Weaver, L.M. The shikimate pathway. *Ann. Rev. Plant Biol.* **1999**, *50*, 473–503. [CrossRef] [PubMed]
2. Nabavi, S.F.; Nabavi, S.M.; Habtemariam, S.; Moghaddam, A.H.; Sureda, A.; Jafari, M.; Latifi, A.M. Hepatoprotective effect of gallic acid isolated from *Peltiphyllum peltatum* against sodium fluoride-induced oxidative stress. *Ind. Crops Prod.* **2013**, *44*, 50–55. [CrossRef]
3. Kim, S.H.; Jun, C.D.; Suk, K.; Choi, B.J.; Lim, H.; Park, S.; Lee, S.H.; Shin, H.Y.; Kim, D.K.; Shin, T.Y. Gallic acid inhibits histamine release and pro-inflammatory cytokine production in mast cells. *Toxicol. Sci.* **2006**, *91*, 123–131. [CrossRef] [PubMed]
4. Daglia, M.; Di Lorenzo, A.; Nabavi, S.F.; Talas, Z.S.; Nabavi, S.M. Polyphenols: Well beyond the antioxidant capacity: Gallic acid and related compounds as neuroprotective agents: You are what you eat! *Curr. Pharm. Biotechnol.* **2014**, *15*, 362–372. [CrossRef] [PubMed]

5. Kaur, M.; Velmurugan, B.; Rajamanickam, S.; Agarwal, R.; Agarwal, C. Gallic acid, an active constituent of grape seed extract, exhibits anti-proliferative, pro-apoptotic and anti-tumorigenic effects against prostate carcinoma xenograft growth in nude mice. *Pharm. Res.* **2009**, *26*, 2133–2140. [CrossRef]

6. Nabavi, S.M.; Habtemariam, S.; Nabavi, S.F.; Sureda, A.; Daglia, M.; Moghaddam, A.H.; Amani, M.A. Protective effect of gallic acid isolated from *Peltiphyllum peltatum* against sodium fluoride-induced oxidative stress in rat's kidney. *Mol. Cell. Biochem.* **2013**, *372*, 233–239. [CrossRef]

7. Shao, D.; Li, J.; Li, J.; Tang, R.; Liu, L.; Shi, J.; Huang, Q.; Yang, H. Inhibition of gallic acid on the growth and biofilm formation of *Escherichia coli* and *Streptococcus mutans*. *J. Food Sci.* **2015**, *80*, M1299–M1305. [CrossRef] [PubMed]

8. Habtemariam, S. Methyl-3-*O*-methyl gallate and gallic acid from the leaves of *Peltiphyllum peltatum*: isolation and comparative antioxidant, prooxidant, and cytotoxic effects in neuronal cells. *J. Med. Food* **2011**, *14*, 1412–1418. [CrossRef]

9. Nabavi, S.F.; Nabavi, S.M.; Habtemariam, S.; Moghaddam, A.H.; Sureda, A.; Mirzaei, M. Neuroprotective effects of methyl-3-*O*-methyl gallate against sodium fluoride-induced oxidative stress in the brain of rats. *Cell. Mol. Neurobiol.* **2013**, *33*, 261–267. [CrossRef]

10. Nabavi, S.M.; Habtemariam, S.; Nabavi, S.F.; Moghaddam, A.H.; Latifi, A.M. Prophylactic effects of methyl-3-*O*-methyl gallate against sodium fluoride-induced oxidative stress in erythrocytes *in vivo*. *J. Pharm. Pharmacol.* **2013**, *65*, 868–873. [CrossRef] [PubMed]

11. Curti, V.; Capelli, E.; Boschi, F.; Nabavi, S.F.; Bongiorno, A.I.; Habtemariam, S.; Nabavi, S.M.; Daglia, M. Modulation of human miR-17-3p expression by methyl 3-*O*-methyl gallate as explanation of its *in vivo* protective activities. *Mol. Nutr. Food Res.* **2014**, *58*, 1776–1784. [CrossRef] [PubMed]

12. Civenni, G.; Iodice, M.; Nabavi, S.F.; Habtemariam, S.; Nabavi, S.M.; Catapano, C.; Daglia, M. Gallic acid and methyl-3-*O*-methyl gallate: A comparative study on their effects on prostate cancer stem cells. *RSC Adv.* **2015**, *5*, 63800–63806. [CrossRef]

13. Roger, V.L.; Go, A.S.; Lloyd-Jones, D.M.; Benjamin, E.J.; Berry, J.D.; Borden, W.B.; Bravata, D.M.; Dai, S.; Ford, E.S.; Fox, C.S.; *et al.* Heart disease and stroke statistics—2012 update a report from the American heart association. *Circulation* **2012**, *125*, e2–e220.

14. Bolaños, J.P.; Moro, M.A.; Lizasoain, I.; Almeida, A. Mitochondria and reactive oxygen and nitrogen species in neurological disorders and stroke: Therapeutic implications. *Adv. Drug Deliv. Rev.* **2009**, *61*, 1299–1315. [CrossRef] [PubMed]

15. Yang, Y.; Rosenberg, G.A. Blood–brain barrier breakdown in acute and chronic cerebrovascular disease. *Stroke* **2011**, *42*, 3323–3328. [CrossRef] [PubMed]

16. Loubinoux, I.; Kronenberg, G.; Endres, M.; Schumann-Bard, P.; Freret, T.; Filipkowski, R.K.; Kaczmarek, L.; Popa-Wagner, A. Post-stroke depression: Mechanisms, translation and therapy. *J. Cell. Mol. Med.* **2012**, *16*, 1961–1969. [CrossRef] [PubMed]

17. World Health Organization WH. In *Promoting Fruit and Vegetable Consumption around the World*; World Health Organization: Geneva, Switzerland, 2010.

18. Nabavi, S.F.; Dean, O.M.; Turner, A.; Sureda, A.; Daglia, M.; Nabavi, S.M. Oxidative stress and post-stroke depression: Possible therapeutic role of polyphenols? *Curr. Med. Chem.* **2015**, *22*, 343–351. [CrossRef]

19. Nabavi, S.F.; Habtemariam, S.; Jafari, M.; Sureda, A.; Nabavi, S.M. Protective role of gallic acid on sodium fluoride induced oxidative stress in rat brain. *Bull. Environ. Contam. Toxicol.* **2012**, *89*, 73–77. [CrossRef] [PubMed]

20. Nabavi, S.F.; Habtemariam, S.; Sureda, A.; Moghaddam, A.H.; Daglia, M.; Nabavi, S.M. *In vivo* protective effects of gallic acid isolated from *Peltiphyllum peltatum* against sodium fluoride-induced oxidative stress in rat erythrocytes. *Arch. Ind. Hygiene Toxicol.* **2013**, *64*, 553–559. [CrossRef]

21. Sarkaki, A.; Fathimoghaddam, H.; Mansouri, S.; Korrani, M.S.; Saki, G.; Farbood, Y. Gallic acid improves cognitive, hippocampal long-term potentiation deficits and brain damage induced by chronic cerebral hypoperfusion in rats. *Pak. J. Biol. Sci.* **2014**, *17*, 978.

22. Chhillar, R.; Dhingra, D. Antidepressant-like activity of gallic acid in mice subjected to unpredictable chronic mild stress. *Fundam. Clin. Pharmacol.* **2013**, *27*, 409–418. [CrossRef] [PubMed]

23. Nagpal, K.; Singh, S.K.; Mishra, D.N. Nanoparticle mediated brain targeted delivery of gallic acid: *In vivo* behavioral and biochemical studies for improved antioxidant and antidepressant-like activity. *Drug Deliv.* **2012**, *19*, 378–391. [CrossRef] [PubMed]

24. Azzolini, M.; Mattarei, A.; La Spina, M.; Marotta, E.; Zoratti, M.; Paradisi, C.; Biasutto, L. Synthesis and evaluation as prodrugs of hydrophilic carbamate ester analogues of resveratrol. *Mol. Pharm.* **2015**, *12*, 3441–3454. [CrossRef]

25. Nabavi, S.F.; Sobarzo-Sanchez, E.; Nabavi, S.M.; Daglia, M.; Moghaddam, A.H.; Silva, A.G. Behavioral effects of 2,3-dihydro-and oxoisoaporphine derivatives in post stroke-depressive like behavior in male balb/c mice. *Curr. Top. Med. Chem.* **2013**, *13*, 2127–2133. [CrossRef]

26. Di Lorenzo, A.; Nabavi, S.F.; Sureda, A.; Moghaddam, A.H.; Khanjani, S.; Arcidiaco, P.; Nabavi, S.M.; Daglia, M. Antidepressive-like effects and antioxidant activity of green tea and GABA green tea in a mouse model of post-stroke depression. *Mol. Nutr. Food Res.* **2015**. [CrossRef]

27. Moghaddam, A.H.; Sobarzo-Sánchez, E.; Nabavi, S.F.; Daglia, M.; Nabavi, S.M. Evaluation of the antipsychotic effects of 2-(dimethylamino)-and 2-(methylamino)-7H-naphtho [1,2,3-de] quinolin-7-one derivatives in experimental model of psychosis in mice. *Curr. Top. Med. Chem.* **2014**, *14*, 229–233. [CrossRef]

28. Bradford, M.M. A rapid and sensitive method for the quantitation of microgram quantities of protein utilizing the principle of protein-dye binding. *Anal. Biochem.* **1976**, *72*, 248–254. [CrossRef]

29. Misra, H.P.; Fridovich, I. The role of superoxide anion in the autoxidation of epinephrine and a simple assay for superoxide dismutase. *J. Biol. Chem.* **1972**, *247*, 3170–3175.

30. Nabavi, S.M.; Nabavi, S.F.; Eslami, S.; Moghaddam, A.H. *In vivo* protective effects of quercetin against sodium fluoride-induced oxidative stress in the hepatic tissue. *Food Chem.* **2012**, *132*, 931–935. [CrossRef]

31. Ellman, G.L. Tissue sulfhydryl groups. *Arch. Biochem. Biophys.* **1959**, *82*, 70–77. [CrossRef]

32. Castagné, V.; Moser, P.; Roux, S.; Porsolt, R.D. Rodent models of depression: Forced swim and tail suspension behavioral despair tests in rats and mice. *Curr. Protoc. Neurosci.* **2011**, *55*, 11–18. [CrossRef]

33. Mansouri, M.T.; Farbood, Y.; Sameri, M.J.; Sarkaki, A.; Naghizadeh, B.; Rafeirad, M. Neuroprotective effects of oral gallic acid against oxidative stress induced by 6-hydroxydopamine in rats. *Food Chem.* **2013**, *138*, 1028–1033. [CrossRef] [PubMed]

34. Sun, J.; Li, Y.Z.; Ding, Y.H.; Wang, J.; Geng, J.; Yang, H.; Ren, J.; Tang, J.Y.; Gao, J. Neuroprotective effects of gallic acid against hypoxia/reoxygenation-induced mitochondrial dysfunctions *in vitro* and cerebral ischemia/reperfusion injury *in vivo*. *Brain Res.* **2014**, *1589*, 126–139. [CrossRef] [PubMed]

35. Ban, J.Y.; Nguyen, H.T.T.; Lee, H.J.; Cho, S.O.; Ju, H.S.; Kim, J.Y.; Bae, K.; Song, K.S.; Seong, Y.H. Neuroprotective properties of gallic acid from *Sanguisorbae* Radix on amyloid. BETA. Protein (25–35)-induced toxicity in cultured rat cortical neurons. *Biol. Pharm. Bull.* **2008**, *31*, 149–153. [CrossRef] [PubMed]

36. Korani, M.S.; Farbood, Y.; Sarkaki, A.; Moghaddam, H.F.; Mansouri, M.T. Protective effects of gallic acid against chronic cerebral hypoperfusion-induced cognitive deficit and brain oxidative damage in rats. *Eur. J. Pharmacol.* **2014**, *733*, 62–67. [CrossRef]

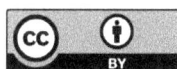

nutrients

MDPI

Article

Mixture of Peanut Skin Extract and Fish Oil Improves Memory in Mice via Modulation of Anti-Oxidative Stress and Regulation of BDNF/ERK/CREB Signaling Pathways

Lan Xiang [1,*], Xue-Li Cao [1], Tian-Yan Xing [2], Daisuke Mori [3], Rui-Qi Tang [1], Jing Li [1], Li-Juan Gao [1] and Jian-Hua Qi [1,*]

[1] College of Pharmaceutical Sciences, Zhejiang University, Hangzhou 310058, China; 11319006@zju.edu.cn (X.-L.C.); ricky.tang@163.com (R.-Q.T.); 11419008@zju.edu.cn (J.L.); gaolijuan04141002@126.com (L.-J.G.)

[2] Hangzhou Napochi Pharmaceutical Co. Ltd., Hangzhou 310018, China; hznqrsw@163.com

[3] Gifu Shellac Mfg. Co., Ltd., 1-27, Kanonishimaru-cho, Gifu 500, Japan; numbermidori@gmail.com

* Correspondence: lxiang@zju.edu.cn (L.X.); qijianhua@zju.edu.cn (J.-H.Q.); Tel.: +86-571-88208631 (L.X.); Tel./Fax: +86-571-88208627 (J.-H.Q.)

Received: 14 March 2016; Accepted: 21 April 2016; Published: 28 April 2016

Abstract: Long-term use of fish oil (FO) is known to induce oxidative stress and increase the risk of Alzheimer's disease in humans. In the present study, peanut skin extract (PSE), which has strong antioxidant capacity, was mixed with FO to reduce its side effects while maintaining its beneficial properties. Twelve-week Institute of Cancer Research (ICR) mice were used to conduct animal behavior tests in order to evaluate the memory-enhancing ability of the mixture of peanut skin extract and fish oil (MPF). MPF significantly increased alternations in the Y-maze and cognitive index in the novel object recognition test. MPF also improved performance in the water maze test. We further sought to understand the mechanisms underlying these effects. A significant decrease in superoxide dismutase (SOD) activity and an increase in malonyldialdehyde (MDA) in plasma were observed in the FO group. The MPF group showed reduced MDA level and increased SOD activity in the plasma, cortex and hippocampus. Furthermore, the gene expression levels of brain-derived neurotrophic factor (BDNF) and cAMP responsive element-binding protein (CREB) in the hippocampus were increased in the MPF group, while phosphorylation of protein kinase B (AKT), extracellular signal-regulated kinase (ERK) and CREB in the hippocampus were enhanced. MPF improves memory in mice via modulation of anti-oxidative stress and activation of BDNF/ERK/CREB signaling pathways.

Keywords: brain-derived neurotrophic factor; fish oil; ERK; oxidative stress; peanut skin extract

1. Introduction

Fish oil (FO) is a widely used nutrition supplement. It is rich in omega-3 fatty acids, specifically docosahexaenoic acid (DHA) and eicosapentaenoic acid (EPA). Previous studies have indicated that FO can reduce blood fat [1] and prevent Alzheimer's disease (AD) [2]. FO also exhibits anti-inflammatory [3], anti-cancer [4], and anti-aging [5] effects. However, negative reports concerning FO consumption have emerged in recent years. The oxidation products of FO are harmful to mitochondria functions [6,7]. Furthermore, FO replaces critical omega-6 metabolites, thus modifying tissue structure, and reducing prostacyclin production, which increases the risk of cardiovascular diseases [8]. Furthermore, prolonged or excessive consumption of FO containing the oxidized product polyunsaturated fatty acid oxide leads to production of free radicals and induction of cellular senescence, which involves senile plaque formation and tissue damage. These problems limit the use of FO as a nutrient supplement. Therefore, reassessment of the function and reliability of FO is imperative.

Oxidative stress, insulin resistance and inflammation interrelate. Oxidative stress can lead to insulin resistance and inflammation. Conversely, both insulin resistance and inflammation can also increase oxidative stress. Several studies have shown that all of these factors can be induced by a high fat diet and can impair cognitive performance and memory decline [9–11]. Therefore, further studies are necessary for improvement of cognitive function of the aging brain by using anti-oxidative, anti-diabetic and anti-inflammatory agents.

Peanut skin is a protective pink-red layer with astringent taste. It is rich in phenolics and other health-promoting compounds. Peanut skin extract (PSE) mainly contains 3-procyanidins, 4-anthocyanins, 2-flavanols, and 5-flavonols. Resveratrol also exists in PSE and its concentration is higher than that in peanut kernels [12]. The anti-inflammatory, anti-cardiovascular disease, anti-cancer, anti-obesity and anti-diabetic properties of many polyphenolic compounds have been investigated recently [13–17]. Peanut skin polyphenols, particularly procyanidine, improve lipid homeostasis, reduce inflammation, and act as natural antioxidants and antimicrobial agents [18–20]. In the current study, we used PSE to alleviate the side effects of FO and sought to determine whether MPF improves memory in mice via its anti-oxidative effects or regulation of gene expression.

2. Materials and Methods

2.1. PSE, FO and MPF

PSE and FO with 20% DHA and 8% EPA were obtained from Gifu Shellac Mfg. Co., Ltd., Gifu, Japan. MPF was composed of PSE and FO at a 1:2 ratio by mass. The vehicle contained 40% glycerin, 6% emulsifier, and 54% water. Samples were prepared by dissolving PSE, FO, and MPF in the vehicle to get final concentrations of 15% PSE, 30% FO, and 15% PSE + 30% FO, respectively. The effective dose of fish oil for use as supplements has been shown to be 20–40 mg/kg for adults. Therefore, 20 mg/kg of FO was used in our study.

2.2. Neurite Outgrowth Assay

Bioassay was performed as described in a previous study [21]. Firstly, 2×10^4 rat pheochromocytoma (PC12) cells were placed in each well of a 24-well microplate and cultured in 5% CO_2 incubator at 37 °C for 24 h. After that, 1 mL of serum-free dulbecco's modified eagle medium that contain test samples (PSE at doses of 0.3, 1 and 3 μg/mL; FO at doses of 0.3, 1 and 3 μg/mL; MPF at doses of 0.3 + 0.3, 0.3 + 1, 0.3 + 3, 1 + 0.3, 1 + 1, 1 + 3 μg/mL) and dimethyl sulfoxide (DMSO) (0.5%) was used to replace old medium and incubated for two days. Nerve growth factor (NGF) was used as positive control. Cells were observed using a phase-contrast microscope (Olympus, Model CKX41, Tokyo, Japan) every 24 h. Approximately 100 cells were counted from a random region of the culture dish. If the outgrowth of a PC12 cell was longer than the diameter of the cell body, the cell was determined to be neurite-bearing. Independent experiments were repeated thrice and the results are expressed as mean ± SEM.

2.3. Animal Study and Experimental Design

Twelve-week-old male ICR mice ($n = 60$) were used as experimental animals (Zhejiang Academy of Medical Sciences, Hangzhou, China). The mice were fed in a clean room at 23 ± 1 °C with a 12:12 light-dark cycle and fed with a commercial diet (Zhejiang Academy of Medical Sciences, Hangzhou, China) *ad libitum*. All experiments were performed according to the Guide by the Animal Ethics Committee of Medical School, Zhejiang University (Permit Number: ZJU201401101005). The mice were divided into six groups. The control group received vehicle treatment. The PSE group received PSE at 10 mg/kg body weight per day. The FO group received FO at 20 mg/kg body weight per day. Three MPF groups received MPF at 0.03, 3 and 30 mg/kg body weight per day with oral administration. The animals were administered with samples for 5 weeks and then subjected to the Y-maze and novel objects recognition (NOR) test. The water maze experiment was performed on the sixth week. After finishing animal behavior experiments, blood was collected from mice orbit with capillary and the treated mice were killed with neck dislocation. Brain and plasma samples of the mice were taken quickly and then frozen at $-20\,°C$.

2.3.1. Y-Maze Memory Test

The mice were tested for spontaneous alternations using the Y-maze as previously reported [22]. The Y-maze used in the present study has three equal arms with $120°$ angle. The mice were placed in the "start" arm of the Y-maze and left to roam freely for 8 min. Three continuous choices in three different arms were considered to be alternations. The average of percentage alternations was plotted.

2.3.2. NOR Memory Tasks

After completion of the Y-maze test, the NOR test was performed. The novel object apparatus consisted of a white plastic box ($46 \times 26 \times 20$ cm), two identical objects (2×12 cm plastic flashlights) and a novel object (5×11 cm coffee can). At first, each mouse was placed in the empty open field of the box for 5 min for habituation on Day 1. The area was cleaned with 75% ethanol solution well ahead of time to ensure that no olfactory cues were present. The next day, the test of the NOR task was performed, which consisted of a training trial and a retention phase. In the training trial, the mice were exposed to the same arena where two identical objects were placed in opposite sides at equal distances for 5 min. The time spent exploring the two objects by each mouse were measured. After 1 h of training trial, one of two identical objects was replaced with a novel object. The animals were removed from the arena and exposed for 5 min again. The time spent exploring each object was recorded. Exploration was fixed as the mice used the nose or forepaws to sniff or touch the objects. A discrimination index (DI) was represented with the percentage of exploring time on the novel object divided by the total time spent exploring both objects.

2.3.3. Morris Water Maze Test

The Morris water maze test was performed after sample administration for 5 weeks. The apparatus comprised of a movable platform (14 cm diameter) and a circular tank (1.2 m diameter, 50 cm depth). In addition, a digital camera connected to a computer hung above the tank and was used to track mice movement. Before the experiment, water was added up to 34 cm depth and warmed to 22 ± 1 $°C$. Black ink was added to make the water opaque and to hide the platform. During training, the tank was divided into four quadrants. Each mouse underwent four trials in four quadrants in 1 day. The mice learned to run away from the water by finding the platform under the water in the center of quadrant 1 in the tank. The experiment was performed in 4 days. The mice which could not locate the platform within 120 s were put on the platform and allowed to stay there for 10 s. The probe trials were done on the fifth day after removing the platform. In every trial, the mouse was placed in the water back to the front from one of four starting points. The time to find the platform in training trials and times of crossing platform in the training trial and probe trial were measured by reviewing the video recordings. Data from four tests conducted each day were averaged for statistical analysis.

2.4. SOD Activity and MDA Level in the Plasma, the Cerebral Cortex and the Hippocampus

Plasma samples were obtained by centrifuging the blood at 10,000 rpm for 10 min at normal temperature and depot at $-20\,°C$ until analysis. Approximately 50 mg of cerebral cortex samples or one hippocampus were homogenized in cold phosphate-buffered saline at a 1:9 volume ratio, sonicated thrice for 1 min each, and then centrifuged at 12,000 rpm for 15 min at 4 $°C$. The supernatants were used for analysis. The samples were assayed for SOD activity and MDA using commercially available T-SOD and MDA assay kits (Bioengineering Institute of Nanjing Jiancheng Company, Nanjing, China) according to the manufacturer's protocols. We selected 5.5 µL of basic plasma solution and 25 µL of 1% cerebral cortex or hippocampus homogenate of each sample as optimal quantities to measure the total SOD activity. Simultaneously, approximately 20 µL of plasma, 20 µL of 10% cerebral cortex and 40 µL of 10% hippocampus homogenate were used to measure MDA. The protein concentrations of the cerebral cortex samples were spectrophotometrically measured using a Bio-Rad protein assay kit (Bio-Rad Laboratories, Hercules, CA, USA) at 595 nm.

2.5. Real-Time PCR Analysis

Approximately 50 mg of the cerebral cortex and hippocampus samples were obtained. Extraction of total RNA, reverse transcription and cDNA synthesis were performed as described in a previous study [23] using CFX96-Touch (Bio-rad, Hercules, CA, USA) and SYBR Premix EX Taq™ (Takara, Otsu, Japan). The mouse BDNF, CREB, activity-regulated cytoskeleton-associated protein (ARC), B-cell lymphoma-X1 (BCL-X1) and 18S RNA primers used for the PCR were as follows-for BDNF: sense, 5'-TTG TTT TGT GCC GTT TAC CA-3', anti-sense, 5'-GGT AAG AGA GCC AGC CAC TG-3'; for CREB: sense, 5'-AAT GGT ACG ATG GGG TAC A-3', anti-sense, 5'-TCC ATC AGT GGT CTG TGC AT-3'; for ARC: sense, 5'-GAG AGC TGA AAG GGT TGC AC-3', anti-sense, 5'-GCC TTG ATG GAC TTC TTC CA-3'; for: BCL-X1: sense, 5'-TTC GGG ATG GAG TAA ACT GG-3', anti-sense, 5'-TGT CTG GTC ACT TCC GAC TG-3'; and for 18S RNA: sense, 5'-TAA CCC GTT GAA CCC CAT T-3', and anti-sense, 5'-CCA TCC AAT CGG TAG TAG CG-3'. We amplified cDNA using the following conditions: 95 °C for 2 min, followed by 40 cycles for 15 s at 95 °C, and 35 s at 60 °C. All results were standardized to 18S RNA gene expression, and relative mRNA transcript levels were determined by the Ct formula. Each sample was run in triplicate, and the average of the three measurements was calculated for every sample.

2.6. Western Blot

Hippocampus samples obtained at the end of the animal experiment were homogenized in lysis buffer containing 1% protease inhibitors. Approximately 15 µg proteins were moved to a new tube and incubated at 100 °C for 5 min for denaturation. Sodium dodecyl sulfate-polyacrylamide gel electrophoresis was run at 120 V for 45 min. The proteins were transferred to polyvinylidene difluoride membranes and then blocked with 5% non-fat dry milk buffer for 60 min at room temperature (RT). Blots were incubated with anti-phospho-p44/42 mitogen-activated protein kinase (MAPK), anti-p44/42 MAPK (ERK1/2), anti-CREB, anti-phospho-CREB, anti-AKT (Cell Signaling Technology, Boston, MA, USA), and anti-phospho-AKT (Abcam, Hong Kong, China) antibodies overnight at 4 °C. After washing three times, the membranes were incubated with secondary antibody for 45 min at RT. ᵉECL Western Blot Kit (Beijing CoWin Biotechnology, Beijing, China) was used to develop the bands.

2.7. Statistical Analysis

All experiments were independently performed twice, and each experiment was conducted using five or ten samples. Data are presented as mean $\pm$ SEM. Significant differences between groups were determined by one-way ANOVA, followed by two-tailed multiple *t*-tests using the Student–Newman–Keuls method in SPSS biostatistics software (IBM, Armonk, NY, USA). Statistical significance was considered at $p < 0.05$.

3. Results

3.1. NGF-Mimicking Effects of PSE, FO, and MPF on PC12 Cells

The NGF-mimicking effects of PSE, FO, and MPF on PC12 cells are displayed in Figure 1A–B. PSE-induced neurite outgrowth in PC12 cells, and the percentages of neurite-bearing cells for those treated with 0.3, 1.0, and 3.0 µg/mL PSE for 48 h reached 37.0% $\pm$ 2.4%, 34.7% $\pm$ 1.3%, and 34.0% $\pm$ 3.3%, respectively. These values were significantly higher than that of the control group (16.0% $\pm$ 2.4%,

$p < 0.001$). FO induced neurite outgrowth, and the percentages of neurite-bearing cells for those treated with 0.3, 1.0 and 3.0 µg/mL FO for 48 h reached 39.0% ± 1.7%, 43.3% ± 2.4%, and 32.5% ± 2.0%, respectively ($p < 0.001$). The percentages of neurite outgrowth after treatment with 0.3 + 0.3, 0.3 + 1.0, 0.3 + 3.0, 1.0 + 0.3, 1.0 + 1.0, and 1.0 + 3.0 µg/mL PSE + FO (MPF) for 48 h reached 50.7% ± 0.6%, 37.0% ± 1.2%, 43.0% ± 2.4%, 43.0% ± 2.5, 39.5% ± 1.2%, and 40.0% ± 1.3%, respectively ($p < 0.01$, $p < 0.001$). These results suggest that PSE, FO and MPF significantly influence neurite outgrowth of PC12 cells.

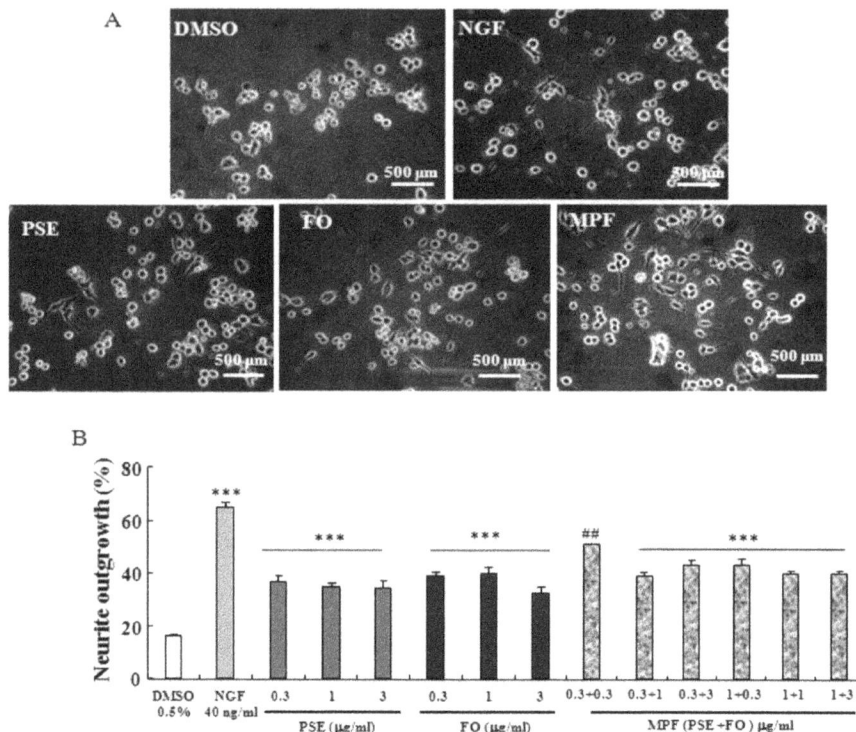

Figure 1. NGF-mimicking effects of PSE, FO and MPF on PC12 cells. (**A**) microphotograph of PC12 cells after treatment with DMSO, NGF, PSE, FO and MPF for 48 h; (**B**) percentage of PC12 cells with neurite outgrowth after treatment with DMSO, NGF, PSE, FO and MPF for 48 h. Cells bearing neurites were identified as those with processes that were at least twice the cell diameter in length. (Control: DMSO, 0.5%; Positive control: NGF, 40 ng/mL). *** Significantly different from the control group at the same time point at $p < 0.001$. ## Significantly different compared to only PSE or FO treated group at a dose of 0.3 µg/mL.

3.2. MPF Improves Learning Ability and Spatial Memory

Examination of animal behavior is a highly important part for functional evaluation. The Y-maze and NOR tests were performed to evaluate the behavior of PSE, FO, MPF treated mice and control mice. The total numbers of enter arms did not change in any of the groups (Figure 2A). Hence, the spontaneous alternation in PSE group at 10 mg/kg (70% ± 3.3%) and MPF treated group at 3 (71% ± 2.6%) and 30 mg/kg (76% ± 3.3%) were obviously higher than that of the control group (58% ± 2.1%, $p < 0.05$, $p < 0.01$ or $p < 0.001$) (Figure 2B). During the NOR test, all animals in the training phase showed similar DIs for recognition of the two familiar objects (Figure 2C). In the trial phase, all treated mice receiving PSE, FO and MPF spent more time exploring the novel object (69% ± 2.7%,

73% $\pm$ 4.8%, 72% $\pm$ 4.1%, 76% $\pm$ 3.2% and 73% $\pm$ 2%) than the control mice (66% $\pm$ 4%). These results reveal that PSE, FO and MPF enhance the learning ability of mice *in vivo*.

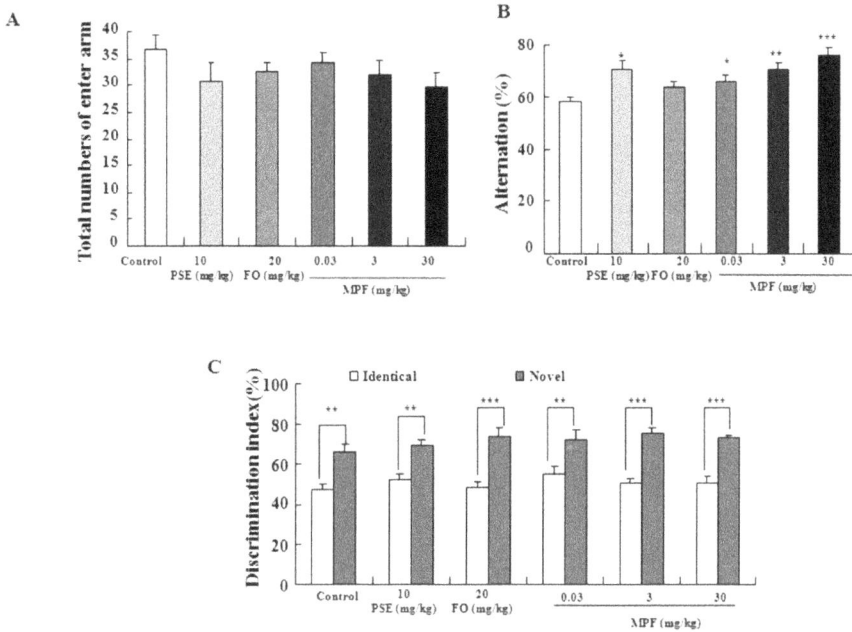

Figure 2. Effects of PSE, FO, and MPF on the learning and memory of mice *in vivo*. (**A**) changes in total numbers of enter arm; (**B**) alternation in the Y-maze test after treating PSE, FO and MPF; (**C**) change in cognitive index in the novel object recognition test after treating PSE, FO and MPF. Y maze and NOR tests were performed after sample administration for five weeks. Each value represents the mean $\pm$ SEM of eight or seven mice. *, ** and *** indicate significant difference relative to the control group at the same time point at $p < 0.05$, $p < 0.01$ and $p < 0.001$, respectively.

To further evaluate spatial memory, the water maze test was used to assess the training over four days using the hidden platform. A probe trial was conducted without a platform on the fifth day. PSE, FO and MPF did not significantly affect the latency time before training for two days. The latency time significantly reduced in the MPF groups at doses of 3 mg/kg on the second (19.88 $\pm$ 2.71) and fourth training day (10.86 $\pm$ 1.64) compared with that in the control group at the same time point (38.59 $\pm$ 6.84, 50.5 $\pm$ 8.3, $p < 0.05$, $p < 0.001$) (Figure 3A). At the same time, the significant reduction of latency time in PSE group was also observed on the fourth training day (28.09 $\pm$ 3.10, $p < 0.05$). The crossing platform times in the PSE at 10 mg/kg and MPF-treated groups at 3 and 30 mg/kg (5.3 $\pm$ 0.7, 6.0 $\pm$ 0.7 and 5.5 $\pm$ 0.8) also significantly increased on the fifth day in the probe trial *versus* the control (2.8 $\pm$ 0.8, $p < 0.05$ and $p < 0.01$) (Figure 3B). These results indicate that MPF can improve the learning ability and spatial memory of normal mice.

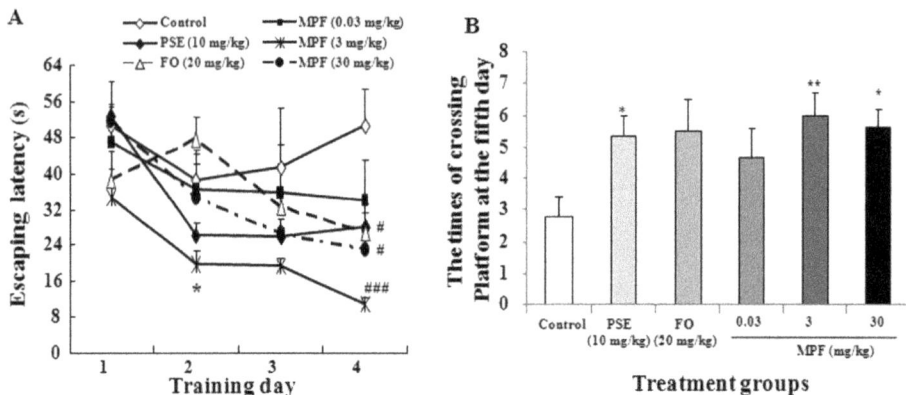

Figure 3. Effects of PSE, FO, and MPF on the spatial memory of mice *in vivo*. (**A**) Escape latency of mice during the training period in water maze test after administrating PSE, FO and MPF; (**B**) Times of crossing platform after training for 4 days in water maze test after administering PSE, FO and MPF. Water maze test was conducted after sample administration for 5 weeks. Each value represents the mean ± SEM of eight or seven mice. [#] and [###] indicate significant difference relative to the control at the same time point at $p < 0.05$ and $p < 0.001$; [*] and [**] indicate significant difference relative to the control at the same time point at $p < 0.05$ and $p < 0.01$, respectively.

3.3. MPF Can Rescue SOD Activity Reduction and Reduce MDA Production Induced by FO in the Plasma

The changes in SOD activity and MDA level in the plasma after administering MPF, PSE, and FO are displayed in Figure 4A,B. The total SOD activity of the FO group (42.8 ± 1.62) was lower than that of the control group (48.8 ± 1.0, $p < 0.05$). However, the reduction in SOD activity in the FO group can be alleviated by adding PSE to FO (MPF) (47.7 ± 0.8, 48.6 ± 0.9; $p < 0.05$, $p < 0.05$, respectively). The MDA level increased in the plasma of the FO group (5.6 ± 0.5) and reduced in the plasma of the PSE group (2.7 ± 0.3), respectively, compared with that in the control group (4.2 ± 0.1, $p < 0.05$, $p < 0.05$, respectively). The plasma MDA level in the MPF groups at 3 and 30 mg/kg (4.8 ± 0.3, 4.1 ± 0.4) was normalized. These results suggest that using a single FO can induce oxidative stress *in vivo* and that PSE can inhibit the oxidative stress caused by FO.

3.4. MPF Increases SOD Activity and Lowers MDA Production in the Cerebral Cortex and Hippocampus

Oxidative stress in the brain impairs the memory and learning ability of mice. Therefore, we also investigated changes in SOD activity and MDA level in the cerebral cortex and hippocampus after treatment. In the cortex, no difference in SOD activity was observed in the FO-treated group (19.3 ± 1.2). However, SOD activity increased in the PSE (23.0 ± 1.2) and MPF groups at 3 and 30 mg/kg (23.8 ± 0.7, 23 ± 0.6) compared with that in the control group (19.4 ± 1.1) (Figure 5A, $p < 0.05$, $p < 0.05$, $p < 0.05$, respectively). The MDA level was significantly lower in the PSE and MPF groups (2.7 ± 0.6, 2.7 ± 0.5, 3.4 ± 0.7) compared with that in the control group (6.8 ± 0.7) (Figure 5B, $p < 0.05$, $p < 0.01$ and $p < 0.01$, respectively). The MDA level in the FO group (4.6 ± 1.0) was decreased but showed no statistically significant differences. In the hippocampus, SOD activity was also significantly increased in PSE (30.7 ± 1.17) and MPF groups at 3 and 30 mg/kg (29.26 ± 0.79, 29.57 ± 0.58) compared with that in the control group (26.1 ± 0.81) (Figure 5C, $p < 0.05$, $p < 0.05$ and $p < 0.05$). The MDA level of the FO group (3.44 ± 0.29) was significantly increased (Figure 5D, $p < 0.05$). Meanwhile, the MDA levels in the PSE and MPF groups at 3 and 30 mg/kg (1.65 ± 0.18, 1.08 ± 0.1, 1.12 ± 0.06) were significantly lowered compared with that of the control group (2.56 ± 0.20) (Figure 5D, $p < 0.01$, $p < 0.001$ and $p < 0.001$, respectively). These results indicate that MPF improves the memory and learning ability of mice by reducing oxidative stress.

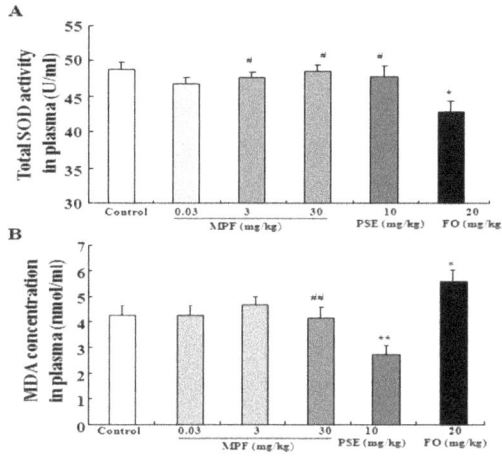

Figure 4. Effects of PSE, FO, and MPF on the SOD activity and MDA level of the plasma. Effects of PSE, FO, and MPF on the SOD activity (**A**) and MDA level (**B**) of the plasma after oral administration of PSE, FO, and MPF for six weeks. Each value represents the mean $\pm$ SEM of eight or seven mice. *, ** indicates significant difference relative to the control group at the same time point at $p < 0.05$ and $p < 0.01$; # and ## indicates significant difference relative to the FO group at the same time point at $p < 0.05$ and $p < 0.01$, respectively.

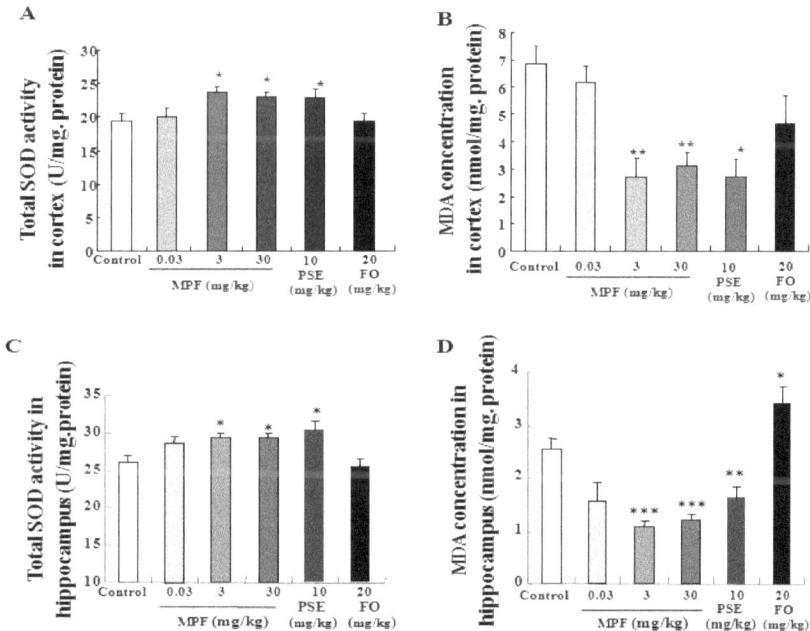

Figure 5. Effects of PSE, FO, and MPF on the SOD activity and MDA level of the cerebral cortex and hippocampus. Effects of PSE, FO, and MPF on the SOD activity and MDA level of the cerebral cortex (**A**, **B**) and hippocampus (**C**, **D**) after oral treatment for six weeks. Each value represents the mean $\pm$ SEM of eight or seven mice. *, ** and *** indicate significant difference relative to the control at the same time point at $p < 0.05$, $p < 0.01$ and $p < 0.001$, respectively.

3.5. MPF Increases BDNF and CREB Gene Expression Levels in the Cerebral Cortex and the Hippocampus

The gene expression levels of BDNF, CREB, ARC, and BCL-X1 in the cerebral cortex are displayed in Figure 6A. MPF did not affect the mRNA expression levels of CREB, ARC, and BCL-X1 in the cerebral cortex. Only BDNF gene expression was significantly increased in the cerebral cortex ($p < 0.05$). However, changes in both BDNF and CREB gene expression levels were observed in the hippocampus (Figure 6B, $p < 0.05$, $p < 0.01$ and $p < 0.001$). These results suggest that MPF can promote the expression of genes related to memory and learning ability in the hippocampus.

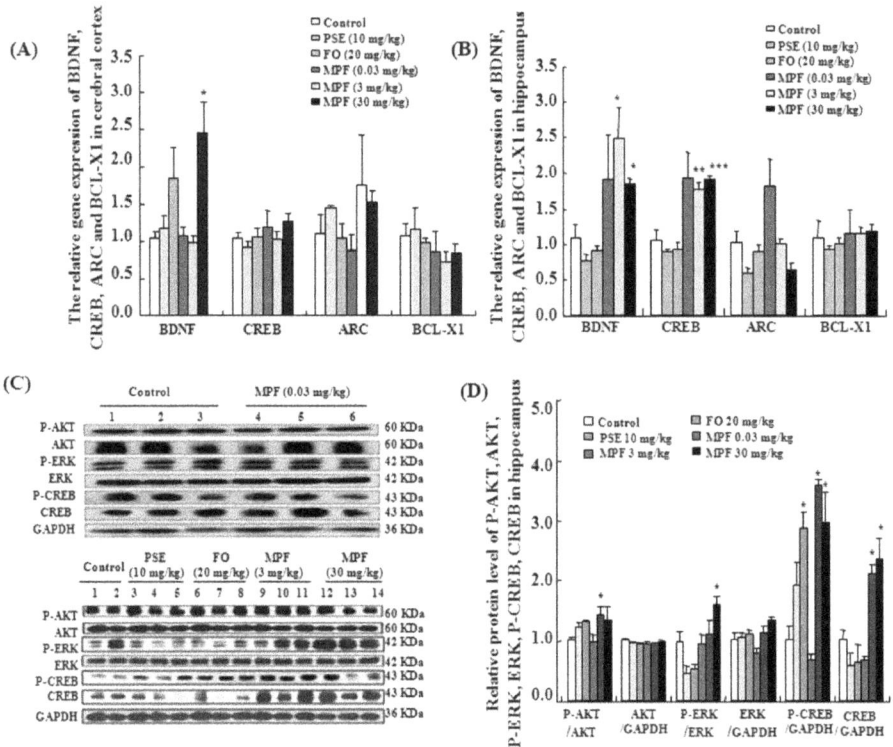

Figure 6. Effects of PSE, FO, and MPF on gene expression, and Western blot analysis in the cerebral cortex and hippocampus. Effects of PSE, FO, and MPF on expression of CREB, BDNF, ARC, and BCL-X1 in the cerebral cortex (**A**) and the hippocampus (**B**), and phosphorylation of AKT, ERK, and CREB proteins in the hippocampus (**C** and **D**). Each value represents mean ± SEM of seven mice. *, ** and *** indicate significant difference relative to the control at the same time point at $p < 0.05$, $p < 0.01$ and $p < 0.001$, respectively.

3.6. MPF Increases Phosphorylation of AKT, ERK and CREB in the Hippocampus

The hippocampus is critically important for memory and learning. It receives sensory information from the five senses and adjusts endocrine activity. Therefore, we investigated phosphorylation of AKT, ERK, and CREB proteins related to memory and learning in the hippocampus. Phosphorylation of AKT, ERK and CREB was found to be significantly increased in the MPF groups (Figure 6C,D, $p < 0.05$, $p < 0.05$ and $p < 0.05$, respectively). These results suggest that MPF may improve the memory and learning ability of mice via the ERK signaling pathway.

4. Discussion

This report demonstrated that PSE, FO and MFP had NGF-mimicking effects on PC12 cells (Figure 1A,B). It is consistent with our previous study [20]. Furthermore, we found that MPF and PSE can enhance both learning and special memory of mice (Figures 2 and 3). However, FO alone can improve the learning ability but not the spatial memory of normal mice (Figures 2 and 3). This result agreed with other reports [24].

In this study, the effects of MPF did not display a dose-dependent relationship; it is possible that normal mice were used to do experiments since we mainly considered the health functions of MPF for healthy people. The index of normal mice was difficult to change by a large margin. Thus, we will investigate the treatment effects of MPF with a pathological model in the future.

Oxidative stress has been implicated in the pathogenesis of dementia and neurodegenerative disorders. Moreover, increases in reactive oxygen species have been implicated in cognitive decline of the aging brain and in AD [25–27]. SOD and MDA are closely related to the redox state of an organism. MDA is a lipid peroxide product that indicates aging. Therefore, we focus on these two points to investigate the mechanisms of action of FO, PSE, and MPF in this study. Administration of FO alone for six weeks significantly reduced SOD activity and increased MDA level in the plasma (Figure 4). These results agree with previous reports [28]. As expected, MPF alleviated this symptom and normalized the MDA level. These results indicate that FO induces oxidative stress after long-term administration *in vivo* and that adding PSE can alleviate the side effects of FO. The observed an increase in SOD activity and reduction of MDA production in the cerebral cortex and hippocampus (Figure 5), after treating the samples suggested that long-term administration of FO alone cannot confer neuroprotection *in vivo* and that PSE can alleviate the side effects of FO. MPF and PSE can also significantly improve the memory of mice via anti-oxidative effects.

Memory is known to be regulated by key genes such as BDNF, CREB and ARC. BDNF and CREB participate in memory formation and storage [29–32]. ARC is an immediate early gene that mediates consolidation of long-term potentiation by altering actin dynamics [30]. Increasing BDNF, CREB, and ARC levels enhance some forms of long-lasting memory. Our observation of elevated expression of BDNF and CREB in the hippocampus (Figure 6B) suggests that BDNF/CREB signaling pathways may have important roles in the enhanced intelligence of MPF-treated mice. We used normal mice in this study, and sensitivity to MPF in the hippocampus was higher than that in the cerebral cortex. PI3K/AKT-signaling pathway is also important for spatial and working memory and amygdala-dependent fear conditioning, whereas the ERK1/2 cascade is involved in an aversively motivated hippocampus and amygdala-dependent learning tasks [33–35]. Thus, we investigated the phosphorylation of AKT, ERK, and CREB proteins in the hippocampus using Western blot analysis. The significant increase in the phosphorylation of AKT, ERK and CREB (Figure 6C) indicates that the ERK signaling pathway is also involved in improving the memory of MPF-treated mice.

5. Conclusions

In conclusion, FO and PSE exhibited NGF-mimicking effects on PC12 cells and improved the learning ability of normal mice. PSE alleviated the side effects of FO produced in the body after long-term administration, and MPF significantly improved the learning ability and spatial memory of mice via modulation of anti-oxidative stress and regulation of BDNF/ERK/CREB signaling pathways.

Acknowledgments: This study is supported in part by International Science and Technology Cooperation Program of China (No. 2014DFG326900), and the Qinglan Plan of Hangzhou, Zhejiang Province, China (Grant No. 20131831k94). All authors read and approved the final manuscript.

Author Contributions: Xueli Cao, Tianyan Xing, Daisuke Mori, Ruiqi Tang, Jing Li and Lijuan Gao conducted the research and analyzed the data; Lan Xiang guided research and wrote the manuscript; Jianhua Qi contributed to the experimental design.

Conflicts of Interest: There are no conflicts of interest.

Abbreviations

The following abbreviations are used in this article:

AD	Alzheimer's disease
AKT	Protein kinase B
ARC	Activity-regulated cytoskeleton-associated protein
BCL-X1	B-cell lymphoma-X1
BDNF	Brain derived-neurophic factor
CREB	cAMP responsive element-binding protein
DHA	Docosahexaenoic acid
DI	Discrimination index
DMSO	Dimethyl sulfoxide
EPA	Eicosapentaenoic acid
ERK	Extracellular signal-regulated kinase
FO	Fish oil
ICR	Institute of Cancer Research
MAPK	Mitogen-activated protein kinase
MDA	Malonyldialdehyde
MPF	Mixture of peanut skin extract and fish oil
NGF	Nerve growth factor
NOR	Novel object recognition
PC12 cells	Rat pheochromocytoma cells
PSE	Peanut skin extract
RT	Room temperature
SOD	Superoxide dismutase

References

1. Schirmer, S.H.; Werner, C.M.; Binder, S.B.; Faas, M.E.; Custodis, F.; Böhm, M.; Laufs, U. Effects of omega-3 fatty acids on postprandial triglycerides and monocyte activation. *Atherosclerosis* **2012**, *225*, 166–172. [CrossRef] [PubMed]

2. Cole, G.M.; Lim, G.P.; Yang, F.; Teter, B.; Begum, A.; Ma, Q.; Harris-White, M.E.; Frautschy, S.A. Prevention of Alzheimer's disease: Omega-3 fatty acid and phenolic anti-oxidant interventions. *Neurobiol. Aging* **2005**, *26*, 133S–136S. [CrossRef] [PubMed]

3. Im, D.S. Omega-3 fatty acids in anti-inflammation (pro-resolution) and GPCRs. *Prog. Lipid Res.* **2012**, *51*, 232–237. [CrossRef] [PubMed]

4. Iagher, F.; de Brito Belo, S.R.; Souza, W.M.; Nunes, J.R.; Naliwaiko, K.; Sassaki, G.L.; Bonatto, S.J.; de Oliveira, H.H.; Brito, G.A.; de Lima, C.; *et al.* Anti-tumor and anti-cachectic effects of shark liver oil and fish oil: Comparison between independent or associative chronic supplementation in walker 256 tumor-bearing rats. *Lipids Health Dis.* **2013**, *12*, 146. [CrossRef] [PubMed]

5. Ishida, S. Lifestyle-related diseases and anti-aging ophthalmology: Suppression of retinal and choroidal pathologies by inhibiting renin-angiotensin system and inflammation. *Nihon Ganka Gakkai Zasshi* **2009**, *113*, 403–422. [PubMed]

6. Albert, B.B.; Cameron-Smith, D.; Hofman, P.L.; Cutfield, W.S. Oxidation of marine omega-3 supplements and human health. *Biomed. Res. Int.* **2013**, *2013*, 464921. [CrossRef] [PubMed]

7. Liu, X.; Shibata, T.; Hisaka, S.; Kawai, Y.; Osawa, T. DHA hydroperoxides as a potential inducer of neuronal cell death: A mitochondrial dysfunction-mediated pathway. *J. Clin. Biochem. Nutr.* **2008**, *43*, 26–33. [CrossRef] [PubMed]

8. Enns, J.E.; Yeganeh, A.; Zarychanski, R.; Abou-Setta, A.M.; Friesen, C.; Zahraska, P.; Taylor, C.G. The impact of omega-3 polyunsaturated fatty acid supplementation on the incidence of cardiovascular events and complications in peripheral arterial disease: A systematic review and meta-analysis. *BMC Cardiovasc. Disord.* **2014**, *14*, 70. [CrossRef] [PubMed]

9. Morrison, C.D.; Pistell, P.J.; Ingram, D.K.; Johnson, W.D.; Liu, Y.; Fernandez-Kim, S.O.; White, C.L.; Purpera, M.N.; Uranga, R.M.; Bruce-Keller, A.J.; *et al.* High fat diet increases hippocampal oxidative

stress and cognitive impairment in aged mice: Implications for decreased Nrf2 signaling. *J. Neurochem.* **2010**, *114*, 1581–1589. [CrossRef] [PubMed]

10. Greenwood, C.E.; Winocur, G. High-fat diets, insulin resistance and declining cognitive function. *Neurobiol. Aging* **2005**, *26*, S42–S45. [CrossRef] [PubMed]

11. Pistell, P.J.; Morrison, C.D.; Gupta, S.; Knight, A.G.; Keller, J.N.; Ingram, D.K.; Bruce-Keller, A.J. Cognitive impairment following high fat diet consumption is associated with brain inflammation. *J. Neuroimmunol.* **2010**, *219*, 25–32. [CrossRef] [PubMed]

12. Sanders, T.H.; McMichael, R.W.; Hendrix, K.W., Jr. Occurrence of resveratrol in edible peanuts. *J. Agric. Food Chem.* **2000**, *48*, 1243–1246. [CrossRef] [PubMed]

13. Georgiev, V.; Ananga, A.; Tsolova, V. Recent advances and uses of grape flavonoids as nutraceuticals. *Nutrients* **2014**, *6*, 391–415. [CrossRef] [PubMed]

14. Khan, N.; Khymenets, O.; Urpí-Sardà, M.; Tulipani, S.; Garcia-Aloy, M.; Monagas, M.; Mora-Cubillos, X.; Llorach, R.; Andres-Lacueva, C. Cocoa polyphenols and inflammatory markers of cardiovascular disease. *Nutrients* **2014**, *6*, 844–880. [CrossRef] [PubMed]

15. Ravishankar, D.; Rajora, A.K.; Greco, F.; Osborn, H.M. Flavonoids as prospective compounds for anti-cancer therapy. *Int. J. Biochem. Cell Biol.* **2013**, *45*, 2821–2831. [CrossRef] [PubMed]

16. Oršolić, N.; Sirovina, D.; Gajski, G.; Garaj-Vrhovac, V.; JazvinšćakJembrek, M.; Kosalec, I. Assessment of DNA damage and lipid peroxidation in diabetic mice: Effects of propolis and epigallocatechingallate (EGCG). *Mutat. Res.* **2013**, *757*, 36–44. [CrossRef] [PubMed]

17. Cordero-Herrera, I.; Martín, M.Á.; Goya, L.; Ramos, S. Cocoa flavonoids attenuate high glucose-induced insulin signalling blockade and modulate glucose uptake and production in human HepG2 cells. *Food Chem. Toxicol.* **2014**, *64*, 10–19. [CrossRef] [PubMed]

18. Sarnoski, P.J.; Johnson, J.V.; Reed, K.A.; Tanko, J.M.; O'Keefe, S.F. Separation and characterization of proanthocyanidins in Virginia type peanut skins by LC-MS. *Food Chem.* **2012**, *131*, 927–939. [CrossRef]

19. Bansode, R.R.; Randolph, P.; Hurley, S.; Ahmedna, M. Evaluation of hypolipidemic effects of peanut skin-derived polyphenols in rats on a western-diet. *Food Chem.* **2012**, *135*, 1659–1666. [CrossRef] [PubMed]

20. Catalan, U.; Fernandez-Castillejo, S.; Angles, N.; Morello, J.R.; Yebras, M.; Solà, R. Inhibition of the transcription factor c-Jun by the MAPK family, and not the NF-κB pathway, suggests that peanut extract has anti-inflammatory properties. *Mol. Immunol.* **2012**, *52*, 125–132. [CrossRef] [PubMed]

21. Gao, L.J.; Xiang, L.; Luo, Y.; Wang, G.F.; Li, J.Y.; Qi, J.H. Gentisides C.-K: Nine new neuritogenic compounds from the traditional Chinese medicine *Gentiana rigescens* Franch. *Bioorg. Med. Chem.* **2010**, *18*, 6995–7000. [CrossRef] [PubMed]

22. Beppe, G.J.; Dongmo, A.B.; Foyet, H.S.; Tsabang, N.; Olteanu, Z.; Cioanca, O.; Hancianu, M.; Dimo, T.; Hritcu, L. Memory-enhancing activities of the aqueous extract of *Albiziaadianthifolia*leaves in the 6-hydroxydopamine-lesion rodent model of Parkinson's disease. *BMC Complement. Altern. Med.* **2014**, *14*, 142. [CrossRef] [PubMed]

23. Sun, K.Y.; Yang, W.; Huang, Y.N.; Wang, Y.F.; Xiang, L.; Qi, J.H. Leu452His mutation in lipoprotein lipase gene transfer associated with hypertriglyceridemia in mice *in vivo*. *PLoS ONE* **2013**, *8*, e75462. [CrossRef] [PubMed]

24. Hashimoto, M.; Katakura, M.; Tanabe, Y. *n*-3 fatty acids effectively improve the reference memory-related learning ability associated with increased brain docosahexaenoic acid-derived docosanoids in aged rats. *Biochim. Biophys. Acta* **2015**, *1851*, 203–209. [CrossRef] [PubMed]

25. Jeong, E.J.; Lee, K.Y.; Kim, S.H.; Sung, S.H.; Kim, Y.C. Cognitive-enhancing and antioxidant activities of iridoid glycosides from *Scrophularia buergeriana* in scopolamine-treated mice. *Eur. J. Pharmacol.* **2008**, *588*, 78–84. [CrossRef] [PubMed]

26. Sano, M.; Ernesto, C.; Thomas, R.G.; Klauber, M.R.; Schafer, K.; Grundman, M. A controlled trial of selegiline, alpha-to copherol, or both as treatment for Alzheimer's disease. The Alzheimer's Disease Cooperative Study. *N. Engl. J. Med.* **1997**, *336*, 1216–1222. [CrossRef] [PubMed]

27. Nade, V.S.; Kanhere, S.V.; Kawale, L.A.; Yadav, A.V. Cognitive enhancing and antioxidant activity of ethyl acetate soluble fraction of the methanol extract of *Hibiscus rosa sinensis* in scopolamine-induced amnesia. *Indian J. Pharmacol.* **2011**, *43*, 137–142. [CrossRef] [PubMed]

28. Piche, L.A.; Draper, H.H.; Cole, P.D. Malondialdehyde excretion by subjects consuming cod liver oil *vs.* a concentrate of *n*-3 fatty acids. *Lipids* **1988**, *23*, 370–371. [CrossRef] [PubMed]

29. Bekinschtein, P.; Cammarota, M.; Katche, C.; Slipczuk, L.; Rossato, J.I.; Goldin, A.; Izquierdo, I.; Medina, J.H. BDNF is essential to promote persistence of long-term memory storage. *Proc. Natl. Acad. Sci. USA* **2008**, *105*, 2711–2716. [CrossRef] [PubMed]

30. Restivo, L.; Vetere, G.; Bontempi, B.; Ammassari-Teule, M. The formation of recent and remote memory is associated with time-dependent formation of dendritic spines in the hippocampus and anterior cingulate cortex. *J. Neurosci.* **2009**, *29*, 8206–8214. [CrossRef] [PubMed]

31. Bramham, C.R.; Alme, M.N.; Bittins, M.; Kuipers, S.D.; Nair, R.R.; Pai, B.; Panja, D.; Schubert, M.; Soule, J.; Tiron, A.; *et al.* The Arc of synaptic memory. *Exp. Brain Res.* **2010**, *200*, 125–140. [CrossRef] [PubMed]

32. Kong, L.B.; Yang, Z.Y.; An, R.; Ding, S.H. Effects of special brain area cerebral blood flow abnormal perfusion on learning and memory function and its molecular mechanism in rats. *Front. Biol. China* **2008**, *3*, 147–153. [CrossRef]

33. Alonso, M.; Medina, J.H.; Pozzo-Miller, L. ERK1/2 activation is necessary for BDNF to increase dendritic spine density in hippocampal CA1 pyramidal neurons. *Learn. Mem.* **2004**, *11*, 172–178. [CrossRef] [PubMed]

34. Mizuno, M.; Yamada, K.; Olariu, A.; Nawa, H.; Nabeshima, T. Involvement of brain-derived neuotrophic factor in spatial memory formation and maintenance in a radial arm maze test in rats. *J. Neurosci.* **2000**, *20*, 7116–7121. [PubMed]

35. Ou, L.C.; Gean, P.W. Regulation of amygdata-dependent learning by brain-derived neurotrophic factor is mediated by extracellular signal-regulated kinase and phosphatidyliostiol-3-kinase. *Neuopsychopharmacology* **2006**, *31*, 287–296. [CrossRef] [PubMed]

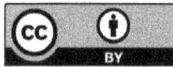

nutrients

MDPI

Article

Impact of Food Components on in vitro Calcitonin Gene-Related Peptide Secretion—A Potential Mechanism for Dietary Influence on Migraine

Margaret Slavin [1,*], Julia Bourguignon [1], Kyle Jackson [1] and Michael-Angelo Orciga [2]

[1] Department of Nutrition and Food Studies, George Mason University, 4400 University Drive, MS 1F8, Fairfax, VA 22030, USA; jbourgu@gmail.com (J.B.); kjacks21@masonlive.gmu.edu (K.J.)
[2] School of Systems Biology, George Mason University, 4400 University Drive, MS 3E1, Fairfax, VA 22030, USA; michaelangelo.orciga@gmail.com
* Correspondence: mslavin@gmu.edu; Tel.: +1-703-993-6106

Received: 16 May 2016; Accepted: 27 June 2016; Published: 1 July 2016

Abstract: Calcitonin gene-related peptide (CGRP) is a pivotal messenger in the inflammatory process in migraine. Limited evidence indicates that diet impacts circulating levels of CGRP, suggesting that certain elements in the diet may influence migraine outcomes. Interruption of calcium signaling, a mechanism which can trigger CGRP release, has been suggested as one potential route by which exogenous food substances may impact CGRP secretion. The objective of this study was to investigate the effects of foods and a dietary supplement on two migraine-related mechanisms in vitro: CGRP secretion from neuroendocrine CA77 cells, and calcium uptake by differentiated PC12 cells. Ginger and grape pomace extracts were selected for their anecdotal connections to reducing or promoting migraine. S-petasin was selected as a suspected active constituent of butterbur extract, the migraine prophylactic dietary supplement. Results showed a statistically significant decrease in stimulated CGRP secretion from CA77 cells following treatment with ginger (0.2 mg dry ginger equivalent/mL) and two doses of grape pomace (0.25 and 1.0 mg dry pomace equivalent/mL) extracts. Relative to vehicle control, CGRP secretion decreased by 22%, 43%, and 87%, respectively. S-petasin at 1.0 µM also decreased CGRP secretion by 24%. Meanwhile, S-petasin and ginger extract showed inhibition of calcium influx, whereas grape pomace had no effect on calcium. These results suggest that grape pomace and ginger extracts, and S-petasin may have anti-inflammatory propensity by preventing CGRP release in migraine, although potentially by different mechanisms, which future studies may elucidate further.

Keywords: calcitonin gene-related peptide; migraine; food trigger; calcium; grape pomace; ginger; butterbur; petasin

1. Introduction

Migraine is a complex primary headache condition that affects 17% of American women and 5.6% of men annually [1]. Worldwide, migraine is responsible for half of all neurological disease-induced disability [2]. Suggestions abound regarding the potential connection between food and migraine, but valid scientific evidence on the subject remains limited.

The current pathophysiological understanding of migraine entails over-sensitization of the brain, which produces a painful response to otherwise normal stimuli, in combination with an inflammatory response. A key inflammatory mediator in neurogenic inflammation of migraine is calcitonin gene-related peptide (CGRP). The connections of CGRP to migraine are numerous. Fibers originating in the trigeminal ganglion terminate in the dura where they release CGRP, and this connection is thought to be central to the genesis of migraine pain [3]. Elevated CGRP levels have been detected in the serum of migraineurs [4,5] and at higher levels in individuals with chronic migraine than in episodic migraineurs [6]; CGRP is capable of precipitating migraine in prone individuals [7]; and sumatriptan, a pharmaceutical intervention used to abort migraine, has been shown to decrease CGRP levels concomitant with symptom relief [8]. Sumatriptan is primarily classified as a 5-HT$_1$ (serotonin) receptor agonist, but has also demonstrated inhibition of action potential signaling by inhibiting N-type Ca^{2+} channels in CGRP fibers [3]. Calcium influx upon depolarization is a fundamental signaling mechanism which, among a host of other functions, stimulates the release of CGRP.

Several lines of evidence indicate that food intake may be capable of altering CGRP levels [9–12], suggesting a potential mechanistic link between diet and migraine whereby some component of food may modulate expression and/or release of CGRP. Conversely, intraperitoneal administration of CGRP is also shown to induce a short term reduction in food intake likely resulting from cAMP/PKA (cyclic adenosine monophosphate/protein kinase A) pathway activation [13]. Foods or components whose ingestion results in a decrease of CGRP would be hypothesized to reduce migraine, whereas those which increase CGRP would be expected to increase migraine.

This project sought to improve our understanding of the potential mechanisms by which grape pomace and ginger may impact migraine. These foods were chosen because of anecdotal connections to migraine. Ginger is renowned for its anti-inflammatory abilities, while anecdotal evidence and traditional medicine connect it with anti-migraine abilities. Grape is viewed suspiciously because of the common belief that red wine triggers migraine events, while the naturally present phenolic compounds have anti-inflammatory qualities. Meanwhile, we have also included a pure compound in our investigations: *S*-petasin is believed to be an active component in the butterbur dietary supplement, which is classified as having "established efficacy" for the prophylaxis of migraine, as reviewed by the American Academy of Neurology and the American Headache Society [14]. Nonetheless, the potential of these foods and supplement for impacting biomechanisms related to migraine have not been sufficiently investigated. We have prepared extractions of ground dried ginger root and two varieties of grape pomace, and tested purified *S*-petasin and these extractions in cell culture models to investigate their ability to modulate CGRP secretion and calcium signaling.

2. Materials and Methods

2.1. Materials

Solvents—methanol, ethanol, acetone, DMSO (dimethyl sulfoxide), and ultrapure water—and syringe filters were obtained through Fisher Scientific (Pittsburgh, PA, USA). Cell culture media and reagents were purchased from Life Technologies (Grand Island, NY, USA), including fetal bovine serum, horse serum, trypsin-EDTA (ethylenediaminetetraacetic acid), HEPES (4-(2-hydroxyethyl)- 1-piperazineethanesulfonic acid) buffer, HBSS (Hank's balanced salt solution) buffer, penicillin-streptomycin, and Lipofectamine 2000. Poly-D-lysine for cell culture adherence was produced by MP Biomedicals (Santa Ana, CA, USA). Methylene blue, glutaraldehyde, Type I Collagen, nerve growth factor, and *S*-petasin (>98% pure) were obtained through Sigma Aldrich (St. Louis, MO, USA). CGRP enzyme immunoassay kits were produced by Bertin Pharma (Montigny le Bretonneux, France) and purchased through Cayman Chemicals. The GCaMP5 plasmid was provided courtesy of Dr. Nadine Kabbani lab at George Mason University, Fairfax, VA, USA. GCAMP5 is a genetically encoded calcium indicator, originated by Janelia Research (Ashburn, VA, USA). Grape pomace samples from Chrysalis Vineyards (Middleburg, VA, USA) were obtained through Dr. John Parry, formerly at the Agricultural Research Station at Virginia State University (Petersburg, VA, USA). Dried, sliced ginger root was obtained commercially through Penzeys Spices (Wauwatosa, WI, USA).

2.2. Extractions

Dried, sliced ginger root was ground in a standard coffee grinder to pass through a 40-mesh sieve, to select for particles of size 0.420 mm or smaller. Ground ginger was extracted at a ratio of 1 g in 10 mL 100% methanol [15]. After 24 h, the combination was centrifuged, liquid extract transferred to a clean tube, and the extraction was repeated twice. The three fractions were combined, filtered with a 0.45 μm nylon syringe filter and evaporated under nitrogen gas stream. Each extraction was performed in triplicate. Average percent yield by weight was 13.1% ± 0.2%.

Two varieties of dried grape pomace (*Tinta cao* and *Cabernet franc*) were ground in a standard coffee grinder to pass through a 40-mesh sieve, to select for particles of size 0.420 mm or smaller. Ground pomace was extracted at a ratio of 1 g in 10 mL solvent (50:50, acetone:water, *v*/*v*) [16,17]. Tubes were vortexed to mix. After 24 h, the combination was centrifuged and the liquid extract transferred to a clean tube, and partially evaporated under nitrogen gas stream, followed by lyophilization to remove water. Each extraction was performed in triplicate.

Dried extracts were stored at −20 °C until further use. Immediately prior to use, extracts were dissolved in DMSO for cell treatments. For cell assays, concentrations of treatments are expressed as mg equivalents of original pomace extracted per mL of cell treatment media (mg PE/mL) or mg dry ginger extracted per mL of cell treatment media (mg PE (pomace equivalent)/mL or mg equivalent/mL).

2.3. Cell Culture Maintenance

The CA77 rat medullary thyroid carcinoma cell line is an in vitro model used to study the modulation of CGRP levels. CA77 cells are neuroendocrine, having originated from the neural crest and retaining neuronal tendencies. Specifically, the cells express a high ratio of CGRP mRNA (90%) relative to the alternately spliced calcitonin mRNA. CA77 cells were received from Dr. Andrew Russo, Department of Molecular Physiology and Biophysics, University of Iowa, Iowa City, IA, USA. CA77 cells are now available through the ATCC repository (Manassas, VA, USA) as product number CRL-3234. Cells were maintained on laminin-coated plates with a DMEM-F12 (Dulbecco's Modified Eagle Medium-Nutrient Mixture F-12) base media, containing 10% fetal bovine serum, 10 mM HEPES, and 50 units/mL penicillin/streptomycin. CA77 cells were passaged via trypsin-EDTA incubation.

Meanwhile, PC-12 cells are rat adrenal pheochromocytoma cells used as a model for sympathetic neurons due to the presence of Ca^{2+} transporters. PC-12 cells are available for purchase from the ATCC repository (Manassas, VA, USA) as product number CRL-1721. PC-12 cells were maintained on collagen-coated plates with a low-glucose DMEM base media, containing 10% horse serum, 5% fetal bovine serum, 10 mM HEPES, and 50 units/mL penicillin/streptomycin. PC-12 cells were passaged by the cell scraping technique. All cells were maintained under humidity at 37 °C, 5% CO_2.

2.4. Cytotoxicity Assay

To determine appropriate doses for further testing, several doses of the grape extracts and spice extracts were tested for cytotoxicity via the Methylene Blue Assay according to a previously published protocol [18]. In short, cells were exposed to treatments for 24 h in a 96-well plate, after which the viable cells were fixed to the plate with glutaraldehyde and dyed with methylene blue. Subsequently, the plate was rinsed and developed by elution of the dye in ethanol. Absorbance at 570 nm was interpreted as representing a linear relationship with the number of viable cells.

2.5. CGRP Assay

CGRP secretion was measured in CA-77 cells according to a method previously reported, with modifications [10]. Cells were seeded in a 96-well, Advanced Tissue Culture coated plates (Greiner Bio-One, Monroe, NC, USA) at 70,000/well. After 24 h, media was removed by gentle aspiration and replaced with treatment solution for 1 h. All treatment solutions, including vehicle control contained 0.1% DMSO. Treatment was immediately followed by incubation with 50 mM KCl to stimulate release of CGRP. After 1 h, media was collected, diluted in buffer as necessary, and assayed for CGRP content using a commercial enzyme immunoassay (EIA) kit, according to manufacturer instructions (Bertin Pharma, Montigny le Bretonneux, France). Samples were diluted with assay buffer as needed to fall within the standard curve. Absorbance readings were taken at 410 nm on a Spectramax M3 multimode plate reader (Molecular Devices, Sunnyvale, CA, USA).

2.6. Calcium Influx

We used the transfected probe, GCaMP5, for measuring cytosolic calcium. The probe was transfected into PC-12 cells using lipofection via incubation of cells in the presence of GCaMP5-encoding plasmid and Lipofectamine 2000 reagent for 6 h, according to manufacturer instructions. Following transfection, cells were seeded on a poly-D-lysine coated glass-bottom, black-sided 96-well plate and incubated in regular growth media with 100 ng/mL nerve growth factor (NGF) for 48 h, to induce neuronal differentiation prior to stimulation and imaging. A Zeiss fluorescence microscope was used for imaging at room temperature with GFP (green fluorescent protein) filter with excitation/emission at 470/525 nm. After 48 h, NGF-containing media was removed by careful aspiration, and wells were immediately treated with 100 μL media with extract for 10 min prior to the calcium challenge. Fluorescence readings were then taken every 70 milliseconds for 50 s. After approximately 10 s of baseline readings, cells were challenged with KCl injection while readings continued, to a final concentration of 50 mM KCl. Image sequence data was processed using PhysImage, a fork of Image J open-source image processing software (imagej.nih.gov), manually selecting the cell body as the area of interest and using the Moving Average Filter set to a 5 frame average. A plot of change in fluorescence compared to baseline ($\Delta F/F_0$) versus time was produced. The maximum $\Delta F/F_0$ value, typically reached as a spike within the first 5 s after KCl injection, was used as an indicator of the extent of calcium influx upon KCl stimulation, and thus the treatment impact on calcium permeability. Vehicle controls were performed for each 96-well plate.

2.7. Statistical Analysis

Statistical analysis was conducted with SPSS for Windows (version 22, SPSS Inc., Chicago, IL, USA). Data in figures is reported as mean ± standard deviation. Differences in means were detected using one-way ANOVA and either Tukey's (dose comparison) or Dunnett's (comparison only to vehicle control) post hoc test. Statistical significance was defined at $P \leqslant 0.05$.

3. Results

3.1. Cytotoxicity Assay

The cytotoxicity assay successfully identified grape pomace extract, ginger extract, and purified S-petasin treatment doses which did not impact cell viability, and thus were acceptable for further testing. Results of the grape pomace cytotoxicity assay with CA-77 cells show that all doses of extracts at or below 1.0 mg equivalents/mL media did not impact cell viability ($P < 0.05$), as compared to the vehicle control (Figure 1). Higher doses could not be tested due to extract solubility and a DMSO solvent maximum of 0.1% total volume in the treatment media. In other words, grape pomace extracts were not toxic to cultured CA-77 cells at achievable doses. Results in PC-12 cells with solvent extractions followed the same pattern.

Meanwhile, ginger extract treatment doses at or below 0.2 mg equivalents/mL did not impact cell viability, and S-petasin treatments at 1 μM also produced no statistical difference. Higher doses of both treatments were observed to reduce cell viability (Figure 1b,c).

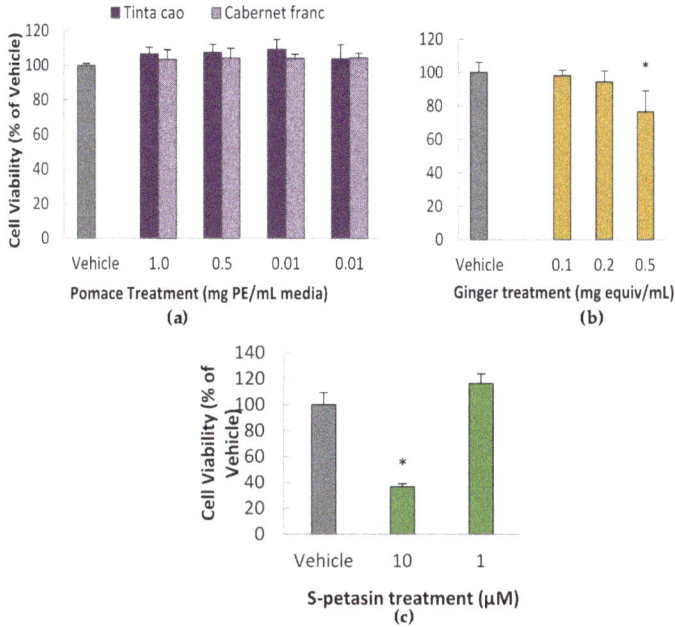

Figure 1. CA77 cell viability after 24-h treatment with extracts: (**a**) *Tinta cao* and *Cabernet franc* grape pomace extract treatments ($n = 8$), (**b**) Ginger root extract treatments ($n = 8$), and (**c**) purified *S*-petasin treatments ($n = 4$). PE = pomace equivalents. Results obtained via the Methylene Blue Cytotoxicity Assay. All treatments contain 0.1% DMSO (dimethyl sulfoxide), including vehicle. * Indicates a value statistically different from the vehicle ($P < 0.05$).

3.2. CGRP Secretion

The CGRP secretion assay demonstrated that grape pomace extracts, ginger extract, and purified *S*-petasin could inhibit CGRP secretion in CA77 cells at various doses. The high and medium dose of both grape pomace extracts produced a significant decrease in CGRP secretion by CA77 cells, upon a 1 h pre-treatment with the extracts. At a dose of 1.0 mg pomace equivalent/mL treatment, the *Tinta cao* extraction resulted in an 87% decrease in CGRP secretion (shown in Figure 2a), which was statistically significant as compared to vehicle control and the lower doses of *Tinta cao* extraction ($P < 0.05$). Varying the concentration produced a dose dependent response, where the medium dose of 0.25 mg PE/mL had approximately half the effect of the high dose, reducing CGRP secretion by 43%. The low *Tinta cao* dose of 0.1 mg PE/mL did not produce a significant change, as compared to the vehicle. *Cabernet franc* extraction treatments produced a similar response, decreasing CGRP secretion by 88% and 73% for the high and medium doses, respectively (Figure 2b). The lowest dose of *C. franc* did not produce a statistical difference in CGRP secretion.

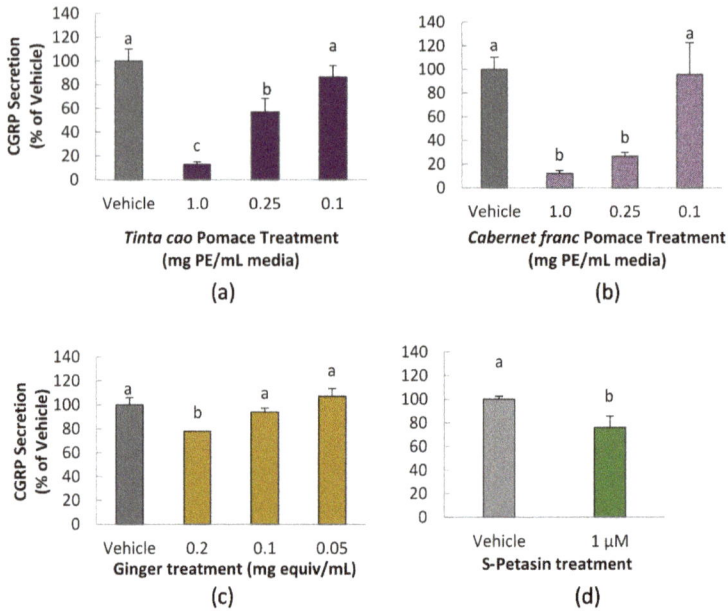

Figure 2. CGRP (Calcitonin gene-related peptide) secretion levels upon treatment with extracts: (a) *Tinta cao* grape pomace extract ($n = 6$), (b) *Cabernet franc* grape pomace extract ($n = 6$), (c) dried ginger root extract ($n = 9$), and (d) purified *S*-petasin ($n = 4$). CA-77 cells were treated for 1 h with extracts at specified final doses. All treatments contain 0.1% DMSO, including vehicle. Results obtained via commercial ELISA kit. Columns of the same sub-figure marked by the same letter are not statistically different ($P < 0.05$).

Upon 1 h pre-treatment with extracts, the high dose of ginger extract produced a significant decrease in CGRP secretion by CA77 cells. At a dose of 0.2 mg equivalent/mL treatment, the ginger methanol extraction resulted in a 22% decrease in CGRP secretion (shown in Figure 2a), which was statistically significant as compared to vehicle control and the lower doses of ginger methanol extracts. *S*-petasin was tested at only one dose of 1.0 μM, which did produce a significant decrease in CGRP secretion by 24%, as compared to the 0.1% DMSO vehicle.

3.3. Effect on Calcium Influx

The impact of treatments on acute KCl-stimulated calcium influx was measured using the fluorescent, genetically-encoded GCaMP5 calcium indicator and fluorescence microscopy. The data shows no statistical difference in maximum fluorescence between grape pomace treatment or the vehicle control (Table 1). Visual images of the observed progression before, immediately after, and 20 s after KCl stimulation are shown in Figure 3.

Table 1. Maximum change in GCaMP5 [1] fluorescence by treatment, relative to vehicle control.

Sample	Treatment Concentration	$\Delta F/F_0$ (% Vehicle) [2]	n	P
Tinta cao extract	1.0 mg PE/mL [3]	66.2 (55.7)	13	0.146
Cabernet franc extract	1.0 mg PE/mL [3]	76.8 (43.2)	14	0.365
Ginger extract	0.2 mg equivalent/mL	60.1 (23.9)	14	0.007
S-Petasin	10 μM	22.3 (8.4)	6	<0.001

[1] GCAMP5 is a genetically encoded calcium indicator originated by Janelia Research (Ashburn, VA, USA).
[2] Data shown as mean (SD); [3] PE = pomace equivalents. Vehicle control for all samples was 0.1% DMSO.

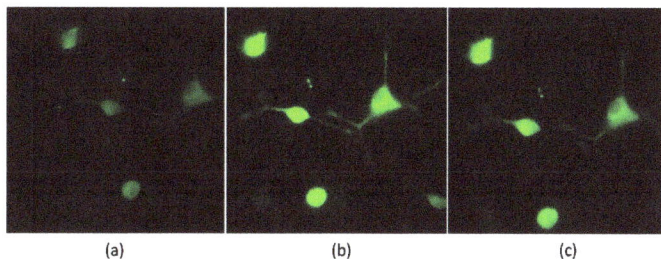

Figure 3. Time lapse of calcium-mediated fluorescence following KCl stimulation. Images depict the fluorescence in GCaMP5 transfected PC-12 cells pre-treated with 0.1% DMSO Vehicle. Images were taken (**a**) before, (**b**) immediately after, and (**c**) 20 s post-KCl injection. Final KCl concentration = 50 mM.

Given that no difference was detected for grape pomace extracts, it is expected that calcium channels remained unobstructed in the presence of these treatments, thus allowing calcium influx into the cell. Therefore, observed decreases in CGRP secretion by grape pomace extracts cannot be attributed to modulation of calcium signals.

The impact of ginger extract on calcium influx is shown in Figure 4. When a decrease of fluorescence is observed as compared to vehicle control—as is seen with the ginger extract ($P = 0.007$, $n = 14$)—it is expected the treatment is blocking one or more type of calcium channel.

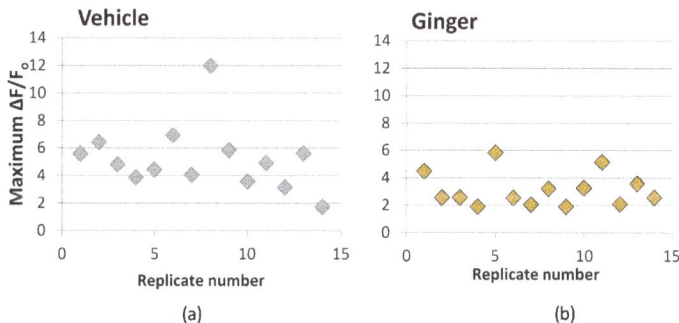

Figure 4. Calcium influx following treatment with methanol ginger extract. PC-12 cells transfected with GCaMP5 fluorescent calcium indicator were pre-treated for 10 min with (**a**) 0.1% DMSO vehicle or (**b**) 0.2 mg equiv/mL ginger extract. Maximum change in fluorescence compared to background ($\Delta F/F_o$) when stimulated with 50 mM KCl is reported. All treatments contain 0.1% DMSO in media, including vehicle. ($P = 0.007$, $n = 14$).

4. Discussion

This study explored the impact of grape pomace and ginger extracts, and purified *S*-petasin on two mechanisms related to migraine inflammation: the release of CGRP by CA-77 neuroendocrine cells and calcium signaling in PC-12 cells. CGRP and its signaling properties are key targets for drug discovery for migraine, thus the ability of food to impact CGRP is of high interest.

Two mechanisms have been observed to cause cellular release of CGRP in trigeminal cells: calcium signal and low pH [19]. In this study, we verified the pH of each prepared cell media plus extract to be approximately 7.2. Interestingly, grape pomace extracts displayed the strongest ability to inhibit CGRP secretion of any of the tested substances. This is notable not only for the scale of the inhibition, but also because the grape pomace extracts did not significantly inhibit calcium uptake upon stimulation. This suggests that inhibition of CGRP release of grape pomace extracts occurs by a mechanism different from calcium channel inhibition. We did not explore the chemical composition of grape pomace extracts in this study, but the phenolic composition of *Tinta Cao* extracts prepared by this extraction procedure is previously reported, and chlorogenic acid was the predominating phenolic acid, followed by ferulic, vanillic, and p-coumaric acids [17]. Total phenolics content was reported at 72.0 mg gallic acid equivalents/g pomace. Presumably, as red grapes, both pomace extracts would also contain anthocyanins, procyanidins, flavonols, and catechins [20]. It is reasonable to propose these phenolic acids and polyphenolics may be responsible for the activity witnessed here.

Cocoa extracts, which are also known to contain high levels of phenolic compounds, showed a similarly dramatic suppression of CGRP secretion, both in cell culture and an in vivo rat feeding study [10,11]. Interestingly, the authors suggest that calcium channel blocking is the likely mechanism, having shown that the cocoa extracts blocked effects of KCl stimulated calcium influx. However, food phenolic bioactivity is an intensely researched area, but no evidence could be found in the literature of calcium channel blockade activity by cocoa phenolics or more generally, cocoa.

Meanwhile, ginger extract at the highest tested dose of 0.2 mg ginger equivalents/mL media demonstrated a mild decrease in calcium uptake as well as a mild reduction in CGRP secretion. While we did not assess composition of the ginger extract, a prior study demonstrated that extracts prepared by this method contain 6-, 8-, and 10-gingerol, as well as 6-shogoal [15]. The proportion of shogoals, the dehydrated form of gingerols, is increased in dried ginger root as compared to fresh, thus we might expect higher shogoals in our dried ginger extracts [21]. The gingerol family of compounds has been identified as calcium channel antagonists [22]. The minor decrease in CGRP secretion may have been mediated by a relative decrease in the intracellular calcium signal caused by the gingerols' calcium channel antagonism. Ginger has been recognized for centuries in traditional medicine for its anti-inflammatory and analgesic properties, which is increasingly corroborated by demonstrations of impact on cell signaling in various models, including inhibition of prostaglandin and leukotriene synthesis, and inhibition of cyclooxygenase-1 (COX-1) and inducible nitric oxide synthase (iNOS) enzyme activity [21]. Interestingly, a randomized placebo-controlled trial successfully relieved acute migraine symptoms with a sublingual feverfew and ginger preparation [23].

In the present study, CGRP secretion from CA-77 cells was mildly but statistically significantly reduced by 1 μM *S*-petasin treatment. Treatment with *S*-petasin also significantly decreased the calcium influx in PC-12 cells. Thus, it is likely that the inhibition of calcium uptake is at least partially responsible for the decrease in CGRP secretion witnessed here. *S*-petasin, an eremophilane sesquiterpenoid, and other petasins are the suspected bioactive components of butterbur (*Petasites hybridus*) extract, the only dietary supplement with Level A "established efficacy" evidence for the prophylaxis of migraine, as reviewed by the American Academy of Neurology and the American Headache Society [14]. It is a known antagonist of L-type voltage-gated calcium channels and has antispasmotic activity at least partially independent of this calcium blocking ability [24–27]. Impact of *S*-petasin or butterbur on CGRP levels has not been previously reported in vitro or in vivo.

Petasites extract, though not specifically petasins, has been demonstrated to inhibit leukotriene synthesis and COX-2 expression in cell models [28]. Petasins other than *S*-petasin have demonstrated ability to inhibit leukotriene synthesis [29]. Thus, reductions in CGRP are only one potential mechanism to explain the anti-migraine activity of the supplement. Importantly, the *Petasites hybridus* plant contains hepatotoxic, mutagenic, and carcinogenic pyrrolizidine alkaloids. Unpurified botanical supplements (i.e., leaves or crude extracts) should be avoided due to these potentially severe side effects. Purified *Petasites* extracts are available, with higher concentrations of the active petasins, and concentrations of toxic alkaloids below 0.1 ppm [30].

There is some in vivo evidence in the literature to support the notion that diet is capable of impacting CGRP levels, both in circulation and specifically in the brain. One study demonstrated that rats orally fed grape seed extract for 14 days had lower basal expression of CGRP in the neurons and microglia of the trigeminal nucleus caudalis than control rats [12]. Furthermore, there is believed to be shared pathology between TMJ disorders and migraine. When rats were injected with Freud's adjuvant to stimulate the tempromandibular joint (TMJ) capsule, those who received the oral grape seed extract experienced repressed levels of phosphorylated-p38, OX-42 and glial fibrillary acidic protein as compared to control rats, suggesting the grape seed extract suppressed sensitization. Another study fed rats diets containing 1% or 10% cocoa, and observed suppression of basal neuronal CGRP expression, in addition to suppression of stimulated iNOS proteins and MAPK p38 [11]. This study confirmed in vivo prior observations from a primary trigeminal ganglia cell model, which secreted less CGRP when pre-treated with a methanol extract of cocoa beans [10]. In humans, meals containing various amounts of macronutrients elicited different responses in plasma CGRP: the high protein meal produced the greatest drop in CGRP, beginning at 30 min post-prandial [31].

A recent publication suggested the link between dietary triggers and oxidative stress [32], including discussion of dietary phenolic "antioxidants". Anecdotal evidence suggests that chocolate and red wine are migraine triggers, yet we present data on red grape pomace and discuss published results of cocoa research, which demonstrate a decrease of CGRP release in response to in vitro or in vivo exposure to these high-phenolic foods. The dual chemical nature of these molecules, functioning as anti- or pro-oxidants depending on their concentration, may warrant further exploration in relation to migraine. It is possible that one concentration eliciting an antioxidant effect may inhibit migraine, whereas a concentration capable of a pro-oxidant effect may provoke it. Alternatively, it is also interesting to note that this discrepancy bears some resemblance to the CGRP levels observed in relation to medication-overuse headaches (MOH). As mentioned in the Introduction, the triptan family of drugs relieves acute migraine symptoms while also decreasing CGRP levels; however, triptans increase circulating CGRP and cause allodynia in animals with chronic exposure, and cause MOH in humans when taken too frequently [33]. This similarity suggests that the presence of the offending food may not alone precipitate migraine, but the repeated presence of the food followed by its absence may contribute to a rebound effect in sensitive patients.

5. Conclusions

CGRP secretion was dramatically and dose-dependently inhibited by treatment with grape pomace extracts, while S-petasin and ginger root extract elicited a minor decrease. Meanwhile, at similar doses, grape pomace did not elicit a significant difference in calcium uptake, whereas S-petasin and ginger extract inhibited calcium influx. Because of their differing impact on calcium signals, grape pomace extract may impact CGRP release by a different mechanism than ginger extract and S-petasin, which inhibit calcium influx to some degree. Overall, if these results were to translate to the in vivo human, the ability of foods to mitigate CGRP release would be considered anti-inflammatory and may decrease occurrence of migraine.

Acknowledgments: Funding for this research was provided by the Herbert D. and Nylda Gemple Research Award and the McCormick Science Institute Award, both issued through the Academy of Nutrition and Dietetics Foundation. The research was also supported by a faculty start-up fund in the College of Health and Human Services at George Mason University.

Author Contributions: M.S. and J.B. conceived and designed the experiments. J.B., M.O., K.J. and M.S. performed the experiments. M.S. and J.B. analyzed the data. M.S. wrote the manuscript and had final approval.

Conflicts of Interest: The authors declare no conflict of interest. The funding sponsors had no role in the design of the study; in the collection, analyses, or interpretation of data; in the writing of the manuscript, and in the decision to publish the results.

References

1. Stewart, W.; Wood, C.; Reed, M.; Roy, J.; Lipton, R. Cumulative lifetime migraine incidence in women and men. *Cephalalgia* **2008**, *28*, 1170–1178. [CrossRef] [PubMed]
2. Vos, T.; Flaxman, A.D.; Naghavi, M.; Lozano, R.; Michaud, C.; Ezzati, M.; Shibuya, K.; Salomon, J.A.; Abdalla, S.; Aboyans, V. Years lived with disability (YLDs) for 1160 sequelae of 289 diseases and injuries

1990–2010: A systematic analysis for the Global Burden of Disease Study 2010. *Lancet* **2013**, *380*, 2163–2196. [CrossRef]

3. Baillie, L.D.; Ahn, A.H.; Mulligan, S.J. Sumatriptan inhibition of N-type calcium channel mediated signaling in dural CGRP terminal fibres. *Neuropharmacology* **2012**, *63*, 362–367. [CrossRef] [PubMed]

4. Recober, A.; Russo, A.F. Calcitonin gene-related peptide: An update on the biology. *Curr. Opin. Neurol.* **2009**, *22*, 241–246. [CrossRef] [PubMed]

5. Gupta, S.; Nahas, S.J.; Peterlin, B.L. Chemical mediators of migraine: Preclinical and clinical observations. *Headache J. Head Face Pain* **2011**, *51*, 1029–1045. [CrossRef] [PubMed]

6. Silberstein, S.D.; Edvinsson, L. Is CGRP a marker for chronic migraine? *Neurology* **2013**, *81*, 1184–1185. [CrossRef] [PubMed]

7. Lassen, L.H.; Haderslev, P.A.; Jacobsen, V.B.; Iversen, H.K.; Sperling, B.; Olesen, J. CGRP may play a causative role in migraine. *Cephalalgia* **2002**, *22*, 54–61. [CrossRef] [PubMed]

8. Goadsby, P.J.; Edvinsson, L. The trigeminovascular system and migraine: Studies characterizing cerebrovascular and neuropeptide changes seen in humans and cats. *Ann. Neurol.* **1993**, *33*, 48–56. [CrossRef] [PubMed]

9. Zelissen, P.M.; Koppeschaar, H.P.; Lips, C.J.; Hackeng, W.H. Calcitonin gene-related peptide in human obesity. *Peptides* **1991**, *12*, 861–863. [CrossRef]

10. Abbey, M.J.; Patil, V.V.; Vause, C.V.; Durham, P.L. Repression of calcitonin gene-related peptide expression in trigeminal neurons by a *Theobroma cacao* extract. *J. Ethnopharmacol.* **2008**, *115*, 238–248. [CrossRef] [PubMed]

11. Cady, R.J.; Durham, P.L. Cocoa-enriched diets enhance expression of phosphatases and decrease expression of inflammatory molecules in trigeminal ganglion neurons. *Brain Res.* **2010**, *1323*, 18–32. [CrossRef] [PubMed]

12. Cady, R.J.; Hirst, J.J.; Durham, P.L. Dietary grape seed polyphenols repress neuron and glia activation in trigeminal ganglion and trigeminal nucleus caudalis. *Mol. Pain* **2010**, *6*, 91. [CrossRef] [PubMed]

13. Sun, J.-Y.; Jing, M.-Y.; Wang, J.-F.; Weng, X.-Y. The approach to the mechanism of calcitonin gene-related peptide-inducing inhibition of food intake: Calcitonin gene-related peptide and food intake. *J. Anim. Physiol. Anim. Nutr.* **2010**, *94*, 552–560. [CrossRef] [PubMed]

14. Holland, S.; Silberstein, S.D.; Freitag, F.; Dodick, D.W.; Argoff, C.; Ashman, E. Evidence-based guideline update: NSAIDS and other complementary treatments for episodic migraine prevention in adults report of the quality standards subcommittee of the American Academy of Neurology and the American Headache Society. *Neurology* **2012**, *78*, 1346–1353. [CrossRef] [PubMed]

15. Mahady, G.B.; Pendland, S.L.; Yun, G.S.; Lu, Z.-Z.; Stoia, A. Ginger (*Zingiber officianale* roscoe) and the Gingerols inhibit the growth of Cag A+ Strains of *Helicobacter pylori*. *Anticancer Res.* **2003**, *23*, 3699–3702. [PubMed]

16. Parry, J.; Su, L.; Moore, J.; Cheng, Z.; Luther, M.; Rao, J.N.; Wang, J.-Y.; Yu, L.L. Chemical compositions, antioxidant capacities, and antiproliferative activities of selected fruit seed flours. *J. Agric. Food Chem.* **2006**, *54*, 3773–3778. [CrossRef] [PubMed]

17. Parry, J.W.; Li, H.; Liu, J.-R.; Zhou, K.; Zhang, L.; Ren, S. Antioxidant activity, antiproliferation of colon cancer cells, and chemical composition of grape pomace. *Food Nutr. Sci.* **2011**, *2*, 530–540. [CrossRef]

18. Yoon, H.; Liu, R.H. Effect of selected phytochemicals and apple extracts on NF-κB activation in human breast cancer MCF-7 cells. *J. Agric. Food Chem.* **2007**, *55*, 3167–3173. [CrossRef] [PubMed]

19. Durham, P.L.; Masterson, C.G. Two mechanisms involved in trigeminal CGRP release: Implications for migraine treatment. *Headache J. Head Face Pain* **2013**, *53*, 67–80. [CrossRef] [PubMed]

20. Yu, J.; Ahmedna, M. Functional components of grape pomace: Their composition, biological properties and potential applications. *Int. J. Food Sci. Technol.* **2013**, *48*, 221–237. [CrossRef]

21. Ali, B.H.; Blunden, G.; Tanira, M.O.; Nemmar, A. Some phytochemical, pharmacological and toxicological properties of ginger (*Zingiber officinale* Roscoe): A review of recent research. *Food Chem. Toxicol.* **2008**, *46*, 409–420. [CrossRef] [PubMed]

22. Cai, Z.-X.; Tang, X.-D.; Wang, F.-Y.; Duan, Z.-J.; Li, Y.-C.; Qiu, J.-J.; Guo, H.-S. Effect of gingerol on colonic motility via inhibition of calcium channel currents in rats. *World J. Gastroenterol.* **2015**, *21*, 13466–13472. [CrossRef] [PubMed]

23. Cady, R.K.; Goldstein, J.; Nett, R.; Mitchell, R.; Beach, M.E.; Browning, R. A double-blind placebo-controlled pilot study of sublingual feverfew and ginger (LipiGesicTMM) in the treatment of migraine: July/August 2011. *Headache J. Head Face Pain* **2011**, *51*, 1078–1086. [CrossRef] [PubMed]

24. Ko, W.-C.; Lei, C.-B.; Lin, Y.-L.; Chen, C.-F. Mechanisms of relaxant action of *S*-Petasin and *S*-Isopetasin sesquiterpenes of *Petasites formosanus*, in isolated guinea pig trachea. *Planta Med.* **2001**, *67*, 224–229. [CrossRef] [PubMed]

25. Wu, S.-N.; Chen, H.; Lin, Y.-L. The mechanism of inhibitory actions of *S*-petasin, a sesquiterpene of *Petasites formosanus*, on L-type calcium current in NG108-15 neuronal cells. *Planta Med.* **2003**, *69*, 118–124. [CrossRef] [PubMed]

26. Wang, G.-J.; Shum, A.Y.-C.; Lin, Y.-L.; Wu, X.-C.; Ren, J.; Chen, C.-F. Calcium channel blockade in vascular smooth muscle cells- major hypotensive mechansim of *S*-petasin, a hypotensive sesquiterpene from *Petasites formosanus*. *J. Pharmacol. Exp. Ther.* **2001**, *297*, 240–247. [PubMed]

27. Sheykhzade, M.; Smajilovic, S.; Issa, A.; Haunso, S.; Christensen, S.B.; Tfelt-Hansen, J. *S*-petasin and butterbur lactones dilate vessels through blockage of voltage gated calcium channels and block DNA synthesis. *Eur. J. Pharmacol.* **2008**, *593*, 79–86. [CrossRef] [PubMed]

28. Fiebich, B.L.; Grozdeva, M.; Hess, S.; Hull, M.; Danesch, U.; Bodensieck, A.; Bauer, R. *Petasites hybridus* extracts in vitro inhibit COX-2 and PGE2 release by direct interaction with the enzyme and by preventing p42/44 MAP kinase activation in rat primary microglial cells. *Planta Med.* **2005**, *71*, 12–19. [CrossRef] [PubMed]

29. Thomet, O.A.R.; Wiesmann, U.N.; Schapowal, A.; Bizer, C.; Simon, H.-U. Thomet 2001—Role of petasin in the potential anti-inflmmatory activity of a plant extract of *petasites hybridus*. *Biochem. Pharmacol.* **2001**, *61*, 1041–1047. [CrossRef]

30. Aydın, A.A.; Zerbes, V.; Parlar, H.; Letzel, T. The medical plant butterbur (*Petasites*): Analytical and physiological (re)view. *J. Pharm. Biomed. Anal.* **2013**, *75*, 220–229. [CrossRef] [PubMed]

31. Pedersen-Bjergaard, U.; Host, U.; Kelbaek, H.; Schifter, S.; Rehfeld, J.F.; Faber, J.; Christensen, N.J. Influence of meal composition on postprandial peripheral plasma concentrations of vasoactive peptides in man. *Scand. J. Clin. Lab. Investig.* **1996**, *56*, 497–503. [CrossRef] [PubMed]

32. Borkum, J.M. Migraine triggers and oxidative stress: A narrative review and synthesis: Headache. *Headache J. Head Face Pain* **2016**, *56*, 12–35. [CrossRef] [PubMed]

33. Srikiatkhachorn, A.; Grand, S.M.; Supornsilpchai, W.; Storer, R.J. Pathophysiology of medication overuse headache—An update. *Headache J. Head Face Pain* **2014**, *54*, 204–210. [CrossRef] [PubMed]

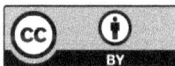

Chapter 4:
Metabolic Syndrome

nutrients

MDPI

Article

Walnut Polyphenol Extract Attenuates Immunotoxicity Induced by 4-Pentylphenol and 3-methyl-4-nitrophenol in Murine Splenic Lymphocyte

Lubing Yang [1,2], Sihui Ma [1,2], Yu Han [1,2], Yuhan Wang [1], Yan Guo [3], Qiang Weng [1,2] and Meiyu Xu [1,2,*]

[1]   Collage of Biological Science and Technology, Beijing Forestry University, Beijing 100083, China; yanglubingo@163.com (L.Y.); masihuikindle@163.com (S.M.); rebeccahan@bjfu.edu.cn (Y.H.); wwangyuhann@163.com (Y.W.); qiangweng@bjfu.edu.cn (Q.W.)
[2]   Beijing Key Laboratory of Forest Food Processing and Safety, Beijing Forestry University, Beijing 100083, China
[3]   College of Basic Medicine, Changchun University of Traditional Chinese Medicine, Changchun 130117, China; ccguoyan@163.com
*   Correspondence: xumeiyu@bjfu.edu.cn; Tel.: +86-10-6233-8221

Received: 23 February 2016; Accepted: 21 April 2016; Published: 12 May 2016

Abstract: 4-pentylphenol (PP) and 3-methyl-4-nitrophenol (PNMC), two important components of vehicle emissions, have been shown to confer toxicity in splenocytes. Certain natural products, such as those derived from walnuts, exhibit a range of antioxidative, antitumor, and anti-inflammatory properties. Here, we investigated the effects of walnut polyphenol extract (WPE) on immunotoxicity induced by PP and PNMC in murine splenic lymphocytes. Treatment with WPE was shown to significantly enhance proliferation of splenocytes exposed to PP or PNMC, characterized by increases in the percentages of splenic T lymphocytes (CD3+ T cells) and T cell subsets (CD4+ and CD8+ T cells), as well as the production of T cell-related cytokines and granzymes (interleukin-2, interleukin-4, and granzyme-B) in cells exposed to PP or PNMC. These effects were associated with a decrease in oxidative stress, as evidenced by changes in OH, SOD, GSH-Px, and MDA levels. The total phenolic content of WPE was $34,800 \pm 200$ mg gallic acid equivalents/100 g, consisting of at least 16 unique phenols, including ellagitannins, quercetin, valoneic acid dilactone, and gallic acid. Taken together, these results suggest that walnut polyphenols significantly attenuated PP and PNMC-mediated immunotoxicity and improved immune function by inhibiting oxidative stress.

Keywords: 3-methyl-4-nitrophenol; 3-methyl-4-nitrophenol; walnut polyphenol extract; attenuates; immunotoxicity; splenic lymphocyte

1. Introduction

Vehicle emissions have been shown to significantly inhibit endocrine [1–3], reproductive [4–7], and immune system [8,9] function through a variety of different mechanisms. Diesel exhaust particles confer toxicity in human neutrophil granulocytes, rat alveolar macrophages, and murine RAW 264.7 macrophages [10,11], and suppress cytokine release [12], significantly diminishing immune function [13,14], while gasoline exhaust particles have also been shown to inhibit T-cell proliferation [15]. Among the bioactive compounds found in vehicle emissions, two chemicals, 4-pentylphenol (PP) and 3-methyl-4-nitrophenol (PNMC), have been shown to significantly inhibit splenocyte viability and cytokine production, indicating immunotoxicity of the two vehicle exhaust [16–18].

Dietary polyphenols have been shown to confer protective activity against a variety of toxins. One such polyphenol, proanthocyanidin, significantly attenuated cadmium-induced renal damage in mice [19], inhibited neurological impairments caused by lead exposure in rats [20], and prevented nodularin-mediated lymphocyte toxicity in *Carassius auratus* [21]. Similarly, another polyphenol, quercetin, protected against male reproductive toxicity caused by PNMC in germ cells of embryonic chickens and mice [22–24], as well as inhibited atrazine-induced damage in the liver, kidney, brain, and heart of adult Wistar rats [25]. However, despite these preliminary observations, little is known about the role of these compounds in preventing the immunotoxicity caused by PP or PNMC.

Walnuts (*Juglans regia* L.) are not only an excellent source of essential unsaturated fatty acids (linoleic and α-linolenic acids) but are also rich in polyphenols [26], ranking second in antioxidant content among 1113 different foods evaluated [27]. Beneficial properties associated with walnut extracts include antibacterial, anticancer, hepatoprotective, antidiabetic, anti-inflammatory, anti-depressive, and antioxidative activities [28]. Walnut polyphenols were shown to protect against CCl_4-induced oxidative damage in rat liver, inflammation and cellular dysfunction in rat primary hippocampal neurons, amyloid beta protein-induced oxidative stress and cell death [29–31], and cisplatin-induced disruptions in motor and cognitive function [32]. However, despite these well-documented activities, the effect of walnut polyphenols on immune toxicity is unknown. Here, we investigated the potential protective effects of walnut polyphenol extract (WPE) on PP- and PNMC-induced immunotoxicity and evaluated the relationship between immunotoxicity and oxidative stress. Finally, we sought to identify the individual phenolic constituents contained within WPE.

2. Materials and Methods

2.1. Materials

Walnuts were obtained from the Jingpin Fruit Industry Co., Ltd (Hebei, China). Quercetin (purity $\geqslant$ 98%) was purchased from Tauto Biotech Co., Ltd. (Shanghai, China), and proanthocyanidin (purity $\geqslant$ 95%) from Jianfeng Natural Product R and D Co., Ltd. (Tianjin, China). PP was purchased from Sigma (St. Louis, MO, USA) and PNMC from TCI Chemicals (Tokyo, Japan). RPMI 1640 medium and phosphate-buffered saline (PBS, pH 7.4) were obtained from Mediatech (Manassas, VA, USA). Pharmingen Stain Buffer (BSA) was obtained from BD (Becton Dickinson, San Diego, CA, USA). 3-(4,5-dimethylthiazol-2-yl)-2,5-diphenyl tetrazolium bromide (MTT) was purchased from Sigma. ELISA kits for IL-2, IL-4, and Granzyme B were purchased from Cusabio Biotech (Wuhan, China). Assay kits of hydroxyl free radical ($\cdot$OH), superoxide dismutase (SOD), glutathione peroxidase (GSH-Px), and malondialdehyde (MDA) were bought from the Nanjing Jiancheng Bioengineering Institute (Nanjing, China). LC–MS grade solvents were obtained from Honeywell Burdick and Jackson (Muskegon, MI, USA). All other commercial reagents were of analytical grade and were purchased from local commercial firms.

The following antibodies purchased from Biogen (San Diego, CA, USA) were used in the phenotypic analysis studies: fluorescein isothiocyanate (FITC)-labeled anti-mouse CD3 (IgG_{2b}) to stain T-cells, FITC-anti-mouse CD4 (IgG_{2b}) and FITC-anti-mouse CD8 (IgG_{2b}) to stain T-cell subsets, and FITC-anti-mouse CD19 (IgG_{2a}) to stain B-cells. FITC-labeled rat IgG_{2a} and IgG_{2b} were used as negative isotype controls.

2.2. Experimental Animals

Specific-pathogen-free Kunming mice (male, eight weeks of age) were purchased from the Military Academy of Medical Sciences Laboratory Animal Center (Beijing, China) to serve as the source of cells for use in all assays herein. The mice were housed in a pathogen-free facility maintained at a temperature of 23–25 °C and a relative humidity at 57%–60% with a 12-h light-dark cycle. All mice had *ad libitum* access to standard sterilized rodent chow and filtered water. All procedures here were carried out in accordance with the Policy on the Care and Use of Animals established by the Ethical

Committee of the Beijing Forestry University and approved by the Department of Agriculture of Hebei Province, China (JNZF11/2007).

2.3. Preparation of WPE

The WPE was prepared by the method of Muthaiyah *et al.* [31]. In brief, walnuts (30 g) were frozen for 24 h; the shelled kernels were ground with a mechanical grinder and then immersed in 240 mL of 100 mM acetate buffer, pH 4.8/acetone (30:70, v/v) at 4 °C for 24 h. This process was repeated. The two extracts were combined and concentrated using a rotary evaporator under reduced pressure at 37 °C until the organic solvent was completely evaporated. The concentrated solution was extracted three times with 75 mL ethyl acetate. The three ethyl acetate extracts were combined and then evaporated to remove ethyl acetate. Powder of WPE was obtained by lyophilizing.

2.4. Preparation of Splenocytes

Based on the protocols of Benencia *et al.* [33], naïve mice were euthanized by cervical dislocation and its spleen was removed. Single cell suspensions were prepared by mincing and tapping spleen fragments on a stainless 200-mesh held in RPMI 1640 medium. Thereafter, erythrocytes present were lysed by incubating the cells in ammonium chloride (0.8%, w/v) solution on ice for 2 min. After centrifugation ($380\times g$, 5 min), the pelleted cells were washed three times with RPMI-1640 and finally re-suspended in RPMI-1640 supplemented with 10% fetal bovine serum, 2 mM L-glutamine, 100 U penicillin/mL, and 100 μg streptomycin/mL (all products from Mediatech). Cell number and viability were determined using a hemocytometer and trypan blue dye. Cell viability always exceeded 95%.

2.5. Cell Viability Assay

Measurement of cell survival was assayed as previously described [34]. In brief, one hundred microliters of splenocyte suspension (5×10^6 cell/mL) was aliquoted into each well of a 96-well flat-bottom microtiter plates. After 4 h incubation, 100 μL PP/PNMC (10^{-4} M final concentration in well, optimal dose as determined by preliminary experiments) alone or in combinations with WPE (0.01, 0.1, 1.0, 2.0, 3.0, 4.0, 5.0, and 10.0 μg/mL final concentration in well), Que (1.0 μg/mL final concentration in well), or PC (1.0 μg/mL final concentration in well) was added to designated wells. Cells treated with RPMI 1640 medium were used as positive control. The cells were then incubated at 37 °C in a humidified atmosphere with 5% CO_2 for another 48 h. At the end of the exposure, 20 μL MTT solution (5 mg/mL) were then added into each well. The samples were incubated a further 4 h. The culture supernatant was carefully removed, and 200 μL DMSO was added to each well. The plate was shaken slightly for 20 min and the absorbance was determined at 570 nm using an ELISA plate reader (BioRad, Hercules, CA, USA). Cell viability (%) = (the absorbance of experiment group/the absorbance of control group) × 100%.

2.6. Cell Staining/Flow Cytometry for Phenotypic Analysis

Cell staining for phenotypic analysis was carried out as described previously [9,35]. In short, the treated spleen cells were harvested, washed with PBS, then diluted to 2.5×10^7 cells/mL in PBS. Re-centrifuged the cells and then re-suspended in 50 μL Ab Block (BD Pharmingen Stain Buffer (BSA)) for 5 min at 4 °C. After blocking, the cells were added a given specific FITC-labeled antibody at 1 μg/mL (optimal dose as determined by preliminary experiments), then incubated for 30 min at 4 °C in the dark. After staining, the cells were washed three times with PBS and centrifugation. After the final washing, the cells were transferred to FACS tubes (in PBS) for phenotypic analysis using a BD FACS Calibur flow cytometer (Becton Dickinson, San Diego, CA, USA) equipped with FloJo software (Emerald Biotech, Hangzhou, China) for data analysis. Cells were excited with a 488 nm argon laser line and the fluorescence of FITC was analyzed on FL1 (530 nm), counting 10,000 events per sample. Splenocytes were electronically gated to exclude any residual platelets, red cells, or dead cell debris.

The results were indicated as the percentage positive cells within a gate which was the same for both exposed and control splenocytes.

2.7. Measurement of Cytokine/Granzyme Production and Determination of ·OH, SOD, GSH-Px, and MDA Levels

For assessment of IL-2, IL-4, granzyme-B, SOD, GSH-Px, ·OH, and MDA levels, splenocytes was treated with the test reagents for 48 h at a density of 5×10^6 cells/mL in 96-well plates. Culture supernatant was then collected and quantified following procedures by commercial ELISA kits. The lower detection limit of the kits was 3.9 pg IL-2/mL, 0.4 pg IL-4/mL, 3.1 pg Granzyme B/mL, 0.5 U SOD/mL, 0.5 U GSH-Px/mL, 0.04 U · OH/mL, and 0.01 mmol MDA/mL.

2.8. Determination of the Total Phenolic Content

The total phenolic content was determined by the Folin–Ciocalteu phenol reagent method prescribed by Wang *et al.* [36]. 200 μL of WPE was transferred to a 10 mL volumetric flask, to which 0.5 mL of Folin–Ciocalteu reagent was added. After 1 min, 1.5 mL of 20% (w/v) Na_2CO_3 was added and the volume was made up to 10 mL with distilled water. After 2 h incubation at 40 °C, the absorbance was measured at 760 nm in a 722 UV-VIS Spectrum Spectrophotometer (ShunYu Constant Scientific Instrument co., Ltd., Shanghai, China). The total phenolic content was calculated on the basis of the standard curve for gallic acid solutions and expressed as g of gallic acid equivalents (GAE)/100 g of sample.

2.9. LC-MS Analyses (HPLC-ESI-IT-TOF-MS)

LC–MS analysis was conducted as described previously [37,38] and with some modifications. LC–MS analysis was performed using a Shimadzu ESI-IT-TOF-MS instrument (Shimadzu, Tokyo, Japan) equipped with a HPLC system (SIL-20A HT autosampler, LC-20AD pump system, SDP-M20A photo diode array detector). The LC separation was performed using a C18 reverse-phase column (Shimpack XR-ODS column, 50 mm × 3.0 mm id × 2.2 μm; Shimadzu Scientific Instruments Inc., Columbia, MD, USA) and maintained at 30 °C with a solvent system comprising of 0.1% formic acid in H_2O (A) and 0.1% formic acid in acetonitrile (B). Prior to the injection, the column was equilibrated for 5 min at initial conditions (5% B). Compounds were eluted into the ion source at a flow rate of 1 mL/min with a step gradient of 5%–95% B over 30 min, isocratic at 95% B over 2 min, and return to 5% B over 1 min. The injection volume was set to 10 μL. The heat block and curved desolvation line of were maintained at 200 °C. Nitrogen gas was used as nebulizer and drying gas with the flow rate set at 1.5 L/min. The ESI source voltage was set at 4.5 kV and the detector was set at 1.5 V. Ionization was performed using a conventional ESI source in negative ionization mode. Data was acquired from m/z 100–1000. Shimadzu's LC-MS Solution software (Shimadzu Scientific Instruments Inc.) was used for system control and data analysis. Each compound was identified by comparison between retention time, compound spectra, as well as mass (m/z), with their counterparts in previous studies (please see reference in Table 1).

Table 1. Identification of phenolic compounds in WPE using HPLC-ESI-IT-TOF-MS in the negative ion mode.

No.	t_R (min)	Measured [M − H]⁻ (m/z)	Predicted [M − H]⁻ (m/z)	λ (nm)	Molecular Formula	Identification	Expressed as	Reference
1	12.663, 12.906	300.9993	300.9990	280	$C_{14}H_6O_8$	Ellagic aci	Ellagitannins	[37–39]
2	11.946	433.0432	433.0412	280	$C_{19}H_{14}O_{12}$	Ellagic acid 4-*O*-xyloside	Ellagitannins	[37–39]
3	12.507	433.1119	433.0772	280	$C_{20}H_{18}O_{11}$	Quercetin pentoside isomer	Quercetin	[38]
4	11.946	456.0383	457.0781	280	$C_{22}H_{17}O_{11}$	Epigallocatechin-3-*O*-gallate	Ellagitannins	[40]
5	13.74	447.0831	447.0938	280	$C_{21}H_{19}O_{11}$	Kaempferol-3-*O*-glucoside	Ellagitannins	[40]
6	12.507, 12.663, 12.906	469.0492	469.0049	280	$C_{21}H_{10}O_{13}$	Valoneic acid dilactone	Valoneic acid dilactone	[38]

Table 1. *Cont.*

No.	t_R (min)	Measured [M − H]⁻ (m/z)	Predicted [M − H]⁻ (m/z)	λ (nm)	Molecular Formula	Identification	Expressed as	Reference
7	11.946	481.5355	481.0620	280	$C_{20}H_{18}O_{14}$	2,3-*O*-HHDP-D-glucoside	Ellagitannins	[38]
8	9.828, 10.020, 10.512, 10.784	483.5192	483.0777	280	$C_{20}H_{20}O_{14}$	Digalloyl-glucose isomer	Gallic acid	[38,39]
9	12.25	615.5905	615.0986	280	$C_{28}H_{24}O_{16}$	Quercetin galloylhexoside isomer	Quercetin	[38]
10	8.382, 8.751, 9.624	633.0720	633.0720	280	$C_{27}H_{22}O_{18}$	Strictinin (galloyl-HHDP-glucose)	Ellagitannins	[37–39]
11	10.784, 11.136	635.0876	635.0877	280	$C_{27}H_{24}O_{18}$	Trigalloyl-glucose isomer	Ellagitannins	[38]
12	8.382, 8.751, 9.003	783.0685	783.0681	280	$C_{34}H_{24}O_{22}$	Pedunculagin (bis-HHDP-glucose)	Ellagitannins	[37–39]
13	10.020, 10.236	785.0808	785.0840	280	$C_{34}H_{26}O_{22}$	Tellimagrandin I isomer(digalloyl-HHDP-glucose)	Ellagitannins	[37–39]
14	11.946, 12.250	787.1144	787.0996	280	$C_{34}H_{28}O_{22}$	Tetragalloyl-glucose	Ellagitannins	[38]
15	10.784, 11.488	933.0316	933.0630	280	$C_{41}H_{26}O_{26}$	Praecoxin D	Ellagitannins	[37–39]
16	11.136	935.0746	935.0786	280	$C_{41}H_{28}O_{26}$	Casuarinin(Galloyl bis HHDP glucose)	Ellagitannins	[37–39]

2.10. Statistical Analysis

All data were expressed as means ± SD. Statistical analyses were performed using one-way analysis of variance (ANOVA) followed by a *post hoc* test, Tukey's test (as part of SPSS software package (IBM, Armonk, NY, USA)). Significance was accepted at a p-value < 0.05.

3. Results

3.1. WPE Attenuates Cytotoxicity in Splenocytes

Splenocyte cells exposed to PP or PNMC were examined by MTT assay to assess the effect of WPE on cell viability. PP and PNMC significantly decreased cell viability to 66% and 88%, respectively, relative to controls. These effects were significantly attenuated in cells treated with WPE (Figure 1A,B), which limited cytotoxicity in a concentration-dependent manner at concentrations of 0.01–1.0 μg/mL. Treatment of splenocytes with 1.0 μg/mL WPE increased cell viability from 66% to 100% and from 88% to 102% in PP- and PNMC-treated cells, respectively, relative to controls. As no additional benefits were seen at concentrations > 1.0 μg/mL WPE, this concentration was chosen for use in all subsequent experiments. Treatment with quercetin or proanthocyanidin (1 μg/mL) increased cell viability (Figure 1C,D), but the protective effects of the two compounds were weaker than those of WPE. These data showed that WPE protected against PP- and PNMC-induced cytotoxicity in splenocytes.

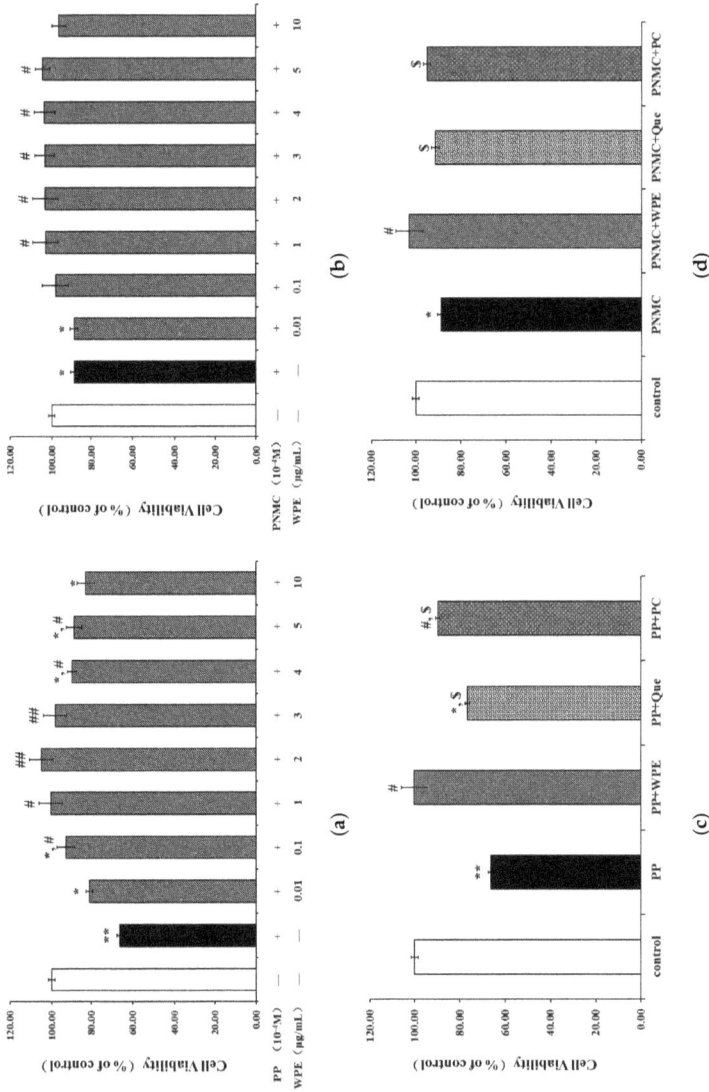

Figure 1. Effect of WPE on cytotoxicity in splenocytes exposed to PP/PNMC. Splenocytes were treated with (**A**) PP (10^{-4} M) or different concentrations (0.01, 0.1, 1.0, 2.0, 3.0, 4.0, 5.0, and 10.0 μg/mL) of WPE together with PP; (**B**) PNMC (10^{-4} M) or different concentrations (0.01, 0.1, 1.0, 2.0, 3.0, 4.0, 5.0, and 10.0 μg/mL) of WPE together with PNMC; (**C**) PP (10^{-4} M) or WPE (1.0 μg/mL), Que (1.0 μg/mL), PC (1.0 μg/mL) together with PP (**D**) PNMC (10^{-4} M) or WPE (1.0 μg/mL), Que (1.0 μg/mL), PC (1.0 μg/mL) together with PNMC for 48 h. Que, quercetin; PC, proanthocyanidin. Results shown are means ± SD of three separate experiments. * $p < 0.05$ or ** $p < 0.01$ *vs.* untreated control; # $p < 0.05$ or ## $p < 0.01$ *vs.* PP or PNMC treatment; $ $p < 0.05$ *vs.* WPE (1.0 μg/mL), together with PP (10^{-4} M) or PNMC (10^{-4} M) treatment.

3.2. WPE Inhibited Decreases in Splenic T Cell Sub-Populations

To determine the effects of WPE on splenic T cell populations exposed to PP and PNMC, splenocytes were stained with FITC-labeled antibodies for 48 h and evaluated by flow cytometry. The percentages of CD3+ T and CD8+ T cells were significantly lower in splenocytes exposed to PP relative to controls (Figure 2A,C). Although PP did not have a significant effect on CD4+ T cells, and decreased the cells populations (Figure 2B), with similar results seen for all CD3+, CD4+, and CD8+ T cells exposed to PNMC (Figure 3A–C). However, neither compound appeared to affect the levels of CD19+ B cells (Figures 2D and 3D). Treatment with WPE resulted in higher proportions of CD3+, CD4+, and CD8+ T cells among splenocytes exposed to PP and PNMC (Figures 2 and 3), with overall T cell population numbers similar to those of controls. These results suggest that WPE may restore T cell sub-populations in splenic cells exposed to PP or PNMC.

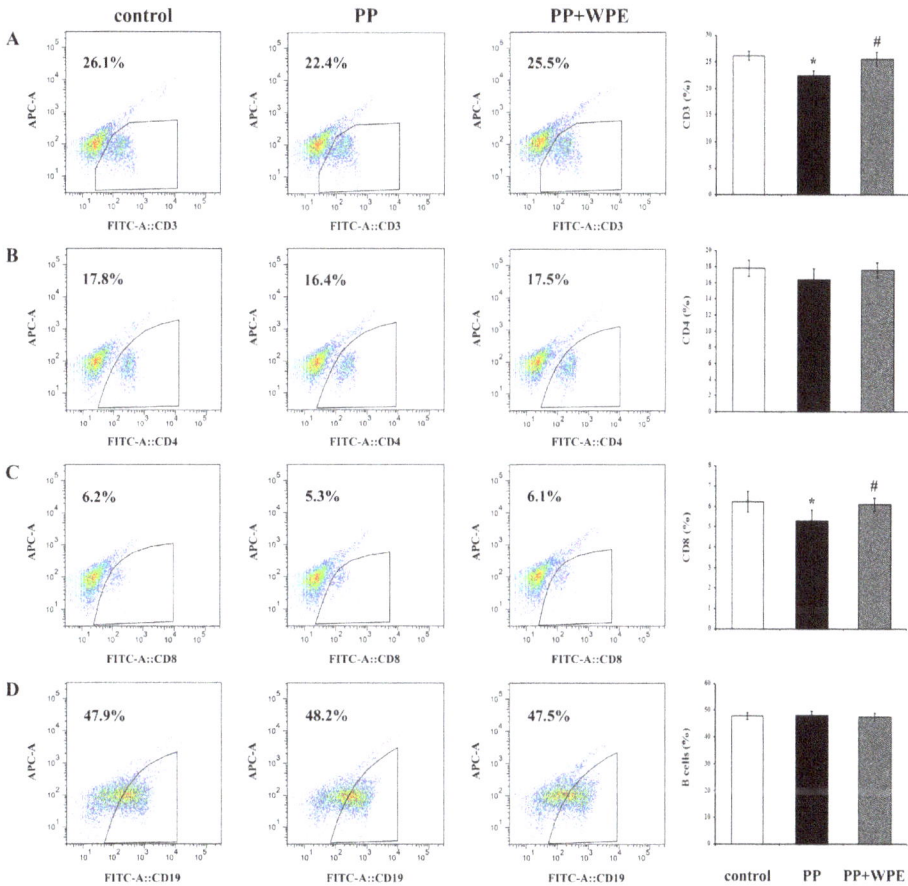

Figure 2. Percentages of various lymphocyte cell types as determined using flow cytometric analysis. (**A**) CD3+ T-cells; (**B**) CD4+ T-cells; (**C**) CD8+ T-cells; and (**D**) B-cells in cells exposed to medium only (control), PP (10^{-4} M), or WPE (1.0 µg/mL), together with PP for 48 h. Results shown are means ± SD of three separate experiments. * $p < 0.05$ *vs.* untreated control; # $p < 0.05$ *vs.* PP treatment.

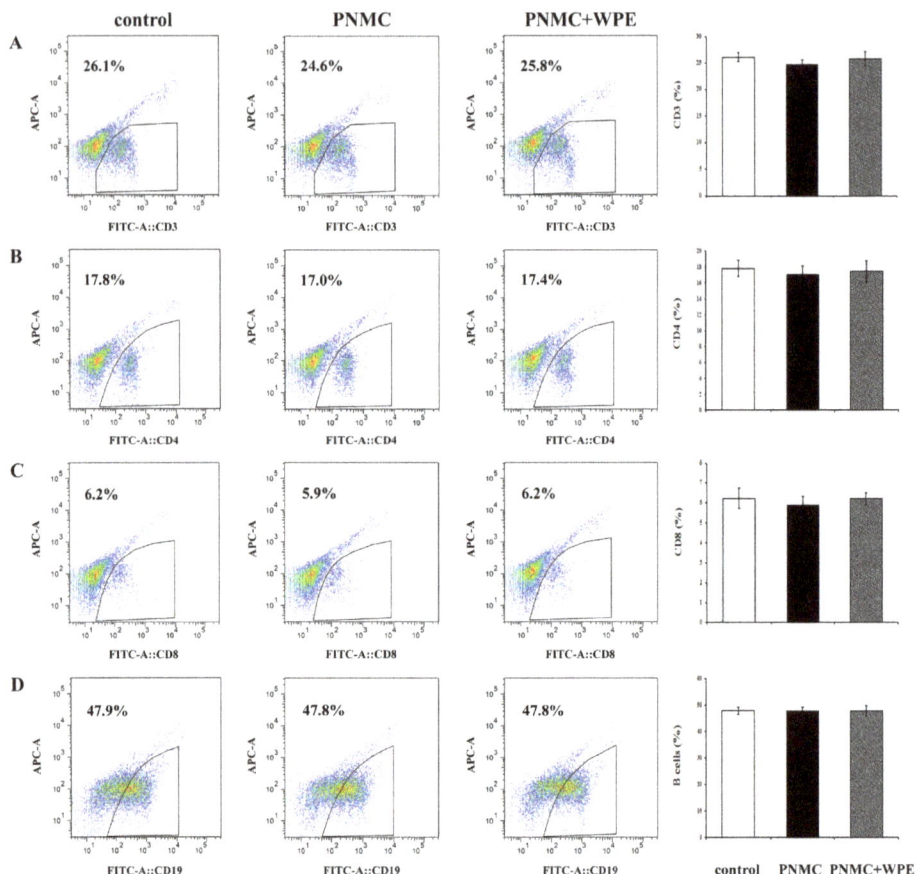

Figure 3. Percentages of various lymphocyte cell types as determined using flow cytometric analysis. (**A**) CD3+ T-cells; (**B**) CD4+ T-cells; (**C**) CD8+ T-cells; and (**D**) B-cells in cells exposed to medium only (control), PNMC (10^{-4} M), or WPE (1.0 µg/mL), together with PNMC for 48 h. Results shown are means ± SD of three separate experiments.

3.3. Treatment with WPE Prevents the Loss of Splenic T Cell Activity

To determine the effect of WPE on T cell activation, cells were exposed to PP or PNMC for 48 h in the presence or absence of WPE and analyzed for cytokine and granzyme production by ELISA: interleukin (IL)-2, IL-4, and granzyme B were chosen as markers for CD4+ TH1 cells, CD4+ TH2 cells, and CD8+ T cells, respectively. Both PP and PNMC inhibited secretion of IL-2, IL-4, and granzyme B relative to controls (Figures 4 and 5). These effects were significantly attenuated in cells treated with WPE: IL-2 increased from 58% to 99% and 36% to 80% in cells exposed to PP and PNMC, respectively; IL-4 increased from 52% to 80% and 77% to 93%, respectively; and granzyme B increased from 27% to 90% and 52% to 93%, respectively, relative to controls (Figures 4 and 5). These results clearly showed that WPE protected splenocytes from the loss of cytokine/granzyme production in cells exposed to PP and PNMC.

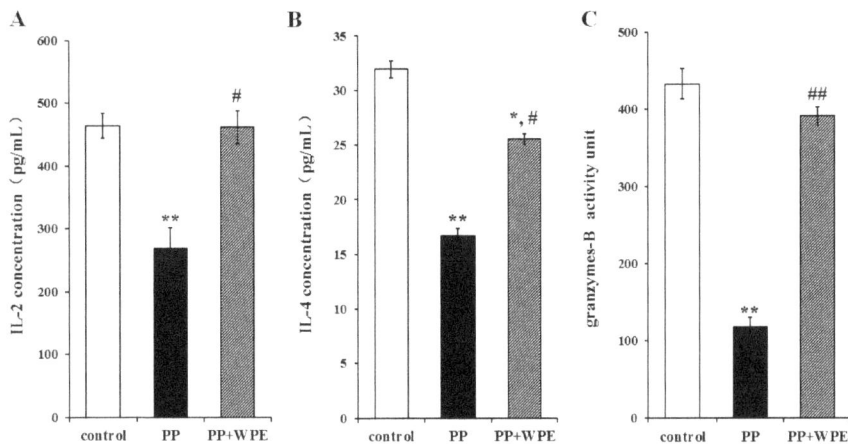

Figure 4. Effect of WPE on select cytokine/granzyme production in splenocytes exposed to PP. Splenocytes were cultured for 48 h in the presence of PP (10^{-4} M) or WPE (1.0 µg/mL) together with PP. Levels of (**A**) IL-2; (**B**) IL-4; and (**C**) granzyme B released into culture media were then measured by ELISA. Results shown are means ± SD of three separate experiments. * $p < 0.05$ or ** $p < 0.01$ *vs.* untreated control; [#] $p < 0.05$ or [##] $p < 0.01$ *vs.* PP treatment.

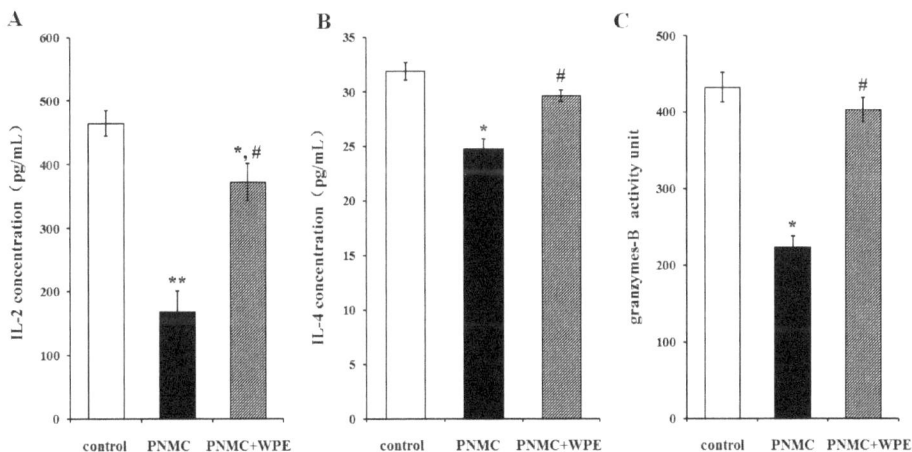

Figure 5. Effects of WPE on select cytokine/granzyme production in splenocytes exposed to PNMC. Splenocytes were cultured for 48 h in the presence of PNMC (10^{-4} M) or WPE (1.0 µg/mL) together with PNMC. Levels of (**A**) IL-2; (**B**) IL-4; and (**C**) granzyme B released into culture media were then measured by ELISA. Results shown are means ± SD of three separate experiments. * $p < 0.05$ or ** $p < 0.01$ *vs.* untreated control; [#] $p < 0.05$ *vs.* PNMC treatment.

3.4. WPE Attenuates PP- and PNMC-Induced Oxidative Damage in Splenocytes

To examine whether WPE can inhibit PP- and PNMC-induced oxidative stress in splenocytes, we examined SOD, GSH-Px, OH, and MDA levels following treatment with PP and PNMC. PP significantly enhanced ·OH and MDA levels in treated cells (Figure 6A,D), while PNMC induced significant increases in ·OH content relative to controls (Figure 7A,D). These levels were significantly attenuated in cells treated with WPE, with decreases in ·OH contents from 923 U/mL to 736 U/mL and 852 U/mL to 761 U/mL in cells treated with PP and PNMC, respectively (Figures 6A and 7A); MDA levels were reduced from 0.63 to 0.53 mmol/mL and 0.60 to 0.48 mmol/mL, respectively (Figures 6D and 7D). In contrast, there were marked decreases in SOD and GSH-Px activity in cells exposed to PP and PNMC. These data are consistent with previous studies that established the effect of PNMC on oxidative stress parameters in several models [22,24]. Treatment with WPE restored SOD activity levels from 76% to 91% and 84% to 90%, relative to controls, in cells exposed to PP and PNMC, respectively (Figures 6B and 7B). Similarly, GSH-Px activity was also increased in WPE-treated cells exposed to PP or PNMC, from 54% or 72% to 125% or 106% of control levels, respectively (Figures 6C and 7C).

Finally, we compared the effects of WPE to those of the polyphenol proanthocyanidin, as this compound has been shown to exhibit strong antioxidant activity [41]. As seen with WPE, proanthocyanidin treatment reduced both ·OH and MDA levels and increased SOD and GSH-Px activities in splenocytes exposed to PP and PNMC; however, the protective effects were lower than those of WPE (Figures 6C and 7C). Taken together, these results indicate that WPE can inhibit both PP- and PNMC-mediated oxidative stress in splenocytes at levels greater than those by proanthocyanidin.

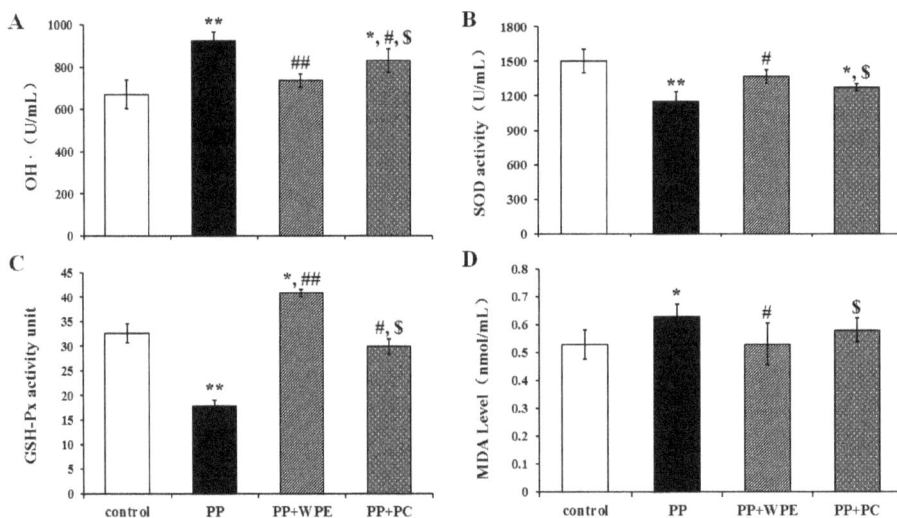

Figure 6. Effects of WPE on levels of ·OH, SOD, GSH-Px, and MDA in splenocytes exposed to PP. Splenocytes were cultured in the presence of PP (10^{-4} M) or WPE (1.0 µg/mL), PC (1.0 µg/mL), together with PP for 48 h. Changes in (**A**) hydroxyl free radical (·OH) activity; (**B**) superoxide dismutase (SOD) activity; (**C**) glutathione peroxidase (GSH-Px) activity; and (**D**) malonaldehyde (MDA) content in the cells were measured using specific assay kits. Results shown are means ± SD of three separate experiments. * $p < 0.05$ or ** $p < 0.01$ vs. untreated control; # $p < 0.05$ or ## $p < 0.01$ vs. PP treatment; $ $p < 0.05$ vs. WPE (1.0 µg/mL) together with PP (10^{-4} M) treatment.

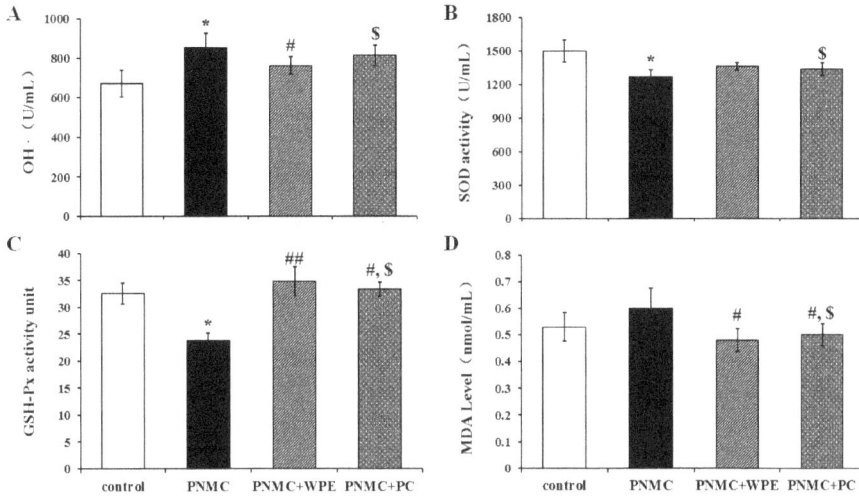

Figure 7. Effects of WPE on levels of · OH, SOD, GSH-Px, and MDA in splenocytes exposed to PNMC. Splenocytes were cultured in the presence of PNMC (10^{-4} M) or WPE(1.0 µg/mL), PC (1.0 µg/mL) together with PNMC for 48 hr. Changes in (**A**) hydroxyl free radical (· OH) activity; (**B**) superoxide dismutase (SOD) activity; (**C**) glutathione peroxidase (GSH-Px) activity; and (**D**) malonaldehyde (MDA) content in the cells were measured using specific assay kits. Results shown are means ± SD of three separate experiments. * $p < 0.05$ *vs.* untreated control; # $p < 0.05$ or ## $p < 0.01$ *vs.* PNMC treatment; $ $p < 0.05$ *vs.* WPE (1.0 µg/mL), together with PNMC (10^{-4} M) treatment.

3.5. Quantification and Characterization of Phenolic Compounds in WPE

Given the strong antioxidant effects of WPE in splenocytes, we next examined the phenolic constituents of WPE. Total phenolic content was quantified using the Folin–Ciocalteu phenol assay, revealing an average content of 34,800 ± 200 mg gallic acid equivalents (GAE)/100 g. Individual compounds were then identified by LC-MS analyses, with the names and m/z scores of each compound listed in Table 1. These results are considered tentative. A total of 16 individual phenolic compounds were identified, including ellagitannins (1,2,4,5,7,10–16), quercetin (3,9), valoneic acid dilactone (6), and gallic acid (8). In-depth studies should be performed to further clarify and characterize the phenolic compounds in WPE, and to determine the specific role of each constituent in the protective effect of WPE.

4. Discussion

The data presented here show that WPE attenuated PP- and PNMC-mediated toxicity in murine splenocytes, characterized by significant increases in cell viability following treatment with WPE, as well as increases in the proportions of splenic CD3+, CD4+, and CD8+ T cells following exposure to the agents. These increases in T cell populations were accompanied by strong increases in the secretion of IL-2, IL-4, and granzyme B in WPE-treated cells, relative to those exposed to PP or PNMC alone. Examination of · OH, SOD, GSH-Px, and MDA levels showed that WPE administration significantly inhibited oxidative damage in treated cells. Finally, we determined the total phenolic content of WPE to be 34,800 ± 200 mg GAE/100 g, consisting of at least 16 phenolic compounds based on LC-MS analyses. Taken together, these findings suggest that WPE may provide protection against PP- and PNMC-mediated immunotoxicity in splenocytes by inhibiting oxidative stress.

In recent years, the ability of natural products to both treat and prevent diseases has gained significant attention. Polyphenols have been shown to protect against certain toxicities caused by vehicle emissions. Two compounds, a polyphenol extract of *Ginkgo biloba* and quercetin were shown to protect against endocrine disruptions caused by diesel exhaust [1], while rosmarinic acid significantly attenuated lung injury caused by diesel exhaust [42]. Similarly, *in vitro* treatment of rat primary neurons with partridgeberry polyphenols significantly attenuated β amyloid-induced cell death and membrane damage [43]. Preliminary studies of walnut polyphenols revealed significant anti-oxidative properties [27], limiting oxidative damage induced by CCl_4 and β amyloid protein [29,31]. In this study, WPE significantly attenuated cytotoxicity caused by PP and PNMC in splenocytes. Furthermore, this protective effect was greater than that seen with two other polyphenols, proanthocyanidin, and quercetin (Figure 1C,D).

Polyphenols may also help maintain proper T cell function. Treatment of normal human peripheral blood lymphocytes with cacao liquor polyphenol *in vitro* regulated T cell proliferation in a concentration-dependent manner [44]. Similarly, the phenolic compounds in *P. glaucum* grains modulated splenic T cell growth in rats [45], while *L. guyonianum* polyphenols are capable of inducing both T and B cell proliferation [46]. In contrast, oligomeric proanthocyanidins from blueberry leaves inhibited the growth of human T cell lymphotropic virus type 1-associated cell lines by inducing apoptosis and cell cycle arrest [47], indicating a more complex regulatory effect for these compounds. Similarly, icariin flavonoid glucoside has been shown to ameliorate autoimmune encephalomyelitis by suppressing the proliferation of T cells and the differentiation of Th1 and Th17 cells among splenocytes and lymph node cells [48]. The results presented here showed that WPE restored the proportion of T cell sub-populations to a level at or near that of controls. This observation is in general agreement with many previous studies suggesting that polyphenols may be useful for maintaining proper T cell function.

Cytokines are essential regulators of both innate and adaptive immune responses, which can be influenced by a variety of dietary antioxidants [49–51]. Supplementation of sea bass fed with polyphenols extracted from red grapes increased their production of interferon (IFN)-γ, which may protect against loss of immune function in animals exposed to continuous antigenic pressure by microbes and environmental agents [50]. Ellagic acid and polyphenols present in walnut kernels increased the secretion of IL-2 in peripheral blood mononuclear cells [51], while the expression of IL-3, IL-4, IL-1R2, IL-6R, and IL-7R2 were all upregulated in response to tea polyphenols following alcohol-induced liver injury in rats [52]. Similarly, green tea polyphenols regulated both IFN-γ and TNF-α secretion in colon and lamina propria lymphocytes in a murine model of inflammatory bowel disease [53]. In the present study, treatment of splenic lymphocytes with WPE led to increases in the production of T cell-related effector molecules in cells exposed to PP and PNMC, consistent with previous studies.

In this study, the total phenolic content of WPE was $34,800 \pm 200$ mg GAE/100 g, which was greater than that seen in other studies (2464–11,500 mg GAE/100 g) [38,54,55]. In total, 16 polyphenolic compounds, including ellagitannins, quercetin, valoneic acid dilactone, and gallic acid, were identified in the extract [37–40]. Ellagitannins have been reported to stimulate the immune system by activating macrophages and promoting the release of Il-1β [56]. Quercetin has been shown to have a protective effect on immune function by decreasing lymphocyte DNA damage *in vivo* [57]. Gallic acid may inhibit murine leukemia WEHI-3 cells *in vivo* and promote macrophage phagocytosis [58]. In this study, the polyphenolic compounds extracted from WPE, including ellagitannins, quercetin, and gallic acid, had a protective effect against immunotoxicity induced by PP and PNMC in murine splenic lymphocytes.

In recent years, several lines of evidence have shown that dietary polyphenols can protect against oxidative damage caused by a variety of substances. The polyphenolic compounds found in raspberry seeds prevented damage to human peripheral blood lymphocytes by reactive oxygen species [59], while green tea polyphenols protected against nicotine-induced oxidative stress by significantly elevating plasma catalase and SOD activities in male rats [60]. Supplementation with quercetin (1.0 µg/mL) attenuated the toxicity of three nitrophenol components of diesel exhaust by limiting the production of ·OH and MDA, while simultaneously increasing GSH-Px and SOD activities in embryonic chicken testicular cells *in vitro* [22,61,62]. Similar effects on MDA levels and SOD activity were also seen in brain tissue following administration of walnut polyphenols, leading to improvements in both learning and memory functions [63].

The data presented here showed that WPE was able to increase SOD and GSH-Px activities, while decreasing the levels of both ·OH and MDA in splenocytes after exposure to PP and PNMC. SOD and GSHPX activities are associated with cellular enzymatic defense against free radical attacks. The ·OH radical is one of the most toxic and harmful ROS, and MDA is an end-product of lipid peroxidation in cells. Although there was no direct evidence in this study that the protective effect of WPE against PP- or PNMC-induced immunotoxicity was due to its activity against oxidative damage, past findings indicate that certain WPE phenolic compounds are able to protect immune cells from oxidative damage by inhibiting the formation of excessive free radicals.

5. Conclusions

Here, we showed that WPE protected against PP- and PNMC-mediated toxicity in splenic lymphocytes, limiting the damaging effects of these compounds on both cell viability and cytokine/granzyme production *in vitro*. The data also support the idea that the protective effect of WPE may at least be partly due to the attenuation of oxidative damage. Further studies will be necessary to identify the active phenolic compounds in WPE and to determine the mechanisms underlying these protective effects.

Acknowledgments: This study was supported by the Beijing Natural Science Foundation (8142029).

Author Contributions: Meiyu Xu and Qiang Weng conceived the study; Lubing Yang, Sihui Ma, Yu Han, Yan Guo worked on experiments performing and data analysis; Lubing Yang, Yan Guo, Qiang Weng and Meiyu Xu wrote the paper. All authors approved the final version.

Conflicts of Interest: The authors declare no conflict of interest.

References

1. Furuta, C.; Suzuki, A.K.; Taneda, S.; Kamata, K.; Hayashi, H.; Mori, Y.; Li, C.; Watanabe, G.; Taya, K. Estrogenic activities of nitrophenols in diesel exhaust particles. *Biol. Reprod.* **2004**, *70*, 1527–1533. [CrossRef] [PubMed]
2. Furuta, C.; Li, C.; Taneda, S.; Suzuki, A.K.; Kamata, K.; Watanabe, G.; Taya, K. Immunohistological study for estrogenic activities of nitrophenols in diesel exhaust particles. *Endocrine* **2005**, *27*, 33–36. [CrossRef]
3. Satoh, K.; Nonaka, R.; Ohyama, K.; Nagai, F. Androgenic and anti-androgenic effects of alkylphenols and parabens assessed using the reporter gene assay with stably transfected CHO-K1 Cells (AR-EcoScreen System). *J. Health Sci.* **2005**, *51*, 557–568. [CrossRef]
4. Li, C.M.; Takahashi, S.; Taneda, S.; Furuta, C.; Watanabe, G.; Suzuki, A.K.; Taya, K. Impairment of testicular function in adult male Japanese quail (*Coturnix japonica*) after a single administration of 3-methyl-4-nitrophenol in diesel exhaust particles. *J. Endocrinol.* **2006**, *189*, 555–564. [CrossRef] [PubMed]
5. Li, C.M.; Takahashi, S.; Taneda, S.; Furuta, C.; Watanabe, G.; Suzuki, A.K.; Taya, K. Effects of 3-methyl-4-nitrophenol in diesel exhaust particles on the regulation of testicular function in immature male rats. *J. Androl.* **2007**, *28*, 252–258. [CrossRef] [PubMed]
6. Meier, S.; Morton, H.C.; Andersson, E.; Geffen, A.J.; Taranger, G.L.; Larsen, M.; Petersen, M.; Djurhuus, R.; Klungsøyr, J.; Svardal, A. Low-dose exposure to alkylphenols adversely affects sexual development of Atlantic cod (*Gadus morhua*): Acceleration of onset of puberty and delayed seasonal gonad development in mature female cod. *Aquat. Toxicol.* **2011**, *105*, 136–150. [CrossRef] [PubMed]
7. Yue, Z.; She, R.P.; Bao, H.H.; Li, W.G.; Wang, D.C.; Zhu, J.F.; Chang, L.L.; Yu, P. Exposure to 3-methyl-4-nitrophenol affects testicular morphology and induces spermatogenic cell apoptosis in immature male rats. *Res. Vet. Sci.* **2011**, *91*, 261–268. [CrossRef] [PubMed]

8. Che, W.J.; Liu, G.M.; Qiu, H.; Zhang, H.; Ran, Y.; Zeng, X.G.; Wen, W.H.; Shu, Y. Comparison of immunotoxic effects induced by the extracts from methanol and gasoline engine exhausts *in vitro*. *Toxicol. Vitro* **2010**, *24*, 1119–1125. [CrossRef] [PubMed]

9. Li, Q.; Kobayashi, M.; Inagaki, H.; Hirata, Y.; Sato, S.; Ishizaki, M.; Okamura, A.; Wang, D.; Nakajima, T.; Kamijima, M.; Kawada, T. Effect of oral exposure to fenitrothion and 3-methyl-4-nitrophenol on splenic cell populations and histopathological alterations in spleen in Wistar rats. *Hum. Exp. Toxicol.* **2010**, *30*, 665–674. [CrossRef] [PubMed]

10. Aam, B.B.; Fonnum, F. ROS scavenging effects of organic extract of diesel exhaust particles on human neutrophil granulocytes and rat alveolar macrophages. *Toxicology* **2007**, *230*, 207–218. [CrossRef] [PubMed]

11. Durga, M.; Nathiya, S.; Rajasekar, A.; Devasena, T. Effects of ultrafine petrol exhaust particles on cytotoxicity, oxidative stress generation, DNA damage and inflammation in human A549 lung cells and murine RAW 264.7 macrophages. *Environ. Toxicol. Pharmacol.* **2014**, *38*, 518–530. [CrossRef] [PubMed]

12. Amakawa, K.; Terashima, T.; Matsuzaki, T.; Matsumaru, A.; Sagai, M.; Yamaguchi, K. Suppressive effects of diesel exhaust particles on cytokine release from human and murine alveolar macrophages. *Exp. Lung Res.* **2003**, *29*, 149–164. [CrossRef] [PubMed]

13. Chiang, D.; Sanjanwala, B.; Nadeau, K.C. Diesel exhaust particles impair regulatory T- cell function. In Proceedings of the International Conference on American Thoracic Society, San Diego, CA, USA, 15–20 May 2009; Abstract 4295.

14. Sasaki, Y.; Ohtani, T.; Ito, Y.; Mizuashi, M.; Nakagawa, S.; Furukawa, T.; Horii, A.; Aiba, S. Molecular events in human T-cells treated with diesel exhaust particles or formaldehyde that underlie their diminished Interferon-γ and Interleukin-10 production. *Int. Arch. Allergy Immunol.* **2009**, *148*, 239–250. [CrossRef] [PubMed]

15. Karakaya, A.; Ates, I.; Yucesoy, B. Effects of occupational polycyclic aromatic hydro-carbon exposure on T-lymphocyte functions and natural killer cell activity in asphalt and coke oven workers. *Hum. Exp. Toxicol.* **2004**, *23*, 317–322. [CrossRef] [PubMed]

16. Mori, Y.; Kamata, K.; Toda, N.; Hayashi, H.; Seki, K.; Taneda, S.; Yoshino, S.; Sakushima, A.; Sakata, M.; Suzuki, A.K. Isolation of nitrophenols from diesel exhaust particles (DEP) as vasodilatation compounds. *Biol. Pharm. Bull.* **2003**, *26*, 394–395. [CrossRef] [PubMed]

17. Murahashi, T.; Sasaki, S.; Nakajima, T. Determination of endocrine disruptors in automobile exhaust particulate matter. *J. Health Sci.* **2003**, *49*, 72–75. [CrossRef]

18. Yang, L.B.; Ma, S.H.; Wan, Y.F.; Duan, S.Q.; Ye, S.Y.; Du, S.J.; Ruan, X.W.; Sheng, X.; Xu, M.Y.; Weng, Q.; Taya, K. *In vitro* effect of 4-pentylphenol and 3-methyl-4-nitrophenol on murine splenic lymphocyte populations and cytokine/granzyme production. *J. Immunotoxicol.* **2016**, *31*, 1–9. [CrossRef] [PubMed]

19. Chen, Q.; Zhang, R.; Li, W.M.; Niu, Y.J.; Guo, H.C.; Liu, X.H.; Hou, Y.C.; Zhao, L.J. The protective effect of grape seed procyanidin extract against cadmium-induced renal oxidative damage in mice. *Environ. Toxicol Pharmcol.* **2013**, *36*, 759–768. [CrossRef] [PubMed]

20. Liu, C.M.; Ma, J.Q.; Liu, S.S.; Zheng, G.H.; Feng, Z.J.; Sun, J.M. Proanthocyanidins improves lead-induced cognitive impairments by blocking endoplasmic reticulum stress and nuclear factor-κB-mediated inflammatory pathways in rats. *Food Chem. Toxicol.* **2014**, *72*, 295–302. [CrossRef] [PubMed]

21. Zhang, H.J.; Fang, W.D.; Xiao, W.F.; Lu, L.P.; Jia, X.Y. Protective role of oligomeric proanthocyanidin complex against hazardous nodularin-induced oxidative toxicity in *Carassius auratus* lymphocytes. *J. Hazard. Mater.* **2014**, *274*, 247–257. [CrossRef] [PubMed]

22. Mi, Y.L.; Zhang, C.Q.; Li, C.M.; Taneda, S.; Watanabe, G.; Suzuki, A.K.; Taya, K. Quercetin protects embryonic chicken spermatogonial cells from oxidative damage intoxicated with 3-methyl-4-nitrophenol in primary culture. *Toxicol. Lett.* **2009**, *190*, 61–65. [CrossRef] [PubMed]

23. Bu, T.L.; Mi, Y.L.; Zeng, W.D.; Zhang, C.Q. Protective effect of quercetin on cadmium-induced oxidative toxicity on germ cells in male mice. *Anat. Rec.* **2011**, *294*, 520–526. [CrossRef] [PubMed]

24. Bu, T.L.; Jia, Y.D.; Lin, J.X.; Mi, Y.L.; Zhang, C.Q. Alleviative effect of quercetin on germ cells intoxicated by 3-methyl-4-nitrophenol from diesel exhaust particles. *J. Zhejiang Univ. Sci. B* **2012**, *13*, 318–326. [CrossRef] [PubMed]

25. Abarikwu, S.O. Protective effect of quercetin on atrazine-induced oxidative stress in the liver, kidney, brain, and heart of adult Wistar rats. *Int. Toxicol.* **2014**, *21*, 148–155. [CrossRef] [PubMed]

26. Kornsteiner, M.; Wagner, K.H.; Elmadfa, I. Tocopherols and total phenolics in 10 different nut types. *Food Chem.* **2006**, *98*, 381–387. [CrossRef]

27. Halvorsen, B.L.; Carlsen, M.H.; Phillips, K.M.; Bøhn, S.K.; Holte, K.; Jacobs, D.R.; Blomhoff, R. Content of redox-active compounds (ie, antioxidants) in foods consumed in the United States. *A. J. Clin. Nutr.* **2006**, *84*, 95–135.

28. Taha, N.A. Utility and importance of walnut, *Juglans regia* Linn: A review. *Afr. J. Microbiol. Res.* **2011**, *5*, 5796–5805.

29. Eidi, A.; Moghadam, J.Z.; Mortazavi, P.; Rezazadeh, S.; Olamafar, S. Hepatoprotective effects of *Juglans regia* extract against CCl₄-induced oxidative damage in rats. *Pharm. Biol.* **2013**, *51*, 558–565. [CrossRef] [PubMed]

30. Carey, A.N.; Fisher, D.R.; Joseph, J.A.; Shukitt, H.B. The ability of walnut extract and fatty acids to protect against the deleterious effects of oxidative stress and inflammation in hippocampal cells. *Nutr. Neurosci.* **2013**, *16*, 13–20. [CrossRef] [PubMed]

31. Muthaiyah, B.; Essa, M.; Chauhan, V.; Chauhan, A. Protective effects of walnut extract against amyloid beta peptide-induced cell death and oxidative stress in PC12 cells. *Neurochem. Res.* **2011**, *36*, 2096–2103. [CrossRef] [PubMed]

32. Shabani, M.; Nazeri, M.; Parsania, S.; Razavinasab, M.; Zangiabadi, N.; Esmaeilpour, K.; Abareghi, F. Walnut consumption protects rats against cisplatin-induced neurotoxicity. *NeuroToxicol* **2012**, *33*, 1314–1321. [CrossRef] [PubMed]

33. Benencia, F.; Courrèges, M.C.; Coulombié, F.C. *In vivo* and *in vitro* immunomodu-latory activities of *Trichilia glabra* aqueous leaf extracts. *J. Ethnopharmacol.* **2000**, *69*, 199–205. [CrossRef]

34. Sun, H.X.; Qin, F.; Pan, Y.J. *In vitro* and *in vivo* immunosuppressive activity of *Spica Prunellae* ethanol extract on the immune responses in mice. *J. Ethnopharmacol.* **2005**, *101*, 31–36. [CrossRef] [PubMed]

35. Li, Q.; Hirata, Y.; Piao, S.; Minami, M. Immunotoxicity of *N,N*-diethylaniline in mice: Effect on natural killer activity, cytotoxic T-lymphocyte activity, lymphocyte proliferation response, and cellular components of the spleen. *Toxicology* **2000**, *150*, 179–189. [CrossRef]

36. Wang, X.; Zhao, M.M.; Su, G.W.; Cai, M.S.; Zhou, C.M.; Huang, J.Y.; Lin, L.Z. The antioxidant activities and the xanthine oxidase inhibition effects of walnut (*Juglans regia* L.) fruit, stem and leaf. *Int. J. Food Sci. Tech.* **2015**, *50*, 233–239. [CrossRef]

37. Grace, M.H.; Warlick, C.W.; Neff, S.A.; Lila, M.A. Efficient preparative isolation and identification of walnut bioactive components using high-speed counter-current chromatography and LC-ESI-IT-TOF-MS. *Food Chem.* **2014**, *158*, 229–238. [CrossRef] [PubMed]

38. Regueiro, J.; Sánchez-González, C.; Vallverdú-Queralt, A.; Simal-Gándara, J.; Lamuela-Raventós, R.; Izquierdo-Pulido, M. Comprehensive identification of walnut polyphenols by liquid chromatography coupled to linear ion trap–Orbitrap mass spectrometry. *Food Chem.* **2014**, *152*, 340–348. [CrossRef] [PubMed]

39. Slatnar, A.; Mikulic-Petkovsek, M.; Stampar, F.; Veberic, R.; Solar, A. Identification and quantification of phenolic compounds in kernels, oil and bagasse pellets of common walnut (*Juglans regia* L.). *Food Res. Int.* **2015**, *67*, 255–263. [CrossRef]

40. Van der Hooft, J.J.; Akermi, M.; Unlu, F.Y.; Mihaleva, V.; Roldan, V.G.; Bino, R.J.; de Vos, R.C.; Vervoort, J. Structural annotation and elucidation of conjugated phenolic compounds in black, green, and white tea extracts. *J. Agric. Food Chem.* **2012**, *60*, 8841–8850. [CrossRef] [PubMed]

41. Ou, K.; Gu, L. Absorption and metabolism of proanthocyanidins. *J. Funct. Foods* **2014**, *7*, 43–53. [CrossRef]

42. Sanbongi, C.; Takano, H.; Osakabe, N.; Sasa, N.; Natsume, M.; Yanagisawa, R.; Inoue, K.; Kato, Y.; Osawa, T.; Yoshikawa, T. Rosmarinic acid inhibits lung injury induced by diesel exhaust particles. *Free Radical. Biol. Med.* **2003**, *34*, 1060–1069. [CrossRef]

43. Bhullar, K.S.; Rupasinghe, H.P.V. Partridgeberry polyphenols protect primary cortical and hippocampal neurons against β-amyloid toxicity. *Food Res. Int.* **2015**, *74*, 237–249. [CrossRef]

44. Sanbongi, C.; Suzuki, N.; Sakane, T. Polyphenols in chocolate, which have antioxidant activity, modulate immune functions in humans in vitro. *Cell. Immunol.* **1997**, *177*, 129–136. [CrossRef] [PubMed]

45. Nani, A.; Belarbi, M.; Ksouri-Megdiche, W.; Abdoul-Azize, S.; Benammar, C.; Ghiringhelli, F.; Hichami, A.; Khan, N.A. Effects of polyphenols and lipids from *Pennisetum glaucum* grains on T-cell activation: Modulation of Ca²⁺ and ERK1/ERK2 signaling. *BMC Complement. Altern. Med.* **2015**, *15*, 1–11. [CrossRef] [PubMed]

46. Krifa, M.; Bouhlel, I.; Ghedira-Chekir, L.; Ghedira, K. Immunomodulatory and cellular anti-oxidant activities of an aqueous extract of *Limoniastrum guyonianum* gall. *J. Ethnopharmacol.* **2013**, *146*, 243–249. [CrossRef] [PubMed]

47. Nagahama, K.; Eto, N.; Sakakibara, Y.; Matsusita, Y.; Sugamoto, K.; Morishita, K.; Suiko, M. Oligomeric proanthocyanidins from rabbiteye blueberry leaves inhibits the proliferation of human T-cell lymphotropic virus type 1-associated cell lines via apoptosis and cell cycle arrest. *J. Funct. Foods* **2014**, *6*, 356–366. [CrossRef]

48. Shen, R.; Deng, W.; Li, C.; Zeng, G. A natural flavonoid glucoside icariin inhibits Th1 and Th17 cell differentiation and ameliorates experimental autoimmune encephalomyelitis. *Int. Immunopharmacol.* **2015**, *24*, 224–231. [CrossRef] [PubMed]

49. Edfeldt, K.; Liu, P.T.; Chun, R.; Fabri, M.; Schenk, M.; Wheelwright, M.; Keegan, C.; Krutzik, S.R.; Adams, J.S.; Hewison, M.; *et al.* T-cell cytokines differentially control human monocyte antimicrobial responses by regulating vitamin D metabolism. *Proc. Natl. Acad. Sci. USA* **2010**, *107*, 22593–22598. [CrossRef] [PubMed]

50. Magrone, T.; Fontana, S.; Laforgia, F.; Dragone, T.; Jirillo, E.; Passantino, L. Administration of a polyphenol-enriched feed to farmed sea bass (*Dicentrarchus labrax* L.) modulates intestinal and spleen immune responses. *Oxid. Med. Cell. Longev.* **2016**, *2016*, 1–11. [CrossRef] [PubMed]

51. Anderson, K.C.; Teuber, S.S. Ellagic acid and polyphenolics present in walnut kernels inhibit *in vitro* human peripheral blood mononuclear cell proliferation and alter cytokine production. *Ann. N. Y. Acad. Sci.* **2010**, *1190*, 86–96. [CrossRef] [PubMed]

52. Zhang, X.G.; Xu, P.; Liu, Q.; Yu, C.H.; Zhang, Y.; Chen, S.H.; Li, Y.M. Effect of tea polyphenol on cytokine gene expression in rats with alcoholic liver disease. *HBPD Int.* **2006**, *5*, 268–272. [PubMed]

53. Varilek, G.W.; Yang, F.; Lee, E.Y.; deVilliers, W.J.; Zhong, J.; Oz, H.S.; Westberry, K.F.; McClain, C.J. Green tea polyphenol extract attenuates inflammation in interleukin-2-deficient mice, a model of autoimmunity. *J. Nutr.* **2001**, *131*, 2034–2039. [PubMed]

54. Pereira, J.A.; Oliveira, I.; Sousa, A.; Ferreira, I.C.F.R.; Bento, A.; Estevinho, L. Bioactive properties and chemical composition of six walnut (*Juglans regia* L.) cultivars. *Food Chem. Toxicol.* **2008**, *46*, 2103–2111. [CrossRef] [PubMed]

55. Vinson, J.A.; Cai, Y. Nuts, especially walnuts, have both antioxidant quantity and efficacy and exhibit significant potential health benefits. *Food Funct.* **2012**, *3*, 134–140. [CrossRef] [PubMed]

56. Clifford, M.N.; Scalbert, A. Ellagitannins—Nature, occurrence and dietary burden. *J. Sci. Food Agric.* **2000**, *80*, 1118–1125. [CrossRef]

57. Chan, S.T.; Lin, Y.C.; Chuang, C.H.; Shiau, R.J.; Liao, J.W.; Yeh, S.L. Oral and intraperitoneal administration of quercetin decreased lymphocyte DNA damage and plasma lipid peroxidation induced by TSA *in vivo*. *Biomed. Res. Int.* **2009**, *15*, 197–243. [CrossRef] [PubMed]

58. Ho, C.C.; Lin, S.Y.; Yang, J.S.; Liu, K.C.; Tang, Y.J.; Yang, M.D.; Chiang, J.H.; Lu, C.C.; Wu, C.L.; Chiu, T.H. Gallic acid inhibits murine leukemia WEHI-3 cells *in vivo* and promotes macrophage phagocytosis. *Vivo* **2009**, *23*, 409–413.

59. Gođevac, D.; Tešević, V.; Vajs, V.; Milosavljević, S.; Stanković, M. Antioxidant properties of raspberry seed extracts on micronucleus distribution in peripheral blood lymphocytes. *Food Chem. Toxicology* **2009**, *47*, 2853–2859.

60. Mosbah, R.; Yousef, M.I.; Mantovani, A. Nicotine-induced reproductive toxicity, oxidative damage, histological changes and haematotoxicity in male rats: The protective effects of green tea extract. *Exp. Toxicol. Pathol.* **2015**, *67*, 253–259. [CrossRef] [PubMed]

61. Mi, Y.L.; Zhang, C.Q.; Li, C.M.; Taneda, S.; Watanabe, G.; Suzuki, A.K.; Taya, K. Quercetin attenuates oxidative damage induced by treatment of embryonic chicken spermatogonial cells with 4-nitro-3-phenylphenol in diesel exhaust particles. *Biosci. Biotechnol. Biochem.* **2010**, *74*, 934–938. [CrossRef] [PubMed]

62. Mi, Y.L.; Zhang, C.Q.; Li, C.M.; Taneda, S.; Watanabe, G.; Suzuki, A.K.; Taya, K. Protective effect of quercetin on the reproductive toxicity of 4-nitrophenol in diesel exhaust particles on male embryonic chickens. *J. Reprod. Dev.* **2010**, *56*, 195–199. [CrossRef] [PubMed]

63. Shi, D.D.; Chen, C.Y.; Zhao, S.L.; Ge, F.; Liu, D.Q.; Hao, S. Effects of walnut polyphenol on learning and memory functions in hypercholesterolemia mice. *J. Food Nutr. Res.* **2014**, *2*, 450–456. [CrossRef]

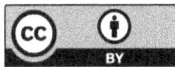

nutrients

MDPI

Article

Apigenin Ameliorates Dyslipidemia, Hepatic Steatosis and Insulin Resistance by Modulating Metabolic and Transcriptional Profiles in the Liver of High-Fat Diet-Induced Obese Mice

Un Ju Jung [1], Yun-Young Cho [2] and Myung-Sook Choi [3],*

[1] Department of Food Science and Nutrition, Pukyong National University, 45 Yongso-ro, Nam-gu, Busan 48513, Korea; jungunju@pknu.ac.kr
[2] Biotech Research Center, AMICOGEN INC., 64, Dongbu-ro 1259 beon-gil, Jinseong-myeon, Jinju-si, Gyeongsangnamdo 660-852, Korea; yycho@amicogen.com
[3] Department of Food Science and Nutrition, Kyungpook National University, 1370 Sankyuk Dong Puk-ku, Daegu 702-701, Korea
* Correspondence: mschoi@knu.ac.kr; Tel.: +82-53-950-7936

Received: 27 April 2016; Accepted: 13 May 2016; Published: 19 May 2016

Abstract: Several *in vitro* and *in vivo* studies have reported the anti-inflammatory, anti-diabetic and anti-obesity effects of the flavonoid apigenin. However, the long-term supplementary effects of low-dose apigenin on obesity are unclear. Therefore, we investigated the protective effects of apigenin against obesity and related metabolic disturbances by exploring the metabolic and transcriptional responses in high-fat diet (HFD)-induced obese mice. C57BL/6J mice were fed an HFD or apigenin (0.005%, w/w)-supplemented HFD for 16 weeks. In HFD-fed mice, apigenin lowered plasma levels of free fatty acid, total cholesterol, apolipoprotein B and hepatic dysfunction markers and ameliorated hepatic steatosis and hepatomegaly, without altering food intake and adiposity. These effects were partly attributed to upregulated expression of genes regulating fatty acid oxidation, tricarboxylic acid cycle, oxidative phosphorylation, electron transport chain and cholesterol homeostasis, downregulated expression of lipolytic and lipogenic genes and decreased activities of enzymes responsible for triglyceride and cholesterol ester synthesis in the liver. Moreover, apigenin lowered plasma levels of pro-inflammatory mediators and fasting blood glucose. The anti-hyperglycemic effect of apigenin appeared to be related to decreased insulin resistance, hyperinsulinemia and hepatic gluconeogenic enzymes activities. Thus, apigenin can ameliorate HFD-induced comorbidities via metabolic and transcriptional modulations in the liver.

Keywords: apigenin; hepatic metabolic and transcriptional responses; hepatic steatosis; high-fat diet-induced obesity; insulin resistance

1. Introduction

The global prevalence of obesity and associated metabolic complications has increased in recent decades [1]. Obesity, especially abdominal obesity, is a main risk factor and a feature of metabolic syndrome, including insulin resistance, type 2 diabetes, dyslipidemia and nonalcoholic fatty liver disease (NAFLD) [2]. Evidence has suggested that inflammation, a hallmark of metabolic syndrome, can trigger obesity and obesity-related metabolic diseases [2,3]. Therefore, the use of anti-inflammatory phytochemicals is one of the strategies for treating obesity and its associated metabolic disturbances [4]. Moreover, obesity is directly associated with NAFLD, which includes a spectrum of disease ranging from simple hepatic steatosis to non-alcoholic steatohepatitis [5]. Excessive hepatic lipid accumulation is associated with systemic and hepatic inflammation, as well as dysregulated lipid metabolism [6].

Some herbal products, including silymarin, a lipophilic extract derived from milk thistle, have been reported to exhibit beneficial effects in NAFLD [7].

Flavonoids are a group of phytochemicals present in various fruits and vegetables. Among the diverse flavonoids, apigenin (5,7-dihydroxy-2-(4-hydroxyphenyl)-4H-1-benzopyran-4-one) is a flavone common in chamomile, parsley, onions, grapefruit and oranges [8]. It has been shown to reduce inflammation and has beneficial effects against cardiovascular disease and cancer [8]. In addition, recent studies have demonstrated the anti-obesity and anti-diabetic effects of apigenin. It suppressed adipogenesis in 3T3-L1 cells by activating $5'$ AMP-activated protein kinase (AMPK) and by inhibiting mitotic clonal expansion [9,10]. It also improved glucose homeostasis, glucose tolerance and hepatic lipid metabolism in mice fed a high-fat diet (HFD) [11]. Moreover, apigenin (0.05%, w/w) slightly reduced food intake and body weight gain for 30 days in HFD-induced obese mice [12]. However, little is known about the long-term supplementary effects of low-dose apigenin on obesity and its associated metabolic disturbances, as well as the molecular mechanisms underlying its actions. Here, we examined the effects of apigenin (0.005%, w/w) on adiposity, insulin resistance, dyslipidemia and NAFLD in mice fed an HFD for 16 weeks and elucidated the metabolic and transcriptional mechanisms involved.

2. Materials and Methods

2.1. Animals

Four-week-old male C57BL/6J mice (n = 24) were purchased from the Jackson Laboratory (Bar Harbor, ME, USA). All mice were individually housed under constant temperature (24 °C) with a 12-h light/dark cycle, fed the AIN-76 (AIN, the American Institute of Nutrition) semi-purified diet for 1 week after arrival and then randomly divided into two groups. The mice were fed an HFD consisting of 20% (w/w) fat and 1% (w/w) cholesterol (n = 12) or HFD with 0.005% (w/w) apigenin (Sigma Chemical, St. Louis, MO, USA, from parsley powder) (n = 12) for 16 weeks. The HFD contains 40 kcal% fat, 17 kcal% protein and 43 kcal% carbohydrate. In the HFD, 85% (w/w) of total fat was from lard, which contains high amounts of saturated fat, and 15% (w/w) of total fat was from soybean oil, an unsaturated fat source. They were provided free access to food and distilled water, and food consumption, body weight and fasting blood glucose levels were measured daily, weekly and every 2 weeks. At the end of the experimental period, all mice were anesthetized with ether after a 12-h fast, and blood was taken from the inferior vena cava for the determination of plasma parameters. The liver and adipose tissue were removed, rinsed with physiological saline, weighed, immediately frozen in liquid nitrogen and stored at -70 °C until analysis. Studies were performed using protocols for animal studies approved by the Ethics Committee at Kyungpook National University (KNU-2010-4-14).

2.2. Levels of Fasting Blood Glucose, Plasma Insulin and Homeostatic Index of Insulin Resistance

Every 2 weeks, 12-h fasting whole blood samples were obtained from the tail veins, and the fasting blood glucose concentration was measured using a glucose analyzer (GlucDr supersensor, Allmedicus, Korea). The plasma insulin level was determined using a commercial radioimmunometric assay (MilliplexTM MAP Mouse endocrine kit, Millipore, Billerica, MA, USA), and the homeostatic index of insulin resistance (HOMA-IR) was calculated as follows: HOMA-IR = (fasting glucose (mmol/L) $\times$ fasting insulin (μL· U/mL))/22.51.

2.3. Plasma Adipocytokines, Lipids, Apolipoproteins and Aminotransferases Levels

Plasma levels of adipocytokines (leptin, monocyte chemoattractant protein-1 (MCP-1), interferon gamma-γ (IFN-γ), tumor necrosis factor-α (TNF-α) and interleukin-6 (IL-6)) were determined with a multiplex detection kit from Bio-Rad (Hercules, CA, USA). Plasma triglyceride, total cholesterol, HDL-cholesterol, alanine aminotransferase (ALT) and aspartate aminotransferase (AST) levels were measured using enzymatic assay kits (Asan Pharm, Seoul, Korea). Plasma free fatty acid (FFA, Wako,

Tokyo, Japan), apolipoprotein A1 (apoA1, Eiken, Tokyo, Japan) and apolipoprotein B (apoB, Eiken, Tokyo, Japan) levels were also determined using enzymatic kits. The ratio of HDL cholesterol to total cholesterol (HTR) and the atherogenic index (AI) were calculated using the following Equations (1) and (2):

$$HTR = ((HDL\text{-}cholesterol)/(total\,cholesterol)) \times 100 \qquad (1)$$

$$AI = ((total\,cholesterol) - (HDL\text{-}cholesterol)/(HDL\text{-}cholesterol)) \qquad (2)$$

2.4. Morphology of Liver

The livers were removed from each mouse, fixed in 10% (*v/v*) paraformaldehyde/phosphate-buffered saline (PBS) and then embedded in paraffin for staining with hematoxylin and eosin. The stained areas were viewed using an optical microscope (Nikon, Tokyo, Japan) with a magnifying power of ×200.

2.5. Hepatic Enzymes Activity

Hepatic cytosolic, mitochondrial and microsomal fractions were prepared as previously described [9]. The activities of cytosolic glucokinase, phosphoenolpyruvate carboxykinase (PEPCK), mitochondrial glucose-6-phosphatase (G6Pase), microsomal phosphatidate phosphohydrolase (PAP), acyl CoA cholesterol acyltransferase (ACAT) and glycogen content were measured according to previously described procedures [13,14].

2.6. RNA Preparation

Total RNA was extracted from the liver using TRIzol RIZOL reagent (Invitrogen, Grand Island, NY, USA), and the RNA purity and integrity were evaluated by microfluidics analysis using the Agilent 2100 Bioanalyzer (Agilent Technologies, Santa Clara, CA, USA). RNA samples were then stored at −70 °C prior to further analysis by microarray and real-time quantitative PCR (RT-qPCR). To reduce variation among individuals within each of the two groups, total RNA from mice of the same group was pooled together in equal amounts to generate a mixed sample. These three pooled RNA sample sets were subsequently used for RT-qPCR and microarray analysis.

2.7. Microarray Analysis and RT-qPCR

Biotinylated cRNA was generated using the Ambion Illumina RNA amplification kit (Ambion, Waltham, MA, USA). A total of 750 ng biotinylated cRNA per sample was hybridized to Illumina MouseWG-6 v2 Expression BeadChips (Illumina, San Diego, CA, USA) for 16–18 h at 58 °C, and hybridized arrays were washed and stained with Amersham fluorolink streptavidin-Cy3 (GE Healthcare Bio-Sciences, Little Chalfont, U.K.) following the standard protocol in the bead array manual. BeadChips were then scanned using an Illumina BeadArray Reader, and raw gene expression data were obtained from the array scanned images using the Illumina BeadStudio software. Probe signal intensities were quantile normalized and log transformed. Limma was used to determine significantly differentially-expressed genes based on a false discovery rate of less than 5%, a Benjamin and Hochberg-adjusted *p*-value of less than 0.05 and a fold change greater than 1 [15]. The DAVID (Database for Annotation, Visualization and Integrated Discovery) Functional Annotation Tool was used to identify enriched biological themes and to cluster redundant annotation terms.

For the validation of microarray data, several randomly-selected genes (Lpl, Pparγ, Srebf1, Dgat2, Scd1 and Cidea) were measured independently by RT-qPCR using the same pooled RNA samples that were hybridized to BeadChips. Total RNA (1 µg) was reverse-transcribed into cDNA using the QuantiTect® reverse transcription kit (Qiagen, Hilden, Germany), and then, mRNA expression was quantified by RT-qPCR using the SYBR green PCR kit (Qiagen, Hilden, Germany) and the CFX96TM real-time system (Bio-Rad, Hercules, CA, USA). Cycle thresholds were determined based on SYBR green emission intensity during the exponential phase. Ct data were normalized using Gapdh, and relative gene expression was calculated with the $2^{-\Delta\Delta Ct}$ method.

2.8. Statistical Analysis

The values were expressed as the means $\pm$ standard error (S.E). Significant differences between two groups were determined by Student's *t*-test or the Wilcoxon *t*-test using the SPSS program (SPSS Inc., Chicago, IL, USA). Results were considered statistically significant at $p < 0.05$.

3. Results

3.1. Apigenin Did Not Alter Food Intake, Body Weight Gain and Fat Accumulation

Supplementation of apigenin did not alter food and energy intake in mice (Figure 1A,B). Initial body weight, final body weight, body weight gain and fat mass also did not differ between the two groups (Figure 1C–E). Moreover, apigenin did not affect circulating levels of leptin, a representative adipokine secreted from adipocytes in proportion to fat mass and involved in the regulation of food intake and energy homeostasis [2].

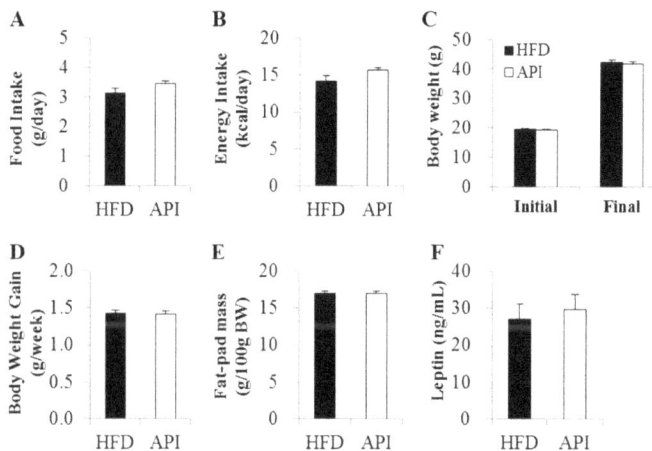

Figure 1. Effects of apigenin on (**A**) food intake; (**B**) energy intake; (**C,D**) body weight; (**E**) fat-pad mass and (**F**) plasma leptin level in C57BL/6J mice fed a high-fat diet. Data are shown as the means $\pm$ S.E. HFD: high-fat diet (20% fat, 1% cholesterol); API: HFD + 0.005% apigenin.

3.2. Apigenin Decreased Fasting Blood Glucose and Plasma Insulin Levels and Ameliorated Insulin Resistance and Inflammation

We next examined whether apigenin influenced HFD-induced insulin resistance and inflammation. Apigenin significantly decreased fasting blood glucose levels after two weeks of supplementation in HFD-fed mice (Figure 2A). Levels of plasma insulin and HOMA-IR, a method used to quantify insulin resistance and β-cell function [16], were also significantly decreased by apigenin (Figure 2B,C). Although hepatic glucokinase activity and glycogen content remained unaffected (Figure 2D,E), hepatic PEPCK and G6Pase activities were decreased in apigenin-supplemented mice. Moreover, plasma levels of pro-inflammatory mediators, such as MCP-1, IFN-γ, TNF-α and IL-6, were significantly decreased by apigenin (Figure 2F).

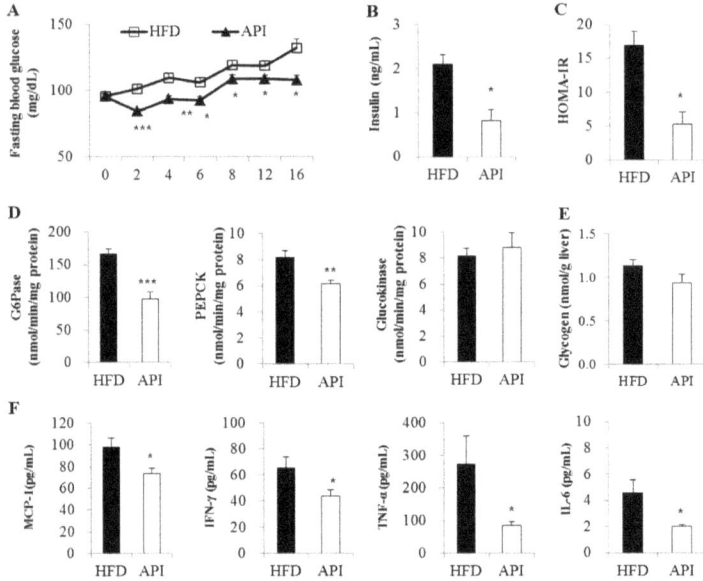

Figure 2. Effects of apigenin on (**A**) fasting blood glucose level; (**B**) plasma insulin level; (**C**) homeostatic index of insulin resistance (HOMO-IR); (**D**) hepatic glucose metabolism-related enzyme activities; (**E**) hepatic glycogen content and (**F**) plasma pro-inflammatory marker levels in C57BL/6J mice fed a high-fat diet. Data are shown as the means ± S.E. Values are significantly different between the high-fat diet and apigenin groups according to Student's *t*-test: * $p < 0.05$; ** $p < 0.01$; *** $p < 0.001$. HFD: high-fat diet (20% fat, 1% cholesterol); API: HFD + 0.005% apigenin.

3.3. Apigenin Improved Dyslipidemia, Hepatic Steatosis and Hepatomegaly

There were no significant differences in plasma triglyceride, HDL-cholesterol and apoA1 levels between the two groups (Figure 3). However, plasma free fatty acid levels were significantly decreased in apigenin-supplemented obese mice. Plasma total-cholesterol levels, as well as plasma apoB levels and the apoB/apoA1 ratio were also markedly decreased by apigenin.

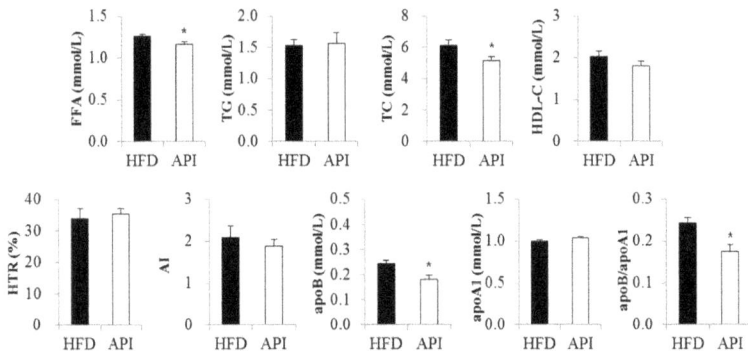

Figure 3. Effect of apigenin on plasma lipids and apolipoproteins in C57BL/6J mice fed a high-fat diet. Data are shown as the means ± S.E. Values are significantly different between the high-fat diet and apigenin groups according to Student's *t*-test: * $p < 0.05$. HFD: high-fat diet (20% fat, 1% cholesterol); API: HFD + 0.005% apigenin.

In addition, apigenin significantly decreased liver weight and hepatic lipid droplets' accumulation along with plasma ALT and AST levels (Figure 4A–C). Hepatic PAP and ACAT activities were also significantly lowered in apigenin-supplemented obese mice (Figure 4D).

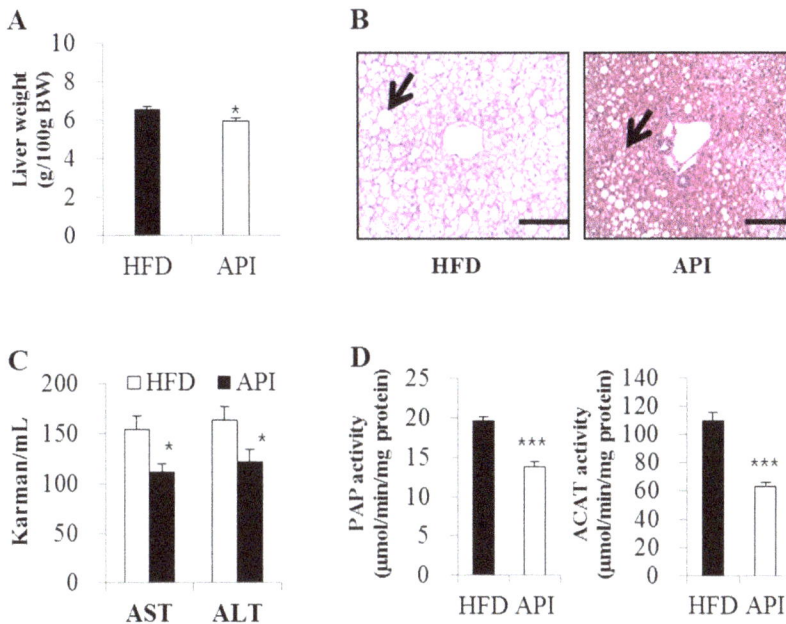

Figure 4. Effect of apigenin on liver weight (**A**), hepatic morphology (**B**), plasma transaminases activities (**C**) and activities of hepatic enzymes controlling the synthesis of triglyceride and cholesterol ester (**D**) in C57BL/6J mice fed a high-fat diet; ((**A**), (**C**), and (**D**)) Data are shown as the means $\pm$ S.E. Values are significantly different between the high-fat diet and apigenin groups according to Student's *t*-test: * $p < 0.05$, ** $p < 0.05$; (**B**) Original magnification $\times 200$. Bar, 50 M. HFD: high-fat diet (20% fat, 1% cholesterol); API: HFD + 0.005% apigenin.

3.4. Liver Gene Expression Profiles in Response to Apigenin

To investigate changes in hepatic gene expression profiles in response to apigenin, we identified differentially-expressed genes in apigenin-supplemented mice compared to HFD control mice using microarray analysis. Of the 281 differentially-expressed genes in the two groups, 271 genes were upregulated, and one gene was downregulated. The top 10 differentially-upregulated genes and one downregulated gene are shown in Figure 5A. Functional annotation clustering using DAVID revealed that the majority of hepatic genes regulated by apigenin in HFD-fed mice were related to oxidative phosphorylation (OXPHOS), the electron transport chain, the tricarboxylic acid (TCA) cycle, fatty acid metabolism and cholesterol homeostasis (Figure 5B).

To further validate the reliability of our microarray data, we performed RT-qPCR on six randomly-selected genes (Lpl, Ppary, Srebf1, Dgat2, Scd1 and Cidea). The results were in agreement with the microarray data, and RT-qPCR was more sensitive to small changes in gene expression compared to the microarray, similar to a previous study [15]. Except for Scd1, mRNA expression of lipolysis- and lipogenesis-related genes (Lpl, Ppary, Srebf1, Dgat2 and Cidea) was downregulated in the livers of apigenin-supplemented mice (Figure 5C).

A

Up-regulated genes	Down-regulated genes
mtDNA_ND4L, Hbb-b1, Hsd17b6, Ugt2b1, Cf b, Pgrmc1, 1200016E24Rik, Pah, LOC1000486 22, Ugt2b34	Bmx

B

ES	GO Term	P-value	No. Gene	
4.23	Oxidative phosphorylation	0.0008	7	
	Electron transport chain	0.0023	6	
2.66	Tricarboxylic acid cycle	0.0014	4	
1.29	Fatty acid metabolic process	0.024	6	
1.15	Cholesterol homeostasis	0.039	3	

C

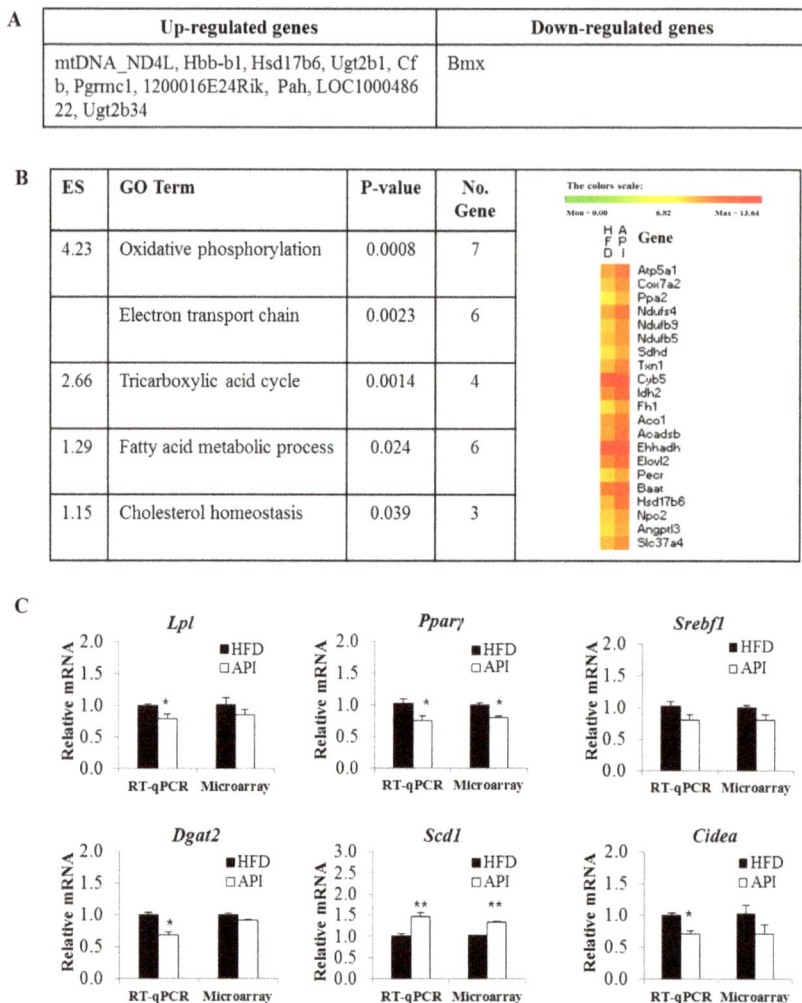

Figure 5. The top 10 most upregulated and downregulated genes in the livers of the apigenin group compared to the control group (**A**); functional gene ontologies associated with the apigenin-responsive genes (**B**); and real-time quantitative PCR validation (**C**); (**A**,**B**) comparison of differentially-expressed genes in the apigenin group vs. the control group using Benjamin–Hochberg adjusted p-value < 0.05, FDR (False Discovery Rate) <5%, fold change >1; (**B**) functional gene ontology terms enriched among apigenin responsive genes are clustered according to biological processes (enrichment score >1) using DAVID. The heatmap shows the expression profiles of the representative apigenin responsive genes in each cluster; (**C**) Data are shown as the means ± S.E. Values are significantly different between the high-fat diet and apigenin groups according to Student's t-test: * p < 0.05; ** p < 0.05. Microarray data based on pooled RNA hybridized to Illumina MouseWG-6 v2.0 BeadChips. HFD: high-fat diet (20% fat, 1% cholesterol); API: HFD + 0.005% Apigenin; Lpl: lipoprotein lipase; Pparγ: peroxisome proliferator-activated receptor γ; Srebf1: sterol regulatory element-binding transcription factor 1; Dgat2: diacylglycerol O-acyltransferase 2; Scd1: stearoyl-CoA desaturase-1; Cidea: cell death activator; ES: Enrichment Score.

4. Discussion

In the present study, supplementation of an HFD with apigenin (0.005%, w/w) for 16 weeks did not alter food intake, body weight gain and fat accumulation in mice. These findings were in disagreement with previous findings, which demonstrated that apigenin (0.05%, w/w) reduced food intake and body weight gain for 30 days in HFD-fed mice [5], and it inhibited adipogenesis in 3T3-L1 cells through downregulation of PPARγ by activating AMPK and the modulation of mitotic clonal expansion [9,10]. The low-dose (0.005%, w/w) of apigenin used in the present study may be insufficient for suppressing food intake, body weight gain and body fat accumulation.

Insulin resistance and hyperinsulinemia are hallmarks of obesity and can induce many of the abnormalities associated with metabolic syndrome [17]. A previous study from our laboratory demonstrated that an HFD for 16 weeks led to increased fasting blood glucose, hyperinsulinemia and insulin resistance in mice compared to a normal diet [15]. In the present study, apigenin significantly decreased levels of fasting blood glucose, plasma insulin and HOMA-IR, a surrogate marker for insulin resistance, in HFD-fed mice. Moreover, it significantly decreased the activities of hepatic PEPCK and G6Pase. These are key enzymes for gluconeogenesis, and controlling hepatic gluconeogenesis is crucial for maintaining glucose homeostasis [18]. Insulin is the most important hormone, which inhibits gluconeogenesis, and it directly suppresses the transcription and activity of hepatic gluconeogenic enzymes [18]. Hepatic insulin resistance results in impaired insulin-induced suppression of gluconeogenesis in obese subjects, and gluconeogenesis closely correlates with the severity of diabetes and the degree of obesity [19]. Therefore, apigenin seems to decrease fasting blood glucose by inhibiting hepatic gluconeogenic enzyme activities, and the changes in hepatic glucose-regulating enzymes may be partly attributed to the apigenin-induced improvements in insulin resistance. Our findings were supported by a previous *in vitro* study that demonstrated the inhibitory effects of apigenin on gene expression of PEPCK and G6Pase in HepG2 cells [20]. Moreover, a significant decrease in fasting blood glucose levels after apigenin consumption was observed in HFD-fed mice [11] and streptozotocin-induced type 1 diabetic rats [21].

Inflammation is one of the main mechanisms of impaired insulin action. The production of adipocytokines is related to ectopic fat accumulation and decreases insulin sensitivity directly and/or indirectly in adipose tissue and the liver, leading to impaired glucose homeostasis [3,22,23]. For example, TNF-α is an important mediator of insulin resistance in obesity owing to its inhibitory effects on insulin receptor signaling. IL-6 also plays a direct role in insulin resistance by inhibiting insulin receptor signal transduction and insulin action in hepatocytes [24]. Their circulating levels were increased in insulin resistance states, such as obesity and type 2 diabetes, while they were decreased in response to weight reduction or anti-diabetic drugs [2,25,26]. IFN-γ is another pro-inflammatory cytokine mainly produced by T-cells, and it regulates insulin resistance in obesity by inducing pro-inflammatory cytokine expression in macrophages [27]. The production of IFN-γ by T-cells in adipose tissue was higher in HFD-induced obese mice than lean mice, and obese IFN-γ-deficient mice showed modest increases in insulin sensitivity [27]. O'Rourke *et al.* [28] also demonstrated a role for IFN-γ in the regulation of inflammation and glucose homeostasis in obesity though multiple mechanisms, including its effects on pro-inflammatory cytokine expression and macrophage phenotype. In addition to cytokines, obese adipose tissue secretes chemokines, such as MCP-1, which contribute to obesity-related insulin resistance [2]. A previous study reported that apigenin exerted anti-inflammatory activity *in vitro* and *in vivo* by inactivating NF-κB, thereby reducing the production of inflammatory mediators [29]. Since we also observed that plasma levels of pro-inflammatory mediators, such as MCP-1, IFN-γ, TNF-α and IL-6, were significantly decreased by apigenin, these changes could be partly associated with the decreased fat accumulation, improved insulin resistance and glucose homeostasis in apigenin-supplemented obese mice.

It is well known that abnormal lipid metabolism in obesity is regarded as a major driving force for dyslipidemia and hepatic steatosis, and insulin resistance and inflammation play an important role in the development of dyslipidemia and hepatic steatosis [2]. In insulin resistance states, the increased lipolysis of stored triglycerides in adipose tissue promotes the production of fatty acids, and the elevation of circulating free fatty acid inhibits the anti-lipolytic action of insulin and favors increased uptake into the liver, leading to dyslipidemia and hepatic steatosis. Free fatty acid can also serve as an endogenous signal to stimulate the production of pro-inflammatory mediators, such as TNF-α and IL-6, and inhibition of pro-inflammatory signaling pathways can prevent free fatty acid-induced insulin resistance [2,30]. Moreover, pro-inflammatory cytokines, including TNF-α and IL-6, increase circulating levels of total cholesterol, LDL-cholesterol and free fatty acid and stimulate over secretion of apoB in the liver [2]. In addition, elevated levels of TNF-α, IL-6 and MCP-1 were associated with the development of NAFLD, and pharmacological and genetic inhibition of these pro-inflammatory mediators ameliorated hepatic steatosis in obese animals [2,31].

In the present study, apigenin markedly decreased plasma total-cholesterol levels, as well as plasma apoB levels and the apoB/apoA1 ratio, indicating its protective role against atherogenic dyslipidemia in HFD-induced obese mice. In addition, plasma free fatty acid levels were significantly decreased in apigenin-supplemented obese mice. As described in the preceding text, increased delivery and uptake of free fatty acids into the liver promote the production of triglycerides, which ultimately leads to hepatic steatosis [2]. Moreover, increased levels of circulating free fatty acids, rather than excessive hepatic lipid accumulation, serve as an indicator of the degree of liver damage [32]. The plasma levels of ALT and AST, useful biomarkers of liver injury, as well as hepatic lipid droplet accumulation were elevated in HFD-induced obese animals [33]. In the present study, apigenin decreased hepatomegaly and hepatic lipid droplets' accumulation along with plasma ALT and AST levels, indicating its beneficial effects on NAFLD.

Lipid droplets are dynamic organelles that govern the storage and turnover of lipids and comprise a core of storage of neutral lipids, *i.e.*, triglycerides and cholesterol esters. PAP is a rate-limiting enzyme for hepatic triglyceride synthesis, and the activity and expression of the lipin-1 gene encoding PAP were increased in HFD-fed obese mice or *ob/ob* mice [15,34], while deficiency of lipin-1 attenuated hepatic steatosis [34]. The esterified cholesterol is also a major component of lipid droplets, and ACAT, a key cholesterol-regulating enzyme involved in the hepatic esterification of cholesterol, facilitates cholesterol ester incorporation into lipid droplets [35]. The activity of ACAT in the livers of HFD-induced obese mice was higher than that of non-obese mice [15], and inhibition of ACAT improved abnormal lipid metabolism and hepatic steatosis in obese mice [36]. Alger *et al.* [37] also demonstrated that the increased accumulation of cholesterol ester in lipid droplets could limit the mobilization of hepatic triglycerides and decrease the release of very-low-density lipoprotein-triglyceride by the liver, leading to cholesterol-associated hepatic steatosis. Interestingly, we observed that hepatic PAP and ACAT activities were significantly lowered by apigenin. Based on these results, apigenin seemed to ameliorate hepatic steatosis by reducing lipid droplet accumulation via a decrease in plasma free fatty acid and an inhibition of hepatic enzyme activities involved in the synthesis of triglycerides and cholesterol esters in HFD-fed mice. Moreover, inhibition of hepatic ACAT may be a possible mechanism for decreased plasma total cholesterol and apoB levels observed in apigenin-supplemented mice, since ACAT inhibitors stimulate bile acid synthesis and inhibit apoB secretion, thus controlling plasma cholesterol levels, as well as hepatic cholesterol biosynthesis and catabolism [38,39].

In aerobic organisms from bacteria to humans, OXPHOS is the major source of energy-rich ATP, and the electron transport chain is responsible for creating the proton gradient that drives the generation of ATP via OXPHOS. The electron transport chain is composed of four protein complexes (complexes I, II, III and IV), which are found in the inner membrane of a mitochondrion. Ndufs4 is a gene encoding the NADH-ubiquinone oxidoreductase subunit of complex I, the first multisubunit enzyme complex of the mitochondrial respiratory chain, which plays a critical role in cellular generation of ATP. In a recent study, a deletion of Ndufs4 led to an inhibition of OXPHOS and increases in circulating free fatty acid and inflammation [40]. In addition to Atp5a1, which encodes a subunit of mitochondrial ATP synthase (complex V), other mitochondrial complex I and II subunit-encoding genes (e.g., Ndufb5, Ndufb9 and Sdhd) were downregulated in obese subjects and type 2 diabetic patients, and impaired mitochondrial OXPHOS was proposed as an etiological mechanism underlying insulin resistance [41]. Interestingly, apigenin upregulated nine genes involved in OXPHOS and the electron transport chain, including Atp5a1, Cox7a2, Ndufs4, Ndufb5, Ndufb9 and Sdhd.

We also observed that TCA cycle genes (Idh2, Fh1, Aco1) and fatty acid oxidation genes (Acadsb, Ehhadh) were upregulated in the livers of apigenin-supplemented obese mice, along with other genes that facilitate fatty acid utilization (e.g., Elovl2 and Pecr) (Figure 5B). Fatty acid oxidation is the catabolic process by which fatty acid molecules are broken down in the mitochondria to produce acetyl coenzyme A, which enters the TCA cycle [42]. The reactions of the TCA cycle generate NADH and FADH2, which are in turn used by the OXPHOS pathway to generate ATP [42]. The mRNA expression of Elovl2, which is involved in the elongation required for the synthesis of docosahexaenoic acid, was reduced in the livers of obese subjects, and an intervention to improve hepatic steatosis and diabetes upregulated hepatic Elovl2 expression along with hepatic fatty acid oxidation [43,44]. Since the synthesis of docosahexaenoic acid from linolenic acid requires one round of peroxisomal β-oxidation in addition to elongation and desaturation [45], the observed upregulation of Elovl2 may be related to the upregulated expression of peroxisomal fatty acid oxidation genes, such as Ehhadh. Hepatic gene expression of Pecr, another fatty acid elongation gene, was also upregulated by a dietary strategy for the treatment of hepatic steatosis [46], and its gene expression was downregulated in mice after acute inhibition of β-oxidation [47]. Taken together, our microarray data suggest that apigenin can upregulate the expression of hepatic genes involved in energy metabolism, such as OXPHOS, electron transport chain, TCA cycle and fatty acid oxidation, which may contribute to improved metabolic abnormalities, such as hepatic steatosis, dyslipidemia and insulin resistance.

The microarray data of the liver also revealed that supplementation of the HFD with apigenin upregulated the expression of genes involved in cholesterol homeostasis. The liver plays a critical role in cholesterol metabolism and in controlling its removal through the bile. Along with cholesterol esterification, the hepatic conversion of cholesterol into bile acid is an important cholesterol-metabolizing pathway for the elimination of excess cholesterol. Approximately 95% of bile acids are reabsorbed in the intestine and transported back to the liver, and the remaining 5% is lost via the feces and compensated via *de novo* bile acid synthesis from cholesterol in the liver. Prior to bile acid secretion, the synthesized bile acids in the liver need to be conjugated to either glycine or taurine to form bile salts. The bile acid conjugation processes can protect against hepatic damage, because glycine/taurine conjugates are generally less toxic and more hydrophilic than the primary bile acids [48]. Baat is implicated in the conjugation of *de novo*-synthesized bile acids from cholesterol in the liver. Defects in Baat can cause intrahepatic cholestasis, which occurs in a subgroup of patients with NAFLD [49]. Similar to our study, hepatic Baat mRNA expression was upregulated by treatment with an agent protecting against diet-induced NAFLD [50]. Moreover, we observed that apigenin upregulated hepatic gene expression of NPC2 encoding a cholesterol-binding protein, Niemann-Pick type C 2, which positively regulates biliary cholesterol secretion via stimulation of ABCG5/ABCG8-mediated cholesterol efflux [51]. Since the amount of cholesterol secreted into the bile each day is comparable to the amounts synthesized in the liver and absorbed from the intestine, the regulation of biliary cholesterol secretion by Npc2 is thought to be important in the maintenance of the whole-body cholesterol level. Moreover, lack of Npc2 increased cellular cholesterol, suggesting the role for Npc2 in the regulation of sterol homeostasis [52].

In addition to bile acid, steroid hormones are generally synthesized from cholesterol. Among the various genes involved in steroid hormone synthesis, the gene expression of Hsd17b6, which is involved in the conversion of testosterone back to androstenedione, was upregulated in the livers of apigenin-supplemented obese mice. The Hsd17b6 is suggested to act as a modifier gene influencing insulin resistance and obesity [53], and obese subjects show lower Hsd17b6 gene expression in the liver [43], whereas its gene expression is increased in the livers of obesity-resistant animals [54]. In the present study, apigenin also upregulated mRNA expression of hepatic Slc37a4 mRNA, whose expression was decreased during the progression of liver fibrosis [55], and suppression of this molecule was associated with stimulation of *de novo* lipogenesis and the development of hepatic steatosis [56]. A recent study suggested that it is involved in processes determining the total plasma cholesterol concentration [57]. In addition, we observed that apigenin increased hepatic gene expression of angiopoietin-like (Angptl) 3, which is exclusively expressed in the liver and is involved in the trafficking and metabolism of lipids. Although genetic deletion of Angptl3 was associated with reduced circulating HDL-cholesterol and triglyceride levels in mice [58], apigenin did not affect these circulating lipid levels in the present study. This may be related to unchanged hepatic Angptl8 mRNA expression, because Quagliarini *et al.* [59] recently demonstrated that the plasma triglyceride level was not altered in mice expressing Angptl3 alone, but coexpression of Angptl8 leads to hypertriglyceridemia despite a reduction in the circulating Angptl3 level. They have suggested that Angptl8 is a paralog of Angptl3, which controls triglyceride metabolism together with Angptl3.

We also observed that mRNA expression of lipolysis- and lipogenesis-related genes (Lpl, Ppary, Srebf1, Dgat2 and Cidea) was downregulated in the livers of apigenin-supplemented mice. The gene expression of Lpl, which controls fatty acid uptake through the hydrolysis of triglyceride-rich lipoproteins, was higher in obese subjects with NAFLD compared to subjects without NAFLD [60], and liver-specific overexpression of Lpl induced hepatic steatosis and insulin resistance in mice [61]. Therefore, it is proposed that upregulation of Lpl can contribute to hepatic steatosis by promoting the incorporation of circulating fatty acids into intrahepatic triglycerides [62]. Similar to Ppary, Srebf1, Dgat2 and Cidea, several lipogenic genes have also been suggested as steatogenic factors in the liver [62]. The hepatic overexpression of Dgat2, which catalyzes the final step of triglyceride synthesis, led to hepatic steatosis in mice [63], and liver-specific disruption of Ppary or Srebf1 protected mice against hepatic steatosis [64]. Moreover, Cidea promoted large lipid droplets' accumulation in the liver [65]. In contrast, a deficiency of hepatic Scd1, which converts saturated fatty acids to monounsaturated fatty acids, provided protection against hepatic steatosis induced by a high-carbohydrate diet, but not HFD [66]. Together, our data indicate that the molecular mechanism of apigenin action involves not only activation of energy metabolism and regulation of cholesterol metabolism, but also reduction of lipolysis and lipogenesis in the liver.

5. Conclusions

Long-term supplementation of apigenin (0.005%, *w/w*) to HFD-fed mice ameliorated dyslipidemia and hepatic steatosis. These beneficial effects were accompanied by decreased activities of hepatic enzymes controlling triglyceride synthesis and cholesterol esterification and by increased expression of hepatic genes involved in fatty acid oxidation, the TCA cycle, OXPHOS, the electron transport chain and cholesterol homeostasis, as well as decreased expression of hepatic lipogenic and lipolytic genes, as summarized in Figure 6. Furthermore, apigenin lowered levels of pro-inflammatory cytokines and chemokines in plasma, and it improved hyperglycemia, hyperinsulinemia and insulin resistance. The improved glucose metabolism by apigenin appeared to be mediated through the inhibition of hepatic gluconeogenic enzyme activities. Taken together, our findings suggest that apigenin may help to ameliorate HFD-induced metabolic disturbances, such as dyslipidemia, hepatic steatosis and insulin resistance.

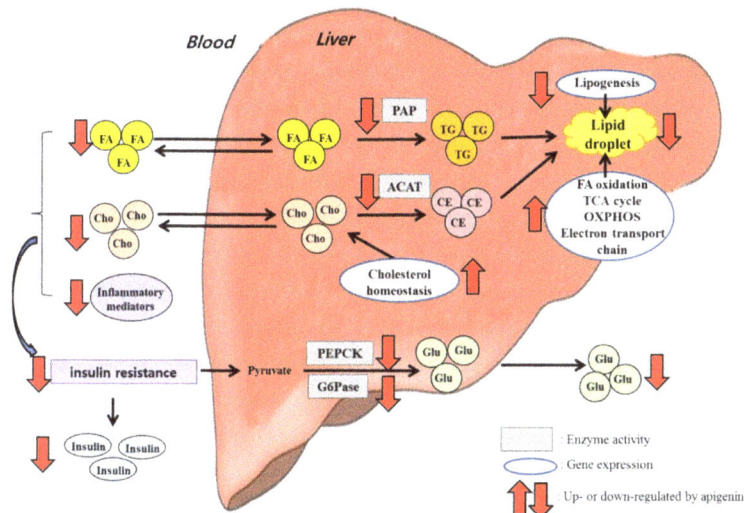

Figure 6. Schematic diagram showing the mechanisms underlying the beneficial effects of apigenin on obesity-related metabolic disturbances. Apigenin decreased the activities of hepatic enzymes controlling triglyceride synthesis and cholesterol esterification and increased the expression of hepatic genes involved in fatty acid oxidation, the TCA cycle, OXPHOS, the electron transport chain and cholesterol homeostasis while decreasing the expression of hepatic lipogenic and lipolytic genes, indicating that these changes may be potential mechanisms for improving dyslipidemia and hepatic steatosis in HFD-fed mice. Moreover, apigenin decreased plasma pro-inflammatory adipocytokines levels and hepatic gluconeogenic enzyme activities, which may be partly associated with the improved hyperglycemia, hyperinsulinemia and insulin resistance.

Acknowledgments: This work was supported by the Science Research Center Project (NRF-2015R1A5A6001906) and the Bio-Synergy Research Project (NRF-2012M3A9C4048818) of the Ministry of Science, ICT and Future Planning through the National Research Foundation of Korea.

Author Contributions: Yun-Young Cho carried out experiments and analyzed data with Un Ju Jung. Un Ju Jung wrote the original manuscript, and Myung-Sook Choi edited the manuscript. All authors approved the final manuscript.

Conflicts of Interest: The authors declare no conflict of interest.

References

1. Padwal, R.S.; Sharma, A.M. Prevention of cardiovascular disease: Obesity, diabetes and the metabolic syndrome. *Can. J. Cardiol.* **2010**, *26* (Suppl. C), 18C–20C. [CrossRef]
2. Jung, U.J.; Choi, M.S. Obesity and its metabolic complications: The role of adipokines and the relationship between obesity, inflammation, insulin resistance, dyslipidemia and nonalcoholic fatty liver disease. *Int. J. Mol. Sci.* **2014**, *15*, 6184–6223. [CrossRef] [PubMed]
3. Schmidt, M.I.; Duncan, B.B.; Sharrett, A.R.; Lindberg, G.; Savage, P.J.; Offenbacher, S.; Azambuja, M.I.; Tracy, R.P.; Heiss, G. Markers of inflammation and prediction of diabetes mellitus in adults (Atherosclerosis Risk in Communities study): A cohort study. *Lancet* **1999**, *353*, 1649–1652. [CrossRef]
4. Yu, R.; Kim, C.S.; Kang, J.H. Inflammatory components of adipose tissue as target for treatment of metabolic syndrome. *Forum Nutr.* **2009**, *61*, 95–103. [PubMed]
5. Abenavoli, L.; di Renzo, L.; Guzzi, P.H.; Pellicano, R.; Milic, N.; de Lorenzo, A. Non-alcoholic fatty liver disease severity, central fat mass and adinopectin: A close relationship. *Clujul Med.* **2015**, *88*, 489–493. [CrossRef] [PubMed]

6. Wang, S.; Miller, B.; Matthan, N.R.; Goktas, Z.; Wu, D.; Reed, D.B.; Yin, X.; Grammas, P.; Moustaid-Moussa, N.; Shen, C.L.; *et al.* Aortic cholesterol accumulation correlates with systemic inflammation but not hepatic and gonadal adipose tissue inflammation in low-density lipoprotein receptor null mice. *Nutr. Res.* **2013**, *33*, 1072–1082. [CrossRef] [PubMed]

7. Milosević, N.; Milanović, M.; Abenavoli, L.; Milić, N. Phytotherapy and NAFLD—From goals and challenges to clinical practice. *Rev. Recent Clin. Trials* **2014**, *9*, 195–203. [CrossRef] [PubMed]

8. Shukla, S.; Gupta, S. Apigenin: A promising molecule for cancer prevention. *Pharm. Res.* **2010**, *27*, 962–978. [CrossRef] [PubMed]

9. Ono, M.; Fujimori, K. Antiadipogenic effect of dietary apigenin through activation of AMPK in 3T3-L1 cells. *J. Agric. Food Chem.* **2011**, *59*, 13346–13352. [CrossRef] [PubMed]

10. Kim, M.A.; Kang, K.; Lee, H.J.; Kim, M.; Kim, C.Y.; Nho, C.W. Apigenin isolated from *Daphne genkwa* Siebold et Zucc. inhibits 3T3-L1 preadipocyte differentiation through a modulation of mitotic clonal expansion. *Life Sci.* **2014**, *101*, 64–72. [CrossRef] [PubMed]

11. Escande, C.; Nin, V.; Price, N.L.; Capellini, V.; Gomes, A.P.; Barbosa, M.T.; O'Neil, L.; White, T.A.; Sinclair, D.A.; Chini, E.N. Flavonoid apigenin is an inhibitor of the NAD+ ase CD38: Implications for cellular NAD+ metabolism, protein acetylation, and treatment of metabolic syndrome. *Diabetes* **2013**, *62*, 1084–1093. [CrossRef] [PubMed]

12. Myoung, H.J.; Kim, G.; Nam, K.W. Apigenin isolated from the seeds of *Perilla frutescens* britton var crispa (Benth.) inhibits food intake in C57BL/6J mice. *Arch. Pharm. Res.* **2010**, *33*, 1741–1746. [CrossRef] [PubMed]

13. Seo, K.I.; Choi, M.S.; Jung, U.J.; Kim, H.J.; Yeo, J.; Jeon, S.M.; Lee, M.K. Effect of curcumin supplementation on blood glucose, plasma insulin, and glucose homeostasis related enzyme activities in diabetic *db/db* mice. *Mol. Nutr. Food Res.* **2008**, *52*, 995–1004. [CrossRef] [PubMed]

14. Cho, S.J.; Jung, U.J.; Choi, M.S. Differential effects of low-dose resveratrol on adiposity and hepatic steatosis in diet-induced obese mice. *Br. J. Nutr.* **2012**, *108*, 2166–2175. [CrossRef] [PubMed]

15. Do, G.M.; Oh, H.Y.; Kwon, E.Y.; Cho, Y.Y.; Shin, S.K.; Park, H.J.; Jeon, S.M.; Kim, E.; Hur, C.G.; Park, T.S.; *et al.* Long-term adaptation of global transcription and metabolism in the liver of high-fat diet-fed C57BL/6J mice. *Mol. Nutr. Food Res.* **2011**, *55* (Suppl. 2), S173–S185. [CrossRef] [PubMed]

16. Wallace, T.M.; Levy, J.C.; Matthews, D.R. Use and abuse of HOMA modeling. *Diabetes Care* **2004**, *27*, 1487–1495. [CrossRef] [PubMed]

17. Singh, B.; Saxena, A. Surrogate markers of insulin resistance: A review. *World J. Diabetes* **2010**, *1*, 36–47. [CrossRef] [PubMed]

18. Barthel, A.; Schmoll, D. Novel concepts in insulin regulation of hepatic gluconeogenesis. *Am. J. Physiol. Endocrinol. Metab.* **2003**, *285*, E685–E692. [CrossRef] [PubMed]

19. Gastaldelli, A.; Baldi, S.; Pettiti, M.; Toschi, E.; Camastra, S.; Natali, A.; Landau, B.R.; Ferrannini, E. Influence of obesity and type 2 diabetes on gluconeogenesis and glucose output in humans: A quantitative study. *Diabetes* **2000**, *49*, 1367–1373. [CrossRef] [PubMed]

20. Bumke-Vogt, C.; Osterhoff, M.A.; Borchert, A.; Guzman-Perez, V.; Sarem, Z.; Birkenfeld, A.L.; Bähr, V.; Pfeiffer, A.F. The flavones apigenin and luteolin induce FOXO1 translocation but inhibit gluconeogenic and lipogenic gene expression in human cells. *PLoS ONE* **2014**, *9*, e104321. [CrossRef]

21. Hossain, C.M.; Ghosh, M.K.; Satapathy, B.S.; Dey, N.S.; Mukherjee, B. Apigenin causes biochemical modulation, GLUT4 and CD38 alterations to improve diabetes and to protect damages of some vital organs in experimental diabetes. *Am. J. Pharmacol. Toxicol.* **2014**, *9*, 39–52. [CrossRef]

22. Polyzos, S.A.; Kountouras, J.; Mantzoros, C.S. Adipokines in nonalcoholic fatty liver disease. *Metabolism* **2015**. [CrossRef]

23. Abenavoli, L.; Peta, V. Role of adipokines and cytokines in non-alcoholic fatty liver disease. *Rev. Recent Clin. Trials* **2014**, *9*, 134–140. [CrossRef] [PubMed]

24. Senn, J.J.; Klover, P.J.; Nowak, I.A.; Mooney, R.A. Interleukin-6 induces cellular insulin resistance in hepatocytes. *Diabetes* **2002**, *51*, 3391–3399. [CrossRef] [PubMed]

25. Ryan, A.S.; Nicklas, B.J. Reductions in plasma cytokine levels with weight loss improve insulin sensitivity in overweight and obese postmenopausal women. *Diabetes Care* **2004**, *27*, 1699–1705. [CrossRef] [PubMed]

26. Grosso, A.F.; de Oliveira, S.F.; Higuchi, M.L.; Favarato, D.; Dallan, L.A.; da Luz, P.L. Synergistic anti-inflammatory effect: Simvastatin and pioglitazone reduce inflammatory markers of plasma and epicardial adipose tissue of coronary patients with metabolic syndrome. *Diabetol. Metab. Syndr.* **2014**, *6*, 47. [CrossRef] [PubMed]

27. Rocha, V.Z.; Folco, E.J.; Sukhova, G.; Shimizu, K.; Gotsman, I.; Vernon, A.H.; Libby, P. Interferon-gamma, a Th1 cytokine, regulates fat inflammation: A role for adaptive immunity in obesity. *Circ. Res.* **2008**, *103*, 467–476. [CrossRef] [PubMed]

28. O'Rourke, R.W.; White, A.E.; Metcalf, M.D.; Winters, B.R. Systemic inflammation and insulin sensitivity in obese IFN-γ knockout mice. *Metabolism* **2012**, *61*, 1152–1161. [CrossRef] [PubMed]

29. Nicholas, C.; Batra, S.; Vargo, M.A.; Voss, O.H.; Gavrilin, M.A.; Wewers, M.D.; Guttridge, D.C.; Grotewold, E.; Doseff, A.I. Apigenin blocks lipopolysaccharide-induced lethality *in vivo* and proinflammatory cytokines expression by inactivating NF-κB through the suppression of p65 phosphorylation. *J. Immunol.* **2007**, *179*, 7121–7127. [CrossRef] [PubMed]

30. Nguyen, M.T.; Satoh, H.; Favelyukis, S.; Babendure, J.L.; Imamura, T.; Sbodio, J.I.; Zalevsky, J.; Dahiyat, B.I.; Chi, N.W.; Olefsky, J.M. JNK and TNF-α mediate free fatty acid-induced insulin resistance in 3T3-L1 adipocytes. *J. Biol. Chem.* **2005**, *280*, 35361–35371. [CrossRef] [PubMed]

31. Braunersreuther, V.; Viviani, G.L.; Mach, F.; Montecucco, F. Role of cytokines and chemokines in non-alcoholic fatty liver disease. *World J. Gastroenterol.* **2012**, *18*, 727–735. [CrossRef] [PubMed]

32. Liu, Q.; Bengmark, S.; Qu, S. The role of hepatic fat accumulation in pathogenesis of non-alcoholic fatty liver disease (NAFLD). *Lipids Health Dis.* **2010**, *9*, 42. [CrossRef] [PubMed]

33. Li, H.; Yokoyama, N.; Yoshida, S.; Tsutsumi, K.; Hatakeyama, S.; Sato, T.; Ishihara, K.; Akiba, S. Alleviation of high-fat diet-induced fatty liver damage in group IVA phospholipase A2-knockout mice. *PLoS ONE* **2009**, *4*, e8089. [CrossRef]

34. Ryu, D.; Oh, K.J.; Jo, H.Y.; Hedrick, S.; Kim, Y.N.; Hwang, Y.J.; Park, T.S.; Han, J.S.; Choi, C.S.; Montminy, M.; *et al.* TORC2 regulates hepatic insulin signaling via a mammalian phosphatidic acid phosphatase, LIPIN1. *Cell Metab.* **2009**, *9*, 240–251. [CrossRef] [PubMed]

35. Anderson, R.A.; Joyce, C.; Davis, M.; Reagan, J.W.; Clark, M.; Shelness, G.S.; Rudel, L.L. Identification of a form of acyl-CoA:cholesterol acyltransferase specific to liver and intestine in nonhuman primates. *J. Biol. Chem.* **1998**, *273*, 26747–26754. [CrossRef] [PubMed]

36. Yamamoto, T.; Yamaguchi, H.; Miki, H.; Shimada, M.; Nakada, Y.; Ogino, M.; Asano, K.; Aoki, K.; Tamura, N.; Masago, M.; *et al.* Coenzyme A: Diacylglycerol acyltransferase 1 inhibitor ameliorates obesity, liver steatosis, and lipid metabolism abnormality in KKAy mice fed high-fat or high-carbohydrate diets. *Eur. J. Pharmacol.* **2010**, *640*, 243–249. [CrossRef] [PubMed]

37. Alger, H.M.; Mark Brown, J.; Sawyer, J.K.; Kelley, K.L.; Shah, R.; Wilson, M.D.; Willingham, M.C.; Rudel, L.L. Inhibition of acyl-coenzyme A: Cholesterol acyltransferase 2 (ACAT2) prevents dietary cholesterol-associated steatosis by enhancing hepatic triglyceride mobilization. *J. Biol. Chem.* **2010**, *285*, 14267–14274. [CrossRef] [PubMed]

38. Post, P.M.; Zoeteweij, J.P.; Bos, M.H.; de Wit, E.C.; Havinga, R.; Kuipers, F.; Princen, H.M. Acyl-coenzyme A: Cholesterol acyltransferase inhibitor, avasimibe, stimulates bile acid synthesis and cholesterol 7alpha-hydroxylase in cultured rat hepatocytes and *in vivo* in the rat. *Hepatolohy* **1999**, *30*, 491–500. [CrossRef] [PubMed]

39. Huff, M.W.; Telford, D.E.; Barrett, P.H.; Billheimer, J.T.; Gillies, P.J. Inhibition of hepatic ACAT decreases ApoB secretion in miniature pigs fed a cholesterol-free diet. *Arterioscler. Thromb.* **1994**, *14*, 1498–1508. [CrossRef] [PubMed]

40. Jin, Z.; Wei, W.; Yang, M.; Du, Y.; Wan, Y. Mitochondrial complex I activity suppresses inflammation and enhances bone resorption by shifting macrophage-osteoclast polarization. *Cell Metab.* **2014**, *20*, 483–498. [CrossRef] [PubMed]

41. Dahlman, I.; Forsgren, M.; Sjögren, A.; Nordström, E.A.; Kaaman, M.; Näslund, E.; Attersand, A.; Arner, P. Downregulation of electron transport chain genes in visceral adipose tissue in type 2 diabetes independent of obesity and possibly involving tumor necrosis factor-alpha. *Diabetes* **2006**, *55*, 1792–1799. [CrossRef] [PubMed]

42. Jaswal, J.S.; Keung, W.; Wang, W.; Ussher, J.R.; Lopaschuk, G.D. Targeting fatty acid and carbohydrate oxidation—A novel therapeutic intervention in the ischemic and failing heart. *Biochim. Biophys. Acta* **2011**, *1813*, 1333–1350. [CrossRef] [PubMed]

43. Elam, M.B.; Cowan, G.S.; Rooney, R.J., Jr.; Hiler, M.L.; Yellaturu, C.R.; Deng, X.; Howell, G.E.; Park, E.A.; Gerling, I.C.; Patel, D.; *et al.* Hepatic gene expression in morbidly obese women: Implications for disease susceptibility. *Obesity* **2009**, *17*, 1563–1573. [CrossRef] [PubMed]

44. Lu, W.D.; Li, B.Y.; Yu, F.; Cai, Q.; Zhang, Z.; Yin, M.; Gao, H.Q. Quantitative proteomics study on the protective mechanism of phlorizin on hepatic damage in diabetic *db/db* mice. *Mol. Med. Rep.* **2012**, *5*, 1285–1294. [PubMed]

45. Sprecher, H. Metabolism of highly unsaturated *n*-3 and *n*-6 fatty acids. *Biochim. Biophys. Acta* **2000**, *1486*, 219–231. [CrossRef]

46. Martín-Pozuelo, G.; Navarro-González, I.; González-Barrio, R.; Santaella, M.; García-Alonso, J.; Hidalgo, N.; Gómez-Gallego, C.; Ros, G.; Periago, M.J. The effect of tomato juice supplementation on biomarkers and gene expression related to lipid metabolism in rats with induced hepatic steatosis. *Eur. J. Nutr.* **2015**, *54*, 933–944. [CrossRef] [PubMed]

47. Van der Leij, F.R.; Bloks, V.W.; Grefhorst, A.; Hoekstra, J.; Gerding, A.; Kooi, K.; Gerbens, F.; te Meerman, G.; Kuipers, F. Gene expression profiling in livers of mice after acute inhibition of beta-oxidation. *Genomics* **2007**, *90*, 680–689. [CrossRef] [PubMed]

48. Perez, M.J.; Briz, O. Bile-acid-induced cell injury and protection. *World J. Gastroenterol.* **2009**, *15*, 1677–1689. [CrossRef] [PubMed]

49. Hadžić, N.; Bull, L.N.; Clayton, P.T.; Knisely, A.S. Diagnosis in bile acid-CoA: Amino acid *N*-acyltransferase deficiency. *World J. Gastroenterol.* **2012**, *18*, 3322–3326. [PubMed]

50. Pircher, P.C.; Kitto, J.L.; Petrowski, M.L.; Tangirala, R.K.; Bischoff, E.D.; Schulman, I.G.; Westin, S.K. Farnesoid X receptor regulates bile acid-amino acid conjugation. *J. Biol. Chem.* **2003**, *278*, 27703–27711. [CrossRef] [PubMed]

51. Yamanashi, Y.; Takada, T.; Yoshikado, T.; Shoda, J.; Suzuki, H. NPC2 regulates biliary cholesterol secretion via stimulation of ABCG5/G8-mediated cholesterol transport. *Gastroenterology* **2011**, *140*, 1664–1674. [CrossRef] [PubMed]

52. Abi-Mosleh, L.; Infante, R.E.; Radhakrishnan, A.; Goldstein, J.L.; Brown, M.S. Cyclodextrin overcomes deficient lysosome-to-endoplasmic reticulum transport of cholesterol in Niemann-Pick type C cells. *Proc. Natl. Acad. Sci. USA* **2009**, *106*, 19316–19321. [CrossRef] [PubMed]

53. Jones, M.R.; Mathur, R.; Cui, J.; Guo, X.; Azziz, R.; Goodarzi, M.O. Independent confirmation of association between metabolic phenotypes of polycystic ovary syndrome and variation in the type 6 17beta-hydroxysteroid dehydrogenase gene. *J. Clin. Endocrinol. Metab.* **2009**, *94*, 5034–5038. [CrossRef] [PubMed]

54. Morita, M.; Oike, Y.; Nagashima, T.; Kadomatsu, T.; Tabata, M.; Suzuki, T.; Nakamura, T.; Yoshida, N.; Okada, M.; Yamamoto, T. Obesity resistance and increased hepatic expression of catabolism-related mRNAs in Cnot3$^{+/-}$ mice. *EMBO J.* **2011**, *30*, 4678–4691. [CrossRef] [PubMed]

55. Takahara, Y.; Takahashi, M.; Wagatsuma, H.; Yokoya, F.; Zhang, Q.W.; Yamaguchi, M.; Aburatani, H.; Kawada, N. Gene expression profiles of hepatic cell-type specific marker genes in progression of liver fibrosis. *World J. Gastroenterol.* **2006**, *12*, 6473–6499. [CrossRef] [PubMed]

56. Bandsma, R.H.; Wiegman, C.H.; Herling, A.W.; Burger, H.J.; ter Harmsel, A.; Meijer, A.J.; Romijn, J.A.; Reijngoud, D.J.; Kuipers, F. Acute inhibition of glucose-6-phosphate translocator activity leads to increased de novo lipogenesis and development of hepatic steatosis without affecting VLDL production in rats. *Diabetes* **2001**, *50*, 2591–2597. [CrossRef] [PubMed]

57. Van de Pas, N.C.; Soffers, A.E.; Freidig, A.P.; van Ommen, B.; Woutersen, R.A.; Rietjens, I.M.; de Graaf, A.A. Systematic construction of a conceptual minimal model of plasma cholesterol levels based on knockout mouse phenotypes. *Biochim. Biophys. Acta* **2010**, *1801*, 646–654. [CrossRef] [PubMed]

58. Shimamura, M.; Matsuda, M.; Yasumo, H.; Okazaki, M.; Fujimoto, K.; Kono, K.; Shimizugawa, T.; Ando, Y.; Koishi, R.; Kohama, T.; *et al.* Angiopoietin-like protein3 regulates plasma HDL cholesterol through suppression of endothelial lipase. *Arterioscler. Thromb. Vasc. Biol.* **2007**, *27*, 366–372. [CrossRef] [PubMed]

59. Quagliarini, F.; Wang, Y.; Kozlitina, J.; Grishin, N.V.; Hyde, R.; Boerwinkle, E.; Valenzuela, D.M.; Murphy, A.J.; Cohen, J.C.; Hobbs, H.H. Atypical angiopoietin-like protein that regulates ANGPTL3. *Proc. Natl. Acad. Sci. USA* **2012**, *109*, 19751–19756. [CrossRef] [PubMed]

60. Pardina, E.; Baena-Fustegueras, J.A.; Catalán, R.; Galard, R.; Lecube, A.; Fort, J.M.; Allende, H.; Vargas, V.; Peinado-Onsurbe, J. Increased expression and activity of hepatic lipase in the liver of morbidly obese adult patients in relation to lipid content. *Obes. Surg.* **2008**, *19*, 894–904. [CrossRef] [PubMed]

61. Kim, J.K.; Fillmore, J.J.; Chen, Y.; Yu, C.; Moore, I.K.; Pypaert, M.; Lutz, E.P.; Kako, Y.; Velez-Carrasco, W.; Goldberg, I.J.; *et al.* Tissue-specific overexpression of lipoprotein lipase causes tissue-specific insulin resistance. *Proc. Natl. Acad. Sci. USA* **2001**, *98*, 7522–7527. [CrossRef] [PubMed]

62. Fabbrini, E.; Sullivan, S.; Klein, S. Obesity and nonalcoholic fatty liver disease: Biochemical, metabolic, and clinical implications. *Hepatology* **2010**, *51*, 679–689. [CrossRef] [PubMed]

63. Monetti, M.; Levin, M.C.; Watt, M.J.; Sajan, M.P.; Marmor, S.; Hubbard, B.K.; Stevens, R.D.; Bain, J.R.; Newgard, C.B.; Farese, R.V., Sr.; *et al.* Dissociation of hepatic steatosis and insulin resistance in mice overexpressing DGAT in the liver. *Cell Metab.* **2007**, *6*, 69–78. [CrossRef] [PubMed]

64. Morán-Salvador, E.; López-Parra, M.; García-Alonso, V.; Titos, E.; Martínez-Clemente, M.; González-Périz, A.; López-Vicario, C.; Barak, Y.; Arroyo, V.; Clària, J. Role for PPARγ in obesity-induced hepatic steatosis as determined by hepatocyte- and macrophage-specific conditional knockouts. *FASEB J.* **2011**, *25*, 2538–2550. [CrossRef] [PubMed]

65. Zhou, L.; Xu, L.; Ye, J.; Li, D.; Wang, W.; Li, X.; Wu, L.; Wang, H.; Guan, F.; Li, P. Cidea promotes hepatic steatosis by sensing dietary fatty acids. *Hepatology* **2012**, *56*, 95–107. [CrossRef] [PubMed]

66. Miyazaki, M.; Flowers, M.T.; Sampath, H.; Chu, K.; Otzelberger, C.; Liu, X.; Ntambi, J.M. Hepatic stearoyl-CoA desaturase-1 deficiency protects mice from carbohydrate-induced adiposity and hepatic steatosis. *Cell Metab.* **2007**, *6*, 484–496. [CrossRef] [PubMed]

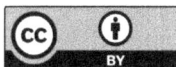

![nutrients logo] *nutrients*

MDPI

Article

Total Flavonoids from *Rosa laevigata* Michx Fruit Ameliorates Hepatic Ischemia/Reperfusion Injury through Inhibition of Oxidative Stress and Inflammation in Rats

Xufeng Tao [1], Xiance Sun [2], Lina Xu [1], Lianhong Yin [1], Xu Han [1], Yan Qi [1], Youwei Xu [1], Yanyan Zhao [1], Changyuan Wang [1] and Jinyong Peng [1,*]

[1] College of Pharmacy, Dalian Medical University, Western 9 Lvshunnan Road, Dalian 116044, China; taoxufengdalian@163.com (X.T.); Linaxu_632@126.com (L.X.); Lianhongyin_1980@163.com (L.Y.); Xuhan2002zs@163.com (X.H.); Yanqi_1976@163.com (Y.Q.); Youweixu_1964@163.com (Y.X.); Yanyanzhao_2009@126.com (Y.Z.); yuhao.1988517zs@163.com (C.W.)
[2] Department of Occupational and Environmental of Health, Dalian Medical University, No. 9 Western Section of Lushun South Road, Dalian 116044, China; qimengdy2020@163.com
*   Correspondence: jinyongpeng2008@126.com; Tel./Fax: +86-411-8611-0411

Received: 1 May 2016; Accepted: 4 July 2016; Published: 8 July 2016

Abstract: The effects of total flavonoids (TFs) from *Rosa laevigata* Michx fruit against liver damage and cerebral ischemia/reperfusion (I/R) injury have been reported, but its action on hepatic I/R injury remains unknown. In this work, the effects and possible mechanisms of TFs against hepatic I/R injury were examined using a 70% partial hepatic warm ischemia rat model. The results demonstrated TFs decreased serum aspartate transaminase (AST), alanine aminotransferase (ALT), myeloperoxidase (MPO), and lactate dehydrogenase (LDH) activities, improved liver histopathology and ultrastructure through hematoxylin-eosin (HE) staining and electron microscope observation. In addition, TFs significantly decreased malondialdehyde (MDA) and increased the levels of superoxide dismutase (SOD) and glutathione peroxidase (GSH-Px), which indicated that TFs alleviated oxidative stress caused by I/R injury. RT-PCR results proved that TFs downregulated the gene levels of inflammatory factors including interleukin-1 beta (IL-1β), interleukin-1 (IL-6), and tumor necrosis factor alpha (TNF-α). Further research indicated that TF-induced hepatoprotection was completed through inhibiting TLR4/MyD88 and activating Sirt1/Nrf2 signaling pathways. Blockade of the TLR4 pathway by TFs inhibited NF-κB and AP-1 transcriptional activities and inflammatory reaction. Activation of Sirt1/Nrf2 pathway by TFs increased the protein levels of HO-1 and GST to improve oxidative stress. Collectively, these findingsconfirmed the potent effects of TFs against hepatic I/R injury, which should be developed as a candidate for the prevention of this disease.

Keywords: hepatic ischemia/reperfusion; inflammation; oxidative stress; *Rosa laevigata* Michx fruit; total flavonoids

1. Introduction

Ischemia/reperfusion (I/R) injury is a pathologic process occurring in the organs that suffer temporary blood flow deprivation (ischemia) and restoration (reperfusion) [1]. Clinically, hepatic I/R injury always occurs in a number of settings, including hepatic transplantation, hepatic resection, and hemorrhagic shock, which can lead to higher incidences of acute and chronic organ failure [2]. Patients who suffer from hepatic I/R are exposed to enormous pain and financial burdens [3]. However, no ideal drugs show good efficiency to cure hepatic I/R injury at the clinical level [4]. Therefore, it is urgent to develop new and effective therapies for the treatment of hepatic I/R injury.

Many basic and clinical experiments have demonstrated that hepatic I/R can induce direct cellular insult and delayed dysfunction, as well as the injury resulting from activating multiple oxidative stress and inflammatory pathways [5–7]. Sirtuin 1 (Sirt1) is a nicotinamide adenine dinucleotide (NAD$^+$)-dependent nuclear class III histone deacetylase that participates in theregulation of metabolic and oxidative stress [8]. Briefly, a transcription factor-nuclear erythroid factor 2-related factorn2 (Nrf2) is anchored in the cytoplasm where it binds to Kelch-like ECH-associated protein 1 (Keap1) under normal circumstances [9]. However, Nrf2 translocates into the nucleus and then activates its target genes through an antioxidant-response element (ARE) when Sirt1 triggers the separation of Nrf2 and Keap1 [10]. Among the target genes of Nrf2, heme oxygenase-1 (HO-1), and glutathione-*S*-transferase (GST) are two anti-oxidative stress representatives [11]. HO-1 can catalyze heme metabolism to eliminate free radicals [12]. GST, one xenobiotic-metabolizing enzyme, can catalyze the nucleophilic attack of reactive oxygen species (ROS) and help to detoxify [13]. Accordingly, Sirt1/Nrf2 signaling can activate some antioxidant enzymes to improve the cellular redox state.

Furthermore, inflammatory response is well known to concern the activation of congenital immunity through binding toll-like receptor 4 (TLR4) with endogenous ligands in the absence of pathogens [14]. Recent reports have shown that activated TLR4 can trigger TNF receptor-associated factor 6 (TRAF6) by its adaptor protein myeloid differentiation primary response gene (88) (MyD88) [15]. Then, TRAF6 increases nuclear factor kappa B (NF-κB) translocation and c-Jun *N*-terminal kinase (JNK) phosphorylation that subsequently stimulates activator protein 1 (AP-1) transcription [16]. Ultimately, these molecules cause the release of a large number of inflammation cytokines including interleukin-1 beta (IL-1β), interleukin-1 (IL-6), and tumor necrosis factor alpha (TNF-α) after warm hepatic I/R [17]. Thus, many studies have focused on regulation of immune function to alleviate hepatic I/R injury.

Rosa laevigata Michx fruit has been used in China for a long history to treat chronic cough, arterial sclerosis, menstrual irregularities, and urinary incontinence [18,19], which mainly contains polysaccharose, flavonoids, and saponins [20,21]. The crude extract of total flavonoids (TFs) from it mainly contains flavones and flavonols, including quercetin, kaempferide, apigenin, and isorhamnetin [22,23]. Our previous investigations have demonstrated that TFs have hepatoprotective effects against high-fat diet and carbon tetrachloride-induced liver damage [24,25]. We also indicated that TFs have potent effects against cerebral I/R injury [26]. Nevertheless, to the best of our knowledge, no work has been investigated to report the actions of TFs against hepatic I/R injury.

Thus, the aim of this paper was to investigate the effects and possible mechanisms of TFs from *R. laevigata* Michx fruit against liver I/R damage.

2. Material and Methods

2.1. Chemicals and Materials

D101 macroporous resin was purchased from the chemical plant of Nankai University (Tianjin, China). Aspartate transaminase (AST, Code No. C010-1), alanine aminotransferase (ALT, Code No. C009-1), myeloperoxidase (MPO, Code No. A044), lactate dehydrogenase (LDH, Code No. A020-1), malondialdehyde (MDA, Code No. A003-1), superoxide dismutase (SOD, Code No. A001-1), and glutathione (GSH, No. A005) kits were obtained from Nanjing Jiancheng Institute of Biotechnology (Nanjing, China). Hematoxylin (Code No. ZLI9606), eosin (Code No. ZLI9612), and diaminobenzidine (DAB, Code No. ZLI9632) staining kits were purchased from Zhongshan Golden Bridge Biotechnology (Beijing, China). Tissue Protein Extraction Kit (Code No. KGP2100) and Nuclear and Cytoplasmic Protein Extraction kit (Code No. KGP150) were obtained from KEYGEN Biotech. Co., Ltd. (Nanjing, China). Bicinchoninic acid Protein Assay Kit (BCA, Code No. P0012S) was purchased from Beyotime Institute of Biotechnology (Shanghai, China). RNAiso Plus (Code No. 9109), PrimeScript™ RT reagent

Kit with gDNA Eraser (Perfect Real Time) (Code No. RR047A) and SYBR® Premix Ex Taq™ II (Tli RNaseH Plus) (Code No. RR820A) were purchased from TaKaRa Biotechnology Co., Ltd. (Dalian, China).

2.2. Herbal Material and Preparation of TFs

R. laevigata Michx fruit was obtained from Yunnan Qiancaoyuan Pharmaceutical Company Co. Ltd. (Yunnan, China) and identified by Dr. Yunpeng Diao (College of Pharmacy, Dalian Medical University, Dalian, China). The crude extract was prepared and the content of TFs was 81.5% according to our previous work [22]. Briefly, the powder (500 g) of the *R. laevigata* Michx fruit was crushed and extracted with 60% aqueous ethanol (4 L) two times and at 2 h for each under heat reflux. The extracted solution was condensed under 60 °C and the produced residue was added into a D101 macroporous resin column. Then, in order to obtain the crude extract, the 40% ethanol fraction was collected and evaporated. Finally, according to the previous methods [27], the content of TFs in the crude extract was detected by colorimetric methods.

2.3. Animals

The TFs weresuspended in 0.5% sodium carboxyl methyl cellulose (CMC-Na). Male SD rats (180–220 g) were purchased from the Experimental Animal Center at Dalian Medical University (Dalian, China) (SCXK: 2013-0003). All experimental procedures were approved by the Animal Care and Use Committee of Dalian Medical University (approval number: SYXK (Liao) 2013-0108; 8 November 2013), and performed in strict accordance with the PR China Legislation Regarding the Use and Care of Laboratory Animals. The rats were allowed to adapt to the new environment for one week before the experiments, which were housed in a room under 12 h light/dark cycles, a relative humidity of 60% ± 10%, and a controlled temperature of 22 ± 3 °C. The rats were group housed and allowed ad libitum access to water and a standard pellet diet throughout the experiment.

2.4. Pharmacological Treatments and I/R

The rats were randomly divided into eight groups: animals (*n* = 32) in vehicle groups were treated with 0.5% CMC-Na; animals (*n* = 32) in TF groups were treated with TFs, which were administered intragastrically (i.g.) to the animals at the doses of 200 mg/kg once daily for seven consecutive days. On the eighth day, the model of 70% partial hepatic ischemia as described previously was performed [28]. Previous studies have implemented a time course to detect the optimal ischemia time period for inducing liver injury [29,30]. The results indicated that less than 60 min of ischemia produced only minimal transaminase elevations, whereas greater than 75 min of ischemia was poorly tolerated with gross evidence of poor reperfusion of the ischemic lobes. Therefore, a reproducible level of liver injury was observed using 1 h of ischemia and, thus, used for the modeling methods in this paper. In addition, the activities of AST and ALT were of greater relevance to the times of reperfusion. Thus, we carried out different times of reperfusion (2 h, 6 h, and 24 h). Briefly, the rats were anesthetized, and the livers were exposed by midline laparotomy, then the inflow of the left lateral and median lobes of the livers were choked by placement of a bulldog clamp, while the right lobes were remained perfused to prevent intestinal congestion occlusion. After 1 h of hepatic ischemia, the bulldog clamp was removed and the liver was reperfused by the blood. Furthermore, the animals in vehicle and TF groups were divided into four groups: the rats in the sham groups underwent similar surgical procedures without I/R; the rats in the I/R groups were subject to 2, 6, and 24 h reperfusion, respectively. At the end of surgery, blood samples of all rats were obtained via the abdominal vein under anaesthesia. The left lateral lobes of livers were obtained after perfusing with 4 °C phosphate-buffered saline (PBS) and then fixed in 4% paraformaldehyde for histological examination. The median lobes were stored at −80 °C for the other assays.

2.5. Biochemical Assay

The activities of serum AST, ALT, MPO, and LDH in each group were measured by using the commercial kits according to the manufacturer's instructions.

2.6. Histopathological Examination

Formalin-fixed liver samples were embedded in paraffin and cut for 5-μm slices, and then stained with hematoxylin and eosin (HE) according to the manufacturer's instructions. The staining images were acquired using a light microscope (Leica DM4000B, Solms, Germany) with 200× magnification.

2.7. Transmission Electron Microscopy (TEM) Assay

The liver tissue (<1 mm^3) samples were harvested and fixed overnight at 4 °C in 2% glutaraldehyde. After washing in 0.1 M sodium cacodylate buffer, the samples were fixed in 1% osmium tetroxide for 2 h, and then dehydrated in gradient ethanol solutions. Finally, pretreated samples were used for ultramicrotomy and collected on copper grids. The obtained sections were then stained and observed using a transmission electron microscope (JEM-2000EX, JEDL, Tokyo, Japan).

2.8. Oxidative Stress Assay

The activities of MDA, SOD, and GSH in liver tissues were measured by using the commercial kits according to the manufacturer's instructions.

2.9. Immunohistochemical Examination

Regarding the histopathological examination, the slices were incubated in 3% hydrogen peroxide (H_2O_2) for 30 min and normal goat serum to block nonspecific protein binding for 30 min. Then, the sections were incubated overnight at 4 °C with rabbit anti-Sirt1 or TLR4 antibody (1:100, dilution), followed by incubating biotin labeled goat anti-rabbit IgG and horseradish peroxidase-conjugated streptavidin for 15 min, respectively. Eventually, the slides were incubated in DAB solution for 10 min at 37 °C, counterstained by hematoxylin and mounted with neutral gum. Images were taken by a light microscope (Leica DM4000B, Solms, Germany) with 100× magnification. The optical density (IOD) of photographs were assayed by using Image-Pro Plus 6.0 (Media Cybernetics, Rockville, MD, USA).

2.10. Quantitative Real-Time PCR Assay

The total RNA samples were extracted by using RNAiso Plus reagent following the manufacturer's protocol. The purity of the extracted RNA was determined, then reverse transcription polymerase chain reaction (RT-PCR) was performed using a PrimeScript® RT reagent Kit following the manufacturer's instructions with a TC-512 PCR system (TECHNE, Staffordshire, UK). The levels of mRNA expression were quantified by real-time PCR with SYBR® PremixEx Taq™ II (Tli RNaseH Plus) and ABI 7500 Real-Time PCR System (Applied Biosystems, Waltham, MA, USA). The sequences of the primers for rats are shown in Table 1. A no-template control was analyzed in parallel for each gene, and the GAPDH gene was selected as the house-keeping gene in our study. Finally, the unknown template was calculated through the standard curve for quantitative analysis.

Table 1. The primer sequences used for real-time PCR assay in rats.

Gene	GenBank Accession	Full Name	Primer (5'–3')
TNF-α	NM_012675.3	Tumour necrosis factor alpha	Forward: TCAGTTCCATGGCCCAGAC; Reverse: GTTGTCTTTGAGATCCATGCCATT
IL-1β	NM_031512.2	Interleukin-1 beta	Forward: CCCTGAACTCAACTGTGAAATAGCA; Reverse: CCCAAGTCAAGGGCTTGGAA
IL-6	NM_012589.1	Interleukin-6	Forward: ATTGTATGAACAGCGATGATGCAC; Reverse: CCAGGTAGAAACGGAACTCCAGA

2.11. Western Blot Assay

Then, total protein, nuclear, and cytolymph proteins were extracted from the tissues using appropriate cold lysis buffer containing 1 mM phenylmethylsulfonyl fluoride (PMSF) based on the manufacturer's instructions. Samples were loaded onto the SDS-PAGE gel (10%–15%), separated electrophoretically, and transferred onto a PVDF membrane (Merck Millipore, Merck KGaA, Darmstadt, Germany). After blocking non-specific binding sites for 3 h with 5% dried skim milk in TTBS at room temperature, the membrane was individually incubated overnight at 4 °C with primary antibodies (Table 2). Then the membrane was incubated at room temperature for 2 h with horseradish peroxidase-conjugated antibodies at a 1:5000 dilution. Protein expression was detected by an enhanced chemiluminescence (ECL) method and imaged using ChemiDoc XRS (BIO-RAD, Hercules, CA, USA). To eliminate the variations of protein expression, the data were adjusted to correspond internal reference expression (IOD value of target protein versus IOD of correspond internal reference).

Table 2. The information of the antibodies used in the present work.

Antibody	Full Name	Source	Dilutions	Company
Nrf2	Nuclear erythroid factor 2-related factorn2	Rabbit	1:1000	Proteintech Group, Chicago, IL, USA
Sirt1	Sirtuin 1	Rabbit	1:1000	Proteintech Group, Chicago, IL, USA
Keap1	Kelch-like ECH-associated protein 1	Rabbit	1:1000	Proteintech Group, Chicago, IL, USA
HO-1	Heme oxygenase-1	Rabbit	1:1000	Proteintech Group, Chicago, IL, USA
GST	Glutathione-S-transferase	Rabbit	1:1000	Proteintech Group, Chicago, IL, USA
TLR4	Toll like receptor 4	Rabbit	1:1000	Proteintech Group, Chicago, IL, USA
MyD88	Myeloid differentiation primary response gene (88)	Rabbit	1:1000	Abcam, Cambridge, UK
TRAF6	TNF receptor-associated factor 6	Rabbit	1:1000	Proteintech Group, Chicago, IL, USA
p-JNK	Phosphorylation of JNK	Rabbit	1:500	Bioworld Technology, San Luis, MN, USA
JNK	c-Jun N-terminal kinase	Rabbit	1:500	Bioworld Technology, San Luis, MN, USA
NF-κB	Nuclear factor kappa B	Rabbit	1:1000	Proteintech Group, Chicago, IL, USA
AP-1	Jun oncogene	Rabbit	1:1000	Proteintech Group, Chicago, IL, USA
β-Tubulin	Tubulin, beta	Rabbit	1:2000	Proteintech Group, Chicago, IL, USA
Lamin B1	Lamin B1	Rabbit	1:2000	Proteintech Group, Chicago, IL, USA
GAPDH	Glyceraldehyde-3-phosphate dehydrogenase	Rabbit	1:5000	Proteintech Group, Chicago, IL, USA

2.12. Statistical Analysis

All of the data were analyzed using statistical software SPSS 18.0 (IBM, Almon grams, NY, USA) and expressed as means $\pm$ SD. Differences among groups were determined using one-way ANOVA, followed by a post hoc least-significant difference (LSD) test. Comparisons between the two groups were performed using an unpaired Student's *t*-test. $p < 0.05$ and $p < 0.01$ were considered to be significant.

3. Results

3.1. TFs Reduces the Levels of ALT, AST, MPO, and LDH after I/R Injury

As shown in Figure 1A, compared to the sham group, severe hepatotoxicity occurred and was quantified by the distinctly increased serum AST activities after 1 h of ischemia and different times of reperfusion (2 h, 6 h, and 24 h) with p-values of 0.003, 0.004, and 0.019, respectively. Similar results occurred in the serum ALT levels (p-values = 0.001, 1.97×10^{-4}, and 0.023, respectively). However, pretreatment with 200 mg/kg of TFs markedly attenuated AST (p-values = 0.026, 0.002, and 0.046) and ALT (p-values = 0.036, 0.009, and 0.021) activities compared with vehicle groups after 2 h, 6 h, and 24 h reperfusion, respectively. In addition, compared to the sham group, 1 h of ischemia and different times of reperfusion (2 h, 6 h, and 24 h) significantly increased MPO (p-values = 0.005, 0.004, and 0.009) and LDH (p-values = 1.86×10^{-8}, 2.43×10^{-11}, and 0.002) levels in serum, respectively. However, TFs could markedly decrease MPO (p-values = 0.022, 0.048, and 0.044) and LDH (p-values = 3.61×10^{-4}, 1.88×10^{-5}, and 0.008) activities compared with the vehicle rats at 2 h, 6 h, and 24 h reperfusion, respectively.

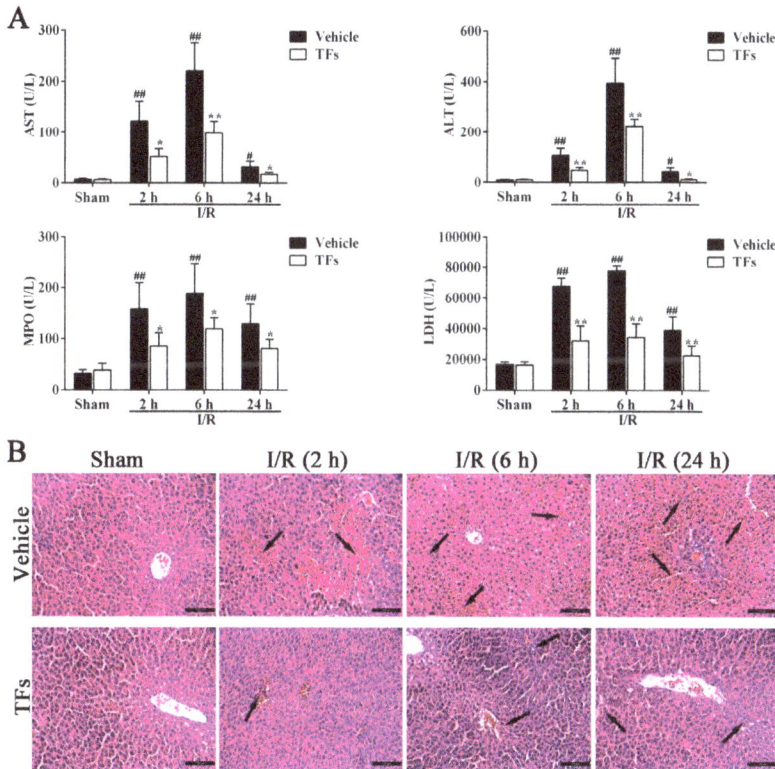

Figure 1. TFs reduced AST, ALT, MPO, and LDH activities after I/R injury. (**A**) Effects of TFs on serum AST, ALT, MPO, and LDH activities after 1 h of ischemia and different times of reperfusion (2 h, 6 h, and 24 h). Data are presented as the mean $\pm$ SD ($n = 6$). # $p < 0.05$ and ## $p < 0.01$ versus sham; * $p < 0.05$ and ** $p < 0.01$ versus vehicle; and (**B**) effects of TFs on HE staining (200$\times$ magnification) after 1 h of ischemia and different times of reperfusion (2 h, 6 h, and 24 h).

3.2. TFs Attenuates I/R-Induced Liver Morphological Changes in Rats

As shown in Figure 1B, H and E staining results indicated that the rats in the model group showed obviously-increased areas of necrotic and inflammatory cell infiltration (the black arrow), correlating with significantly worsened hepatic functions compared with the vehicle group. In addition, there was sparing of the periportal area with progressively increased injury approaching the central vein. However, TFs (200 mg/kg) attenuated the I/R-induced morphological variations after 2 h, 6 h, and 24 h reperfusion.

3.3. TFs Improves I/R-Induced Cellular Structure Changes in Rats

As shown in Figure 2, the ultrastructure of hepatic cells was observed by TEM ($15,000\times$ magnification). The cell in I/R groups displayed nucleus chromatin condensation and marginalization, mitochondrial cristae break-down, and swelling after 2 h, 6 h, and 24 h reperfusion. However, TFs (200 mg/kg) improved I/R-induced cellular structure changes in rats.

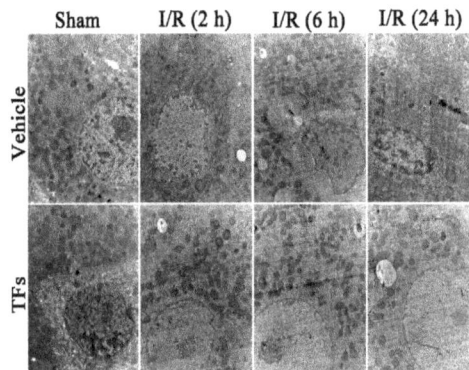

Figure 2. TFs improved I/R-induced cellular structure changes in rats. Effects of TFs on the ultrastructure ($15,000\times$ magnification) of hepatic cells after 1 h of ischemia and different times of reperfusion (2 h, 6 h, and 24 h).

3.4. TFs Improves I/R-Induced Oxidative Stress

As shown in Figure 3A, in I/R-treated group, the levels of MDA were increased compared with sham rats after 2 h (p-value = 5.04×10^{-5}), 6 h (p-value = 1.57×10^{-4}), and 24 h (p-value = 0.001) reperfusion. However, TFs significantly decreased the MDA levels (p-values = 0.046, 0.006, and 1.39×10^{-5}) compared with the vehicle group after 2 h, 6 h, and 24 h reperfusion, respectively. In addition, the decreased levels of SOD (p-values = 0.002, 0.001, and 0.004) and GSH (p-values = 0.009, 0.004, and 0.021) were observed in I/R rats compared with sham group after 2 h, 6 h, and 24 h reperfusion, respectively. However, TFs (200 mg/kg) markedly decreased SOD (p-values = 0.151, 0.041, and 0.027) and GSH (p-values = 0.093, 0.049, and 0.029) levels after 2 h, 6 h, and 24 h reperfusion, respectively.

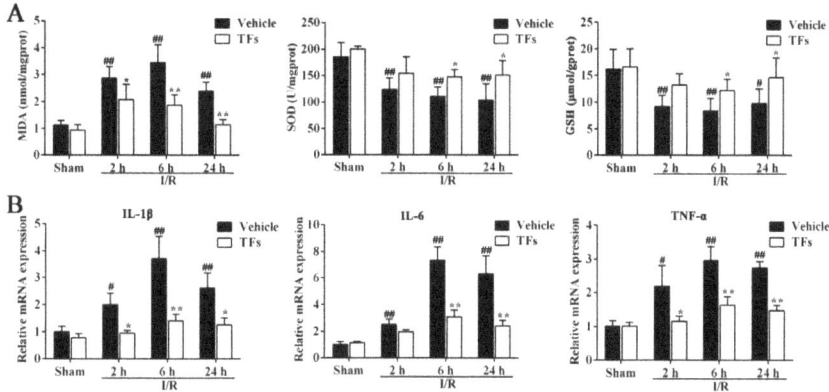

Figure 3. TFs inhibited I/R-induced oxidative stress and inflammation after I/R injury. (**A**) Effects of TFs on MDA, SOD, and GSH activities in liver tissue after 1 h of ischemia and different times of reperfusion (2 h, 6 h, and 24 h); and (**B**) effects of TFs on the mRNA levels of IL-1β, IL-6, and TNF-α in liver tissue after 1 h of ischemia and different times of reperfusion (2 h, 6 h, and 24 h). Data are presented as the mean ± SD (*n* = 6). [#] $p < 0.05$ and [##] $p < 0.01$ versus sham; * $p < 0.05$ and ** $p < 0.01$ versus vehicle.

3.5. TFs Inhibits Liver Inflammation after I/R Injury

As shown in Figure 3B, in I/R-treated group, the mRNA levels of IL-1β (*p*-values = 0.020, 0.005, and 0.009), IL-6 (*p*-values = 0.004, 4.20×10^{-4} and 0.003) and TNF-α (*p*-values = 0.008, 0.002 and 3.03×10^{-4}) were significantly increased compared with sham rats after 2 h, 6 h, and 24 h reperfusion, respectively, which were significantly downregulated by TFs.

3.6. TFs Downregulates SIRT1 and Upregulates TLR4 Protein Levels after I/R Injury

As shown in Figure 4A,B, fewer Sirt1-positive areas (brown areas) and decreased IOD values ($p = 0.002$, 0.003, and 0.002, respectively) were observed in I/R group compared with sham group after 2 h, 6 h, and 24 h reperfusion. However, compared to the vehicle group, TFs markedly increased Sirt1 protein levels (*p*-values = 0.002, 0.006, and 0.022, respectively) after 2 h, 6 h, and 24 h reperfusion. Immunohistochemical analysis also revealed that the protein levels of TLR4 (brown areas) and IOD values (*p*-values = 0.003, 3.98×10^{-4}, and 0.001, respectively) were considerably increased in the I/R group, which were also significantly decreased by TFs (*p*-values = 0.009, 0.001, and 0.001, respectively) compared with vehicle group after 2 h, 6 h, and 24 h reperfusion (Figure 4C,D).

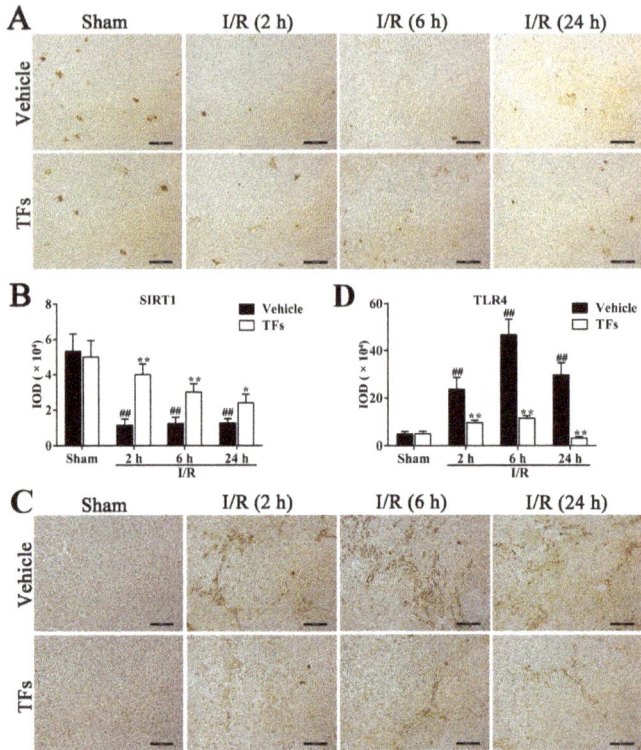

Figure 4. TFs downregulated Sirt1 and upregulated TLR4 protein levels after I/R injury. (**A**) Effects of TFs on Sitr1 protein level (brown areas) in liver tissue after 1 h of ischemia and different times of reperfusion (2 h, 6 h, and 24 h); (**B**) statistical analysis of the IOD values of Sitr1 protein level; (**C**) effects of TFs on TLR4 protein level (brown areas) in liver tissue after 1 h of ischemia and different times of reperfusion (2 h, 6 h, and 24 h); and (**D**) statistical analysis of the IOD values of TLR4 protein levels. Data are presented as the mean $\pm$ SD (n = 6). [#] $p < 0.05$ and [##] $p < 0.01$ versus sham; [*] $p < 0.05$ and [**] $p < 0.01$ versus vehicle.

3.7. TFs Activate SIRT1/Nrf2-Mediated Signaling Pathway

As shown in Figure 5, in I/R-treated group, the total Nrf2 (p-values = 2.57 $\times$ 10^{-4}, 0.002, and 0.015, respectively) and nuclear Nrf2 (nNrf2, p-values = 0.009, 0.009, and 0.009, respectively) levels were downregulated, and cytoplasmic Nrf2 (cyNrf2, p-values = 0.001, 2.77 $\times$ 10^{-4}, and 5.84 $\times$ 10^{-5}, respectively) levels were upregulated compared with sham rats after 2 h, 6 h, and 24 h reperfusion. However, compared to vehicle group, TFs significantly increased the total Nrf2 (p-values = 0.005, 0.007, and 0.020) and nNrf2 (p-values = 0.018, 4.35 $\times$ 10^{-4}, and 0.008) levels, and decreased cyNrf2 level (p-values = 0.003, 0.001, and 3.25 $\times$ 10^{-4}) after 2 h, 6 h, and 24 h reperfusion, respectively. Furthermore, compared with sham rats, the protein levels of Sirt1 (p-values = 0.001, 0.189, and 0.006), Keap1 (p-values = 0.002, 0.072, and 0.684), HO-1 (p-values = 0.005, 0.021, and 0.108), and GST (p-values = 0.001, 0.001, and 0.015) were downregulated after 2 h, 6 h, and 24 h reperfusion. However, TFs at the dose of 200 mg/kg dramatically upregulated the levels of Sirt1 (p-values = 0.002, 0.049, 0.557), Keap1 (p-values = 0.001, 0.008, 0.013), HO-1 (p-values = 0.071, 0.016, and 0.009), and GST (p-values = 0.001, 0.001, and 0.601) compared with vehicle groups after 2 h, 6 h, and 24 h reperfusion, respectively. These findings showed that TFs increased the antioxidant enzyme activities via activating Sirt1/Nrf2 signals.

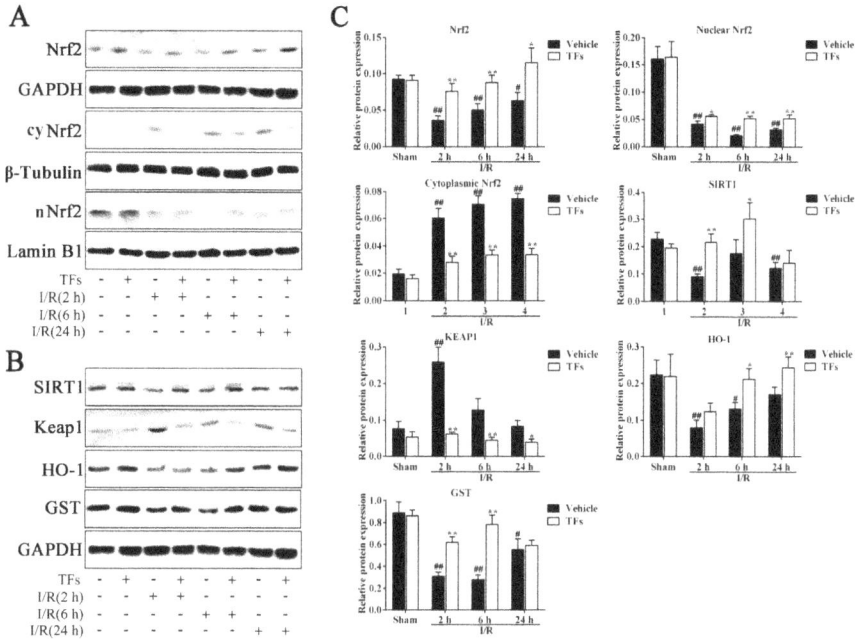

Figure 5. TFs activated the Sirt1/Nrf2-mediated signaling pathway. (**A**) Effects of TFs on Nrf2, nNrf2 (nucleus Nrf2), and cyNrf2 (cytoplasm Nrf2) proteins expression in liver tissue after 1 h of ischemia and different times of reperfusion (2 h, 6 h, and 24 h); (**B**) effects of TFs on Sirt1, KEAP1, HO-1, and GSH protein expression in liver tissue after 1 h of ischemia and different times of reperfusion (2 h, 6 h, and 24 h); and (**C**) statistical analysis of the Western blot assay. Data are presented as the mean $\pm$ SD (n = 6). [#] $p < 0.05$ and [##] $p < 0.01$ versus sham; [*] $p < 0.05$ and [**] $p < 0.01$ versus vehicle.

3.8. TFs Inhibits TLR4 Signaling Pathway after I/R Injury

As shown in Figure 6, compared with sham rats, I/R significantly induced TLR4 levels (p-values = 0.014, 0.003, and 0.011) and suppressed the subsequent activation of its signaling effectors, reflected by the increased levels of MyD88 (p-values = 0.001, 0.001, and 4.39 $\times$ 10^{-4}), TRAF6 (p-values = 0.001, 0.003, and 0.006), p-JNK (p-values = 0.001, 0.018 and 0.001), AP-1 (p-values = 0.001, 0.021, and 0.004) and NF-κB (p-values = 0.001, 0.027, and 0.003), respectively. However, 200 mg/kg TFs pretreatment notably decreased the protein levels of TLR4 (p-values = 0.023, 2.98 $\times$ 10^{-4}, and 0.001), MyD88 (p-values = 0.012, 0.018, and 0.032), TRAF6 (p-values = 0.003, 0.006, and 0.004), p-JNK (p-values = 0.006, 0.016, and 0.004), AP-1 (p-values = 0.003, 0.022, and 0.034), and NF-κB (p-values = 0.005, 0.019, and 0.007) compared with vehicle groups after 2 h, 6 h, and 24 h reperfusion, respectively. Furthermore, after 2 h, 6 h, and 24 h reperfusion, the protein levels of cytoplasmic NF-κB (cyNF-κB, p-values = 0.001, 0.013, and 0.012) in ischemic liver were notably up-regulated, whereas nucleus NF-κB (nNF-κB, p-values = 0.001, 0.001, and 0.001) levels were markedly decreased. Compared with the vehicle group after 2 h, 6 h, and 24 h reperfusion, TFs obviously downregulated cyNF-κB (p-values = 0.006, 0.003, and 0.007), and upregulated nNF-κB (p-values = 0.026, 0.007, and 0.003) protein levels. The results also suggested that TFs inhibited the nuclear translocation from nucleus to cytoplasm of NF-κB in ischemic liver cells.

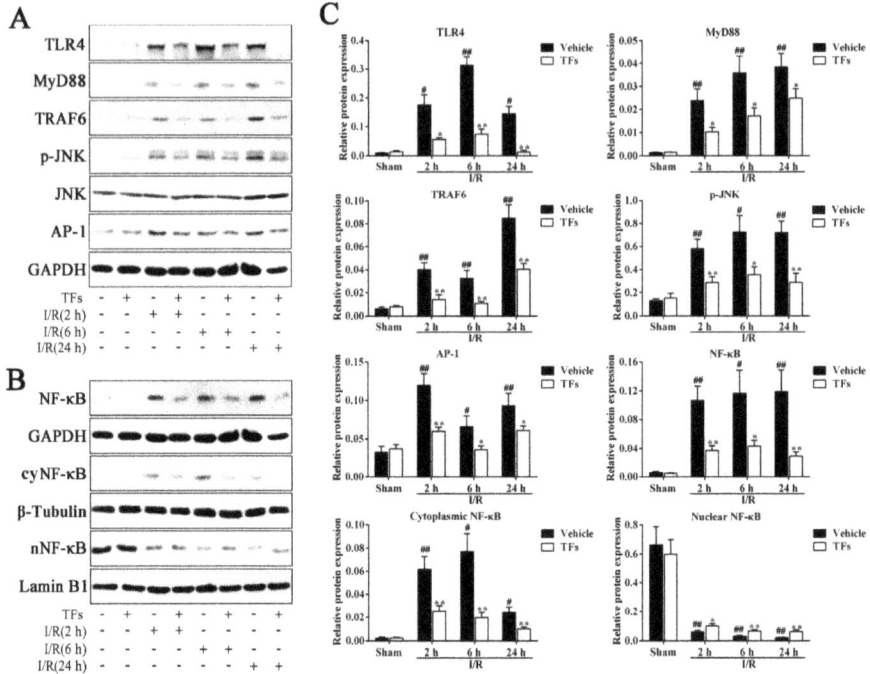

Figure 6. TFs inhibited the TLR4 signaling pathway after I/R injury. (**A**) Effects of TFs on TLR4, MyD88, TRAF6, p-JNK, and AP-1 protein expression in liver tissue after 1 h of ischemia and different times of reperfusion (2 h, 6 h, and 24 h); (**B**) effects of TFs on NF-κB, nNF-κB (nucleus NF-κB), and cyNF-κB (cytoplasm NF-κB) proteins expression in liver tissue after 1 h of ischemia and different times of reperfusion (2 h, 6 h, and 24 h); and (**C**) statistical analysis of the Western blot assay. Data are presented as the mean $\pm$ SD ($n = 6$). [#] $p < 0.05$ and [##] $p < 0.01$ versus sham; [*] $p < 0.05$ and [**] $p < 0.01$ versus vehicle.

4. Discussion

Hepatic I/R injury, a frequent cause of liver failure, is related with liver transplantation, vascular surgery, and stroke [31,32]. A large number of studies have been carried out in the past several decades, but the pathogenesis of hepatic I/R injury has not been completely illuminated, and few medicines are available [33].

Previous studies have shown that liver reperfusion can increase cell injury by oxidative stress and inflammatory reactions [6]. Briefly, the early phase of hepatic I/R insult (within 2 h after reperfusion) involves the release of ROS and pro-inflammatory mediators [17]. The late phase (6–24 h after reperfusion) is featured with neutrophil-mediated inflammatory reaction [4]. ROS may result in lipid peroxidation, and activate signal transduction pathways, mitochondrial permeability transition, necrosis, and apoptosis of hepatocytes [8]. Larger amounts of complement factors, such as chemokines and cytokines, recruit neutrophils into the liver, which will insult hepatocytes through ROS release [3]. Therefore, the modulation of oxidative stress and inflammatory reactions represent promising therapeutic strategies to alleviate hepatic I/R injury.

TFs with potent anti-oxidative stress and anti-inflammatory actions have been shown in our previous research [24,34]. In the present work, a rat hepatic I/R model significantly increased serum AST, ALT, and LDH levels. However, pretreatment with TFs considerably reversed the alternations of these enzyme activities. The richest protein in neutrophils-MPO can be used as a quantitative measure of neutrophil infiltration [7]. Our results proved that TFs notably decreased neutrophil infiltration. In addition, HE staining results indicated that TFs exerted the protective action by decreasing coagulation necrosis with massive inflammatory cell infiltration in the liver. Furthermore, TEM assay results showed that TFs improved I/R-induced cellular structure changes in rats. Altogether, these results suggested that TFs have potent action for the prevention of hepatic I/R injury in rats.

High levels of SOD and GSH can protect hepatic I/R injury. SOD can catalytically reduce superoxide anion (O_2^-) to hydrogen peroxide, and GSH can catalyze the reduction of hydrogen peroxide [13]. MDA is an end-product of lipid hydroperoxide and an indicator of ROS [25]. The present paper indicated that SOD and GSH activities in the liver were markedly increased after TFs pretreatment compared with the model group, and MDA activity was dramatically decreased. Further results presented in this paper suggested that TFs significantly decreased the mRNA levels of IL-1β, IL-6, and TNF-α in the liver. These results proved the inhibition of oxidative stress and inflammatory response may be the potential mechanisms of TFs against hepatic I/R injury.

A number of studies have shown that Sirt1 possesses a potent anti-oxidative effect, which can enhance transcriptional activity of Nrf2 [8]. Nrf2 plays a vital role in the inhibition of cellular oxidative stress by regulating intracellular redox homeostasis, which can also activate phase II antioxidants including HO-1 and GST [10]. Nrf2 can translocate from cytosol to nucleus when it is triggered, and lead to the increased antioxidant enzymes activities and decreased ROS induced insult [9,35]. In this paper, we found that TFs increased the levels of Sirt1, total Nrf2, nuclear Nrf2, HO-1, GST, and decreased cytoplasmic Nrf2 level in liver tissue. These results suggested that the anti-I/R effect of TFs might be through increasing the Sirt1 level and activating the Nrf2/ARE pathway (Figure 7).

The latest evidence suggests that TLR4 signaling plays a vital role in the progress of liver inflammation after I/R [36]. In detail, the activation of TLR4 signaling at the plasma membrane triggers NF-κB and AP-1 signaling, which are the vital regulators of some genes involved in inflammation [37]. Western blotting results in the present work proved that TFs downregulated TLR4 and downstream protein levels, including MyD88, TRAF6, p-JNK, NF-κB, and AP-1. In addition, TFs also inhibited the level and translocation of NF-κB. These findings indicated that the effects of TFs against hepatic I/R damage may be through inhibiting inflammation via adjusting TLR4 signaling (Figure 7).

Our previous studies have shown that the main chemicals of the product were flavonoids, with a content of 80.5% based on the chemical reactions and colorimetric method. The HPLC analysis results further proved that the contents of quercetin, kaempferide, and isorhamnetin in TFs were 3.11%, 2.72%, and 1.49%, respectively. These flavonoid constituents form in the pathophysiology, signaling, and the subsequent hepatic protection. However, other flavonoid substances in the crude extract were still unknown, and we will perform a deep investigation into the chemicals of TFs in our future work.

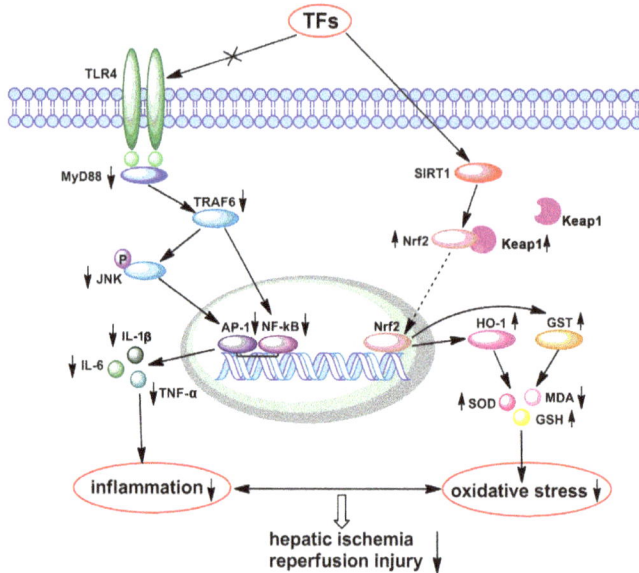

Figure 7. Proposed model for the protective effects of TFs against hepatic I/R injury. TFs alleviated liver I/R damage by regulating oxidative stress and inflammatory reactions through the inhibition of TLR4/MyD88 signaling and the activation of Sirt1/Nrf2 signaling.

5. Conclusions

In summary, TFs have good protective effects against hepatic I/R injury by inhibiting oxidative stress and inflammation. Accordingly, TFs represent a novel and potent candidate for the treatment of I/R-induced liver injury in the future. Of course, further investigations are needed to deeply elucidate the mechanisms and clinical applications of the natural product.

Acknowledgments: This work was supported by the Program for Liaoning Innovative Research Team in University (LT2013019).

Author Contributions: Jinyong Peng conceived and designed the study. Xufeng Tao contributed to the design of the study and performed the experiments. Xiance Sun, Lina Xu, Lianhong Yin, Xu Han and Yan Qi performed the animal experiments and analyzed the data. Youwei Xu, Yanyan Zhao and Changyuan Wang provided statistical consultation and analysis. Jinyong Peng and Xufeng Tao wrote and edited the paper.

Conflicts of Interest: The authors declare no conflicts of interests.

References

1. Peralta, C.; Jimenez-Castro, M.B.; Gracia-Sancho, J. Hepatic ischemia and reperfusion injury: Effects on the liver sinusoidal milieu. *J. Hepatol.* **2013**, *59*, 1094–1106. [CrossRef] [PubMed]
2. Bahde, R.; Spiegel, H.U. Hepatic ischaemia-reperfusion injury from bench to bedside. *Br. J. Surg.* **2010**, *97*, 1461–1475. [CrossRef] [PubMed]
3. Mukhopadhyay, P.; Rajesh, M.; Horvath, B.; Batkai, S.; Park, O.; Tanchian, G.; Gao, R.Y.; Patel, V.; Wink, D.A.; Liaudet, L.; et al. Cannabidiol protects against hepatic ischemia/reperfusion injury by attenuating inflammatory signaling and response, oxidative/nitrative stress, and cell death. *Free Radic. Biol. Med.* **2011**, *50*, 1368–1381. [CrossRef] [PubMed]
4. Hide, D.; Ortega-Ribera, M.; Garcia-Pagan, J.C.; Peralta, C.; Bosch, J.; Gracia-Sancho, J. Effects of warm ischemia and reperfusion on the liver microcirculatory phenotype of rats: Underlying mechanisms and pharmacological therapy. *Sci. Rep.* **2016**, *6*, 22107. [CrossRef] [PubMed]

5. Jaeschke, H.; Woolbright, B.L. Current strategies to minimize hepatic ischemia-reperfusion injury by targeting reactive oxygen species. *Transplant. Rev.* **2012**, *26*, 103–114. [CrossRef] [PubMed]

6. Jaeschke, H. Reactive oxygen and mechanisms of inflammatory liver injury: Present concepts. *J. Gastroenterol. Hepatol.* **2011**, *26*, 173–179. [CrossRef] [PubMed]

7. Xia, Y.; Gong, J.P. Impact of recombinant globular adiponectin on early warm ischemia-reperfusion injury in rat bile duct after liver transplantation. *Sci. Rep.* **2014**, *4*, 6426. [CrossRef] [PubMed]

8. Do, M.T.; Kim, H.G.; Choi, J.H.; Jeong, H.G. Metformin induces microRNA-34a to downregulate the SIRT1/Pgc-1α/Nrf2 pathway, leading to increased susceptibility of wild-type p53 cancer cells to oxidative stress and therapeutic agents. *Free Radic. Biol. Med.* **2014**, *74*, 21–34. [PubMed]

9. Ge, M.; Yao, W.; Wang, Y.; Yuan, D.; Chi, X.; Luo, G.; Hei, Z. Propofol alleviates liver oxidative stress via activating Nrf2 pathway. *J. Surg. Res.* **2015**, *196*, 373–381. [CrossRef] [PubMed]

10. Chi, X.; Zhang, R.; Shen, N.; Jin, Y.; Alina, A.; Yang, S.; Lin, S. Sulforaphane reduces apoptosis and oncosis along with protecting liver injury-induced ischemic reperfusion by activating the Nrf2/ARE pathway. *Hepatol. Int.* **2015**, *9*, 321–329. [CrossRef] [PubMed]

11. Rao, J.; Qian, X.; Li, G.; Pan, X.; Zhang, C.; Zhang, F.; Zhai, Y.; Wang, X.; Lu, L. ATF3-Mediated NRF2/HO-1 signaling regulates TLR4 innate immune responses in mouse liver ischemia/reperfusion injury. *Am. J. Transplant.* **2015**, *15*, 76–87. [CrossRef] [PubMed]

12. Huang, J.; Shen, X.D.; Yue, S.; Zhu, J.; Gao, F.; Zhai, Y.; Busuttil, R.W.; Ke, B.; Kupiec-Weglinski, J.W. Adoptive transfer of heme oxygenase-1 (HO-1)-modified macrophages rescues the nuclear factor erythroid 2-related factor (Nrf2) anti-inflammatory phenotype in liver ischemia/reperfusion injury. *Mol. Med.* **2014**, *20*, 448–455. [CrossRef] [PubMed]

13. Shah, N.M.; Rushworth, S.A.; Murray, M.Y.; Bowles, K.M.; MacEwan, D.J. Understanding the role of Nrf2-regulated mirnas in human malignancies. *Oncotarget* **2013**, *4*, 1130–1142. [CrossRef] [PubMed]

14. Gill, R.; Tsung, A.; Billiar, T. Linking oxidative stress to inflammation: Toll-like receptors. *Free Radic. Biol. Med.* **2010**, *48*, 1121–1132. [CrossRef] [PubMed]

15. Tong, Y.; Ding, X.B.; Chen, Z.X.; Jin, S.Q.; Zhao, X.; Wang, X.; Mei, S.Y.; Jiang, X.; Wang, L.; Li, Q. WISP1 mediates hepatic warm ischemia reperfusion injury via TLR4 signaling in mice. *Sci. Rep.* **2016**, *6*, 20141. [CrossRef] [PubMed]

16. Wang, J.; He, G.Z.; Wang, Y.K.; Zhu, Q.K.; Chen, W.; Guo, T. TLR4-HMGB1-, MyD88-and TRIF-dependent signaling in mouse intestinal ischemia/reperfusion injury. *World J. Gastroenterol.* **2015**, *21*, 8314–8325. [CrossRef] [PubMed]

17. Abu-Amara, M.; Yang, S.Y.; Tapuria, N.; Fuller, B.; Davidson, B.; Seifalian, A. Liver ischemia/reperfusion injury: Processes in inflammatory networks—A review. *Liver Transplant.* **2010**, *16*, 1016–1032. [CrossRef] [PubMed]

18. Zhang, T.Y.; Nie, L.W.; Wu, B.J.; Yang, Y.; Zhao, S.S.; Jin, T. Hypolipedemic activity of the polysaccharose from *Rosa laevigata* Michx fruit. *Chin. J. Public Health* **2004**, *20*, 829–830.

19. Gao, P.Y.; Li, L.Z.; Peng, Y.; Piao, S.J.; Zeng, N.; Lin, H.W.; Song, S.J. Triterpenes from fruits of *Rosa Laevigata*. *Biochem. Syst. Ecol.* **2010**, *38*, 457–459. [CrossRef]

20. Dong, D.S.; Yin, L.H.; Qi, Y.; Xu, L.N.; Peng, J.Y. Protective effect of the total saponins from *Rosa laevigata* Michx fruit against carbon tetrachloride-induced liver fibrosis in rats. *Nutrients* **2015**, *7*, 4829–4850. [CrossRef] [PubMed]

21. Dong, D.S.; Qi, Y.; Xu, L.N.; Yin, L.H.; Xu, Y.W.; Han, X.; Zhao, Y.Y.; Peng, J.Y. Total saponins from *Rosa laevigata* Michx fruit attenuates hepatic steatosis induced by high-fat diet in rats. *Food Funct.* **2014**, *5*, 3065–3075. [CrossRef] [PubMed]

22. Zhang, S.; Zheng, L.L.; Xu, L.N.; Sun, H.J.; Li, H.; Yao, J.H.; Liu, K.X.; Peng, J.Y. Subchronic toxicity study of the total flavonoids from *Rosa laevigata* Michx fruit in rats. *Regul. Toxicol. Pharmacol.* **2012**, *62*, 221–230. [CrossRef] [PubMed]

23. Li, X.; Wei, L. Chemical components from *Rosa laevigata* Michx. *China J. Chin. Mater. Med.* **1997**, *22*, 298–299.

24. Zhang, S.; Zheng, L.L.; Dong, D.S.; Xu, L.N.; Yin, L.H.; Qi, Y.; Han, X.; Lin, Y.; Liu, K.X.; Peng, J.Y. Effects of flavonoids from *Rosa laevigata* Michx fruit against high-fat diet-induced non-alcoholic fatty liver disease in rats. *Food Chem.* **2013**, *141*, 2108–2116. [CrossRef] [PubMed]

25. Cao, Y.W.; Jiang, Y.; Zhang, D.Y.; Wang, M.; Chen, W.S.; Su, H.; Wang, Y.T.; Wan, J.B. Protective effects of *Penthorum chinense* Pursh against chronic ethanol-induced liver injury in mice. *J. Ethnopharmacol.* **2015**, *161*, 92–98. [CrossRef] [PubMed]

26. Zhang, S.; Qi, Y.; Xu, Y.W.; Han, X.; Peng, J.Y.; Liu, K.X.; Sun, C.K. Protective effect of flavonoid-rich extract from *Rosa laevigata* Michx on cerebral ischemia-reperfusion injury through suppression of apoptosis and inflammation. *Neurochem. Int.* **2013**, *63*, 522–532. [CrossRef] [PubMed]

27. Liu, Y.T.; Lu, B.N.; Peng, J.Y. Hepatoprotective activity of the total flavonoids from *Rosa laevigata* Michx fruit in mice treated by paracetamol. *Food Chem.* **2011**, *125*, 719–725. [CrossRef]

28. Lee, V.G.; Johnson, M.L.; Baust, J.; Laubach, V.E.; Watkins, S.C.; Billiar, T.R. The roles of iNOS in liver ischemia-reperfusion injury. *Shock* **2001**, *16*, 355–360. [CrossRef] [PubMed]

29. Tsung, A.; Stang, M.T.; Ikeda, A.; Critchlow, N.D.; Izuishi, K.; Nakao, A.; Chan, M.H.; Jeyabalan, G.; Yim, J.H.; Geller, D.A. The transcription factor interferon regulatory factor-1 mediates liver damage during ischemia-reperfusion injury. *Am. J. Physiol.* **2006**, *290*, 1261–1268. [CrossRef] [PubMed]

30. Tao, X.F.; Wan, X.; Xu, Y.W.; Xu, L.N.; Qi, Y.; Yin, L.H.; Han, X.; Lin, Y.H.; Peng, J.Y. Dioscin attenuates hepatic ischemia-reperfusion injury in rats through inhibition of oxidative-nitrative stress, inflammation and apoptosis. *Transplantation* **2014**, *98*, 604–611. [CrossRef] [PubMed]

31. Yuan, X.; Theruvath, A.J.; Ge, X.; Floerchinger, B.; Jurisch, A.; Garcia-Cardena, G.; Tullius, S.G. Machine perfusion or cold storage in organ transplantation: Indication, mechanisms, and future perspectives. *Transpl. Int.* **2010**, *23*, 561–570. [CrossRef] [PubMed]

32. Zhang, M.; Ueki, S.; Kimura, S.; Yoshida, O.; Castellaneta, A.; Ozaki, K.S.; Demetris, A.J.; Ross, M.; Vodovotz, Y.; Thomson, A.W.; et al. Roles of dendritic cells in murine hepatic warm and liver transplantation-induced cold ischemia/reperfusion injury. *Hepatology* **2013**, *57*, 1585–1596. [CrossRef] [PubMed]

33. Clavien, P.A.; Petrowsky, H.; DeOliveira, M.L.; Graf, R. Strategies for safer liver surgery and partial liver transplantation. *N. Engl. J. Med.* **2007**, *356*, 1545–1559. [CrossRef] [PubMed]

34. Zhang, S.; Lu, B.N.; Han, X.; Xu, L.N.; Qi, Y.; Yin, L.H.; Xu, Y.W.; Zhao, Y.Y.; Liu, K.X.; Peng, J.Y. Protection of the flavonoid fraction from *Rosa laevigata* Michx fruit against carbon tetrachloride-induced acute liver injury in mice. *Food Chem. Toxicol.* **2013**, *55*, 60–69. [CrossRef] [PubMed]

35. Ke, B.; Shen, X.D.; Zhang, Y.; Ji, H.; Gao, F.; Yue, S.; Kamo, N.; Zhai, Y.; Yamamoto, M.; Busuttil, R.W.; et al. KEAP1-NRF2 complex in ischemia-induced hepatocellular damage of mouse liver transplants. *J. Hepatol.* **2013**, *59*, 1200–1207. [CrossRef] [PubMed]

36. Vasques, E.R.; Cunha, J.E.; Coelho, A.M.; Sampietre, S.N.; Patzina, R.A.; Abdo, E.E.; Nader, H.B.; Tersariol, I.L.; Lima, M.A.; Godoy, C.M.; et al. Trisulfate disaccharide decreases calcium overload and protects liver injury secondary to liver ischemia/reperfusion. *PLoS ONE* **2016**, *11*, e0149630. [CrossRef] [PubMed]

37. He, G.Z.; Zhou, K.G.; Zhang, R.; Chen, X.F. The effects of *n*-3 PUFA and intestinal lymph drainage on high-mobility group box 1 and Toll-like receptor 4 mRNA in rats with intestinal ischaemia-reperfusion injury. *Br. J. Nutr.* **2012**, *108*, 883–892. [CrossRef] [PubMed]

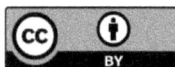

Article

Barley Sprouts Extract Attenuates Alcoholic Fatty Liver Injury in Mice by Reducing Inflammatory Response

Yun-Hee Lee [1,†], Joung-Hee Kim [2,†], Sou Hyun Kim [3], Ji Youn Oh [3], Woo Duck Seo [4], Kyung-Mi Kim [5], Jae-Chul Jung [5] and Young-Suk Jung [3,*]

[1] College of Pharmacy, Yonsei University, Incheon 21983, Korea; yunhee.lee@yonsei.ac.kr
[2] Department of Bio Health Science, College of Natural Science, Changwon National University, Changwon 51140, Korea; k9i1h@naver.com
[3] College of Pharmacy, Pusan National University, Busan 46241, Korea; hyunie9808@naver.com (S.H.K.); pooh7282@naver.com (J.Y.O.)
[4] Crop Foundation Division, National Institute of Crop Science, Rural Development Administration, Wanju-Gun, Jeollabuk-do 54875, Korea; swd@korea.kr
[5] Life Science Research Institute, Novarex Co., Ltd, Ochang, Cheongwon, Cheongju 28126, Korea; kkm3507@novarex.co.kr (K.-M.K.); jcjung@novarex.co.kr (J.-C.J.)
* Correspondence: youngjung@pusan.ac.kr; Tel.: +82-51-510-2816
† These authors contributed equally to this work.

Received: 8 May 2016; Accepted: 15 July 2016; Published: 21 July 2016

Abstract: It has been reported that barley leaves possess beneficial properties such as antioxidant, hypolipidemic, antidepressant, and antidiabetic. Interestingly, barley sprouts contain a high content of saponarin, which showed both anti-inflammatory and antioxidant activities. In this study, we evaluated the effect of barley sprouts on alcohol-induced liver injury mediated by inflammation and oxidative stress. Raw barley sprouts were extracted, and quantitative and qualitative analyses of its components were performed. The mice were fed a liquid alcohol diet with or without barley sprouts for four weeks. Lipopolysaccharide (LPS)-stimulated RAW 264.7 cells were used to study the effect of barley sprouts on inflammation. Alcohol intake for four weeks caused liver injury, evidenced by an increase in serum alanine aminotransferase and aspartate aminotransferase activities and tumor necrosis factor (TNF)-α levels. The accumulation of lipid in the liver was also significantly induced, whereas the glutathione (GSH) level was reduced. Moreover, the inflammation-related gene expression was dramatically increased. All these alcohol-induced changes were effectively prevented by barley sprouts treatment. In particular, pretreatment with barley sprouts significantly blocked inducible nitric oxide synthase (iNOS) and cyclooxygenase (COX)-2 expression in LPS-stimulated RAW 264.7. This study suggests that the protective effect of barley sprouts against alcohol-induced liver injury is potentially attributable to its inhibition of the inflammatory response induced by alcohol.

Keywords: barley sprouts; alcohol-induced liver injury; glutathione; TNF-α; inflammation

1. Introduction

Fatty liver or hepatic steatosis is defined as the accumulation of triglycerides in the liver, leading to more than 5% of the hepatic cells containing either micro- or macrovesicular lipid droplets. Multiple factors are involved in the induction of fatty liver; however, obesity, diabetes, and dyslipidemia, as well as excessive alcohol drinking, are the most frequent causes of fatty liver. Especially, alcoholic liver disease (ALD), one of the major chronic liver diseases, is characterized by a complex spectrum ranging from simple steatosis to cirrhosis. Although it is highly prevalent and holds a high rank in the causes of death worldwide, preventive and therapeutic approaches have yet to be discovered [1,2].

A well-known mechanism of alcohol-induced hepatotoxicity is its ability to induce inflammatory responses and oxidative stress following free radical formation [3]. The liver cells have various sources of reactive oxygen species (ROS) which are activated by chronic alcohol consumption, leading to an increase in the generation of oxidants [4]. In detail, they are generated by a complex pathway by metabolic enzyme-mediated oxidation, abnormal mitochondrial function, Kupffer cell activation, disruption of lipid metabolism, and cytokine production [3,5,6]. Notably, alcohol consumption increases the permeability of intestinal mucosa and sensitizes Kupffer cells to activation by endotoxins via Toll-like receptor 4 (TLR4). The harmful paracrine effects of Kupffer cell activation include the production of various inflammatory mediators as well as ROS, which contribute to the pathological progression of ALD from simple fat accumulation to steatohepatitis [7–10]. Indeed, Li et al. [11] evaluated whether steatosis has inflammatory biomarkers using clinical and experimental approaches. In this study, the group with fatty liver showed a significantly higher level of serum tumor necrosis factor (TNF)-α than the control group did, which correlated with the pathological severity of the hepatic lesions [11].

Barley (*Hordeum vulgare* L.) has been used as a food material since ancient times and was one of the first cultivated grains, particularly in Eurasia, as far back as 13,000 years ago. It has also been used as animal fodder, a source of fermentable material for beer and certain distilled beverages, and a component of numerous health foods. Barley sprouts, which are the young leaves of barley harvested approximately 10 days after sowing the seeds, have recently received much attention as a functional food in numerous countries, especially Japan and Korea. It has been reported that barley leaves possess beneficial properties such as antioxidant, hypolipidemic, antidepressant, and antidiabetic [12–14]. Interestingly, barley sprouts contain a high content of saponarin (Figure 1), which is a member of the flavonoid family, in addition to policosanol polyphenol series, various minerals, and free amino acids. Among these, saponarin is the major compound in barley sprouts, and it shows both anti-inflammatory and antioxidant activities. LPS-induced inflammation in RAW 264.7 cells was significantly inhibited by treatment with saponarin isolated from barley sprouts, and this effect is mediated by the inhibition of nuclear factor kappa-light-chain-enhancer of activated B cells (NF-κB), extracellular signal-regulated kinase (ERK), and p38 signaling [15]. In addition, saponarin prevented cocaine or paracetamol-induced hepatotoxicity by inducing the hepatic antioxidant capacity [16,17]. Based on these reports, we hypothesized that the extract of barley sprouts could have the potential to ameliorate chronic alcohol-induced liver injury mediated by an inflammatory response and, therefore, we investigated our hypothesis in this study.

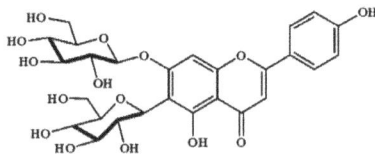

Figure 1. Structure of saponarin, an active compound in barley sprouts extract.

2. Materials and Methods

2.1. Extraction

The barley sprouts were cultivated in Yeonggwang-gun, Jeollanam-do Province, Korea. The original grain of barley used was the saechalssal (hulled barley), and the extract was prepared from the barley sprouts after they had grown to a length of approximately 20 cm. The raw material was provided by Saeddeumwon Co., Ltd. (Yeonggwang, Korea) in 2015 and the extract was produced by Novarex Co., Ltd. (Ochang, Korea). The analysis of the biological component and microbiological test were confirmed by Novarex Co., Ltd. All other chemicals were purchased from Sigma-Aldrich Chemical Corp. (St. Louis, MO, USA) and Wako Pure Chemical Industries (Osaka, Japan). The raw barley sprouts plant material was extracted for 9 h at 25 °C by exposing it to circulating 30% aqueous fermented ethanol. Then, the extract was filtered through a 75-µm cartridge, and the residue was removed by using centrifugation. The supernatant was vacuum-concentrated under reduced pressure (10 atm, 55–58 °C) to attain 35 brix materials. Then, it was blended with dextrin, sterilized at 95 °C for 30 min, followed by spray-drying (liquid temperature, 75–80 °C; blowing temperature, 180 °C; atomizer, 18,000 rpm) to obtain a barley sprouts extract powder. To establish the bulk scale production of the barley sprouts extract we optimized the manufacturing process based on experimental pilot conditions (Figure 2).

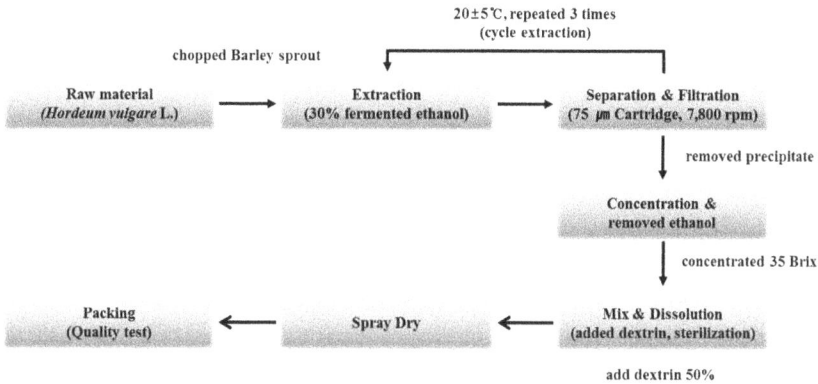

Figure 2. Manufacturing process for production of barley sprouts extract powder.

2.2. Analysis of Saponarin Using Liquid Chromatography-Tandem Mass Spectrometry (LC-MS/MS)

We performed the material separation using the LUNA C_{18} column (2.0 × 150 mm, 5-µm). Solvent A was water with 0.1% formic acid, and solvent B was acetonitrile with 0.1% formic acid. The gradients of the solvents were as follows: 0 min, 10% B; 1 min, 10% B; 7 min, 70% B; 8.5 min, 70% B; 9 min, 10% B; and 15 min, 10% B. The samples were dissolved in 50% acetonitrile and the injection volume was 5 µL. We used digoxin as the internal standard to quantify saponarin in barley sprouts extract, and the detailed conditions for the liquid chromatography-tandem mass spectrometry (LC-MS/MS) analysis are shown in Table 1.

Table 1. Condition for LC-MS/MS analysis of barley sprouts extract.

HPLC Condition	
Column	Luna C_{18} RP column (2.0 × 150 mm, 5 µm)
Flow rate	0.3 mL/min
Injection volume	5 µL
Column temperature	40 °C
Autosampler temperature	4 °C
Mass Condition	
Ion source	Turbo spray (Negative)
Curtain Gas	10 psi
Collision Gas	N_2 (Medium)
Ion spray Voltage	−4.2 kV
Source temperature	400 °C
Gas 1	40 psi
Gas 2	50 psi

2.3. Animals and Treatments

Male C57BL/6 mice were obtained from Orient Bio (Sungnam, Korea). The use of the animals was in compliance with the guidelines established and approved by the Institutional Animal Care and Use Committee of Pusan National University (PNU-2015-1027). The animals were allowed to acclimate to temperature (22 ± 2 °C)- and humidity (55% ± 5%)-controlled rooms with a 12 h light/dark cycle for one week prior to use. The mice were fed a Lieber–DeCarli liquid alcohol diet (Dyets Inc., Bethlehem, PA, USA) with or without barley sprouts for four weeks. For the control diet, 35% of the energy was derived from fat, 18% from protein, and 47% from carbohydrates, while the alcohol diet contained 35% of energy from fat, 18% from protein, 11% from carbohydrates, and 36% from ethanol (Table 2). The barley sprouts were administered by gavage daily, and silymarin (Sigma-Aldrich Chemical Corp., St. Louis, MO, USA) was treated as the positive control.

Table 2. Composition of the alcohol liquid diet.

Component	Standard Diet		Alcohol Diet	
	g/L	kcal/L	g/L	kcal/L
Casein	41.4	176.778	41.4	176.778
L-Cystine	0.5	2	0.5	2
DL-Methionine	0.3	1.2	0.3	1.2
Corn oil	8.5	75.14	8.5	75.14
Olive oil	28.4	251.056	28.4	251.056
Safflower oil	2.7	23.868	2.7	23.868
Dextrin maltose	115.2	456.192	24.72	97.89
Choline barbiturate	0.53	0	0.53	0
Fiber	10.0	0	10.0	0
Xanthan gum	3.0	0	3.0	0
mineral	8.75	4.1125	8.75	4.1125
vitamin	2.5	9.5	2.5	9.5
Ethanol	0	0	51.3	358.46
Total energy		1000 kcal/L		1000 kcal/L

Each diet used the vitamin mix at 2.5 g/L diet (g/kg vitamin mix); thiamine HCl, 0.6; riboflavin, 0.6; pyridoxine HCl, 0.7; niacin, 3.0; calcium pantothenate, 1.6; folic acid, 0.2; biotin, 0.02; vitamin B12 (0.1%), 10; vitamin A acetate (500,000 IU/g), 4.8; vitamin D3 (400,000 IU/g), 0.4; vitamin E acetate (500 IU/g), 24.0; menadione sodium bisulfite, 0.08; *p*-amino benzoic acid, 5.0; inositol, 10.00; dextrose 939.0. Each diet also used the mineral mix at 8.75 g/L diet (g/kg mineral mix); calcium phosphate, 500; sodium chloride, 74; potassium citrate, 220; potassium sulfate, 52; magnesium oxide, 24; manganous sulfate, 4.6; ferrous sulfate, 4.95; zinc carbonate, 1.6; cupric carbonate, 0.3; potassium iodate, 0.01; sodium selenite, 0.01; chromium potassium sulfate, 0.55; sodium fluoride, 0.06; sucrose, 117.92.

2.4. Hematological and Histopathological Evaluation of Liver Injury

The serum activities of alanine aminotransferase (ALT) and aspartate aminotransferase (AST) and total triglyceride (TG) levels were determined by using an automated chemistry analyzer (Prestige 24I, Tokyo Boeki Medical System, Tokyo, Japan). The serum concentration of TNF-α was measured by using an enzyme-linked immunosorbent assay (ELISA) using a commercially available kit (R & D Systems, Minneapolis, MN, USA) according to the manufacturer's instruction. The serum endotoxin level was assessed using the Limulus Amebocyte Lysate chromogenic endotoxin quantitation kit (Thermo Scientific, Sunnyvale, CA, USA). To evaluate the lipid accumulation in the liver tissue, 5-μm cross sections of the left lateral lobe of the liver were sliced, immersed in propylene glycol for 5 min, and then stained with Oil red O. After washing with 85% propylene glycol and distilled water, the sections were counterstained with hematoxylin for 2 min before microscopic examination.

2.5. Determination of Hepatic TG Content

The total lipids were extracted from 100 mg of liver tissue using a mixture of chloroform/methanol (2:1, *v/v*). To determine the TGs content of the total lipids, a commercially available enzymatic kit (Sigma-Aldrich Chemical Corp., St. Louis, MO, USA) was used according to the manufacturer's instruction.

2.6. Measurement of Hepatic Glutathione (GSH)

The liver homogenate was prepared by using a 4-fold volume of ice-cold 1 M perchloric acid. After centrifugation at $10,000\times g$ for 10 min to remove the denatured protein, the total GSH level in the supernatant was measured by using a high-performance liquid chromatography (HPLC) separation/fluorometric detection method [18].

2.7. Cell Culture and Viability Assay

The RAW 264.7 cells were obtained from the American Type Culture Collection (ATCC, Manassas, VA, USA) and were grown in Dulbecco's modified Eagle's medium (DMEM) containing 10% fetal bovine serum (FBS), 2 mM glutamine, 100 U/mL penicillin, and 100 µg/mL streptomycin (GenDEPOT, Barker, TX, USA) at 37 °C in a humidified incubator with 5% CO_2. Cell viability was determined by EZ-CyTox (Daeil Lab Service, Seoul, Korea). After 24 h incubation of cells with barely sprouts extract, EZ-CyTox solution was added to each well and it was measured at a 450 nm. The results were expressed as a percentage compared to the vehicle treated cells.

2.8. Determination of Nitric Oxide (NO) Production

After stimulating the cells with 200 ng/mL of LPS (Sigma-Aldrich, St. Louis, MO, USA) for 24 h, the culture medium was collected and assayed for NO production. A 50 µL aliquot of the medium was mixed with 50 µL Griess reagent (1% sulfanilamide in 5% phosphoric acid and 0.1% naphthylethlyenediamene dihydrochloride) and then incubated for 20 min. The absorbance was measured at 540 nm using a microplate reader (Multiskan™ GO microplate spectrophotometer, Thermo Scientific, Sunnyvale, CA, USA). The NO concentration was determined by using a sodium nitrite standard curve.

2.9. Western Blotting

Cells were lysed with ice-cold PRO-PREP™ protein extract solution (iNtRON, Sungnam, Gyunggi, Korea) and the protein concentration was determined by using the bicinchoninic acid (BCA) procedure (Thermo Scientific, Sunnyvale, CA, USA). Equal amounts of protein were separated by using sodium dodecyl sulfate-polyacrylamide gel electrophoresis (SDS-PAGE) and then transferred onto a polyvinylidene difluoride (PVDF) membrane (Millipore, Billerica, MA, USA). The membrane was blocked with 5% skim milk in 100 mM Tris-hydrochloride (HCl, pH 7.5), 150 mM sodium chloride (NaCl), and 0.2% Tween-20 (TBST) for 1 h at room temperature. The membranes were incubated with TBST containing 5% milk and the primary antibodies against anti-inducible nitric oxide synthase (iNOS), anti-cyclooxygenase (COX)-2, and β-actin (Santa Cruz Biotechnology, Santa Cruz, CA, USA). After washing with TBST, the blot was incubated with the appropriate horseradish peroxidase (HRP)-conjugated secondary antibodies. The antigen was detected by using a Western Bright enhanced chemiluminescence (ECL) HRP substrate kit (Advansta, Menlo Park, CA, USA).

2.10. Real-Time Reverse Transcription-Polymerase Chain Reaction (RT-PCR)

The total RNA was isolated from liver tissue and cells using the RNeasy kit (Qiagen, Valencia, CA, USA). Then, the cDNA was synthesized by using the iScript™ cDNA Synthesis system (Bio-Rad, Hercules, CA, USA). The real-time RT-PCR was performed by using the SensiFAST SYBR qPCR mix (Bioline, London, UK) according to the manufacturer's protocol. The relative values of gene expression were normalized to 18S ribosomal RNA. The primer sequences and full gene names are provided in Table 3.

Table 3. List of mouse primer used for real-time reverse transcription-polymerase chain reaction (RT-PCR).

Genes	Primer Sequences	
TNF-α	F: GGCCTCTCTACCTTGTTGCC	R: CAGCCTGGTCACCAAATCAG
IL-1β	F: TTCACCATGGAATCCGTGTC	R: GTCTTGGCCGAGGACTAAGG
IL-6	F: TTGCCTTCTTGGGACTGATG	R: CCACGATTTCCCAGAGAACA
CD14	F: AAACTCGCTCAATCTGTCTTTCACT	R: TCCTATCCAGCCTGTTGTAACTGA
iNOS	F: CGAAACGCTTCACTTCCAA	R: TGAGCCTATATTGCTGTGGCT
COX2	F: GCATTCTTTGCCCAGCACTT	R: AGACCAGGCACCAGACCAAAG
18S	F: CAGCCACCCGAGATTGAGCA	R: TAGTAGCGACGGGCGGTGTG

2.11. Statistical Analysis

All the results are expressed as mean $\pm$ standard deviation (SD) and were analyzed by using a one-way analysis of variance (ANOVA) followed by the Newman–Keuls multiple range test (parametric). The acceptable level of significance was established at $p < 0.05$.

3. Results

3.1. Analysis of Barley Sprouts Extract Composition

We prepared the calibration curves for saponarin according to a concentration-dependent electrospray ionization-mass spectrometer (ESI-MS) method. We found that the correlation coefficient (r^2) value was 0.9997, which showed good linearity of the calibration curves. The limits of detection and quantification were 2.32 and 7.03 ng/mL, respectively. The condition of the multiple-reaction-monitoring (MRM) mode was m/z 593.2 (precursor ion) → 311.2 (product ion) for saponarin (Figure 3). For the quantitative analysis, we used the calibration curves to calculate the ratios of compounds in the analyzed material to their respective standards. We diluted the barley sprouts extract 1/5 to ensure that the concentration of its components was within the quantitative range of the calibration curves and then multiplied the obtained concentration by 5 (the dilution factor). The quantitative result of saponarin was 14.74 $\pm$ 0.27 μg/mg in the barley sprouts extract.

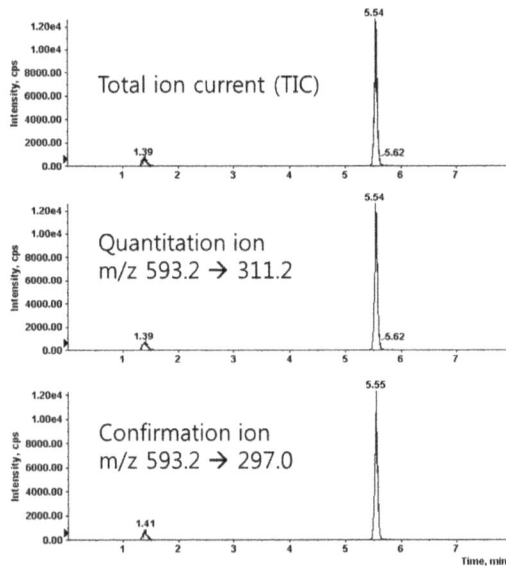

Figure 3. Liquid chromatography-tandem mass spectrometry (LC-MS/MS) spectrum of saponrin.

3.2. Preventive Effect of Barley Sprouts on Alcohol-Induced Liver Injury

To test the effect of barley sprouts on the alcohol-induced liver injury, a study was performed in mice fed a standard Lieber–DeCarli liquid diet supplemented with ethanol for four weeks to determine the potential dose-dependency of the extract. Different doses of the barley sprouts extract ranging from 50 to 200 mg/kg body weight were orally administered daily from the beginning of the liquid diet. We compared the effect of the barley sprouts extract on the alcoholic liver injury with that of silymarin (100 mg/kg body weight), a well-known compound that alleviates alcohol-induced liver injury, as a positive control. The serum ALT and AST activities and TNF-α level in the alcohol-fed mice were all significantly higher than those in the control diet-fed mice were (Figure 4A–C). Whereas the hepatic GSH concentration in the alcohol-treated mice was significantly decreased compared with that of the control mice (Figure 4E). All these alcohol-induced changes were prevented significantly by supplementation with barley sprouts extract at doses exceeding 100 mg/kg. Interestingly, the increased serum level of endotoxin in the alcohol-fed mice was not changed by treatment of barley sprouts extract (Figure 4D). The lipid content of the liver of the alcohol-treated mice showed dramatic accumulation when examined by using both the oil red O staining (Figure 5A) and triglyceride content determination (Figure 5B). Furthermore, supplementation with more than 100 mg/kg of barley sprouts extract significantly reversed the hepatic lipid accumulation (Figure 5). These results were comparable with those obtained with silymarin treatment, indicating that the barley sprouts extract could be a promising candidate to protect against liver injury induced by chronic alcohol ingestion.

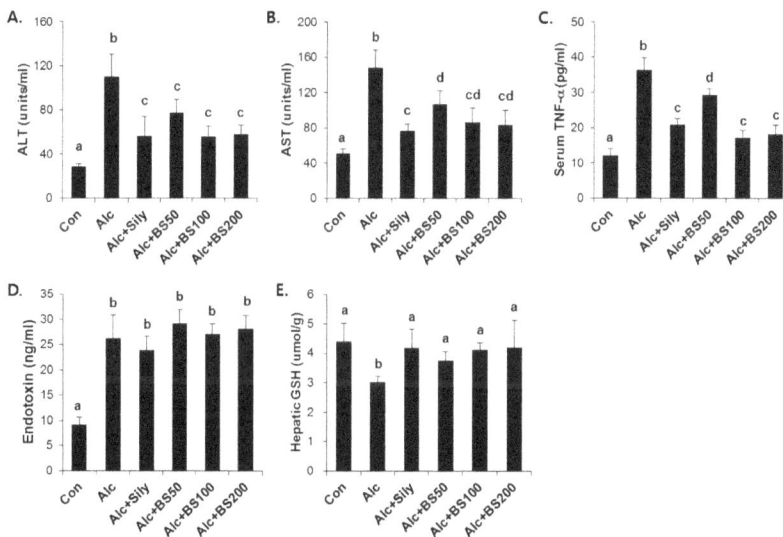

Figure 4. Dose-dependent effect of barley sprouts extract on alcohol-induced liver injury. Serum (**A**) ALT and (**B**) AST activities; (**C**) TNF-α; and (**D**) endotoxin level in the serum; and (**E**) GSH concentration in the liver. Each value is mean $\pm$ standard deviation (SD) of six mice. Values with different letters are significantly different by analysis of variance (ANOVA) followed by Newman–Keuls multiple range test ($p < 0.05$). ALT, alanine aminotransferase; AST, aspartate aminotransferase; TNF, tumor necrosis factor; Con, control diet fed mice; Alc, alcohol diet fed mice; Alc + Sily, Alc fed mice treated with 100 mg/kg silymarin; Alc + BS50, Alc fed mice treated with 50 mg/kg barley sprouts extract; Alc + BS100, Alc fed mice treated with 100 mg/kg barley sprouts extract; Alc + BS200, Alc fed mice treated with 200 mg/kg barley sprouts extract.

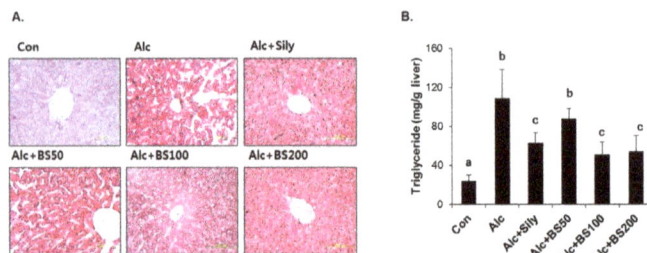

Figure 5. Lipid accumulation in liver of mice treated with alcohol with or without barley sprouts extract. (**A**) Oil red O staining of liver at same magnification (400×) and (**B**) liver triglyceride (TG). Each value is mean ± standard deviation (SD) of six mice. Values with different letters are significantly different by analysis of variance (ANOVA) followed by Newman–Keuls multiple range test ($p < 0.05$). Con, control diet fed mice; Alc, alcohol diet fed mice; Alc + Sily, Alc fed mice treated with 100 mg/kg silymarin; Alc + BS50, Alc fed mice treated with 50 mg/kg barley sprouts extract; Alc + BS100, Alc fed mice treated with 100 mg/kg barley sprouts extract; Alc + BS200, Alc fed mice treated with 200 mg/kg barley sprouts extract.

3.3. Inhibitory Effect of Barley Sprouts Extract on Inflammatory Response-Related Gene Expression in Liver of Alcohol-Treated Mice

The importance of the inflammatory response in alcoholic liver injury has been suggested. Increased circulating endotoxin activates Kupffer cells, which are the resident liver macrophage, and leads to the induction of cytokines, chemokines, and ROS. Here, we determined the expression level of inflammation-related genes using qPCR. The hepatic mRNA expression of TNF-α, interleukin (IL)-1β, IL-6, a cluster of differentiation (CD) 14, iNOS, and COX2 was induced significantly in the liver of the alcohol-treated mice (Figure 6). Supplementation with the barley sprouts extract for the entire alcohol consumption period effectively inhibited the increase of all the mRNAs determined in this experiment (Figure 6).

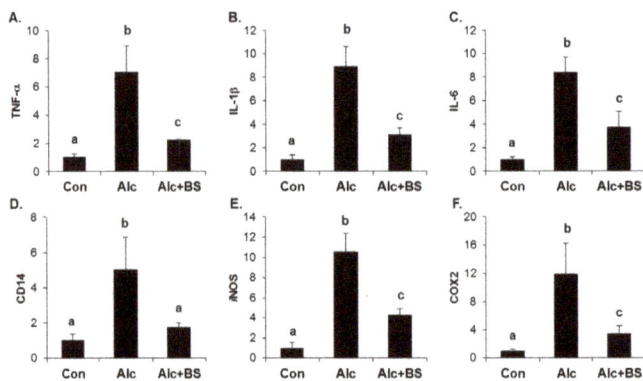

Figure 6. Effect of barley sprouts extracts on inflammation-related gene expression in liver of alcohol-treated mice. mRNA expression of liver (**A**) TNF-α; (**B**) IL-1β; (**C**) IL-6; (**D**) CD14; (**E**) iNOS; and (**F**) COX2 using real-time RT-PCR. Each value is mean ± standard deviation (SD) of six mice. Values with different letters are significantly different by analysis of variance (ANOVA) followed by Newman–Keuls multiple range test ($p < 0.05$). TNF, tumor necrosis factor; IL, interleukin; CD, cluster of differentiation; iNOS, inducible nitric oxide synthase; COX, cyclooxygenase; RT-PCR, reverse transcription-polymerase chain reaction; Con, control diet fed mice; Alc, alcohol diet fed mice; Alc + BS, Alc fed mice with 200 mg/kg barley sprouts extract.

3.4. Anti-Inflammatory Effect of Barley Sprouts Extract in LPS-Activated Raw 264.7 Cells

To investigate whether the barley sprouts extract regulates NO production, cells were pretreated with the extract for 1 h before treatment with LPS for 24 h. As shown in Figure 7A, no cytotoxic effects of barley sprouts extract were observed. Treatment with LPS significantly upregulated the nitrite production (17.7 ± 0.4 μM) compared to that of the untreated control (5.1 ± 0.1 μM, Figure 7B). However, RAW 264.7 cells pretreated with barley sprouts extract displayed a marked decrease in nitrite in a dose-dependent manner after stimulation with LPS. Next, we investigated whether barley sprouts extract regulates iNOS protein expression. Consistent with the suppression of nitrite production, the barley sprouts extract dose-dependently inhibited iNOS protein expression (Figure 7C,D). In addition, the protein expression of COX2 also showed the same pattern as that of iNOS (Figure 7C,D). These data indicate that the barley sprouts extract attenuated the upregulation of LPS-induced COX2 and iNOS expression. Next, we determined the effect of barley sprouts extract on the mRNA expression of TNF-α, iNOS, and COX2 in LPS-stimulated RAW 264.7 cells. Treatment with LPS for 6 h dramatically increased the mRNA expression of TNF-α, iNOS, and COX2 (Figure 8). However, 1 h pretreatment with barley sprouts extract before LPS stimulation significantly blocked the expression of mRNA (Figure 8). These results clearly support the inhibitory effect of barley sprouts extract on inflammatory gene expression in the liver of alcohol-treated mice.

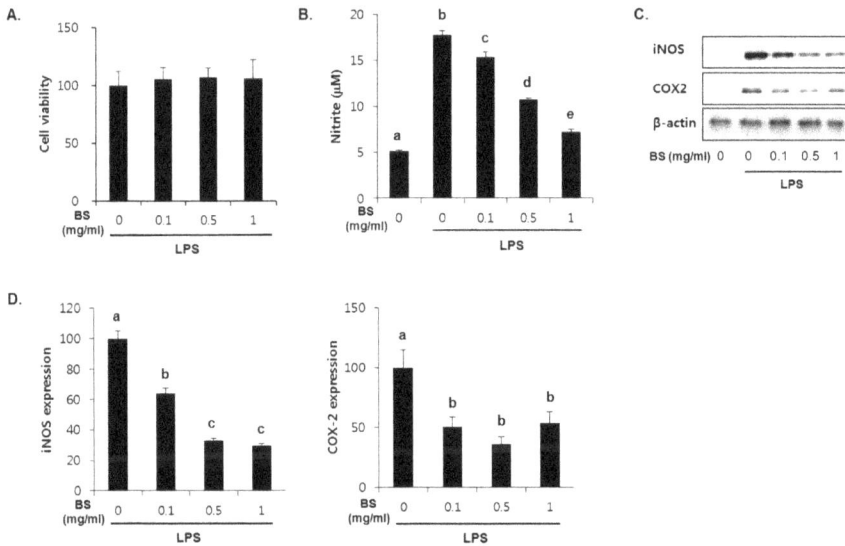

Figure 7. Dose-dependent effect of barley sprouts extract on nitric oxide (NO) generation and protein expression of inducible nitric oxide synthase (iNOS) and cyclooxygenase (COX)-2 in lipopolysaccharide (LPS)-stimulated Raw 264.7 cells. (**A**) Cell viability was determined after treatment with barley sprouts extract for 24 h. Cells were pretreated with barley sprouts extract for 1 h before treatment with 200 ng/mL LPS for 24 h; (**B**) NO generation in medium and (**C**) protein expression of iNOS and COX2 in whole cell lysates; (**D**) Quantitative analysis of blots. Each value is mean ± standard deviation (SD) of triplicates in three independent experiments. Values with different letters are significantly different by analysis of variance (ANOVA) followed by Newman–Keuls multiple range test ($p < 0.05$). BS, barley sprouts extract; iNOS, inducible nitric oxide synthase; COX, cyclooxygenase.

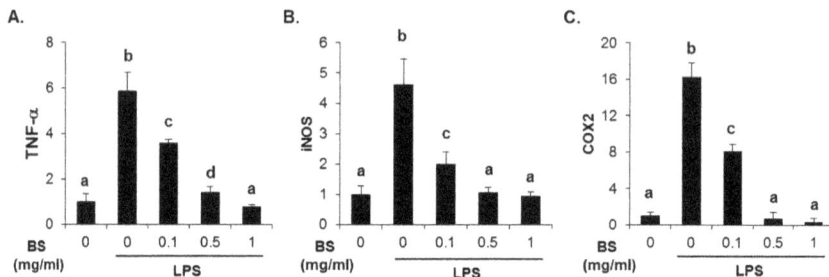

Figure 8. Effect of barley sprouts extract on inflammation-related gene expression in lipopolysaccharide (LPS)-stimulated Raw 264.7 cells. Cells were pretreated with barley sprouts extract for 1 h before treatment with 200 ng/mL LPS for 6 h. mRNA expression of (**A**) TNF-α; (**B**) iNOS; and (**C**) COX2 using real-time RT-PCR. Each value is mean ± standard deviation (SD) of triplicates in three independent experiments. Values with different letters are significantly different by analysis of variance (ANOVA) followed by Newman–Keuls multiple range test ($p < 0.05$). BS, barley sprouts extract; iNOS, inducible nitric oxide synthase; COX, cyclooxygenase; RT-PCR, reverse transcription-polymerase chain reaction.

4. Discussion

In the present study, barley sprouts extract supplementation in the mice fed alcohol for four weeks significantly inhibited the progression of the alcoholic liver injury. Furthermore, the increased levels of the liver injury markers such as hepatic lipid accumulation, as well as serum activities of ALT and AST in alcohol-fed mice were almost completely blocked by treatment with barley sprouts extract. Moreover, its effect on anti-alcoholic liver injury was accompanied by the preservation of hepatic GSH and normalization of the increased serum TNF-α level. This observation suggests that the barley sprouts extract may mechanistically manage the alcohol-induced liver injury.

Accumulating evidence indicates that the role of oxidative stress and inflammation is critical in the pathogenesis of alcohol-induced liver injury [19–21]. Chronic exposure to alcohol generates ROS, mainly hydrogen peroxide and superoxide anion in several metabolic steps, which initiate the peroxidation of membrane phospholipids and lipoproteins. The main sources of ROS include the ethanol-inducible cytochrome P450 (CYP) 2E1, aldosterone dehydrogenase (ADH), mitochondrial respiratory chain, iNOS, and peroxisomal β-oxidation of free fatty acids [19]. Moreover, alcohol depletes GSH, which sensitizes the liver to oxidative stress and TNF-α [20]. Meanwhile, alcohol increases the permeability of the intestinal mucosa and subsequently enhances the level of bacterial-derived endotoxin that stimulates Kupffer cells to produce both ROS by nicotinamide adenine dinucleotide phosphate (NADPH) oxidase (NOX) and cytokines [21]. The oxidants generated activate NF-κB in Kupffer cells, which produces of TNF-α and enhances the inflammatory pathway cascade, ultimately leading to tissue injury [19].

GSH is a thiol-containing tripeptide found in high levels, particularly in the liver. It plays a central role in detoxification and serves as a major antioxidant. It is well known that alcohol intake generates excessive ROS and reactive metabolites, accompanied by a profound depletion of hepatic GSH [22]. Consequently, alcohol administration abrogates the balance between antioxidant and oxidant, and oxidative stress is considered as one of the key mechanisms that cause alcohol-induced liver injury. Several studies have focused on the increase in the antioxidant capacity to prevent oxidative liver damage by alcohol. One study showed that the overexpression of SOD, an enzyme that catalyzes the partitioning of superoxide radical, inhibited the lipid accumulation in the liver, whereas deletion of both glutathione peroxidase-1 and catalase promoted alcohol-induced liver injury [23–25]. The administration of GSH precursor or antioxidants also reduced the liver injury in alcohol-fed mice by decreasing oxidative stress [26–29]. In this study, the alcohol-induced reduction in the GSH

Nutrients **2016**, *8*, 440

levels of the liver of the treated mice was significantly prevented by supplementation with barley sprouts extracts. This result indicates that the improvement of the antioxidant capacity in the liver of alcohol-fed mice via maintenance of hepatic GSH by the barley sprouts extract could make it a potentially valuable treatment strategy for alcoholic liver disease.

The increase in the circulating LPS levels caused by abnormal gut permeability is known to be a key mediator of the inflammatory process in alcoholic liver injury. LPS activates and stimulates Kupffer cells by binding to the CD14 receptor on the cell membrane to release pro-inflammatory cytokines, chemokines, and ROS [19,30,31]. Notably, TNF-α generated in activated Kupffer cells is considered to be one of the most harmful cytokines involved in alcoholic liver injury [30,32]. In the lipid regulatory processes in the body, TNF-α induces lipolysis in adipose tissue, followed eventually by fat accumulation in the liver. Several studies showed that TNF-α causes the release of free fatty acid from adipocytes, and stimulates lipogenesis via sterol regulatory element-binding protein (SREBP)-1c, whereas it inhibits β-oxidation of free fatty acids in the liver [33–36].

In agreement with these reports, the deletion of TNF-receptor 1 (TNFR1) almost completely inhibits the development of alcohol-induced fatty liver [30]. In the present study, chronic alcohol consumption resulted in a significant inflammatory response accompanied by increased circulating TNF-α level, which was significantly inhibited by supplementation with barley sprouts extract. The anti-inflammatory effect of the barley sprouts extract was also demonstrated in the LPS-stimulated RAW 264.7 macrophages.

5. Conclusions

In conclusion, our results indicate that the suppression of TNF-α secretion and maintenance of hepatic GSH by barley sprouts extract contributed to its overall preventive effects against alcohol-induced liver injury.

Acknowledgments: This research was supported by the National Research Foundation of Korea (NRF) grant funded by the Korea government (MSIP) (No. 2009-0083538) and the Foundation of Agri. Tech. Commercialization & Transfer (FACT) through the R & D Results Commercialization Support Project (No. PJ011567) on 2015.

Author Contributions: Y.H.L., J.H.K., W.D.S., J.C.J. and Y.S.J. designed the study. Y.H.L., J.H.K., S.H.K., J.Y.O. and K.M.K. carried out experiment. Y.H.L., J.H.K. and Y.S.J. analyzed experimental results. Y.H.L., J.H.K. and Y.S.J. prepared and Y.S.J. finalized the manuscript. All authors have read and approved the final version of this manuscript.

Conflicts of Interest: The authors declare no conflict of interests.

References

1. Kumar, R.; Rastogi, A.; Sharma, M.K.; Bhatia, V.; Garg, H.; Bihari, C.; Sarin, S.K. Clinicopathological characteristics and metabolic profiles of non-alcoholic fatty liver disease in indian patients with normal body mass index: Do they differ from obese or overweight non-alcoholic fatty liver disease? *Indian J. Endocrinol. Metab.* **2013**, *17*, 665–671. [CrossRef] [PubMed]
2. Rehm, J.; Samokhvalov, A.V.; Shield, K.D. Global burden of alcoholic liver diseases. *J. Hepatol.* **2013**, *59*, 160–168. [CrossRef] [PubMed]
3. Nagata, K.; Suzuki, H.; Sakaguchi, S. Common pathogenic mechanism in development progression of liver injury caused by non-alcoholic or alcoholic steatohepatitis. *J. Toxicol. Sci.* **2007**, *32*, 453–468. [CrossRef] [PubMed]
4. Jones, D.P. Redefining oxidative stress. *Antioxid. Redox Signal.* **2006**, *8*, 1865–1879. [CrossRef] [PubMed]
5. Bailey, S.M.; Mantena, S.K.; Millender-Swain, T.; Cakir, Y.; Jhala, N.C.; Chhieng, D.; Pinkerton, K.E.; Ballinger, S.W. Ethanol and tobacco smoke increase hepatic steatosis and hypoxia in the hypercholesterolemic ApoE(-/-) mouse: Implications for a "multihit" hypothesis of fatty liver disease. *Free Radic. Biol. Med.* **2009**, *46*, 928–938. [CrossRef] [PubMed]
6. Albano, E.; Clot, P.; Morimoto, M.; Tomasi, A.; Ingelman-Sundberg, M.; French, S.W. Role of cytochrome p4502e1-dependent formation of hydroxyethyl free radical in the development of liver damage in rats intragastrically fed with ethanol. *Hepatology* **1996**, *23*, 155–163. [CrossRef] [PubMed]

7. McClain, C.J.; Shedlofsky, S.; Barve, S.; Hill, D.B. Cytokines and alcoholic liver disease. *Alcohol. Health Res. World* **1997**, *21*, 317–320. [PubMed]
8. Tilg, H.; Moschen, A.R.; Kaneider, N.C. Pathways of liver injury in alcoholic liver disease. *J. Hepatol.* **2011**, *55*, 1159–1161. [CrossRef] [PubMed]
9. Miller, A.M.; Horiguchi, N.; Jeong, W.I.; Radaeva, S.; Gao, B. Molecular mechanisms of alcoholic liver disease: Innate immunity and cytokines. *Alcohol. Clin. Exp. Res.* **2011**, *35*, 787–793. [CrossRef] [PubMed]
10. Tsukamoto, H.; Lu, S.C. Current concepts in the pathogenesis of alcoholic liver injury. *FASEB J.* **2001**, *15*, 1335–1349. [CrossRef] [PubMed]
11. Li, Y.; Liu, L.; Wang, B.; Wang, J.; Chen, D. Simple steatosis is a more relevant source of serum inflammatory markers than omental adipose tissue. *Clin. Res. Hepatol. Gastroenterol.* **2014**, *38*, 46–54. [CrossRef] [PubMed]
12. Kamiyama, M.; Shibamoto, T. Flavonoids with potent antioxidant activity found in young green barley leaves. *J. Agric. Food Chem.* **2012**, *60*, 6260–6267. [CrossRef] [PubMed]
13. Yu, Y.M.; Wu, C.H.; Tseng, Y.H.; Tsai, C.E.; Chang, W.C. Antioxidative and hypolipidemic effects of barley leaf essence in a rabbit model of atherosclerosis. *Jpn. J. Pharmacol.* **2002**, *89*, 142–148. [CrossRef] [PubMed]
14. Seo, W.D.; Yuk, H.J.; Curtis-Long, M.J.; Jang, K.C.; Lee, J.H.; Han, S.I.; Kang, H.W.; Nam, M.H.; Lee, S.J.; Lee, J.H.; et al. Effect of the growth stage and cultivar on policosanol profiles of barley sproutss and their adenosine 5'-monophosphate-activated protein kinase activation. *J. Agric. Food Chem.* **2013**, *61*, 1117–1123. [CrossRef] [PubMed]
15. Seo, K.H.; Park, M.J.; Ra, J.E.; Han, S.I.; Nam, M.H.; Kim, J.H.; Lee, J.H.; Seo, W.D. Saponarin from barley sproutss inhibits NF-kappab and mapk on LPS-induced raw 264.7 cells. *Food Funct.* **2014**, *5*, 3005–3013. [CrossRef] [PubMed]
16. Vitcheva, V.; Simeonova, R.; Krasteva, I.; Yotova, M.; Nikolov, S.; Mitcheva, M. Hepatoprotective effects of saponarin, isolated from gypsophila trichotoma wend. on cocaine-induced oxidative stress in rats. *Redox Rep.* **2011**, *16*, 56–61. [CrossRef] [PubMed]
17. Simeonova, R.; Vitcheva, V.; Kondeva-Burdina, M.; Krasteva, I.; Manov, V.; Mitcheva, M. Hepatoprotective and antioxidant effects of saponarin, isolated from gypsophila trichotoma wend. on paracetamol-induced liver damage in rats. *Biomed. Res. Int.* **2013**, *2013*, 757126. [CrossRef] [PubMed]
18. Neuschwander-Tetri, B.A.; Roll, F.J. Glutathione measurement by high-performance liquid chromatography separation and fluorometric detection of the glutathione-orthophthalaldehyde adduct. *Anal. Biochem.* **1989**, *179*, 236–241. [CrossRef]
19. Arteel, G.E. Oxidants and antioxidants in alcohol-induced liver disease. *Gastroenterology* **2003**, *124*, 778–790. [CrossRef] [PubMed]
20. Colell, A.; Garcia-Ruiz, C.; Miranda, M.; Ardite, E.; Mari, M.; Morales, A.; Corrales, F.; Kaplowitz, N.; Fernandez-Checa, J.C. Selective glutathione depletion of mitochondria by ethanol sensitizes hepatocytes to tumor necrosis factor. *Gastroenterology* **1998**, *115*, 1541–1551. [CrossRef]
21. Bode, C.; Bode, J.C. Activation of the innate immune system and alcoholic liver disease: Effects of ethanol per se or enhanced intestinal translocation of bacterial toxins induced by ethanol? *Alcohol. Clin. Exp. Res.* **2005**, *29*, 166S–171S. [CrossRef] [PubMed]
22. Fernandez-Checa, J.C.; Kaplowitz, N.; Garcia-Ruiz, C.; Colell, A.; Miranda, M.; Mari, M.; Ardite, E.; Morales, A. GSH transport in mitochondria: Defense against TNF-induced oxidative stress and alcohol-induced defect. *Am. J. Physiol.* **1997**, *273*, G7–G17. [PubMed]
23. Wheeler, M.D.; Kono, H.; Yin, M.; Rusyn, I.; Froh, M.; Connor, H.D.; Mason, R.P.; Samulski, R.J.; Thurman, R.G. Delivery of the Cu/Zn-superoxide dismutase gene with adenovirus reduces early alcohol-induced liver injury in rats. *Gastroenterology* **2001**, *120*, 1241–1250. [CrossRef] [PubMed]
24. Wheeler, M.D.; Nakagami, M.; Bradford, B.U.; Uesugi, T.; Mason, R.P.; Connor, H.D.; Dikalova, A.; Kadiiska, M.; Thurman, R.G. Overexpression of manganese superoxide dismutase prevents alcohol-induced liver injury in the rat. *J. Biol. Chem.* **2001**, *276*, 36664–36672. [CrossRef] [PubMed]
25. Kim, S.J.; Lee, J.W.; Jung, Y.S.; Kwon do, Y.; Park, H.K.; Ryu, C.S.; Kim, S.K.; Oh, G.T.; Kim, Y.C. Ethanol-induced liver injury and changes in sulfur amino acid metabolomics in glutathione peroxidase and catalase double knockout mice. *J. Hepatol.* **2009**, *50*, 1184–1191. [CrossRef] [PubMed]
26. Kono, H.; Rusyn, I.; Bradford, B.U.; Connor, H.D.; Mason, R.P.; Thurman, R.G. Allopurinol prevents early alcohol-induced liver injury in rats. *J. Pharmacol. Exp. Ther.* **2000**, *293*, 296–303. [PubMed]

27. Kono, H.; Arteel, G.E.; Rusyn, I.; Sies, H.; Thurman, R.G. Ebselen prevents early alcohol-induced liver injury in rats. *Free Radic. Biol. Med.* **2001**, *30*, 403–411. [CrossRef]

28. Kono, H.; Rusyn, I.; Uesugi, T.; Yamashina, S.; Connor, H.D.; Dikalova, A.; Mason, R.P.; Thurman, R.G. Diphenyleneiodonium sulfate, an NADPH oxidase inhibitor, prevents early alcohol-induced liver injury in the rat. *Am. J. Physiol. Gastrointest. Liver Physiol.* **2001**, *280*, G1005–G1012. [PubMed]

29. McKim, S.E.; Konno, A.; Gabele, E.; Uesugi, T.; Froh, M.; Sies, H.; Thurman, R.G.; Arteel, G.E. Cocoa extract protects against early alcohol-induced liver injury in the rat. *Arch. Biochem. Biophys.* **2002**, *406*, 40–46. [CrossRef]

30. Yin, M.; Wheeler, M.D.; Kono, H.; Bradford, B.U.; Gallucci, R.M.; Luster, M.I.; Thurman, R.G. Essential role of tumor necrosis factor α in alcohol-induced liver injury in mice. *Gastroenterology* **1999**, *117*, 942–952. [CrossRef]

31. Rao, R. Endotoxemia and gut barrier dysfunction in alcoholic liver disease. *Hepatology* **2009**, *50*, 638–644. [CrossRef] [PubMed]

32. Ji, C.; Deng, Q.; Kaplowitz, N. Role of TNF-α in ethanol-induced hyperhomocysteinemia and murine alcoholic liver injury. *Hepatology* **2004**, *40*, 442–451. [CrossRef] [PubMed]

33. Feingold, K.R.; Grunfeld, C. Tumor necrosis factor-α stimulates hepatic lipogenesis in the rat in vivo. *J. Clin. Investig.* **1987**, *80*, 184–190. [CrossRef] [PubMed]

34. Hardardottir, I.; Doerrler, W.; Feingold, K.R.; Grunfeld, C. Cytokines stimulate lipolysis and decrease lipoprotein lipase activity in cultured fat cells by a prostaglandin independent mechanism. *Biochem. Biophys. Res. Commun.* **1992**, *186*, 237–243. [CrossRef]

35. Nachiappan, V.; Curtiss, D.; Corkey, B.E.; Kilpatrick, L. Cytokines inhibit fatty acid oxidation in isolated rat hepatocytes: Synergy among TNF, IL-6, and IL-1. *Shock* **1994**, *1*, 123–129. [CrossRef] [PubMed]

36. Endo, M.; Masaki, T.; Seike, M.; Yoshimatsu, H. TNF-α induces hepatic steatosis in mice by enhancing gene expression of sterol regulatory element binding protein-1c (srebp-1c). *Exp. Biol. Med.* **2007**, *232*, 614–621.

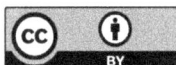

nutrients

MDPI

Review

Natural Phyto-Bioactive Compounds for the Treatment of Type 2 Diabetes: Inflammation as a Target

Sivapragasam Gothai [1], Palanivel Ganesan [2,3], Shin-Young Park [3], Sharida Fakurazi [1,4], Dong-Kug Choi [2,3] and Palanisamy Arulselvan [1,*]

[1] Laboratory of Vaccines and Immunotherapeutics, Institute of Bioscience, Universiti Putra Malaysia, Serdang 43400, Malaysia; gothai_86@yahoo.com (S.G.); sharida.fakurazi@gmail.com (S.F.)

[2] Nanotechnology Research Center and Department of Applied Life Science, College of Biomedical and Health Science, Konkuk University, Chungju 380-701, Korea; palanivel67@gmail.com (P.G.); choidk@kku.ac.kr (D.-K.C.)

[3] Department of Biotechnology, College of Biomedical and Health Science, Konkuk University, Chungju 380-701, Korea; ifresha@nate.com

[4] Department of Human Anatomy, Faculty of Medicine and Health Sciences, Universiti Putra Malaysia, Serdang 43400, Malaysia

* Correspondence: arulbio@gmail.com; Tel.: +603-8947-2331

Received: 19 May 2016; Accepted: 15 July 2016; Published: 4 August 2016

Abstract: Diabetes is a metabolic, endocrine disorder which is characterized by hyperglycemia and glucose intolerance due to insulin resistance. Extensive research has confirmed that inflammation is closely involved in the pathogenesis of diabetes and its complications. Patients with diabetes display typical features of an inflammatory process characterized by the presence of cytokines, immune cell infiltration, impaired function and tissue destruction. Numerous anti-diabetic drugs are often prescribed to diabetic patients, to reduce the risk of diabetes through modulation of inflammation. However, those anti-diabetic drugs are often not successful as a result of side effects; therefore, researchers are searching for efficient natural therapeutic targets with less or no side effects. Natural products' derived bioactive molecules have been proven to improve insulin resistance and associated complications through suppression of inflammatory signaling pathways. In this review article, we described the extraction, isolation and identification of bioactive compounds and its molecular mechanisms in the prevention of diabetes associated complications.

Keywords: type 2 diabetes mellitus; insulin resistance; polyphenols; inflammatory mediators; diabetic complications

1. Introduction

Presently, there are more than 415 million people affected by diabetes mellitus worldwide, according to the International Diabetes Federation, and this figure is projected to rise to over 642 million or more by 2040. Around 90% of diabetic patients in the worldwide are diagnosed with type 2 diabetes mellitus (T2DM). The cost of health care related to diabetes and its secondary complications continues to expand and is a massive economic burden for afflicted diabetic patients and particularly developing countries (Diabetes Atlas, 7th edition, International Diabetes Federation, 2015). T2DM represents a major global health issue and incidence of diseases increases with various genetic and other associated factors such as age, obesity, stress, diet, ethnicity, lack of exercise and inflammation. The burden of type 2 diabetes and its major complications are rising worldwide [1].

Inflammation has been recognized as a key player in the pathophysiology of both type 1 and type 2 diabetes and its secondary complications [2]. Chronic low-grade inflammation and an activation of the various immune reactions are particularly involved in the pathogenesis of obesity-linked insulin resistance and type 2 diabetes. Activated inflammatory markers are major factors to initiate and develop diabetes-associated complications including retinopathy, nephropathy, neuropathy, ischemic heart disease, peripheral vascular disease, and cerebrovascular disease, etc. [3,4]. Therefore, targeting the inflammation and its signaling pathways may be an active target to prevent/manage diabetes mellitus and its associated complications. Existing therapeutic drugs used for diabetes, which increase various secondary complications including cardiovascular disease, kidney failure, liver injury, dizziness, mental disorders, weight gain, and skin diseases [5].

Natural products and its derived active compounds may be achievable alternatives for the treatment of type 2 diabetes and its complications without any adverse effects. There are a huge number of active medicinal plants and its natural bioactive molecules that have already reported the therapeutic nature against diabetes [6]. Several medicinal plants have been used since ancient times to manage and prevent diabetes and associated conditions [7].

Looking into the list of drugs approved within the last decades demonstrates that plant ingredients are still of importance in drug discovery. Plant compounds have been shown to confer some protection against the pathology of diabetes mellitus through the attenuation of inflammatory mediators. Therefore, this paper intends to review the most salient recent reports on the anti-inflammatory associated diabetes mellitus properties of phytochemicals and the molecular mechanisms underlying these properties.

2. Inflammation Status in Diabetes Mellitus

Insulin resistance or T2DM has been well-defined as a state of universal inflammation condition involving both innate and adaptive immunity [3]. Preclinical and clinical studies have demonstrated that various anti-inflammatory agents can improve blood glucose level and pancreatic beta cell function in T2DM [8,9]. Thus, inflammatory associated pathways are one of the principal pathways in the pathogenesis of T2DM and its complications.

T2DM are associated with increased expressions of complete markers of chronic inflammation and the primary molecular link between inflammation and T2DM are macrophage mediators, tumor necrosis factor-α (TNF α), interleukin-1β (IL-1β) and interleukin-6 (IL-6). Elevated amounts of these pro-inflammatory cytokines have been confirmed in diabetes mellitus [10]. The trend of diabetic patients to have higher amounts of inflammation status has serious consequences that contribute to both microvascular and macrovascular complications [11]. Among both types of complications, macrovascular complications are critical for human life, namely, cardiovascular disease and also around 80% of diabetic patients die from coronary artery diseases and its related complications [12].

Monocyte chemoattractant protein-1 (MCP-1) is a key chemokine produced by mainly adipocytes upon recruitment of macrophages and endothelial cells [13]. The augmented release of circulating MCP-1 during adiposity, promotes the expression of pro-inflammatory cytokines thereby, it impairs the inflammation associated with type 2 diabetes. Adiponectin is one of the most important anti-inflammatory cytokines secreted by white adipose tissue. The level of adiponectin mainly reduces in obesity, and inflammation associated type 2 diabetic conditions; meanwhile, the increased level of adiponectin was observed during type 1 diabetes mellitus (T1DM) [14].

Toll-like receptors (TLRs) are playing a central role in innate immunity by their capability to sense pathogens across the pathogen-associated molecular patterns (PAMPs) and to notice tissue injury through the danger-associated molecular patterns (DAMPs) [15]. Among different types of TLRS, TLRs 1,2,4,5,6, and 11 are plasma membrane proteins, while TLRs 3,7,8 and 9 exist in intracellular compartments. Various factors including microbial constituents provoke the activation of the TLR (excluding for TLR3) signaling through a MyD88 (myeloid differentiation factor)-dependent pathway, principal to the activation of the signaling transcription factor NF-κB and the production of inflammatory mediators. These TLR signaling pathways might activate through the production of numerous factors including endogenous HMGB1 (High-Mobility Group Box 1), and advanced glycation end products (AGEs) [15,16].

HMGB1 is also one of the ligands for activation for TLR2 and 4, and it has also been elevated in an experimental diabetic animal model. It was previously recognized as one of the transcription factor regulator, and it was later confirmed as a cytokine produced through cell damage and immune cells like macrophages, thus HMGB1 actively stimulates a NF-κB signaling cascade [17,18].

Advanced glycation end products (AGEs), which were principally believed as oxidative derivatives, due to from diabetic hyperglycemia conditions, and these are gradually realized as a possible risk factor for pancreatic islet β-cell injury and type 2 diabetes. These AGEs significantly elevated the inflammatory markers as well as oxidative markers in diabetic conditions; meanwhile, it impairs the production and action of insulin [19].

Numerous preclinical and clinical studies have clearly established that adipose tissue, livers, muscles and pancreases are major sites of inflammation of the occurrence of obesity and T2DM [2]. An infiltration of macrophages into adipose tissue, liver, muscle and pancreas are seen in obesity and diabetes-induced animal models and in obese human individuals with T2DM. Macrophages are essential for the production of pro-inflammatory cytokines [20], including TNFα, IL-6, IL-1β and other inflammatory mediators. These inflammatory mediators act in an autocrine and paracrine way to stimulate insulin resistance by interfering with insulin signaling in peripheral tissues through activation of various inflammatory associated pathways such as nuclear factor-kappa B (NF-κB) and c-JUN N-terminal kinase (JNK) pathways [21,22]. These pathways are responsible for promoting the tissue inflammation in obesity and diabetic condition.

At the molecular level, signaling pathway, NF-κB is the inflammation principal switch that controls the synthesis of numerous active proteins series such as IκB, IL-1β, IL-1, and TNF-α for the activation and maintenance of the inflamed state. In obesity condition, it stimulates the NF-κB activation and associated pathways in adipose tissue, livers, and pancreases, thus promoting insulin resistance and T2DM. Researchers have proven that inflammation is not only a marker, but it is also a mediator of disease that was confirmed earlier.

The immune cells' macrophages can be categorized into two distinct subtypes: the "classically activated macrophages" phenotype, termed M1, which produce major pro-inflammatory cytokines including TNF-α, IL-6, IL-1β and the "alternatively activated macrophages" phenotype, termed M2, which produces major anti-inflammatory cytokines, IL-10 [20]. Furthermore, macrophage infiltration in to adipose tissue and obesity causes a phenotypic switch from the M2 to M1 phenotype, connecting with insulin resistance in animals and humans [23]. The M1 phenotype of macrophages can alter insulin signaling pathways and adipogenesis in adipocytes while M2 macrophages appear to safeguard against obesity-induced insulin resistance [20].

Increased expression/production of TNFα in adipose tissue was observed in obese individuals, and it is playing the vital role in obesity-induced insulin resistance [24]. Previous findings have been confirmed a specific up-regulation of inflammatory genes and an over-production of numerous pro-inflammatory cytokines and chemokines in inflamed adipose tissue [2]. Furthermore, improvement in insulin sensitivity induced by weight loss was accompanied by a reduction in the expression of multiple pro-inflammatory genes [2,25]; hence, inflammation in adipose tissue was considered as a crucial consequence leading to T2DM and its complications.

In the conclusion, previous investigations reveal a complex interaction between cells of innate and adaptive immunity system and the equilibrium among these immune cells turns out to be essential for the homeostasis and control of tissue inflammation in obesity and T2DM (Figure 1).

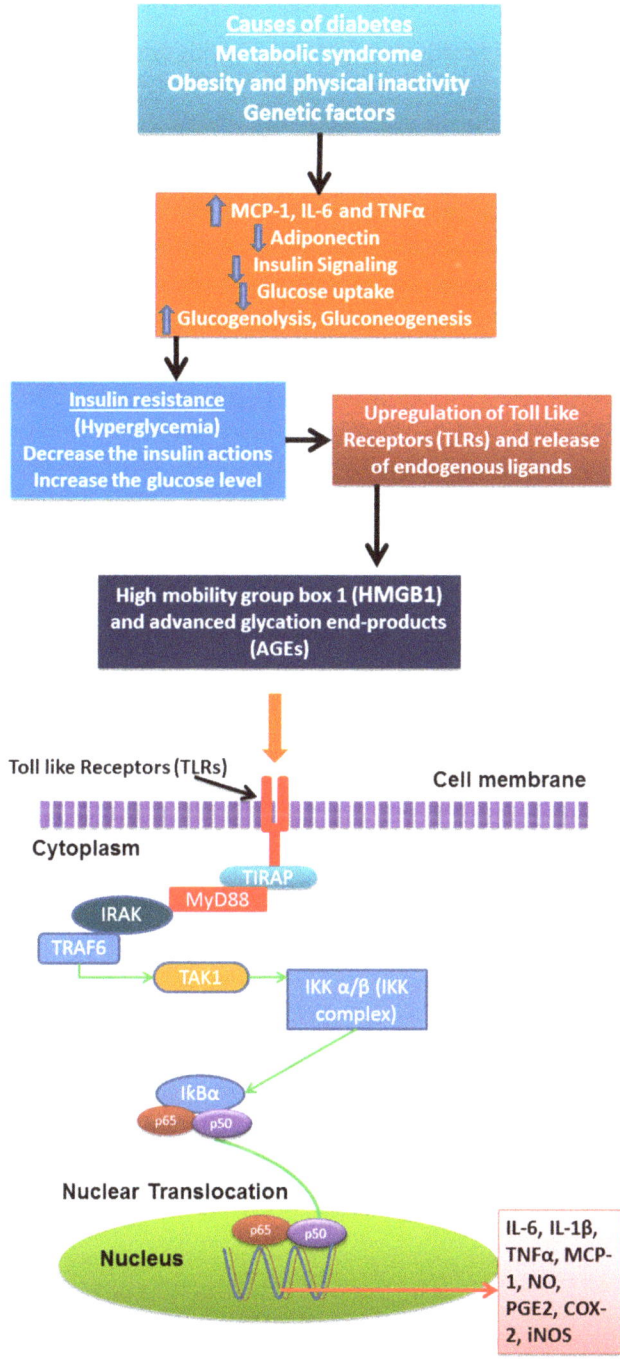

Figure 1. Activation of inflammatory pathway and inflammatory mediators in diabetic condition.

3. Anti-Inflammatory Based Therapeutics for Diabetes

Several therapeutic interventions are very effective in reducing acute and chronic inflammation and improving diabetes and its complications via indirect or pleiotropic mechanisms. Issues that reduce the inflammation (particularly, key inflammatory markers such as pro-inflammatory mediators TNFα, IL-6, IL-1β and CRP) could offer a vital public health tool to reduce the burden of diabetes and associated complications including cardiovascular diseases in the general population. The probability of regulating innate immunity-related inflammation as an important experimental approach for the management/prevention of T2DM is based on findings that investigated the therapeutic efficacy of anti-inflammatory agents [26].

Nowadays, the key therapeutic agents to treat T2DM and its complications, sulfonylureas, metformin, and insulin-sensitizing glitazones all improve metabolic control and lead to control of various circulating inflammation mediators through innate immunity-related signaling pathways. Sulfonylureas and metformin are main drugs to prevent the T2DM, and sulfonylureas increase insulin production from pancreatic β-cells, while metformin suppresses glucose production in the liver and meanwhile increases insulin sensitivity in peripheral tissues [27]. Glitazones, another anti-diabetic drug, binds to peroxisome proliferator-activated receptors (PPARs), beginning a transcriptional activity that leads to improved insulin action through reducing the secretion of inflammatory markers. Consequently, glitazones reduced levels of CRP, PAI-1, TNF-α and other inflammatory markers. These drugs showed better anti-diabetic nature and also have the comparable anti-inflammatory potential [26,28].

Other therapeutic approaches for T2DM that would act as principals in the inflammatory system have been proposed in the form of salicylates, an anti-inflammatory therapeutic that inhibits IκB kinase (IKK), and also lowering the glucose level through improvement of beta cell function [29]. Various well established non-steroidal anti-inflammatory drugs (NSAIDs) and cyclooxygenase inhibitors (e.g., ibuprofen, naproxen) are able to improve glucose-mediated insulin release, glucose tolerance, and reduce the insulin resistance in diabetic patients [30,31].

In clinical studies, treatment with NSAIDs enhanced many biochemical indices such as blood glucose level, glucose uptake, insulin clearance, CRP, lipid profile associated with obesity, and T2DM [32]. Though these findings support the notion that inflammation plays a key role in T2DM and its complications, attenuating inflammation as a strategy for disease prevention in a public health setting will demand a markedly different perspective. In this case, an approach that can be introduced into the population with the minimal side effects and the maximal therapeutic result should be adopted. In this connection, natural products based therapeutic approach would be a better opportunity to treat inflammatory associated chronic diseases like T2DM and its complications, since natural products derived agents are generally safer, lower cost and more highly available in the world.

4. Natural Phyto Bioactive Compounds Role in Anti-Diabetics

Natural phyto bioactive compounds are currently more in demand than the synthetic medicines for the treatment of diabetes owing to the rich availability, efficacy and fewer side effects [33,34]. The higher amount of these phyto bioactive compounds rich foods can be consumed on the daily basis that can enhance the antidiabetic activities. It also performed well in various traditional medicines includes Indian Ayurvedic and Chinese traditional medicines and showed enhanced bioactivity of those phyto compounds [35,36]. These phyto bioactive compounds rich extracts either as a single or combination of the multiple extracts showed enhanced anti-diabetic activities. These combination extract therapy aids in multiple actions of those bioactive compounds by single therapies thereby enhance the beneficiary activities, which, in turn, reduces the drug load to the patients. Among the drugs approved for the anti-diabetic activities in the last 10 years, 49% derived from the plant origin. Overall, 1200 phyto bioactive compound rich plants were reported for their better antidiabetic activities, among them 400 phyto bioactive rich plant extracts showed type 2 anti-diabetic activities [34–36]. Phyto bioactive compounds include saponin, myrcelin, flavonoids, pectin, and glucosides rich in various parts of the plants showed enhanced antidiabetic activities. The antidiabetic activities of these phytocompounds can be varied based on mechanisms of their actions for lowering the glucose including glucose absorption, target insulin resistance and pancreatic functions.

Phyto bioactive compounds rich in extracts of safflower and Japanese kelp showed higher suppress-glucosidase activity, thereby regulating the glucose absorption in the gut [37,38]. In another study, Inulin, the soluble fiber showed regulation of GLp-1 homeostasis [39]. Further regulation of insulin resistance was reported by various phyto bioactive compounds rich plants such as Dioscorea polysaccharides, blueberry anthocyanins, cinnamon and fenugreek seeds [40–43]. In addition, several phyto extracts showed combinational effect of these bioactivities and its include chili peppers, bitter melon, ginseng, turmeric and tea extracts [44–49]. Therefore, the combinational intake of these foods or synergistic efficacy of these phyto compounds will be a future research area in the diabetic disease models. Even though these phyto compounds showed multiple beneficial effects in various in vitro studies, their extraction method limits their actions in their bioactivity of these compounds. A few of those novel technologies used in the extraction of those bioactive compounds and their roles in the anti-diabetic activity are discussed below.

5. Extraction, Identification and Characterization of Bioactive Compounds from Natural Products

World Health Organization (WHO) reported that more than 25,000 medicinally valuable plants exist in different countries including in both developing and developed countries. The principal steps to exploit the bioactive phyto-compounds from natural resources are solvent extraction, bioassays, isolation, and characterization, toxicological, preclinical and clinical investigation of bioactive phyto-compound.

We need to establish the different appropriate methods to investigate the biological properties of phyto compounds from the natural products, and these biological assays are required to identify and isolate the bioactive compounds present in the extract. The entire in vitro biological assay is very reliable and a simple method to get to know the biological activities of extracts, and it may differ based on the targeted diseases like anti-cancer, anti-diabetes, anti-inflammation, anti-malarial, anti-microbial and toxicity studies.

5.1. Extraction

Extraction from the natural products is the first step to screen the biological activities of extracts and identify the bioactive compounds for further isolation, identification and characterization. These steps include washing and drying the raw materials, and blending to obtain the powder and using a different solvent system to extract the crude extract to investigate its biological activities [50,51].

Appropriate extraction methods should be used to ensure that potential bioactive constituents are not lost, distorted or destroyed during the preparation of the crude extract from samples [40]. The selection of a suitable solvent system basically depends on the physical nature of the bioactive compound being targeted as various solvent systems are available to extract/identify the bioactive compound from natural products. The hydrophilic compound extraction, mainly of polar solvents including methanol, ethanol or ethyl-acetate, and for lipophilic compounds extraction, dichloromethane or mixtures of dichloromethane/methanol in the ratio of 1:1, was used to identify the compounds [52].

Recently, various modern extraction techniques were used by natural products based researchers, which include solid-phase micro-extraction, supercritical-fluid extraction, pressurized-liquid extraction, microwave-assisted extraction, and surfactant-mediated techniques. These modern extraction techniques have a lot of advantages including the decrease in organic solvent consumption and in sample stability, removal of unwanted samples clean-up and solvent concentration steps before chromatographic separation, improvement in extraction productivity, selectivity, kinetics of extraction. The exhaustive extraction method is also one of the most efficient extraction methods, and it is mostly carried out with different solvent systems of increasing polarity in order to extract the most bioactive components with significant biological properties. Based on the advantages of these modern techniques, researchers have used these techniques to identify the bioactive compounds more efficiently [53].

Effective identification and isolation of bioactive compounds from natural products are mainly subject to the type of solvent used in the extraction methods. The solvent selection will also depend on the polarity of targeted bioactive compounds to be extracted from natural products [54]. Moreover, the molecular similarity between solvent and solute, mass transfer, use of co-solvent method, toxicity nature, ease of solvent evaporation at low temperature, stability, and inability to cause the extract to composite or dissociate. The choice of solvent selection was affected by other factors such as the amount of phytocompounds to be extracted, the frequency of extraction, the variety of phytocompounds to be extracted, ease of successive handling of the crude extracts and cost effectiveness.

5.2. Novel Technologies Used in Extraction of Phyto Based Antidiabetic Compounds

Extraction of the bioactive compounds from the anti-diabetic plants showed a crucial step in determining the antidiabetic activity of the phyto extracts with higher yield and greater potency of those extracts. For the higher yield extraction of the compounds, several factors need to be considered in conventional technologies such as the type of sample, solvent, mixture of those solvents [55]. In order to overcome several difficulties in conventional technologies includes higher use of organic solvents and sample degradation, several modern technologies serve as an alternative for the extraction of those bioactive compounds from antidiabetic plants. Those technologies include but are not limited to ultrasound extraction, microwave-assisted extraction and supercritical extraction. These technologies overcome the conventional technologies by reducing organic solvents usages, higher yield and elimination of unwanted compounds from the extract and showed the greater antidiabetic efficiency of those phyto bioactive compounds [53].

5.3. Ultra Sound Extraction of Phyto Compounds from Anti-Diabetic Plants

Ultra sound extraction technology is one of the most modern technologies frequently used in the extraction of phyto bioactive compounds from antidiabetic plants with enhanced anti-diabetic bioactivities [56]. This technology enhances the extraction yield with many highly stable bioactive compounds from the antidiabetic plants by the enhanced cell penetrating effect of solvents and breaking of the intramolecular forces through high intensity sound waves [56,57]. The main advantage of these techniques is that they can able to extract the maximum bioactive compounds with limited raw material and shorter time. Recently, polysaccharides from mulberry fruits were extracted using ultrasound technology at an extraction time of about 75 min, produced an extraction yield of about 3.13%, and showed higher anti-glycemic activity by stronger α-glucosidase inhibition activity [58]. Similarly, higher extraction yield of total polyphenol was also obtained by ultrasound assisted extraction of guava leaves extract with higher anti-hyperglycemic activity than acarbose [56]. Likewise, the higher extraction yield of α-glucosidase enzyme was also obtained in the guava leaves with maximum antihyperglycemic activities. Similarly anthocyanins extraction yield increases using ultrasound assisted extraction of bilberry, blackberry and mulberry fruits. The extraction yield of those anthocyanins reached a maximum of up to 2800 mg/L. These extracts showed enhanced anti hyperglycemic activity in the diabetic rats [57]. In another study, the antidiabetic activity of the *Pterocarpus marsupium* Roxb. Heartwood can be enhanced with ultrasound extraction with the higher protection of the phyto bioactive compounds than other conventional methods in alloxan induced antidiabetic rats [59]. From all of these studies, it was confirmed that extraction yield of the phyto bioactive compounds can be enhanced through the ultrasound extraction technologies, and it also opens ways for the researchers to use these non-conventional technologies for the higher extraction of the bioactive compounds from the anti-diabetics plants.

5.4. Microwave Assisted Extraction of Phyto Compounds from Antidiabetic Plants

Microwave assisted extraction is another novel technology currently used in the extraction of phyto bioactive compounds from various medicinal plants like ginger, tea, mango, sapotta [60–65] and other herbs proven to have antidiabetic activities. The microwave technology is highly used in the extraction of phyto bioactive compounds with lesser degradation of those compounds, higher extraction yield and cost effectiveness than other conventional technologies. Recently, antidiabetic activity of microwave assisted extraction of *Solanum nigrum* leaves was studied and found that higher extraction yield of *Solanum nigrum* leaves extract were obtained using microwave assisted extraction with a yield of 64%. The antidiabetic activities of those extracts were found to be dose dependent. Higher and medium doses were found to have a greater antidiabetic effect. In addition, for the extraction of the bioactive compounds, drying using the microwave technology also enhances the extraction yield of the phyto bioactive compounds. Recently, leaves of *Aquilaria subintegra* and *Aquilaria malaccensis* were dried using microwaves and were found to increase the yield of bioactive compounds with enhancing antidiabetic activity [66]. In addition to the extraction and antidiabetic study of the phyto bioactive compounds, several phyto bioactive compounds were studied for the effective extraction using microwave assisted extraction technology with higher extraction yield [67,68]. However, their efficacy in various diabetic models is still limited. This will provide a new research scope about the role of microwave technology in extraction and bioactivity against various diabetic models in near future.

5.5. Supercritical Fluid Extraction of Bioactive Compounds from Antidiabetic Plants

Supercritical fluid extraction technology is one of the novel technologies for the extraction of phyto bioactive compounds from the antidiabetic plants [69–72] with possible application of those ingredients in the developments of the functional foods and pharmaceutical industries. This technology has several advantages over conventional technologies like higher yield, and multiple compounds can be extracted from this technology, and it can ultimately lead to multiple health benefits of those products developed using these extracts. In addition, this technology has several other advantages including the low viscosity of supercritical fluid that leads to multiple extractions, less solvent residue, and faster extraction process [72]. Recently, various non-polar constituents from *Toona sinensis* leaves were extracted using supercritical fluid extraction technology and found 24 different active compounds. The major compound in those extractions was that of phytol which possesses greater antidiabetic activity along with the prevention of hepatosteatosis [72]. The same research group also checked for the commercial essential oils obtained by a supercritical extraction process showed greater antidiabetic activity owing to the higher non polar constituents. Similarly, bixin, a colored pigment that possesses anti-hyperglycemic activity, was obtained by a supercritical extraction process with higher yield [73]. Several bioactive compounds can also be effectively extracted from the anti-diabetic plants such as ginseng, turmeric, but their active role in the diabetic model of supercritical extracted compounds is still yet to be elucidated.

Overall, modern extraction processes such as ultrasounds, microwaves, and supercritical fluid extraction process can efficiently extract various phyto bioactive compounds with higher extraction yield, faster process, and lesser thermal degradation, possessing multiple benefits in anti-diabetic activity. However, certain modern equipment is cost effective such as the supercritical fluid extraction process, requires much space, and needs to be considered in future. Table 1 illustrates the modern extraction techniques used for the preparation of bioactive compounds from medicinal plants.

Table 1. Novel extraction methods of extracting bioactive compounds from anti-diabetic plants.

Serial No.	Extraction Methods	Phyto Bioactive Compounds	Plant Parts	Antidiabetic Activities	Reference
1	Ultrasound assisted extraction	Polysaccharides	Mulberry fruits	α-glucosidase inhibition	[62]
		Polyphenols	Guava leaves	Anti-hyperglycemic	[60]
		Anthocyanins	Berry fruits	Anti-hyperglycemic	[61]
		Crude extract	Heart woods	Anti-diabetic	[63]
2	Microwave assisted extraction	Crude extracts	Night shade leaves	Anti-diabetic	[74]
		Dried leaves extracts	Aquilaria leaves	Anti-diabetic	[70]
3	Supercritical fluid extraction	Phytol	Toona sinensis leaves	Antidiabetic	[75]
		Bixin	Annatoo seeds	Anti-hyperglycemic	[76]

5.6. Purification of Bioactive Compounds

Purification of bioactive compounds from crude extracts is an important task, as purified compounds are much more therapeutically effective. Recent modern techniques have created numerous ways for the purification and large-scale production of several bioactive compounds [77]. The plant crude extracts generally occur as a combination of various categories of bioactive compounds with different polarities, hence different levels of chromatographic separations are used to purify the bioactive compounds including Thin Layer Chromatography (TLC), Column Chromatography and High Performance Liquid Chromatography (HPLC). These chromatographic techniques are still used to purify/isolate the bioactive compounds due to various advantages including convenience, and availability of the variety of stationary phases for separation of active phytochemicals [75,76].

Mainly, TLC has been used to the fraction of different components from natural products and this technique shortens the process of isolation and identification of bioactive compound [74]. HPLC is one of the important widely used purification techniques for the isolation of natural products followed by TLC and other chromatographic techniques [78]. Presently, HPLC is gaining popularity among other analytical chromatographic techniques as the key choice for phytocompound fingerprinting. The bioactive molecules are often existing only as a minor component in the crude extract and the determination ability of HPLC is ideally suited to the quick processing of multicomponent natural products based samples on both an analytical and preparative scale [79].

Apart from HPLC, there are other alternative analytical methods employed to identify phytocompounds, among which is the diode array detector (DAD) coupled with a mass spectrometer (MS), liquid chromatography and gas chromatography coupled with mass spectrometry (LC/MS and GC/MS) [79,80]. These alternative analytical methods provide abundant useful information for structural elucidation and identification of the bioactive compounds when tandem mass spectrometry (MS) is applied. Thus, the combination of HPLC with MS facilitates prompt and more accurate identification of phytocompounds from natural products sample.

LC-NMR is the combination of chromatographic separation and structural elucidation of an unknown compound and mixture. It is the one of the most powerful and a time saving method to isolate the structures of interested molecules [81]. The current introduction of a pulsed field gradient technique in high resolution NMR, together with a three-dimensional technique enhances application in structure elucidation and molecular weight information. These new hyphenated techniques are valuable in the regions of pharmacokinetics, toxicity studies, drug metabolism and drug discovery process [82].

5.7. Structural Characterization of Purified Compounds

The isolated and purified phytocompound needs to be structurally determined to analyze the chemical properties of the compound. This process involves accumulating information from a wide range of spectroscopic techniques, including UV-visible spectroscopy, Infra-Red (IR), and NMR, which provides a certain clue regarding the structure of the isolated/purified molecule. Characteristics of the isolated phyto-compound can be analyzed by UV-visible spectroscopy and the IR spectroscopy technique has proven to be a precious tool for the characterization and identification of compounds and/or its functional groups (chemical bonds) present in an unidentified mixture of the natural products extract [83]. The identification of functional groups in a compound may be detected using IR by analyzing the different bonds present.

NMR spectroscopy is the most unswerving tool for the elucidation of molecular structures. An NMR microscope defines the number and types of nuclei in an organic molecule, describing the individual chemical environment and their interconnection. Swotting the molecule of interest with NMR spectroscopy permits the determination of differences in the magnetic properties of the various magnetic nuclei present and atoms are present in neighboring groups [84,85].

6. Natural Anti-Diabetic/Inflammatory Bioactive Compounds and Their Mechanisms of Action

The chemical substances from living organisms are identified as natural compounds. The primary sources of natural compounds are plants. Plant synthesize diverse groups of natural compounds, commonly referred to as secondary metabolites and their function in plants is now attracting attention because of their use as dyes, glues, oils, waxes, flavoring agents, drugs and perfumes, and they are noticed as potential sources of natural drugs, antibiotics, insecticides and herbicides, etc. [7,86]. Currently, the role of some secondary metabolites as protective dietary elements has become a progressively vital area in human nutrition based research. Evidence affirms that modest long-term intakes can have favorable impacts on the incidence of many chronic inflammatory associated diseases/disorders, including T2DM (Table 2) [7,87].

Based on their biosynthetic origins, plant secondary metabolites can be divided into three major groups such as (i) phenolic compounds; (ii) terpenoids and (iii) nitrogen-containing alkaloids and sulphur-containing compounds. Compared to another group of secondary metabolites, phenolic compounds are largely responsible for beneficial effects on human health [88], and these naturally occurring compounds are found largely in fruits, vegetables, cereals and beverages [89]. The content of the polyphenols in a plant is greatly affected by environmental factors like sun exposure, soil types, rainfall and stress, etc. [90,91]. Phenolics that are not soluble are found in cell walls, while soluble phenolics are present within the plant cell vacuoles (Figure 2) [92]. Phenols are classified into different groups as a function of the number of phenol rings in the structure and their main classes include phenolic acids, flavonoids, stilbenes and lignans.

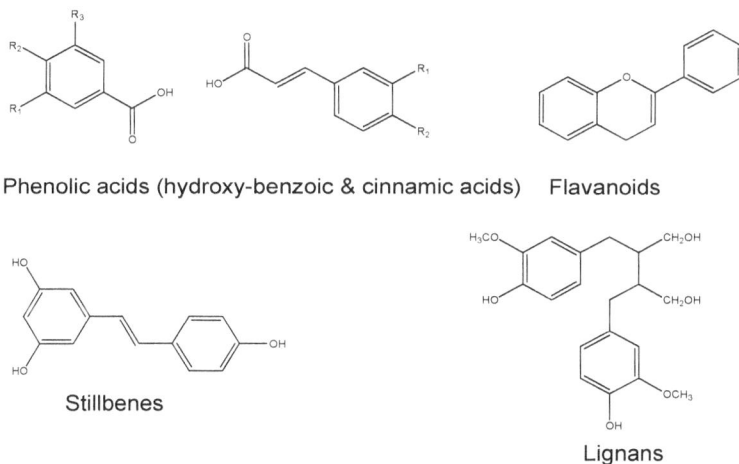

Figure 2. Chemical structures of the different classes of polyphenols.

Two classes of phenolic acids are derivatives of benzoic acid and cinnamic acid. The hydroxybenzoic acid content of edible plants is generally very low, with the exception of certain red fruits, black radishes, and onions. Because these hydroxybenzoic acids, both free and esterified, are found in only a few plants eaten by humans, they have not been extensively studied and are not currently considered to be of great nutritional interest. The hydroxycinnamic acids are more common than are the hydroxybenzoic acids and consist chiefly of *p*-coumaric, caffeic, ferulic, and sinapic acids. These acids are rarely found in the free form, except in processed food that has undergone freezing, sterilization, or fermentation [93].

Favonoids comprise the most studied group of polyphenols. Flavonoids may be divided into six subclasses: flavonols, flavones, flavanones, flavanols, anthocyanins and isoflavones based on the variation in the type of heterocycle involved. They are typically found in the form of glycosides and sometimes as acylglycosides, while acylated, methylated and sulfate molecules are less frequent and in lower concentrations. They are water-soluble and accumulate in cell vacuoles [88].

Stilbenes are a subgroup of non-flavonoid polyphenols with two phenyl moieties connected by a two-carbon methylene bridge and are found in low quantities in the human diet. One of these is resveratrol, and the protective effect of this molecule is unlikely at normal nutritional intakes [94].

Lignins fall under the subgroup of non-flavonoid polyphenols. They are diphenolic compounds that contain a 2,3-dibenzylbutane structure that is formed by the dimerization of two cinnamic acid residues. Several lignans, such as secoisolariciresinol, are the richest dietary source of linseed. They are considered to be phytoestrogens [95].

Table 2. Classification of bioactive compounds and their major plant sources with therapeutic targets for inflammation associated diabetes.

Class	Compounds	Plant Sources	Mechanism of Actions	Reference
Flavone	Apigenin	Parsley Celery Rosemary Oregano Thyme Basil Coriander Chamomile Cloves	1. Activation of ERK1/2 2. Attenuates the production of pro-inflammatory cytokines such as IL-6, IL-1β, and TNF-α	[96,97]
	Diosmin	Lemon Orange Buddha fingers	1. Deactivation of NF-κB targets 2. Suppression of monocyte chemoattractant protein-1 (MCP-1), tumor necrosis factor (TNF-α), and interleukins (IL-1β and 6)	[98]
Flavonol	Quercetin	Capers Onions Cranberries Blueberrie Chokeberris	1. Inhibition of NF-κB system 2. Reduction in serum level of both TNF-α and CRP	[99,100]
	Kaempferol	Tomatoes Green Tea Potatoes Broccoli Brussels Sprouts Squash	1. AMPK activation 2. Decrease the fasting blood glucose, and improved insulin resistance	[101,102]
	Eriodictyol	Lemons Mountain balm	1. Suppress the activation of NF-κB system 2. Reduce TNF-α, intercellular adhesion molecule 1 (ICAM-1), vascular endothelial growth factor (VEGF), and endothelial NOS (eNOS)	[103,104]

Table 2. *Cont.*

Class	Compounds	Plant Sources	Mechanism of Actions	Reference
Flavanone	Naringenin	Grapefruit oranges tomatoes	1. Activation of AMPK and suppression of NF-κB pathways 2. Increases the glucose tolerance and insulin sensitivity	[105,106]
	Hesperetin	LemonOrange Peppermint Tangerine	1. Suppress the activation of NF-κB system 2. Down-regulation of pro-inflammatory cytokines and oxidative stress markers	[107,108]
	Baicalein	ParsleyCellery Capsicum Pepper	1. Activation of AMPK pathway 2. Suppresses fatty acid synthesis, gluconeogenesis and increases the mitochondrial β-oxidation	[109–111]
	Chrysin	Skullcap Honey	1. Suppression of TNF-α production and activation of NF-κB activation 2. Reduce the serum levels of pro-inflammatory cytokines, IL-1β and IL-6	[112]
Flavanol	Catechin	Green tea Chocholate Beans Cherry	Suppress the activation of NF-κB system through the inhibiton of pro-inflammatory cytkines productions	[113,114]
	Morin	Indian guava Green tea extract Almond	1. Modulation of SphK1/S1P signaling pathway 2. Reduce the elevation of inflammatory cytokines IL-1β, IL-6 and TNF-α	[115–117]
Isoflavonoid	Genistein 4′,5,7-OH	Soy flour Soy milk Soy beans	1. Represses the release of TNF-α production 2. Inhibits the activation of ERK and P38 phosphorylation	[118]
Phenolic acid	Curcumin	*Turmeric Curry powder Mango Ginger*	1. Suppression of ICAM-1 expressions & ROS 2. Improves Vascular inflammation Inhibits MCP-1 & ICAM-1 expressions	[119,120]
	Colchicine	Saffron Colchicum	1. Mitigates inflammatory cell infiltration 2. Suppression of MCP-1 and ICAM-1 expression	[121]
Stilbene	Resveratrol	Grapes Wine Grape Peanuts Cocoa Berries	1. Suppress the activation of NF-κB signaling pathway 2. Downregulates the COX-2 gene expression which increase the release of pro-inflammatory mediators	[122,123]
	Emodin	Japanese knotweed Rhubarb Buckthorn	1. Suppress the activation of NF-κB system 2. Down-modulated the adhesion molecules including ICAM-1, and VCAM-1.	[124,125]

Diabetes has been recognized as an oxidative stress based disorder caused by an imbalance between the cellular production of reactive oxygen species and the counteracting antioxidant mechanisms by body's natural antioxidants [126]. Studies have suggested that oxidative stress are enacted in systemic inflammation, endothelial dysfunction, impaired secretion of pancreatic β-cells and glucose utilization in peripheral tissues that lead to long-term secondary complications [127]. Growing evidence from epidemiological studies suggests a positive association between reduction in the incidence diabetes and the consumption of a diet rich in phenols [128]. Several biological beneficial properties have been documented for dietary phenols including antioxidant [129], anti-allergic [130], anti-viral [131], anti-microbial [132], anti-proliferative [133], anti-carcinogenic [134], free radical scavenging [135] and regulation of cell cycle arrest [136].

Phenol-rich foods increase plasma antioxidant capacity, and this incidence may be explained by acceptance of electron from reactive oxygen species (ROS), thus forming relatively stable phenoxyl radicals (Clifford). ROS are considered to be a toxic byproduct, pose a threat to cells by causing peroxidation of lipids, oxidation of proteins, and damage to nucleic acids, enzyme inhibition, activation of a programmed cell death (PCD) pathway, and ultimately lead to death of the cells [137].

Phenols, therefore, protect cell constituents against oxidative damage and limit the risk of various degenerative diseases associated with oxidative stress. Likewise, inflammation and stress are both responsible for the pathogenesis of T2DM, suggesting the potential importance of antioxidants and anti-inflammatory alternatives [138]. The phenolic compounds with potent anti-oxidant activity are capable of exhibiting anti-inflammatory activity, with the potential to prevent DM and its complications. The current review is an attempt to provide a description of various plants' derived phenolic compounds currently used for treatment, and inhibition of inflammatory pathways that are important in diabetic prevention strategies.

Apigenin is a natural flavonoid abundantly present in common fruits and vegetables (Figure 3) [139]. Apigenin as a therapeutic agent for various inflammatory diseases inhibits TNF-α and IL-1β-induced activation of NF-κB via ERK1/2 activation. Apigenin attenuates production of pro-inflammatory cytokines such as IL-6, IL-1β, and TNF-α through modulating multiple intracellular signaling pathways in macrophages, which ameliorated hyperglycemic and improved antioxidants via oxidative stress-related signaling [97].

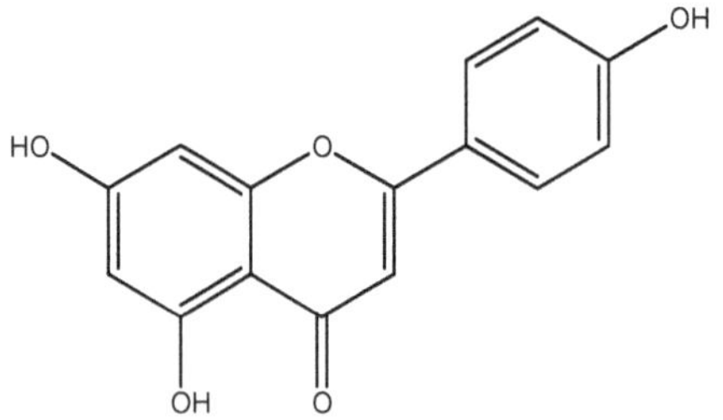

Figure 3. Chemical structure of Apigenin.

Diosmin is a naturally occurring flavonoid, abundant in the pericarp of various citrus fruits (Figure 4) [140]. Excessive production of free fatty acids (hyperglycaemia) has previously been shown to cause inflammation leading to mitochondrial DNA damage and pancreatic cell malfunctioning [141]. Antioxidant supplementation by diosmin suppressed diabetes induced ROS resulting in deactivation of NF-κB associated pro-inflammatory chemokines and cytokines such as macrophage chemotactic protein (MCP-1), tumor necrosis factor (TNF-α), and interleukins (IL-1β and 6) [98].

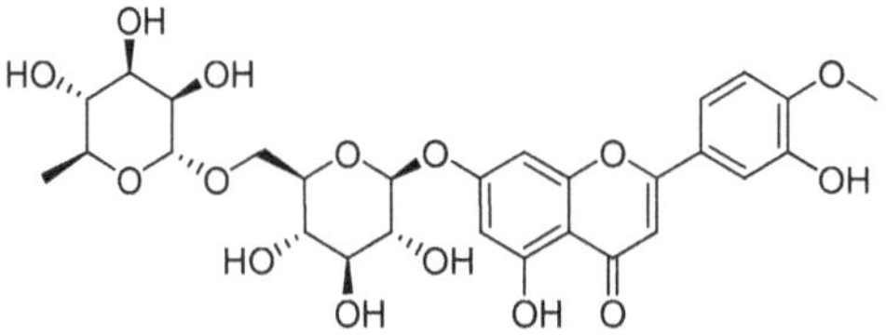

Figure 4. Chemical structure of Diosmin.

Quercetin is found in a great variety of food, including vegetables, tea, apples, grapevines, berries, broccoli, red onions and capers (Figure 5) [142]. Inflammatory mediators can activate a number of receptors, which subsequently result in pancreatic β-cell dysfunction, insulin signaling impairment, endothelial dysfunction and altered vascular flow that lead to diabetic vascular complications [143]. CRP, a marker of systemic inflammation, and markers of endothelial dysfunction have been reported in both type 1 and type 2 diabetic patients [144]. Quercetin administrations protect against diabetes-induced exaggerated vasoconstriction. These effects resulted from the reduction in serum level of both TNF-α and CRP and inhibition of aortic NF-kβ in both models of diabetes [100].

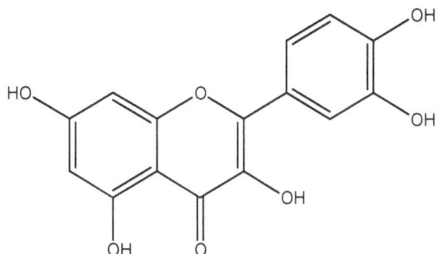

Figure 5. Chemical structure of Quercetin.

Kaempferol is a natural flavonol, relatively abundant in grapefruit, tea cruciferous vegetables and some edible berries (Figure 6) [145]. Previous findings showed that antioxidant content of Kaempferol reduced IL-1β, TNF-α [101], and kaempferol was also reported to significantly decrease the fasting blood glucose and improve insulin resistance. Anti-inflammatory and anti-diabetic effects of kaempferol are mediated by through AMPK activation [102].

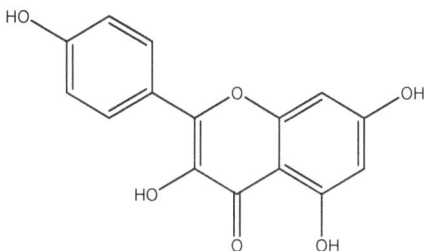

Figure 6. Chemical structure of Kaempferol.

Eriodictyol is a bitter-masking flavanone extracted from lemon, Indian beech and rose hips. Eriodictyol has been reported to possess anti-inflammatory properties, by significantly lower retinal TNF-α, intercellular adhesion molecule 1 (ICAM-1), vascular endothelial growth factor (VEGF), and endothelial NOS (eNOS) (Figure 7) [104]. Supplementation with eriodictyol suppressed diabetes with upregulation of mRNA expression of PPARγ2 and adipocyte-specific fatty acid-binding protein as well as the protein levels of PPARγ2 in differentiated 3T3-L1 adipocytes. Furthermore, eriodictyol reactivated Akt in HepG2 cells with HG-induced insulin resistance [103].

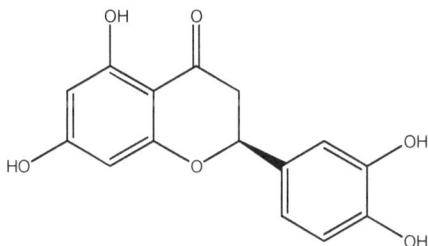

Figure 7. Chemical structure of Eriodictyol.

Naringenin is a flavonoid found in fruits including grapefruit, oranges, and tomatoes with robust antioxidant potential (Figure 8) [146]. Naringenin was also found to prevent reactivity in diabetic via upregulation of both 5′ AMPK. Stimulation of innate immunity by high blood glucose, induce inflammation and lead to type 2 diabetes [147]. Naringenin administration upregulates the activation of the AMPK pathway and then increases glucose tolerance and insulin sensitivity [106].

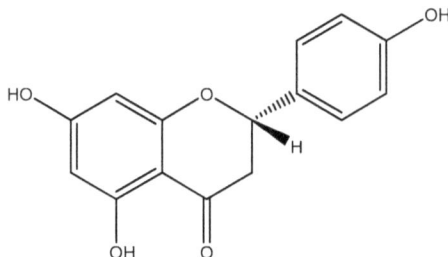

Figure 8. Chemical structure of Naringenin.

Hesperidin is a flavanone glycoside found in citrus fruits, orange, and lemon (Figure 9) [148]. Hesperidin attenuates the diabetic condition through control over hyperglycemia and hyperlipidemia by downregulation of free radical generation, and the release of pro-inflammatory cytokines. Reduced oxidative stress by hesperidin due to strong antioxidant capacity was also found to be helpful in the prevention of damage caused by oxygen free radicals of cellular organelles and its related enzymes and development of insulin resistance [108].

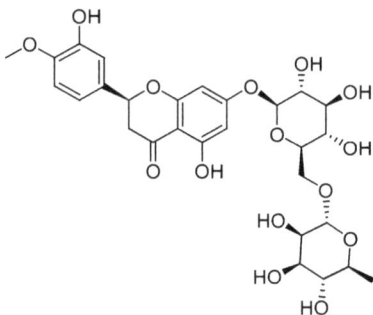

Figure 9. Chemical structure of Hesperidin.

Baicalein, a flavonoid, was originally isolated from the roots of *Scutellaria baicalensis*, *Scutellaria lateriflora* and fruits of *Oroxylum indicum* (Figure 10) [149]. Baicalein was reported to suppress the activation of NF-κB, and decrease expression of iNOS and TGF-β1, which support its anti-inflammatory property [110]. Baicalein displayed significant improvement in hyperglycemia, glucose tolerance, and insulin levels. Mechanism of its action was by upregulation of AMPK and its related signal pathway, a regulator of metabolic homeostasis involving inflammation and oxidative stress. Activated AMPK could abolish inflammation through the MAPK signaling pathway. Activated AMPK could attenuate insulin resistance by phosphorylating IRS-1, AKT and dephosphorylate ERK, JNK and NF-κB. It also suppresses fatty acid synthesis, gluconeogenesis and increases mitochondrial β-oxidation [111].

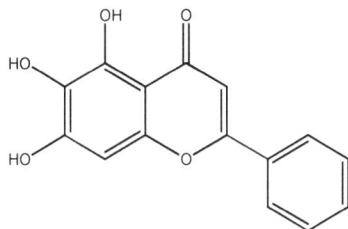

Figure 10. Chemical structure of Baicalein.

Chrysin is a naturally occurring flavonoid and is found in honey, propolis, fruits, vegetables, beverages and medicinal plants such as *Passiflora caerulea*, *Pelargonium peltatum* and *Tilia tomentosa* Moench (Figure 11) [150]. According to Ahad et al. [112], treatment with chrysin reduced the serum levels of pro-inflammatory cytokines, IL-1β and IL-6. Consequently, chrysin prevents the development of diabetes through anti-inflammatory effects, specifically targeting the TNF-α pathway.

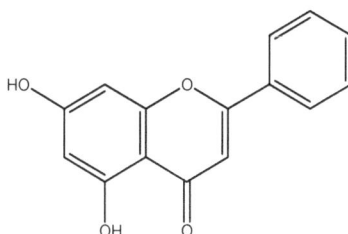

Figure 11. Chemical structure of Chrysin.

Catechin is a flavonol, and high concentrations of catechin can be found in grapes, berries, apples, dark chocolate, ginger, tea and cocoa (Figure 12) [151]. Chronic nutrient surplus and excessive energy balance activate stress in adipose tissue leading to stimulation of the innate immunity defense [152], and provoke inflammation to protect the organism against cellular damage and pathogen invasion. Chronic inflammation can aggravate diseases like obesity, type 2 diabetes, and atherosclerosis [147]. Catechin effectively suppresses the activation of NF-κB system through inhibition of the secretion of pro-inflammatory cytokines (TNF-α and IL-6), specifically into the adipose tissue [114,153,154]. The inhibitory effects of Catechin on the oxidative-inflammatory loop contribute to its therapeutic efficacies against diabetes.

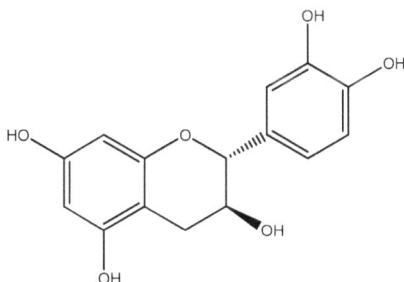

Figure 12. Catechin is a crystalline four molecule flavonoid compound ($C_{15}H_{14}O_6$).

Morin, a major active component of traditional medicinal herbs from almond, guajava (common guava) and wine (Figure 13) [155]. A study demonstrates that management of diabetes with morin reduced the elevation of inflammatory cytokines IL-1β, IL-6 and TNF-α via a SphK1/S1P signaling pathway. This activity supports its anti-inflammatory property and possible beneficial effects in diabetes [116]. Subsequently, treatment with morin expressively abridged the blood glucose, glucose metabolic enzymes and improved the production of insulin levels in the diabetes model [117].

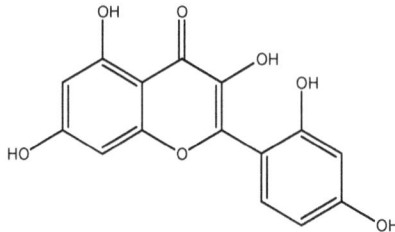

Figure 13. Chemical structure of Morin.

Genisteins are mainly isolated from soybeans and other legumes, such as chickpeas, contain small amounts of genistein (Figure 14) [156]. Diabetic retinopathy is affiliate with microglial activation and increased levels of inflammatory cytokines (TNF-α). This inflammatory signal involves the activation of tyrosine kinase and its subsequent events, ERK and p38 MAPK pathways. These effects of diabetes in retinas were reduced by intervention treatment with genistein. Genistein, a tyrosine kinase inhibitor, represses the release of TNF-α and significantly inhibits ERK and P38 phosphorylation in activated microglial cells [118,157,158].

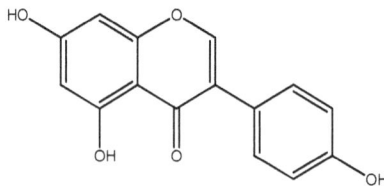

Figure 14. Chemical structure of Genistein.

Curcumin is the major active component of turmeric, and it is one of the polyphenol compounds that exhibits antioxidant, anti-inflammatory, anti-tumorigenic, and antimicrobial properties (Figure 15). Hyperglycemia-induced ROS can stimulate NF-κB activation which then causes the increase in vascular adhesion molecule expression (ICAM-1), which plays a central role in diabetic vascular inflammation [159]. Overexpression of their adhesive capability (ICAM-1) is considered as the main event in the development of atherosclerosis associated diabetes [160]. Curcumin supplementation ameliorates diabetic vascular inflammation through the decrease in ROS overproduction and ICAM-1 expressions [120].

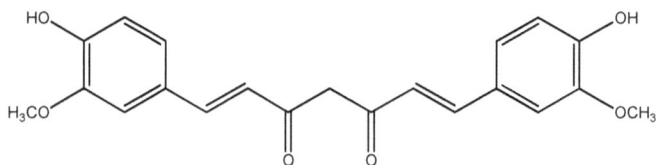

Figure 15. Chemical structure of Curcumin.

Colchicine was originally extracted from the *Colchicum autumnale* (Colchicaceae) plant and also contained in the corms of *Colchicum luteum,* and the seeds of *Gloriosa superba* (Figure 16). Colchicine is traditionally considered the staple therapy for inflammatory diseases such as gout and pericarditis [161]. Elevated infiltration of inflammatory cells in renal tubulointerstitium is commonly seen in diabetic nephropathy patients [162]. Chemokines and adhesion molecules such as monocyte chemotactic protein (MCP)-1 and intercellular adhesion molecule (ICAM-1) expression are increased in diabetes nephropathy. Colchicine supplementation mitigates inflammatory cell infiltration in diabetic nephropathy by inhibiting MCP-1 and ICAM-1 expression [121].

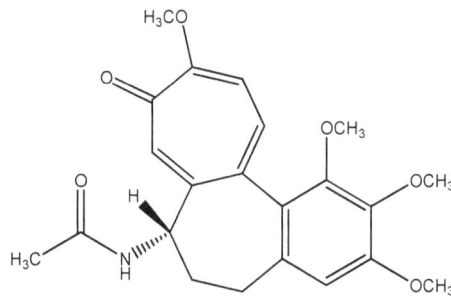

Figure 16. Chemical structure of Colchicine.

Resveratrol is a type of natural phenol compound, and a high concentration of resveratrol is found in the skin and seeds of grapes, peanuts and ground nuts (Figure 17) [161]. Diabetes is usually associated with inflammation, and an excess level of glucose is shunted via alternative pathways, which, in turn, leads to an increase in TGF-β1 and NF-κB (inflammatory mediators). Upregulation of NF-κB is convoyed by the COX-2 [163] enzyme, and it is responsible for the production of prostaglandins, inflammatory mediators produced by activated macrophages/monocytes as well as microglia in the neuroinflammatory diseases [164]. Administration of resveratrol significantly ameliorated diabetes inflammation [123] by acting as a potent scavenger of ROS, which deters lipid peroxidation, which is induced by oxidative stress [165]. In addition, resveratrol attenuates the activation of immune cells and release of pro-inflammatory mediators through the inhibition of NF-κB, followed by downregulated COX-2 gene expression in the diabetic model [123].

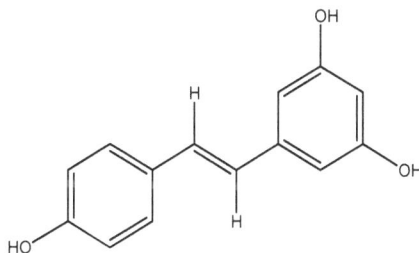

Figure 17. Chemical structure of Resveratrol.

Emodin is a major active component from *Aloe vera*, kiwi fruits, lettuce and banana. Emodin exerts anti-inflammatory effect via suppressing the activation of NF-κB in human umbilical vein endothelial cells (Figure 18) [166]. In addition, Emodin proved to have antidiabetic properties via inhibiting the degradation of IκB, an inhibitory subunit of NF-κB. When added, emodin also downmodulated adhesion molecules like ICAM-1, and VCAM-1 contains NF-κB binding sites in their promoter region in endothelial cells that could reduce the impact of type 2 diabetes [124,125].

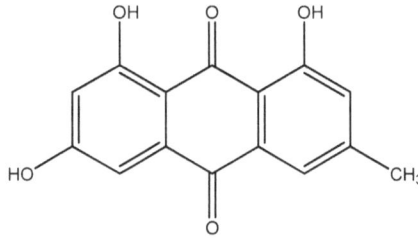

Figure 18. Chemical structure of Emodin.

7. Phytochemicals Bioavailability and Their Effect on Human Metabolism

Bioavailability is defined as substances obtained from ingested materials that reach circulatory systems for further delivery into designated tissues so that the beneficial compounds are biologically available for exerting healthy functions. The normal routes of dietary phytochemicals thus include ingestion, digestions, and transport across gastrointestinal epithelium prior to circulatory vessels. Phytochemicals are located inside vacuoles and cell walls of plant cells. Most cell wall materials are indigestible by human enzymic systems. Therefore, digestibility of the phytochemicals is of great interest or reveals how the phytochemicals can affect human health and fight or prevent diseases [167].

7.1. Digestibility of Phytochemicals

The processing factors (food texture, e.g., heat, temperature, or pressure application) can impinge on the bioaccessibility (fraction of a compound that is released from the matrix and potentially available for further uptake and absorption) of bioactivity [168]. The elimination of a natural barrier of the cell wall yields a better release of phytocompounds. For example, more phenolic is obtained from tomato juice than those from dried and fresh tomato, indicating that the natural barrier of the cell wall has been eliminated. In contrast, chlorogenic acid is present in fresh products, but it gradually disappears in juice. This could be caused by the different extractability due to different matrices of the products or by chemical changes due to processing and digestion environments [169].

Compounds that are free from cell wall materials show clearer responses during gastrointestinal digestion. Phenolic stability is strongly affected by pH. For example, flavonols and proanthocyanidins remain intact, but they may also be broken down when pH is sufficiently low in the stomach. pH higher than 7.4 is unfavorable for phenolics, and the effects of high pH are worsened by lengthy exposures. This results from oxidation further into diketones and other degradation products. The number of –OH groups in benzene rings of simple phenolics can also be critical clues for phenolic stability [170].

7.2. Absorption of Phytochemicals

Most absorptive tissues are comprised of epithelial cells that protect the human body from hazardous components in ingested foods. There is no well-established molecular form of absorbed substances in the gastrointestinal tract, i.e., whether they are absorbed intact or as metabolites. The influence of enzyme concentrations, solubility, pH, and time of digestion all play a role and influence bioaccessibility and absorption [171].

For example, the release of carotenoids increases significantly in intestinal digestion where bile extract and pancreatic secretions exist. Consecutive gastrointestinal digestions do not help with higher release of carotenoids. This is more likely due to insufficient emulsifier–water ratios to provide emulsification of carotenoids that are fat-soluble [172].

7.3. Bioavailability of Phytochemicals

Phytochemicals bioavailability is strongly dependent on cell wall compositions of the food matrices they originate from, the structural chemistry of the phytochemicals, history of processing, and the individual human gastrointestinal system. This factor greatly alters the structure and profile and thus the potential bioactivity of many plant compounds that are not absorbed in the small intestine. These complexities determine the dietary phytochemicals plan that should be recommended in order to reach biologically-safe active dosages [173].

8. Conclusions

Inflammation emerges to contribute to the pathogenesis of T2DM and its secondary complications, particularly in cardiovascular disease. Various researchers have investigated the underlying mechanisms that initiate inflammation and link it to insulin resistance and associated complications. These investigations may provide new opportunities for treating type 2 diabetic patients and its complications. Most of the anti-diabetic drugs have the ability to control the glucose level and improve insulin secretion through anti-inflammatory mechanisms, but they have few undesirable effects based on the preclinical and clinical investigations. The current investigations have suggested that natural products derived bioactive compounds act as a therapeutic tool in chronic inflammatory diseases. Mostly, polyphenols appear to be significant metabolic modulators by virtue of their capability to influence various cellular and molecular pathway targets, which have been proven as potential targets for the polyphenolic group of compounds. Nevertheless, clinical use of natural products based active compounds has not yet been investigated properly through intracellular signaling pathways. Further research will be needed to fully explain the cellular and molecular mechanisms of actions of natural products' derived compounds and their analogues in several physiological processes, in order to yield essential insights into their prophylactic and therapeutic uses.

Acknowledgments: The manuscript was supported by a grant (Project No.: GP-1/2014/9443700) from the Research Management Center, Universiti Putra Malaysia (UPM), Malaysia.

Author Contributions: S.G., P.G. and P.A. collected the literature review and drafted the manuscript; S.-Y.P. revised the manuscript; S.F., D.-K.C. and P.A. critically reviewed and revised the manuscript.

Conflicts of Interest: The authors declare no conflict of interest.

References

1. Wu, Y.; Ding, Y.; Tanaka, Y.; Zhang, W. Risk Factors Contributing to Type 2 Diabetes and Recent Advances in the Treatment and Prevention. *Int. J. Med. Sci.* **2014**, *11*, 1185–1200. [CrossRef] [PubMed]
2. Jung, U.; Choi, M.-S. Obesity and its metabolic complications: The role of adipokines and the relationship between obesity, inflammation, insulin resistance, dyslipidemia and nonalcoholic fatty liver disease. *Int. J. Mol. Sci.* **2014**, *15*, 6184–6223. [CrossRef] [PubMed]
3. Das, A.; Mukhopadhyay, S. The evil axis of obesity, inflammation and type-2 diabetes. *Endocr. Metab. Immune Disord. Drug Targets* **2011**, *11*, 23–31. [CrossRef] [PubMed]
4. Donath, M.Y.; Shoelson, S.E. Type 2 diabetes as an inflammatory disease. *Nat. Rev. Immunol.* **2011**, *11*, 98–107. [CrossRef] [PubMed]
5. Mohammed, S.; Yaqub, A.; Nicholas, A.; Arastus, W.; Muhammad, M.; Abdullahi, S. Review on diabetes, synthetic drugs and glycemic effects of medicinal plants. *J. Med. Plants Res.* **2013**, *7*, 2628–2637.
6. Patel, D.; Prasad, S.; Kumar, R.; Hemalatha, S. An overview on antidiabetic medicinal plants having insulin mimetic property. *Asian Pac. J. Trop. Biomed.* **2012**, *2*, 320–330. [CrossRef]
7. Arulselvan, P.; Ghofar, H.A.A.; Karthivashan, G.; Halim, M.F.A.; Ghafar, M.S.A.; Fakurazi, S. Antidiabetic therapeutics from natural source: A systematic review. *Biomed. Prev. Nutr.* **2014**, *4*, 607–617. [CrossRef]
8. Wang, X.; Bao, W.; Liu, J.; Ouyang, Y.Y.; Wang, D.; Rong, S.; Xiao, X.; Shan, Z.L.; Zhang, Y.; Yao, P.; et al. Inflammatory markers and risk of type 2 diabetes: A systematic review and meta-analysis. *Diabetes Care* **2013**, *36*, 166–175. [CrossRef] [PubMed]
9. Goldfine, A.B.; Fonseca, V.; Jablonski, K.A.; Pyle, L.; Staten, M.A.; Shoelson, S.E. The effects of salsalate on glycemic control in patients with type 2 diabetes: A randomized trial. *Ann. Intern. Med.* **2010**, *152*, 346–357. [CrossRef] [PubMed]

10. Spranger, J.; Kroke, A.; Möhlig, M.; Hoffmann, K.; Bergmann, M.M.; Ristow, M.; Boeing, H.; Pfeiffer, A.F. Inflammatory cytokines and the risk to develop type 2 diabetes results of the prospective population-based european prospective investigation into cancer and nutrition (epic)-potsdam study. *Diabetes* **2003**, *52*, 812–817. [CrossRef] [PubMed]

11. Forbes, J.M.; Cooper, M.E. Mechanisms of diabetic complications. *Physiol. Rev.* **2013**, *93*, 137–188. [CrossRef] [PubMed]

12. Chiquette, E.; Chilton, R. Cardiovascular disease: Much more aggressive in patients with type 2 diabetes. *Curr. Atheroscler. Rep.* **2002**, *4*, 134–142. [CrossRef] [PubMed]

13. Deshmane, S.L.; Kremlev, S.; Amini, S.; Sawaya, B.E. Monocyte chemoattractant protein-1 (MCP-1): An overview. *J. Interferon Cytokine Res.* **2009**, *29*, 313–326. [CrossRef] [PubMed]

14. Karamifar, H.; Habibian, N.; Amirhakimi, G.; Karamizadeh, Z.; Alipour, A. Adiponectin is a good marker for metabolic state among type 1 diabetes mellitus patients. *Iran. J. Pediatr.* **2013**, *23*, 295–301. [PubMed]

15. Mogensen, T.H. Pathogen recognition and inflammatory signaling in innate immune defenses. *Clin. Microbiol. Rev.* **2009**, *22*, 240–273. [CrossRef] [PubMed]

16. Piccinini, A.; Midwood, K. Dampening inflammation by modulating TLR signalling. *Mediat. Inflamm.* **2010**, *2010*. [CrossRef] [PubMed]

17. Kim, J.; Sohn, E.; Kim, C.-S.; Jo, K.; Kim, J.S. The role of high-mobility group box-1 protein in the development of diabetic nephropathy. *Am. J. Nephrol.* **2011**, *33*, 524–529. [CrossRef] [PubMed]

18. Chen, Y.; Qiao, F.; Zhao, Y.; Wang, Y.; Liu, G. HMGB1 is activated in type 2 diabetes mellitus patients and in mesangial cells in response to high glucose. *Int. J. Clin. Exp. Pathol.* **2015**, *8*, 6683. [PubMed]

19. Vlassara, H.; Uribarri, J. Advanced glycation end products (AGE) and diabetes: Cause, effect, or both? *Curr. Diabetes Rep.* **2014**, *14*, 1–10. [CrossRef] [PubMed]

20. Chawla, A.; Nguyen, K.D.; Goh, Y.P. Macrophage-mediated inflammation in metabolic disease. *Nat. Rev. Immunol.* **2011**, *11*, 738–749. [CrossRef] [PubMed]

21. Chen, L.; Chen, R.; Wang, H.; Liang, F. Mechanisms linking inflammation to insulin resistance. *Int. J. Endocrinol.* **2015**, *2015*, 508409. [CrossRef] [PubMed]

22. Baker, R.G.; Hayden, M.S.; Ghosh, S. Nf-κb, inflammation, and metabolic disease. *Cell Metab.* **2011**, *13*, 11–22. [CrossRef] [PubMed]

23. Chinetti-Gbaguidi, G.; Staels, B. Macrophage polarization in metabolic disorders: Functions and regulation. *Curr. Opin. Lipidol.* **2011**, *22*, 365–372. [CrossRef] [PubMed]

24. McArdle, M.A.; Finucane, O.M.; Connaughton, R.M.; McMorrow, A.M.; Roche, H.M. Mechanisms of obesity-induced inflammation and insulin resistance: Insights into the emerging role of nutritional strategies. *Front. Endocrinol.* **2013**, *4*, 52. [CrossRef] [PubMed]

25. Cancello, R.; Henegar, C.; Viguerie, N.; Taleb, S.; Poitou, C.; Rouault, C.; Coupaye, M.; Pelloux, V.; Hugol, D.; Bouillot, J.L.; et al. Reduction of macrophage infiltration and chemoattractant gene expression changes in white adipose tissue of morbidly obese subjects after surgery-induced weight loss. *Diabetes* **2005**, *54*, 2277–2286. [CrossRef] [PubMed]

26. Badawi, A.; Klip, A.; Haddad, P.; Cole, D.E.; Bailo, B.G.; El-Sohemy, A.; Karmali, M. Type 2 diabetes mellitus and inflammation: Prospects for biomarkers of risk and nutritional intervention. *Diabetes Metab. Syndr. Obes.* **2010**, *3*, 173–186. [CrossRef] [PubMed]

27. Rendell, M. The role of sulphonylureas in the management of type 2 diabetes mellitus. *Drugs* **2004**, *64*, 1339–1358. [CrossRef] [PubMed]

28. Krentz, A.J.; Bailey, C.J. Oral antidiabetic agents: Current role in type 2 diabetes mellitus. *Drugs* **2005**, *65*, 385–411. [CrossRef] [PubMed]

29. Shoelson, S.E.; Lee, J.; Yuan, M. Inflammation and the ikk beta/i kappa b/nf-kappa b axis in obesity- and diet-induced insulin resistance. *Int. J. Obes. Relat. Metab. Disord.* **2003**, *27* (Suppl. S3), S49–S52. [CrossRef] [PubMed]

30. Hundal, R.S.; Petersen, K.F.; Mayerson, A.B.; Randhawa, P.S.; Inzucchi, S.; Shoelson, S.E.; Shulman, G.I. Mechanism by which high-dose aspirin improves glucose metabolism in type 2 diabetes. *J. Clin. Investig.* **2002**, *109*, 1321–1326. [CrossRef] [PubMed]

31. Hotamisligil, G.S. Inflammation and metabolic disorders. *Nature* **2006**, *444*, 860–867. [CrossRef] [PubMed]

32. Wilcox, G. Insulin and insulin resistance. *Clin. Biochem. Rev.* **2005**, *26*, 19. [PubMed]

33. Atanasov, A.G.; Waltenberger, B.; Pferschy-Wenzig, E.-M.; Linder, T.; Wawrosch, C.; Uhrin, P.; Temml, V.; Wang, L.; Schwaiger, S.; Heiss, E.H. Discovery and resupply of pharmacologically active plant-derived natural products: A review. *Biotechnol. Adv.* **2015**, *33*, 1582–1614. [CrossRef] [PubMed]

34. Chang, C.L.; Lin, Y.; Bartolome, A.P.; Chen, Y.-C.; Chiu, S.-C.; Yang, W.-C. Herbal therapies for type 2 diabetes mellitus: Chemistry, biology, and potential application of selected plants and compounds. *Evid. Based Complement. Alternat. Med.* **2013**, *2013*, 378657. [CrossRef] [PubMed]

35. Patwardhan, B.; Vaidya, A.D.; Chorghade, M. Ayurveda and natural products drug discovery. *Curr. Sci.* **2004**, *86*, 789–799.

36. Coman, C.; Rugina, O.D.; Socaciu, C. Plants and natural compounds with antidiabetic action. *Not. Bot. Horti Agrobot. Cluj-Napoca* **2012**, *40*, 314.

37. Zhang, Z.; Luo, A.; Zhong, K.; Huang, Y.; Gao, Y.; Zhang, J.; Gao, H.; Xu, Z.; Gao, X. A-glucosidase inhibitory activity by the flower buds of *Lonicera japonica* Thunb. *J. Funct. Foods* **2013**, *5*, 1253–1259. [CrossRef]

38. Takahashi, T.; Miyazawa, M. Potent α-glucosidase inhibitors from safflower (*Carthamus tinctorius* L.) seed. *Phytother. Res.* **2012**, *26*, 722–726. [CrossRef] [PubMed]

39. Kim, W.; Egan, J.M. The role of incretins in glucose homeostasis and diabetes treatment. *Pharmacol. Rev.* **2008**, *60*, 470–512. [CrossRef] [PubMed]

40. Kim, S.; Jwa, H.; Yanagawa, Y.; Park, T. Extract from *Dioscorea batatas* ameliorates insulin resistance in mice fed a high-fat diet. *J. Med. Food* **2012**, *15*, 527–534. [CrossRef] [PubMed]

41. Grace, M.H.; Ribnicky, D.M.; Kuhn, P.; Poulev, A.; Logendra, S.; Yousef, G.G.; Raskin, I.; Lila, M.A. Hypoglycemic activity of a novel anthocyanin-rich formulation from lowbush blueberry, vaccinium angustifolium aiton. *Phytomedicine* **2009**, *16*, 406–415. [CrossRef] [PubMed]

42. Park, S.; Kim, D.S.; Kang, S. Gastrodia elata blume water extracts improve insulin resistance by decreasing body fat in diet-induced obese rats: Vanillin and 4-hydroxybenzaldehyde are the bioactive candidates. *Eur. J. Nutr.* **2011**, *50*, 107–118. [CrossRef] [PubMed]

43. Kho, M.C.; Lee, Y.J.; Cha, J.D.; Choi, K.M.; Kang, D.G.; Lee, H.S. *Gastrodia elata* ameliorates high-fructose diet-induced lipid metabolism and endothelial dysfunction. *Evid. Based Complement. Alternat. Med.* **2014**, *2014*, 101624. [CrossRef] [PubMed]

44. Sen, S.; Chen, S.; Feng, B.; Wu, Y.; Lui, E.; Chakrabarti, S. Preventive effects of north American ginseng (*Panax quinquefolium*) on diabetic nephropathy. *Phytomedicine* **2012**, *19*, 494–505. [CrossRef] [PubMed]

45. Islam, M.; Choi, H. Dietary red chilli (*Capsicum frutescens* L.) is insulinotropic rather than hypoglycemic in type 2 diabetes model of rats. *Phytother. Res.* **2008**, *22*, 1025–1029. [CrossRef] [PubMed]

46. Madkor, H.R.; Mansour, S.W.; Ramadan, G. Modulatory effects of garlic, ginger, turmeric and their mixture on hyperglycaemia, dyslipidaemia and oxidative stress in streptozotocin–nicotinamide diabetic rats. *Br. J. Nutr.* **2011**, *105*, 1210–1217. [CrossRef] [PubMed]

47. Kumar, G.S.; Shetty, A.; Sambaiah, K.; Salimath, P. Antidiabetic property of fenugreek seed mucilage and spent turmeric in streptozotocin-induced diabetic rats. *Nutr. Res.* **2005**, *25*, 1021–1028. [CrossRef]

48. Haidari, F.; Omidian, K.; Rafiei, H.; Zarei, M.; Mohamad Shahi, M. Green tea (*Camellia sinensis*) supplementation to diabetic rats improves serum and hepatic oxidative stress markers. *Iran. J. Pharm. Res.* **2013**, *12*, 109–114. [PubMed]

49. Aybar, M.J.; Riera, A.N.S.; Grau, A.; Sanchez, S.S. Hypoglycemic effect of the water extract of *Smallantus sonchifolius* (yacon) leaves in normal and diabetic rats. *J. Ethnopharmacol.* **2001**, *74*, 125–132. [CrossRef]

50. Abascal, K.; Ganora, L.; Yarnell, E. The effect of freeze-drying and its implications for botanical medicine: A review. *Phytother. Res.* **2005**, *19*, 655–660. [CrossRef] [PubMed]

51. Asami, D.K.; Hong, Y.-J.; Barrett, D.M.; Mitchell, A.E. Comparison of the total phenolic and ascorbic acid content of freeze-dried and air-dried marionberry, strawberry, and corn grown using conventional, organic, and sustainable agricultural practices. *J. Agric. Food Chem.* **2003**, *51*, 1237–1241. [CrossRef] [PubMed]

52. Xu, B.; Chang, S. A comparative study on phenolic profiles and antioxidant activities of legumes as affected by extraction solvents. *J. Food Sci.* **2007**, *72*, S159–S166. [CrossRef] [PubMed]

53. Dai, J.; Mumper, R.J. Plant phenolics: Extraction, analysis and their antioxidant and anticancer properties. *Molecules* **2010**, *15*, 7313–7352. [CrossRef] [PubMed]

54. Joana Gil-Chávez, G.; Villa, J.A.; Fernando Ayala-Zavala, J.; Basilio Heredia, J.; Sepulveda, D.; Yahia, E.M.; González-Aguilar, G.A. Technologies for extraction and production of bioactive compounds to be used as nutraceuticals and food ingredients: An overview. *Compr. Rev. Food Sci. Food Saf.* **2013**, *12*, 5–23. [CrossRef]

55. Robards, K. Strategies for the determination of bioactive phenols in plants, fruit and vegetables. *J. Chromatogr. A* **2003**, *1000*, 657–691. [CrossRef]
56. Liu, C.-W.; Wang, Y.-C.; Lu, H.-C.; Chiang, W.-D. Optimization of ultrasound-assisted extraction conditions for total phenols with anti-hyperglycemic activity from *Psidium guajava* leaves. *Process Biochem.* **2014**, *49*, 1601–1605. [CrossRef]
57. Ştefănuţ, M.N.; Căta, A.; Pop, R.; Tănasie, C.; Boc, D.; Ienaşcu, I.; Ordodi, V. Anti-hyperglycemic effect of bilberry, blackberry and mulberry ultrasonic extracts on diabetic rats. *Plant Foods Hum. Nutr.* **2013**, *68*, 378–384. [CrossRef] [PubMed]
58. Chen, C.; You, L.-J.; Abbasi, A.M.; Fu, X.; Liu, R.H. Optimization for ultrasound extraction of polysaccharides from mulberry fruits with antioxidant and hyperglycemic activity in vitro. *Carbohydr. Polym.* **2015**, *130*, 122–132. [CrossRef] [PubMed]
59. Devgan, M.; Nanda, A.; Ansari, S.H. Comparative evaluation of the anti-diabetic activity of *Pterocarpus marsupium* Roxb. Heartwood in alloxan induced diabetic rats using extracts obtained by optimized conventional and non conventional extraction methods. *Pak. J. Pharm. Sci.* **2013**, *26*, 973–976. [PubMed]
60. Spigno, G.; De Faveri, D. Microwave-assisted extraction of tea phenols: A phenomenological study. *J. Food Eng.* **2009**, *93*, 210–217. [CrossRef]
61. Rojas, R.; Contreras-Esquivel, J.C.; Orozco-Esquivel, M.T.; Muñoz, C.; Aguirre-Joya, J.A.; Aguilar, C.N. Mango peel as source of antioxidants and pectin: Microwave assisted extraction. *Waste Biomass Valorization* **2015**, *6*, 1095–1102. [CrossRef]
62. Rahath Kubra, I.; Kumar, D.; Rao, L.J.M. Effect of microwave-assisted extraction on the release of polyphenols from ginger (*Zingiber officinale*). *Int. J. Food Sci. Technol.* **2013**, *48*, 1828–1833. [CrossRef]
63. Policegoudra, R.; Aradhya, S.; Singh, L. Mango ginger (*Curcuma amada* Roxb.)—A promising spice for phytochemicals and biological activities. *J. Biosci.* **2011**, *36*, 739–748. [CrossRef] [PubMed]
64. Maran, J.P.; Swathi, K.; Jeevitha, P.; Jayalakshmi, J.; Ashvini, G. Microwave-assisted extraction of pectic polysaccharide from waste mango peel. *Carbohydr. Polym.* **2015**, *123*, 67–71. [CrossRef] [PubMed]
65. Pandit, S.G.; Vijayanand, P.; Kulkarni, S. Pectic principles of mango peel from mango processing waste as influenced by microwave energy. *LWT Food Sci. Technol.* **2015**, *64*, 1010–1014. [CrossRef]
66. Yunus, S.; Zaki, M.; Asyikin, N.; Ku Hamid, K.H. Microwave Drying Characteristics and Antidiabetic Properties of *Aquilaria subintegra* and *Aquilaria malaccensis* Leaves. *Adv. Mater. Res.* **2015**, *1113*, 352–357. [CrossRef]
67. Zou, T.; Wu, H.; Li, H.; Jia, Q.; Song, G. Comparison of microwave-assisted and conventional extraction of mangiferin from mango (*Mangifera indica* L.) leaves. *J. Sep. Sci.* **2013**, *36*, 3457–3462. [PubMed]
68. Salomon, S.; Sevilla, I.; Betancourt, R.; Romero, A.; Nuevas-Paz, L.; Acosta-Esquijarosa, J. Extraction of mangiferin from *Mangifera indica* L. Leaves using microwave-assisted technique. *Emir. J. Food Agric.* **2014**, *26*, 616. [CrossRef]
69. Veggi, P.C.; Cavalcanti, R.N.; Meireles, M.A.A. Production of phenolic-rich extracts from Brazilian plants using supercritical and subcritical fluid extraction: Experimental data and economic evaluation. *J. Food Eng.* **2014**, *131*, 96–109. [CrossRef]
70. Herrero, M.; del Pilar Sánchez-Camargo, A.; Cifuentes, A.; Ibáñez, E. Plants, seaweeds, microalgae and food by-products as natural sources of functional ingredients obtained using pressurized liquid extraction and supercritical fluid extraction. *TrAC Trends Anal. Chem.* **2015**, *71*, 26–38. [CrossRef]
71. Liau, B.-C.; Shen, C.-T.; Liang, F.-P.; Hong, S.-E.; Hsu, S.-L.; Jong, T.-T.; Chang, C.-M.J. Supercritical fluids extraction and anti-solvent purification of carotenoids from microalgae and associated bioactivity. *J. Supercrit. Fluids* **2010**, *55*, 169–175. [CrossRef]
72. Hsieh, T.-J.; Tsai, Y.-H.; Liao, M.-C.; Du, Y.-C.; Lien, P.-J.; Sun, C.-C.; Chang, F.-R.; Wu, Y.-C. Anti-diabetic properties of non-polar *Toona sinensis* roem extract prepared by supercritical-co 2 fluid. *Food Chem. Toxicol.* **2012**, *50*, 779–789. [CrossRef] [PubMed]
73. Silva, G.; Gamarra, F.; Oliveira, A.; Cabral, F. Extraction of bixin from annatto seeds using supercritical carbon dioxide. *Braz. J. Chem. Eng.* **2008**, *25*, 419–426. [CrossRef]
74. Sasidharan, S.; Chen, Y.; Saravanan, D.; Sundram, K.; Latha, L.Y. Extraction, isolation and characterization of bioactive compounds from plants' extracts. *Afr. J. Tradit. Complement. Altern. Med.* **2011**, *8*, 1–10. [CrossRef] [PubMed]

75. Queiroz, E.F.; Ioset, J.R.; Ndjoko, K.; Guntern, A.; Foggin, C.M.; Hostettmann, K. On-line identification of the bioactive compounds from *Blumea gariepina* by HPLC-UV-MS and HPLC-UV-NMR, combined with HPLC-micro-fractionation. *Phytochem. Anal.* **2005**, *16*, 166–174. [CrossRef] [PubMed]

76. Ek, S.; Kartimo, H.; Mattila, S.; Tolonen, A. Characterization of phenolic compounds from Lingonberry (*Vaccinium vitis-idaea*). *J. Agric. Food Chem.* **2006**, *54*, 9834–9842. [CrossRef] [PubMed]

77. Kingston, D.G. Modern natural products drug discovery and its relevance to biodiversity conservation. *J. Nat. Prod.* **2010**, *74*, 496–511. [CrossRef] [PubMed]

78. Bucar, F.; Wube, A.; Schmid, M. Natural product isolation—How to get from biological material to pure compounds. *Nat. Prod. Rep.* **2013**, *30*, 525–545. [CrossRef] [PubMed]

79. Tsao, R.; Deng, Z. Separation procedures for naturally occurring antioxidant phytochemicals. *J. Chromatogr. B* **2004**, *812*, 85–99. [CrossRef]

80. Cai, Z.; Lee, F.S.; Wang, X.R.; Yu, W.J. A capsule review of recent studies on the application of mass spectrometry in the analysis of Chinese medicinal herbs. *J. Mass Spectrom.* **2002**, *37*, 1013–1024. [CrossRef] [PubMed]

81. Daffre, S.; Bulet, P.; Spisni, A.; Ehret-Sabatier, L.; Rodrigues, E.G.; Travassos, L.R. Bioactive natural peptides. *Stud. Nat. Prod. Chem.* **2008**, *35*, 597–691.

82. Bobzin, S.C.; Yang, S.; Kasten, T.P. Application of liquid chromatography–nuclear magnetic resonance spectroscopy to the identification of natural products. *J. Chromatogr. B* **2000**, *748*, 259–267. [CrossRef]

83. Koehn, F.E.; Carter, G.T. The evolving role of natural products in drug discovery. *Nat. Rev. Drug Discov.* **2005**, *4*, 206–220. [CrossRef] [PubMed]

84. Thitilertdecha, N.; Teerawutgulrag, A.; Kilburn, J.D.; Rakariyatham, N. Identification of major phenolic compounds from *Nephelium lappaceum* L. And their antioxidant activities. *Molecules* **2010**, *15*, 1453–1465. [PubMed]

85. Bouallagui, Z.; Bouaziz, M.; Han, J.; Boukhris, M.; Rigane, G.; Friha, I.; Jemai, H.; Ghorbel, H.; Isoda, H.; Sayadi, S. Valorization of olive processing by-products-characterization, investigation of chemico-biological activities and identification on active compounds. *J. Arid Land Stud.* **2012**, 22–21.

86. Dewick, P.M. *Medicinal Natural Products: A Biosynthetic Approach*; John Wiley & Sons: New York, NY, USA, 2002.

87. Roglic, G.; Unwin, N.; Bennett, P.H.; Mathers, C.; Tuomilehto, J.; Nag, S.; Connolly, V.; King, H. The burden of mortality attributable to diabetes realistic estimates for the year 2000. *Diabetes Care* **2005**, *28*, 2130–2135. [CrossRef] [PubMed]

88. Pandey, K.B.; Rizvi, S.I. Plant polyphenols as dietary antioxidants in human health and disease. *Oxid. Med. Cell. Longev.* **2009**, *2*, 270–278. [CrossRef] [PubMed]

89. Scalbert, A.; Manach, C.; Morand, C.; Rémésy, C.; Jiménez, L. Dietary polyphenols and the prevention of diseases. *Crit. Rev. Food Sci. Nutr.* **2005**, *45*, 287–306. [CrossRef] [PubMed]

90. Manach, C.; Scalbert, A.; Morand, C.; Rémésy, C.; Jiménez, L. Polyphenols: Food sources and bioavailability. *Am. J. Clin. Nutr.* **2004**, *79*, 727–747. [PubMed]

91. Parr, A.J.; Bolwell, G.P. Phenols in the plant and in man. The potential for possible nutritional enhancement of the diet by modifying the phenols content or profile. *J. Sci. Food Agric.* **2000**, *80*, 985–1012. [CrossRef]

92. Wink, M. Compartmentation of secondary metabolites and xenobiotics in plant vacuoles. *Adv. Bot. Res.* **1997**, *25*, 141–170.

93. Clifford, M.; Scalbert, A. Ellagitannins, occurrence in food, bioavailability and cancer prevention. *J. Food Sci. Agric.* **2000**, *80*, 1118–1125. [CrossRef]

94. Vitrac, X.; Monti, J.-P.; Vercauteren, J.; Deffieux, G.; Mérillon, J.-M. Direct liquid chromatographic analysis of resveratrol derivatives and flavanonols in wines with absorbance and fluorescence detection. *Anal. Chim. Acta* **2002**, *458*, 103–110. [CrossRef]

95. Adlercreutz, H.; Mazur, W. Phyto-oestrogens and western diseases. *Ann. Med.* **1997**, *29*, 95–120. [CrossRef] [PubMed]

96. Ohno, M.; Shibata, C.; Kishikawa, T.; Yoshikawa, T.; Takata, A.; Kojima, K.; Akanuma, M.; Kang, Y.J.; Yoshida, H.; Otsuka, M. The flavonoid apigenin improves glucose tolerance through inhibition of microRNA maturation in miRNA103 transgenic mice. *Sci. Rep.* **2013**. [CrossRef] [PubMed]

97. Zhang, X.; Wang, G.; Gurley, E.C.; Zhou, H. Flavonoid apigenin inhibits lipopolysaccharide-induced inflammatory response through multiple mechanisms in macrophages. *PLoS ONE* **2014**, *9*, e107072. [CrossRef] [PubMed]

98. Jain, D.; Bansal, M.K.; Dalvi, R.; Upganlawar, A.; Somani, R. Protective effect of diosmin against diabetic neuropathy in experimental rats. *J. Integr. Med.* **2014**, *12*, 35–41. [CrossRef]

99. Mahmoud, M.F.; Hassan, N.A.; El Bassossy, H.M.; Fahmy, A. Quercetin protects against diabetes-induced exaggerated vasoconstriction in rats: Effect on low grade inflammation. *PLoS ONE* **2013**, *8*, e63784.

100. Nair, M.P.; Mahajan, S.; Reynolds, J.L.; Aalinkeel, R.; Nair, H.; Schwartz, S.A.; Kandaswami, C. The flavonoid quercetin inhibits proinflammatory cytokine (tumor necrosis factor α) gene expression in normal peripheral blood mononuclear cells via modulation of the NF-$\kappa\beta$ system. *Clin. Vaccine Immunol.* **2006**, *13*, 319–328. [PubMed]

101. Abo-Salem, O.M. Kaempferol attenuates the development of diabetic neuropathic pain in mice: Possible anti-inflammatory and anti-oxidant mechanisms. *Maced. J. Med. Sci.* **2014**, *7*, 424–430. [CrossRef]

102. Zang, Y.; Zhang, L.; Igarashi, K.; Yu, C. The anti-obesity and anti-diabetic effects of kaempferol glycosides from unripe soybean leaves in high-fat-diet mice. *Food Funct.* **2015**, *6*, 834–841. [CrossRef] [PubMed]

103. Zhang, W.-Y.; Lee, J.-J.; Kim, Y.; Kim, I.-S.; Han, J.-H.; Lee, S.-G.; Ahn, M.-J.; Jung, S.-H.; Myung, C.-S. Effect of eriodictyol on glucose uptake and insulin resistance in vitro. *J. Agric. Food Chem.* **2012**, *60*, 7652–7658. [CrossRef] [PubMed]

104. Bucolo, C.; Leggio, G.M.; Drago, F.; Salomone, S. Eriodictyol prevents early retinal and plasma abnormalities in streptozotocin-induced diabetic rats. *Biochem. Pharmacol.* **2012**, *84*, 88–92. [CrossRef] [PubMed]

105. Tsai, S.-J.; Huang, C.-S.; Mong, M.-C.; Kam, W.-Y.; Huang, H.-Y.; Yin, M.-C. Anti-inflammatory and antifibrotic effects of naringenin in diabetic mice. *J. Agric. Food Chem.* **2011**, *60*, 514–521. [CrossRef] [PubMed]

106. Choi, J.S.; Yokozawa, T.; Oura, H. Improvement of hyperglycemia and hyperlipemia in streptozotocin-diabetic rats by a methanolic extract of *Prunus davidiana* stems and its main component, prunin. *Planta Med.* **1991**, *57*, 208–211. [CrossRef] [PubMed]

107. Kumar, B.; Gupta, S.K.; Srinivasan, B.; Nag, T.C.; Srivastava, S.; Saxena, R.; Jha, K.A. Hesperetin rescues retinal oxidative stress, neuroinflammation and apoptosis in diabetic rats. *Microvasc. Res.* **2013**, *87*, 65–74. [CrossRef] [PubMed]

108. Akiyama, S.; Katsumata, S.; Suzuki, K.; Ishimi, Y.; Wu, J.; Uehara, M. Dietary hesperidin exerts hypoglycemic and hypolipidemic effects in streptozotocin-induced marginal type 1 diabetic rats. *J. Clin. Biochem. Nutr.* **2010**, *46*, 87–92. [CrossRef] [PubMed]

109. Yang, L.-P.; Sun, H.-L.; Wu, L.-M.; Guo, X.-J.; Dou, H.-L.; Tso, M.O.; Zhao, L.; Li, S.-M. Baicalein reduces inflammatory process in a rodent model of diabetic retinopathy. *Investig. Ophthalmol. Vis. Sci.* **2009**, *50*, 2319–2327. [CrossRef] [PubMed]

110. Ahad, A.; Mujeeb, M.; Ahsan, H.; Siddiqui, W.A. Prophylactic effect of baicalein against renal dysfunction in type 2 diabetic rats. *Biochimie* **2014**, *106*, 101–110. [CrossRef] [PubMed]

111. Pu, P.; Wang, X.-A.; Salim, M.; Zhu, L.-H.; Wang, L.; Xiao, J.-F.; Deng, W.; Shi, H.-W.; Jiang, H.; Li, H.-L. Baicalein, a natural product, selectively activating AMPKα 2 and ameliorates metabolic disorder in diet-induced mice. *Mol. Cell. Endocrinol.* **2012**, *362*, 128–138. [CrossRef] [PubMed]

112. Ahad, A.; Ganai, A.A.; Mujeeb, M.; Siddiqui, W.A. Chrysin, an anti-inflammatory molecule, abrogates renal dysfunction in type 2 diabetic rats. *Toxicol. Appl. Pharmacol.* **2014**, *279*, 1–7. [CrossRef] [PubMed]

113. Mostafa, U.E.-S. Effect of green tea and green tea rich with catechin on blood glucose levels, serum lipid profile and liver and kidney functions in diabetic rats. *Biological* **2014**, *7*, 7–12. [CrossRef]

114. Stofkova, A. Leptin and adiponectin: From energy and metabolic dysbalance to inflammation and autoimmunity. *Endocr. Regul.* **2009**, *43*, 157–168. [PubMed]

115. Kapoor, R.; Kakkar, P. Protective role of morin, a flavonoid, against high glucose induced oxidative stress mediated apoptosis in primary rat hepatocytes. *PLoS ONE* **2012**, *7*, e41663. [CrossRef] [PubMed]

116. Abuohashish, H.M.; Al-Rejaie, S.S.; Al-Hosaini, K.A.; Parmar, M.Y.; Ahmed, M.M. Alleviating effects of morin against experimentally-induced diabetic osteopenia. *Diabetol. Metab. Syndr.* **2013**, *5*, 5. [CrossRef] [PubMed]

117. Vanitha, P.; Uma, C.; Suganya, N.; Bhakkiyalakshmi, E.; Suriyanarayanan, S.; Gunasekaran, P.; Sivasubramanian, S.; Ramkumar, K. Modulatory effects of morin on hyperglycemia by attenuating the hepatic key enzymes of carbohydrate metabolism and β-cell function in streptozotocin-induced diabetic rats. *Environ. Toxicol. Pharmacol.* **2014**, *37*, 326–335. [CrossRef] [PubMed]

118. Gupta, S.K.; Dongare, S.; Mathur, R.; Mohanty, I.R.; Srivastava, S.; Mathur, S.; Nag, T.C. Genistein ameliorates cardiac inflammation and oxidative stress in streptozotocin-induced diabetic cardiomyopathy in rats. *Mol. Cell. Biochem.* **2015**, *408*, 63–72. [CrossRef] [PubMed]

119. Young, N.A.; Bruss, M.S.; Gardner, M.; Willis, W.L.; Mo, X.; Valiente, G.R.; Cao, Y.; Liu, Z.; Jarjour, W.N.; Wu, L.-C. Oral administration of nano-emulsion curcumin in mice suppresses inflammatory-induced NF-κB signaling and macrophage migration. *PLoS ONE* **2014**, *9*, e111559. [CrossRef] [PubMed]

120. Wongeakin, N.; Bhattarakosol, P.; Patumraj, S. Molecular mechanisms of curcumin on diabetes-induced endothelial dysfunctions: Txnip, ICAM-1, and NOX2 expressions. *Biomed. Res. Int.* **2014**, *2014*. [CrossRef] [PubMed]

121. Li, J.J.; Lee, S.H.; Kim, D.K.; Jin, R.; Jung, D.-S.; Kwak, S.-J.; Kim, S.H.; Han, S.H.; Lee, J.E.; Moon, S.J. Colchicine attenuates inflammatory cell infiltration and extracellular matrix accumulation in diabetic nephropathy. *Am. J. Physiol. Ren. Physiol.* **2009**, *297*, F200–F209. [CrossRef] [PubMed]

122. Guo, R.; Liu, B.; Wang, K.; Zhou, S.; Li, W.; Xu, Y. Resveratrol ameliorates diabetic vascular inflammation and macrophage infiltration in db/db mice by inhibiting the NF-κB pathway. *Diabete Vasc. Dis. Res.* **2014**, *11*, 92–102. [CrossRef] [PubMed]

123. Prabhakar, O. Cerebroprotective effect of resveratrol through antioxidant and anti-inflammatory effects in diabetic rats. *Naunyn Schmiedebergs Arch. Pharmacol.* **2013**, *386*, 705–710. [CrossRef] [PubMed]

124. Zhang, X.; Zhang, R.; Lv, P.; Yang, J.; Deng, Y.; Xu, J.; Zhu, R.; Zhang, D.; Yang, Y. Emodin upregulates glucose metabolism, decreases lipolysis, and attenuates inflammation in vitro. *J. Diabetes* **2015**, *7*, 360–368. [CrossRef] [PubMed]

125. Lee, W.; Ku, S.K.; Lee, D.; Lee, T.; Bae, J.S. Emodin-6-o-β-D-glucoside inhibits high-glucose-induced vascular inflammation. *Inflammation* **2014**, *37*, 306–313. [CrossRef] [PubMed]

126. Salim, S. Oxidative stress and psychological disorders. *Curr. Neuropharmacol.* **2014**, *12*, 140–147. [CrossRef] [PubMed]

127. Zatalia, S.R.; Sanusi, H. The role of antioxidants in the pathophysiology, complications, and management of diabetes mellitus. *Acta Med. Indones.* **2013**, *45*, 141–147. [PubMed]

128. Arts, I.C.; Hollman, P.C. Polyphenols and disease risk in epidemiologic studies. *Am. J. Clin. Nutr.* **2005**, *81*, 317S–325S. [PubMed]

129. Michalak, A. Phenolic compounds and their antioxidant activity in plants growing under heavy metal stress. *Pol. J. Environ. Stud.* **2006**, *15*, 523.

130. Medeiros, K.; Figueiredo, C.; Figueredo, T.; Freire, K.; Santos, F.; Alcantara-Neves, N.; Silva, T.; Piuvezam, M. Anti-allergic effect of bee pollen phenolic extract and myricetin in ovalbumin-sensitized mice. *J. Ethnopharmacol.* **2008**, *119*, 41–46. [CrossRef] [PubMed]

131. Chavez, J.H.; Leal, P.C.; Yunes, R.A.; Nunes, R.J.; Barardi, C.R.; Pinto, A.R.; Simoes, C.M.; Zanetti, C.R. Evaluation of antiviral activity of phenolic compounds and derivatives against rabies virus. *Vet. Microbiol.* **2006**, *116*, 53–59. [CrossRef] [PubMed]

132. Nohynek, L.J.; Alakomi, H.-L.; Kähkönen, M.P.; Heinonen, M.; Helander, I.M.; Oksman-Caldentey, K.-M.; Puupponen-Pimiä, R.H. Berry phenolics: Antimicrobial properties and mechanisms of action against severe human pathogens. *Nutr. Cancer* **2006**, *54*, 18–32. [CrossRef] [PubMed]

133. Lee, K.W.; Hur, H.J.; Lee, H.J.; Lee, C.Y. Antiproliferative effects of dietary phenolic substances and hydrogen peroxide. *J. Agric. Food Chem.* **2005**, *53*, 1990–1995. [CrossRef] [PubMed]

134. Wahle, K.W.; Brown, I.; Rotondo, D.; Heys, S.D. Plant phenolics in the prevention and treatment of cancer. In *Bio-Farms for Nutraceuticals*; Springer: Aberdeen, UK, 2010; pp. 36–51.

135. Prakash, D.; Singh, B.N.; Upadhyay, G. Antioxidant and free radical scavenging activities of phenols from onion (*Allium cepa*). *Food Chem.* **2007**, *102*, 1389–1393. [CrossRef]

136. Catanzaro, D.; Vianello, C.; Ragazzi, E.; Caparrotta, L.; Montopoli, M. Cell cycle control by natural phenols in cisplatin-resistant cell lines. *Nat. Prod. Commun.* **2014**, *9*, 1465–1468. [PubMed]

137. Maheshwari, R.; Dubey, R. Nickel-induced oxidative stress and the role of antioxidant defence in rice seedlings. *Plant Growth Regul.* **2009**, *59*, 37–49. [CrossRef]

138. Montane, J.; Cadavez, L.; Novials, A. Stress and the inflammatory process: A major cause of pancreatic cell death in type 2 diabetes. *Diabetes Metab. Syndr. Obes.* **2014**, *7*, 25–34. [PubMed]

139. Ross, J.A.; Kasum, C.M. Dietary flavonoids: Bioavailability, metabolic effects, and safety. *Annu. Rev. Nutr.* **2002**, *22*, 19–34. [CrossRef] [PubMed]

140. Campanero, M.A.; Escolar, M.; Perez, G.; Garcia-Quetglas, E.; Sadaba, B.; Azanza, J.R. Simultaneous determination of diosmin and diosmetin in human plasma by ion trap liquid chromatography-atmospheric pressure chemical ionization tandem mass spectrometry: Application to a clinical pharmacokinetic study. *J. Pharm. Biomed. Anal.* **2010**, *51*, 875–881. [CrossRef] [PubMed]

141. Giacco, F.; Brownlee, M. Oxidative stress and diabetic complications. *Circ. Res.* **2010**, *107*, 1058–1070. [CrossRef] [PubMed]

142. Hertog, M.; Bueno-de-Mesquita, H.B.; Fehily, A.M.; Sweetnam, P.M.; Elwood, P.C.; Kromhout, D. Fruit and vegetable consumption and cancer mortality in the caerphilly study. *Cancer Epidemiol. Biomark. Prev.* **1996**, *5*, 673–677.

143. Navarro-González, J.F.; Mora-Fernández, C.; de Fuentes, M.M.; García-Pérez, J. Inflammatory molecules and pathways in the pathogenesis of diabetic nephropathy. *Nat. Rev. Nephrol.* **2011**, *7*, 327–340. [CrossRef] [PubMed]

144. Tan, K. Dyslipidaemia, Inflammation and Endothelial Dysfunction in Diabetes Mellitus. *Int. Congr. Ser.* **2004**, *1262*, 511–514. [CrossRef]

145. Häkkinen, S.H.; Kärenlampi, S.O.; Heinonen, I.M.; Mykkänen, H.M.; Törrönen, A.R. Content of the flavonols quercetin, myricetin, and kaempferol in 25 edible berries. *J. Agric. Food Chem.* **1999**, *47*, 2274–2279. [CrossRef] [PubMed]

146. Wilcox, L.J.; Borradaile, N.M.; Huff, M.W. Antiatherogenic properties of naringenin, a citrus flavonoid. *Cardiovasc. Drug Rev.* **1999**, *17*, 160–178. [CrossRef]

147. Hotamisligil, G.S.; Erbay, E. Nutrient sensing and inflammation in metabolic diseases. *Nat. Rev. Immunol.* **2008**, *8*, 923–934. [CrossRef] [PubMed]

148. Emim, J.A.D.S.; Oliveira, A.B.; Lapa, A.J. Pharmacological evaluation of the anti-inflammatory activity of a citrus bioflavonoid, hesperidin, and the isoflavonoids, duartin and claussequinone, in rats and mice. *Pharm. Pharmacol.* **1994**, *46*, 118–122. [CrossRef]

149. Kim, Y.O.; Leem, K.; Park, J.; Lee, P.; Ahn, D.-K.; Lee, B.C.; Park, H.K.; Suk, K.; Kim, S.Y.; Kim, H. Cytoprotective effect of *Scutellaria baicalensis* in CA1 hippocampal neurons of rats after global cerebral ischemia. *J. Ethnopharmacol.* **2001**, *77*, 183–188. [CrossRef]

150. Dhawan, K.; Kumar, S.; Sharma, A. Beneficial effects of chrysin and benzoflavone on virility in 2-year-old male rats. *J. Med. Food* **2002**, *5*, 43–48. [CrossRef] [PubMed]

151. Zheng, L.T.; Ryu, G.-M.; Kwon, B.-M.; Lee, W.-H.; Suk, K. Anti-inflammatory effects of catechols in lipopolysaccharide-stimulated microglia cells: Inhibition of microglial neurotoxicity. *Eur. J. Pharmacol.* **2008**, *588*, 106–113. [CrossRef] [PubMed]

152. Hummasti, S.; Hotamisligil, G.S. Endoplasmic reticulum stress and inflammation in obesity and diabetes. *Circ. Res.* **2010**, *107*, 579–591. [CrossRef] [PubMed]

153. Yan, J.; Zhao, Y.; Suo, S.; Liu, Y.; Zhao, B. Green tea catechins ameliorate adipose insulin resistance by improving oxidative stress. *Free Radic. Biol. Med.* **2012**, *52*, 1648–1657. [CrossRef] [PubMed]

154. Tanti, J.-F.; Ceppo, F.; Jager, J.; Berthou, F. Implication of inflammatory signaling pathways in obesity-induced insulin resistance. *Front. Endocrinol.* **2013**, *3*, 6–20. [CrossRef] [PubMed]

155. Ricardo, K.F.S.; Oliveira, T.T.D.; Nagem, T.J.; Pinto, A.D.S.; Oliveira, M.G.A.; Soares, J.F. Effect of flavonoids morin; quercetin and nicotinic acid on lipid metabolism of rats experimentally fed with triton. *Braz. Arch. Boil. Technol.* **2001**, *44*, 263–267. [CrossRef]

156. Messina, M.; Messina, V. The role of soy in vegetarian diets. *Nutrients* **2010**, *2*, 855–888. [CrossRef] [PubMed]

157. Vinayagam, R.; Xu, B. Antidiabetic properties of dietary flavonoids: A cellular mechanism review. *Nutr. Metab.* **2015**, *12*, 60. [CrossRef] [PubMed]

158. Liu, D.; Zhen, W.; Yang, Z.; Carter, J.D.; Si, H.; Reynolds, K.A. Genistein acutely stimulates insulin secretion in pancreatic β-cells through a CAMP-dependent protein kinase pathway. *Diabetes* **2006**, *55*, 1043–1050. [CrossRef] [PubMed]

159. Yamawaki, H.; Pan, S.; Lee, R.T.; Berk, B.C. Fluid shear stress inhibits vascular inflammation by decreasing thioredoxin-interacting protein in endothelial cells. *J. Clin. Investig.* **2005**, *115*, 733–738. [CrossRef] [PubMed]

160. Kannel, W.B.; McGee, D.L. Diabetes and cardiovascular disease: The Framingham study. *JAMA* **1979**, *241*, 2035–2038. [CrossRef] [PubMed]
161. Fürst, R.; Zündorf, I. Plant-derived anti-inflammatory compounds: Hopes and disappointments regarding the translation of preclinical knowledge into clinical progress. *Mediat. Inflamm.* **2014**, 2014. [CrossRef] [PubMed]
162. Chow, F.; Ozols, E.; Nikolic-Paterson, D.J.; Atkins, R.C.; Tesch, G.H. Macrophages in mouse type 2 diabetic nephropathy: Correlation with diabetic state and progressive renal injury. *Kidney Int.* **2004**, *65*, 116–128. [CrossRef] [PubMed]
163. Edwards, J.L.; Vincent, A.M.; Cheng, H.T.; Feldman, E.L. Diabetic neuropathy: Mechanisms to management. *Pharmacol. Ther.* **2008**, *120*, 1–34. [CrossRef] [PubMed]
164. Rock, R.B.; Peterson, P.K. Microglia as a pharmacological target in infectious and inflammatory diseases of the brain. *J. Neuroimmune Pharmacol.* **2006**, *1*, 117–126. [CrossRef] [PubMed]
165. Yousuf, S.; Atif, F.; Ahmad, M.; Hoda, N.; Ishrat, T.; Khan, B.; Islam, F. Resveratrol exerts its neuroprotective effect by modulating mitochondrial dysfunctions and associated cell death during cerebral ischemia. *Brain Res.* **2009**, *1250*, 242–253. [CrossRef] [PubMed]
166. Aggarwal, B.B.; Prasad, S.; Reuter, S.; Kannappan, R.; Yadev, V.R.; Park, B.; Kim, J.H.; Gupta, S.C.; Phromnoi, K.; Sundaram, C.; et al. Identification of novel anti-inflammatory agents from ayurvedic medicine for prevention of chronic diseases: "Reverse pharmacology" and "bedside to bench" approach. *Curr. Drug Targets* **2011**, *12*, 1595–1653. [CrossRef] [PubMed]
167. Bohn, T.; McDougall, G.J.; Alegría, A.; Alminger, M.; Arrigoni, E.; Aura, A.M.; Brito, C.; Cilla, A.; El, S.N.; Karakaya, S. Mind the gap—Deficits in our knowledge of aspects impacting the bioavailability of phytochemicals and their metabolites—A position paper focusing on carotenoids and polyphenols. *Mol. Nutr. Food Res.* **2015**, *59*, 1307–1323. [CrossRef] [PubMed]
168. Svelander, C.A.; Lopez-Sanchez, P.; Pudney, P.D.; Schumm, S.; Alminger, M.A. High pressure homogenization increases the in vitro bioaccessibility of α-and β-carotene in carrot emulsions but not of lycopene in tomato emulsions. *J. Food Sci.* **2011**, *76*, H215–H225. [CrossRef] [PubMed]
169. Epriliati, M.I. Nutriomic Analysis of Fresh and Processed Fruits through the Development of an In Vitro Model of Human Digestive System. Ph.D. Thesis, The University of Queensland, St Lucia, Australia, February 2008.
170. Williams, A.W.; Boileau, T.W.; Erdman, J.W. Factors influencing the uptake and absorption of carotenoids. *Exp. Biol. Med.* **1998**, *218*, 106–108. [CrossRef]
171. Panozzo, A.; Lemmens, L.; Van Loey, A.; Manzocco, L.; Nicoli, M.C.; Hendrickx, M. Microstructure and bioaccessibility of different carotenoid species as affected by high pressure homogenisation: A case study on differently coloured tomatoes. *Food Chem.* **2013**, *141*, 4094–4100. [CrossRef] [PubMed]
172. Manners, G.D.; Jacob, R.A.; Andrew, P., III; Schoch, T.K.; Hasegawa, S. Bioavailability of citrus limonoids in humans. *J. Agric. Food Chem.* **2003**, *51*, 4156–4161. [CrossRef] [PubMed]
173. Johnson, E.J. Human studies on bioavailability and plasma response of lycopene. *Exp. Biol. Med.* **1998**, *218*, 115–120. [CrossRef]

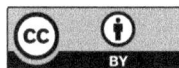

nutrients

MDPI

Article

Hepatoprotective Effect of *Opuntia robusta* and *Opuntia streptacantha* Fruits against Acetaminophen-Induced Acute Liver Damage

Herson Antonio González-Ponce [1,5], María Consolación Martínez-Saldaña [2],
Ana Rosa Rincón-Sánchez [3], María Teresa Sumaya-Martínez [4], Manon Buist-Homan [5,6],
Klaas Nico Faber [5,6], Han Moshage [5,6] and Fernando Jaramillo-Juárez [1,*]

[1] Department of Physiology and Pharmacology, Basic Science Center, Universidad Autónoma de Aguascalientes, Aguascalientes 20131, Mexico; herson_qfbd@hotmail.com
[2] Department of Morphology, Basic Science Center, Universidad Autónoma de Aguascalientes, Aguascalientes 20131, Mexico; mcmtzsal@correo.uaa.mx
[3] Department of Physiology, University Center of Health Sciences, Universidad de Guadalajara, Guadalajara 44340, Mexico; anarosarincon@yahoo.com.mx
[4] Food Technology Unit, Secretary of Research and Graduate Studies, Universidad Autónoma de Nayarit, Tepic 63160, Mexico; teresumaya@hotmail.com
[5] Department of Gastroenterology and Hepatology, University Medical Center Groningen, University of Groningen, Groningen 9713 GZ, The Netherlands; m.buist-homan@umcg.nl (M.B.-H.); k.n.faber@umcg.nl (K.N.F.); a.j.moshage@umcg.nl (H.M.)
[6] Department of Laboratory Medicine, University Medical Center Groningen, University of Groningen, Groningen 9713 GZ, The Netherlands
* Correspondence: jara@att.net.mx; Tel.: +52-449-9910-7400 (ext. 345)

Received: 4 July 2016; Accepted: 20 September 2016; Published: 4 October 2016

Abstract: Acetaminophen (APAP)-induced acute liver failure (ALF) is a serious health problem in developed countries. *N*-acetyl-L-cysteine (NAC), the current therapy for APAP-induced ALF, is not always effective, and liver transplantation is often needed. *Opuntia* spp. fruits are an important source of nutrients and contain high levels of bioactive compounds, including antioxidants. The aim of this study was to evaluate the hepatoprotective effect of *Opuntia robusta* and *Opuntia streptacantha* extracts against APAP-induced ALF. In addition, we analyzed the antioxidant activities of these extracts. Fruit extracts (800 mg/kg/day, orally) were given prophylactically to male Wistar rats before intoxication with APAP (500 mg/kg, intraperitoneally). Rat hepatocyte cultures were exposed to 20 mmol/L APAP, and necrosis was assessed by LDH leakage. *Opuntia robusta* had significantly higher levels of antioxidants than *Opuntia streptacantha*. Both extracts significantly attenuated APAP-induced injury markers AST, ALT and ALP and improved liver histology. The *Opuntia* extracts reversed APAP-induced depletion of liver GSH and glycogen stores. In cultured hepatocytes, *Opuntia* extracts significantly reduced leakage of LDH and cell necrosis, both prophylactically and therapeutically. Both extracts appeared to be superior to NAC when used therapeutically. We conclude that *Opuntia* extracts are hepatoprotective and can be used as a nutraceutical to prevent ALF.

Keywords: *Opuntia* fruits; acetaminophen; acute liver failure; antioxidants; hepatoprotective; nutraceutical

1. Introduction

Non-steroidal anti-inflammatory drugs (NSAID) are widely used for the alleviation of pain, fever and inflammation. NSAID are the most widely prescribed medications in the world and are used by millions of patients on a daily basis. However, excessive consumption of NSAID has been related to severe side effects caused by oxidative stress, resulting in considerable morbidity and mortality [1,2].

Acetaminophen (APAP), a non-prescription drug, is a safe and effective analgesic and antipyretic drug when used at therapeutic doses [3]. However, an acute or cumulative overdose can cause severe liver injury that may progress to acute liver failure (ALF). In fact, APAP is the most common cause of ALF in developed countries [4,5].

The liver is the main organ involved in the metabolism of APAP. At therapeutic doses, APAP is eliminated via glucuronidation and sulfation reactions. However, at high doses, the conjugation pathways are saturated, and part of the drug is converted by cytochrome P450 2E1 (CYP2E1) to the highly reactive metabolite *N*-acetyl-*p*-benzoquinone imine (NAPQI) that reacts with sulfhydryl groups. Reduced glutathione (GSH) initially traps NAPQI, and the GSH adduct is excreted. However, when GSH is depleted, NAPQI reacts with cellular proteins, including a number of mitochondrial proteins, to form NAPQI adducts. Consequences of this process are the inhibition of mitochondrial respiration and ATP depletion, as well as mitochondrial oxidative stress [6–8].

This results in increased susceptibility to liver injury by reactive oxygen species (ROS), including hydrogen peroxide (H_2O_2), superoxide anions ($O_2^{\bullet-}$) and hydroxyl radicals ($\cdot OH$). In addition to reducing the GSH level, the APAP overdose also reduces the antioxidant enzyme activities, increases lipid peroxidation and causes hepatic DNA fragmentation, which ultimately leads to cellular necrosis [9,10].

Currently, the treatment of choice for APAP overdose is *N*-acetyl-L-cysteine, a precursor of intracellular cysteine and GSH that counteracts the depletion of GSH and allows the excretion of NAPQI as the GSH-adduct. This reduces oxidative stress and, consequently, liver injury [11]. Unfortunately, *N*-acetyl-L-cysteine is not always effective, and there is an urgent need for more effective interventions.

Medicinal benefits from plants have been recognized for centuries. Vegetables and fruits are very important in human nutrition and as sources of phytochemicals that reduce disease risks, like oxidative stress, inflammation and DNA damage [12,13]. The protective effects of diets rich in fruits and vegetables are not only due to fibers, vitamins and minerals, but also to secondary metabolites of plant products [14]. In recent years, many antioxidant compounds, such as vitamins, pigments and phenolic phytochemicals from fruits, vegetables and herbs, have received special attention due to their protective actions against oxidative damage and genotoxicity [15,16].

Cactus (*Opuntia* spp.) is used as a common vegetable and medicinal plant on the American continent. There are about 200 recognized species of *Opuntia*, and at least 84 are found in México [17,18]. Cactus pears are sweet edible fruits from the cactus (*Opuntia* spp.) that belong to the Cactaceae family [19]. These fruits have been used in traditional medicine for the treatment of several diseases [20] and contain a wide variety of trace elements, sugars and other bioactive compounds, such as betalains, carotenoids, ascorbic acid, flavonoids and other phenolic compounds [21]. Cactus pear fruits are now recognized as a rich source of nutritional compounds with health-promoting activities, including antioxidant [22–26], neuroprotective, anti-inflammatory, cardioprotective, anti-diabetic [27], anti-clastogenic [28] and anti-genotoxic actions [16]. In addition, they have protective effects on erythrocyte membranes [29] and on acute gastric lesions [30], and they improve platelet function [31] and cancer chemoprevention [18]. Interestingly, APAP-induced liver injury is one of the most widely-used models to evaluate the hepatoprotective potential of natural products [32].

The aim of this study was to investigate the hepatoprotective effect of *Opuntia robusta* and *Opuntia streptacantha* fruits from a semi-arid region of Mexico in a model of APAP-induced liver injury and to perform an initial characterization of the main bioactive compounds in these fruits.

2. Experimental Procedures

2.1. Chemicals and Materials

Stock solutions of acetaminophen (APAP, 2 mol/L), reduced glutathione (GSH, 50 mmol/L) and *N*-acetyl-L-cysteine (NAC, 1 mol/L) were prepared in the appropriate solvents (phosphate-buffered saline for in vivo experiments and culture medium for the in vitro experiments). All reagents were from Sigma Aldrich, St. Louis, MO, USA. Sytox green nucleic acid stain, gentamycin, William's E medium and fetal calf serum were obtained from Invitrogen (Breda, The Netherlands); penicillin-streptomycin-fungizone (PSF) was from Lonza (Verviers, Belgium); microplate readers Biotek PowerWave XS and Biotek Synergy HT were from BioTek Instruments Inc. (Winooski, VT, USA).

2.2. Animals

Adult male Wistar rats (200–250 g) were used for the in vivo and in vitro studies. The animals were kept in polypropylene cages at room temperature (25 ± 2 °C) with food and water ad libitum. Experiments were approved by and performed following the guidelines of the local Committee for Care and Use of laboratory animals (Permission No. 6415A of the Committee for Care and Use of laboratory animals of the University of Groningen and Mexican governmental guideline NOM 033 ZOO 1995).

2.3. Plant Materials and Extracts Preparation

Ripe fruits of *Opuntia robusta* and *Opuntia streptacantha* were collected from randomly-selected plants of the same species in the semi-arid region of Aguascalientes, México ($21°46'55.86''$ N, $102°6'16.08''$ O, and 1994 meters above sea level). The juice of each batch of peeled fruits was extracted and mixed in a single procedure using a Braun J500 juice extractor (Braun GmbH, Taunus, Germany). The collected juice of each batch was aliquoted into 50-mL dark tubes, centrifuged at 5000 rpm for 15 min at 4 °C, filtered through Whatman 40 filter paper (8-μm pore size), stored at -80 °C and lyophilized in a Labconco FreeZone Freeze Dry System (Labconco Corp, Kansas City, MO, USA) [26,28]. Extracts of one batch were used for the entire study. Lyophilized extracts were reconstituted with 50 mL of deionized water.

2.4. Determination of the Main Bioactive Compounds of Fruit Extracts

The reconstituted extract of each *Opuntia* species was clarified ($12,000 \times g$ for 15 min at 15 °C) and used to determine the bioactive compounds. Flavonoids were quantified by the colorimetric method of Zhishen et al. [33], and values were expressed as μg quercetin equivalents/mL. The total content of betalains (betacyanins and betaxanthins) was determined according to the methods described by Stintzing et al. [34] and Sumaya-Martínez et al. [26], and results were expressed as mg of betacyanin or betaxanthin equivalents/L. Ascorbic acid content in the extracts was determined by the method of Dürüst et al. [35], and the results were expressed as mg ascorbic acid equivalents/L. The total phenolic content was determined by the Folin-Ciocalteu method described by Georgé et al. [36] and was expressed as mg gallic acid equivalents/L. All measurements were performed in triplicate on a Biotek PowerWave XS microplate reader.

2.5. Determination of Free Radical Scavenging and Chelating Activities

The antioxidant activity of the *Opuntia* fruit extracts was determined by different methods. The DPPH (2,2-diphenyl-1-picrylhydrazyl) method was performed according to Morales and Jimenez [37], and the antioxidant activity was expressed as mmol Trolox equivalents/L. The ABTS (2,2'-azino-bis(3-ethylbenzothiazoline-6-sulphonic acid)) method was performed according to Re et al. [38] and Kuskoski et al. [39], and the results were expressed as mg ascorbic acid (AA)/100 mL. FRAP (ferric reducing antioxidant power) was determined as described by Hinneburg et al. [40], and the results were expressed as mg ascorbic acid (AA)/100 mL. The assay to determine the chelating activity was performed as described by Gulcin et al. [41] and was expressed as mol EDTA equivalent/L. All measurements were performed in triplicate on a Biotek PowerWave XS microplate reader. The ORAC (oxygen radical absorbance capacity) was determined as described by Huang [42], and the results were expressed as mmol Trolox equivalents/L. This assay was performed in triplicate on a Biotek Synergy HT microplate reader.

2.6. Rat Hepatocyte Isolation

Hepatocytes were isolated from male Wistar rats by two-step collagenase perfusion as described by Conde de la Rosa et al. [43] and Vrenken et al. [44]. The cell viability was determined by trypan blue exclusion assay and was always higher than 85%. After isolation, the hepatocytes were plated on 6-well coated plates in William's E medium supplemented with 50 µg/mL gentamycin, 1% penicillin-streptomycin-fungizone and 10% fetal calf serum. Cells were cultured for 4 h to attach in a humidified incubator at 37 °C and 5% CO_2.

2.7. Experimental Design

2.7.1. In Vivo Study

Animals were randomly divided into seven groups (n = 12): (1) control (C); (2) acetaminophen treated (APAP); (3) *Opuntia robusta* treated (*Or*); (4) *Opuntia streptacantha* treated (*Os*); (5) *Or* + APAP treated; (6) *Os* + APAP treated; and (7) GSH + APAP treated. Rats were pretreated with daily oral doses of cactus extract (800 mg/kg), according to the protocol of Kim et al. [30] with some modifications) or GSH (50 mg/kg, intraperitoneally) for five days before APAP treatment (500 mg/kg intraperitoneally; single dose). Samples of blood and liver tissue were collected 4 h after APAP intoxication for assessment of liver damage markers [45]. Some animals were sacrificed 24 h after APAP intoxication, and liver tissue was obtained for histological evaluation.

Liver damage was assessed by measurement of alanine aminotransferase (ALT), aspartate aminotransferase (AST) and alkaline phosphatase (ALP) serum activities using a commercial spectrophotometrical method (SPINREACT, Girona, Spain). The values represent the mean of three measurements (±standard deviation) and are expressed as IU/L.

The GSH content in liver tissue homogenates was determined according to Hissin and Hilf [46], using *o*-phtaldehyde (OPT) as the fluorescent reagent. The fluorescence intensity was measured at 420 nm using 350 nm as the excitation wavelength, using a Luminescence Spectrophotometer (Model LS-50B, PerkinElmer Inc., Waltham, MA, USA).

For histological studies, animals were anesthetized with sodium pentobarbital and perfused via the portal vein with saline solution (sodium chloride 0.9%), containing 0.5% heparin and 0.1% procaine and fixed in situ with neutral formalin (10%). The hepatic tissue was embedded in paraffin blocks, and sections of 5 µm were prepared with a microtome (Leica RM2125RT). The sections were stained with periodic acid Schiff (PAS) reagent. Liver tissue images were captured using a Carl Zeiss microscope (Axioskope 40) and processed using Image-Pro Plus software.

2.7.2. In Vitro Study

After the attachment period of 4 h, the medium was changed for medium without fetal calf serum. Monolayer cultures were exposed to a toxic dose of acetaminophen (20 mmol/L). A single dose of 125 µL (8% v/v) of *Opuntia streptacantha* or *Opuntia robusta* reconstituted extract or 5 mmol/L N-acetyl-L-cysteine (NAC) was added 30 min before (prophylactic regimen) or 30 min, 1, 2, 4 and 8 h after the addition of acetaminophen (therapeutic regimen).

To quantitatively assess hepatocyte injury, LDH leakage into medium was evaluated. LDH activity was measured spectrophotometrically at 340 nm by determining NADH oxidation in the presence of sodium pyruvate in a microplate reader (BioTek EL808) for 30 min at 37 °C and expressed as fold induction versus control values [47]. Hepatocyte necrosis was also assessed by Sytox Green staining to confirm the LDH leakage results. Sytox green binds to nuclear DNA, but can only enter cells with ruptured plasma membranes, as occurs in necrotic, but not in apoptotic cell death. Necrosis of hepatocytes was determined by incubation for 15 min with Sytox green (1:40,000) nucleic acid stain as described by Woudenberg-Vrenken et al. [48]. Necrosis was quantified by counting fluorescent nuclei and the total number of cells in three randomly chosen high power fields. Fluorescent nuclei were visualized using a Leica microscope DMI 6000B at 450–490 nm.

2.8. Statistical Analysis of Data

For the analysis of the components and antioxidant activities of cactus fruit extracts, the unpaired *t*-test was carried out with a confidence level of 99%. The analysis of biochemical results was done using the one-way ANOVA test, and the means of the different experimental groups were compared using the Tukey test with a confidence level of 95%. GraphPad Prism 5 software was used for the statistical analysis (La Jolla, CA, USA).

3. Results

3.1. Yields of the Juice Extraction Method

Depending on the size and ripeness stage, approximately three fruits of *Opuntia robusta* and six fruits of *Opuntia streptacantha* were used to obtain 50 mL of juice extract. After lyophilization of 50 mL of each fruit juice, 6.89 ± 0.80 g of *Opuntia robusta* and 6.68 ± 0.63 g of *Opuntia streptacantha* powder were obtained (Figure 1). The difference in yield between the two cactus species was not statistically significant ($p > 0.05$). For the in vivo experiments, a dose of 800 mg/kg in rats (200–250 g b.w.) corresponded to approximately 1.5 mL of the reconstituted extract. For the in vitro experiments, a dose of 8% v/v in primary rat hepatocytes corresponded to approximately 125 μL of the reconstituted extract.

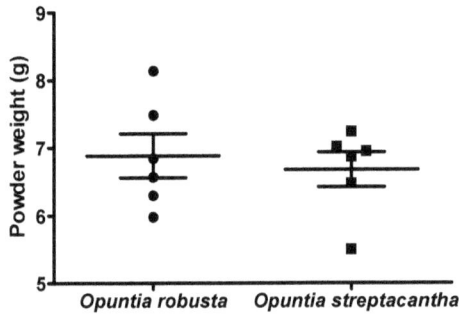

Figure 1. Yield (gram powder) obtained after lyophilization of 50 mL of juice. Each scatter column represents the mean of six samples $\pm$ SEM. $p > 0.05$.

3.2. Bioactive Compounds of Cactus Pear Fruit Extracts

The extracts of *Opuntia robusta* and *Opuntia streptacantha* ripe fruits contain a high quantity of bioactive compounds. *Opuntia robusta* had a significantly higher amount of flavonoids, ascorbic acid and total phenolic compounds than *Opuntia streptacantha* (Table 1). *Opuntia robusta* contained a significantly higher amount of betacyanin than *Opuntia streptacantha*. In addition, both *Opuntia* fruit extracts had more betacyanin than betaxanthin, causing the red-purple color of the fruits (Table 2). Similar values of these compounds have been reported in other *Opuntia* species [26,34].

Table 1. Total amount of bioactive compounds in the *Opuntia* fruit extracts.

Fruit	Flavonoids (μg eq. Quercetin/mL)	Ascorbic Acid (mg eq. Ascorbic Acid/L)	Total Phenolic Compounds (mg eq. Gallic Acid/L)
Opuntia robusta	89.19 ± 2.84 *	328.83 ± 28.47 *	573.73 ± 24.99 *
Opuntia streptacantha	54.48 ± 0.93	65.86 ± 12.33	343.12 ± 9.72

Values are the mean of three measurements $\pm$ SD. *Opuntia robusta* vs. *Opuntia streptacantha* * $p < 0.01$. eq.: equivalent.

Table 2. Betacyanin and betaxanthin content and total amount of betalains in the two *Opuntia* fruit extracts.

Fruit	Betacyanin (mg eq. Betacyanin/L)	Betaxanthin (mg eq. Betaxanthin/L)	Total Betalains (mg eq. Betalains/L)
Opuntia robusta	333.27 ± 11.46 *	133.66 ± 4.83 *	466.93 ± 16.29 *
Opuntia streptacantha	87.24 ± 1.54	36.47 ± 1.07	123.70 ± 2.61

Values are the mean of three measurements ± SD. *Opuntia robusta* vs. *Opuntia streptacantha* * $p < 0.01$.

3.3. Free Radical Scavenging and Chelating Activities of Opuntia Extracts

Both *Opuntia* species demonstrated free radical scavenging capacity, but to different extents (Table 3). *Opuntia robusta* had superior antioxidant activity compared to *Opuntia streptacantha*, which might be due to its chemical composition since *Opuntia robusta* contains higher amounts of bioactive compounds (Tables 1 and 2). On the other hand, extracts of *Opuntia streptacantha* contained more chelating activity than *Opuntia robusta* (Table 4).

Table 3. Free radical scavenging activity of *Opuntia* fruit extracts.

Fruit	DPPH (mmol eq. Trolox®/L)	FRAP (mg eq. Ascorbic Acid/100 mL)	ABTS (mg eq. Ascorbic Acid/100 mL)	ORAC (mmol eq. Trolox®/L)
Opuntia robusta	5.77 ± 0.33 *	73.24 ± 3 *	92.62 ± 5 *	41.78 ± 1.89 *
Opuntia streptacantha	1.31 ± 0.94	28.82 ± 2	61.69 ± 3	31.42 ± 0.43

DPPH, 2,2-diphenyl-1-picrylhydrazyl; FRAP, ferric reducing antioxidant power; ABST, 2,2′-azino-bis (3-ethylbenzothiazoline-6-sulphonic acid); ORAC, oxygen radical absorbance capacity. Values are the mean of three measurements ± SD. *Opuntia robusta* vs. *Opuntia streptacantha* * $p < 0.01$.

Table 4. Chelating activity of *Opuntia* fruit extracts.

Fruit	Ferrous Ion Scavenging (mol eq. EDTA/L)
Opuntia robusta	3.69 ± 0.9
Opuntia streptacantha	6.09 ± 0.8 *

Values are the mean of three measurements ± SD. *Opuntia robusta* vs. *Opuntia streptacantha* * $p < 0.01$.

3.4. In Vivo Experiments

The plasma levels of transaminases and alkaline phosphatase, as well as the GSH content in liver homogenates of experimental animals 4 h after APAP intoxication are shown in Table 5. APAP treatment significantly increased plasma levels of transaminases and ALP compared to control animals ($p < 0.05$). The prophylactic administration of both *Opuntia* fruit extracts (Or + APAP and Os + APAP) in APAP-treated animals significantly decreased all markers of liver cell injury compared to APAP-intoxicated animals ($p < 0.05$). The extracts alone did not cause any changes in these plasma markers (Table 5). GSH appeared to be less effective in attenuating liver damage compared to the *Opuntia* extracts (Table 5).

GSH was almost completely depleted after APAP overdose. *Opuntia robusta* extract completely and *Opuntia streptacantha* extract partially prevented the depletion of GSH induced by APAP treatment. *Opuntia* extracts alone did not change hepatic GSH levels. GSH administration partially prevented the depletion of hepatic GSH levels, comparable to *Opuntia streptacantha*. Thus, *Opuntia robusta* had superior protective effects than *Opuntia streptacantha* in acute APAP intoxication.

In the APAP group, an extensive hydropic vacuolation was observed (Figure 2B), as well as glycogen depletion (Figure 2C) and focal necrosis of cells with pyknotic nuclei (Figure 2D) of the hepatocytes nearest to the central vein compared to the control group (Figure 2A). *Opuntia* extracts alone did not cause morphological changes, glycogen depletion or necrosis (Figure 3A,B). Both *Opuntia* extracts attenuated the histological changes induced by APAP alone and maintained cytoplasmic glycogen stores, without signs of vacuolation or necrosis in the hepatic acinus (Figure 3C,D). GSH supplementation also prevented vacuolation and necrosis, although some hepatocytes lost glycogen stores (Figure 3E).

Table 5. Effect of *Opuntia* fruit extracts on acetaminophen-induced acute liver injury. Levels of transaminases in plasma and reduced glutathione in liver homogenates.

Group	ALT (IU/L)	AST (IU/L)	ALP (IU/L)	GSH (µg/g)
Control	37.9 ± 0.7 *	79.5 ± 4.2 *	319 ± 15.4 *	1797 ± 28 *
APAP	82.4 ± 8.8	320 ± 48.0	512 ± 36.6	198 ± 4
Or	37.3 ± 3.8 *	75.2 ± 2.8 *	285 ± 36.2 *	1709 ± 23 *
Os	39.9 ± 3.3 *	84.5 ± 5.8 *	251 ± 35.2 *	1519 ± 101 *
Or + APAP	41.9 ± 3.3 *	129 ± 10.3 *	246 ± 11.2 *	1608 ± 31 *
Os + APAP	58.1 ± 6.1 *	151 ± 33.3 *	459 ± 28.6	666 ± 47 *
GSH + APAP	69.8 ± 5.5	289 ± 42.2	309 ± 15.4 *	604 ± 26 *

APAP: acetaminophen; *Or*: *Opuntia robusta*; *Os*: *Opuntia streptacantha*; GSH: reduced glutathione. Values are the mean of six measurements (±SEM). * $p < 0.05$ regarding the APAP group.

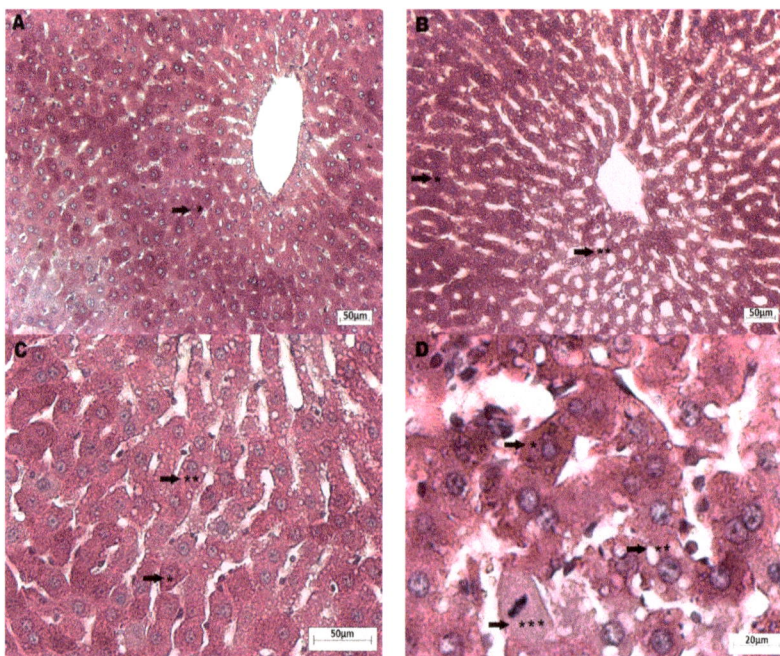

Figure 2. Histopathological images of liver tissue of non-treated control animals and APAP-treated animals. (**A**) Control: normal morphology in all zones of the hepatic acinus with positive PAS staining, indicating glycogen stores (black arrow *); magnification 100×; (**B**) APAP group: intense cytoplasmic vacuolation of hepatocytes nearest to the central vein (Zones II and III; black arrow **); magnification 100×; (**C**) PAS staining of APAP group indicating depletion of cytoplasmic glycogen stores and vacuolation of the hepatocytes near the central vein (black arrow **); magnification 200×; (**D**) APAP group: focal necrosis of hepatocytes (black arrow ***); magnification 400×.

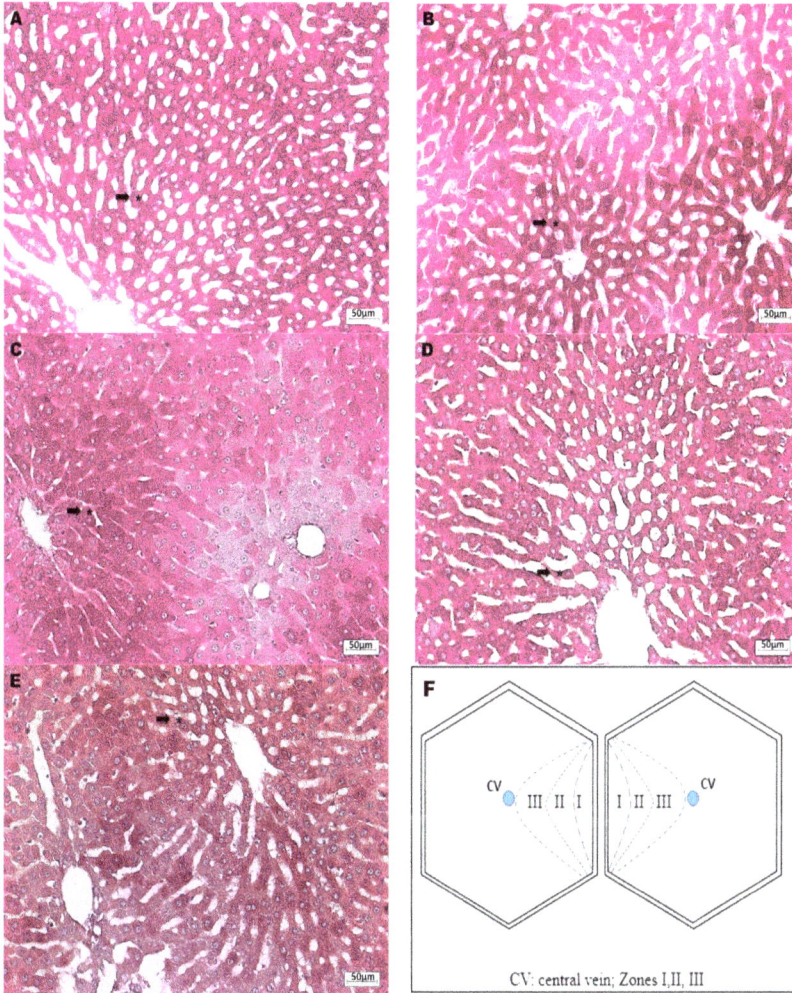

Figure 3. Histopathological images of liver tissue of APAP-intoxicated rats, prophylactically treated with *Opuntia* extracts. (**A**) *Opuntia robusta*-treated group and (**B**) *Opuntia streptacantha*-treated group: hepatocytes of Zones II and III to hepatic acinus showed normal morphology and PAS positive reaction (black arrow *); magnification 100×; (**C**) *Opuntia robusta* + APAP group; (**D**) *Opuntia streptacantha* + APAP; and (**E**) GSH + APAP group: normal morphology and PAS positive staining of pericentral (Zones II and III) hepatocytes (black arrow *); magnification 100×; (**F**) Zones of the hepatic acinus.

3.5. In Vitro Experiments

Both *Opuntia* extracts protected the hepatocytes against APAP-induced cell necrosis when added prior to APAP (prophylactic regimen), as shown in Figure 4. NAC was also protective, but tended to be less potent than the *Opuntia* extracts. In the therapeutic regimen, both *Opuntia* extracts protected against APAP-induced toxicity when added up to 4 h after APAP, whereas NAC was only protective when added up to 1–2 h after APAP (Figure 4).

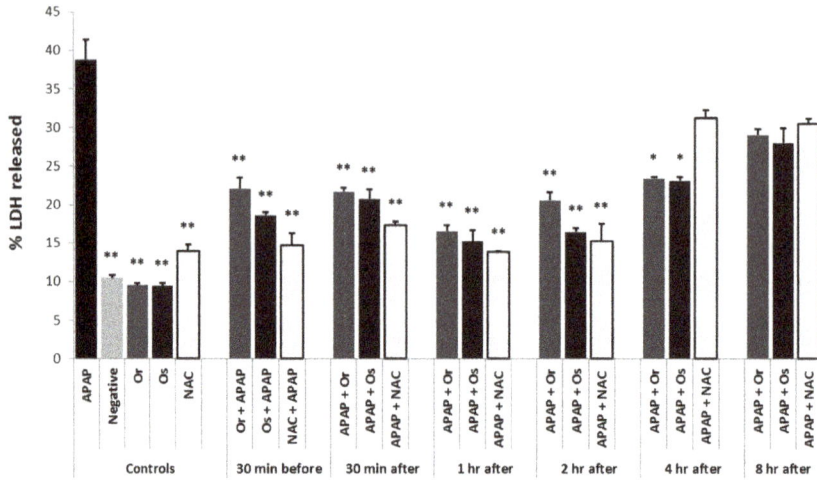

Figure 4. *Opuntia* extracts protect against APAP-induced toxicity in primary cultures of rat hepatocytes. Cell toxicity is represented as LDH released into medium 24 h after the addition of 20 mmol/L APAP. *Opuntia* extracts and NAC were added at different time points before and after APAP intoxication. *Or, Opuntia robusta*; *Os, Opuntia streptacantha*; APAP, acetaminophen; NAC, *N*-acetyl-L-cysteine. Results are expressed as fold-increase relative to control group; * $p < 0.05$, ** $p < 0.01$ compared to the APAP group.

To confirm the results obtained by determining the LDH release, we also used Sytox green as a fluorescent dye for necrotic cells. APAP (20 mmol/L) induced significant cell necrosis in primary cultures of rat hepatocytes (Figure 5B) in comparison to the Control (Figure 5A), which was almost completely abolished by the *Opuntia* extracts (Figure 5F,G). NAC (Figure 5H) showed a similar protective effect as the *Opuntia* extracts. These results confirm the data obtained with the LDH determinations.

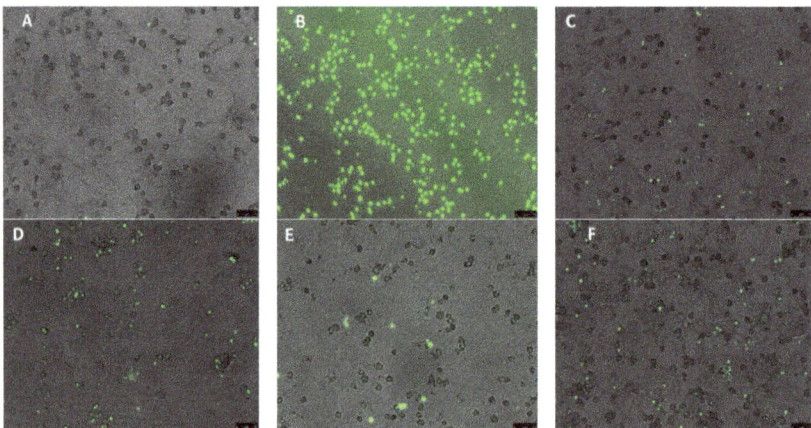

Figure 5. *Cont.*

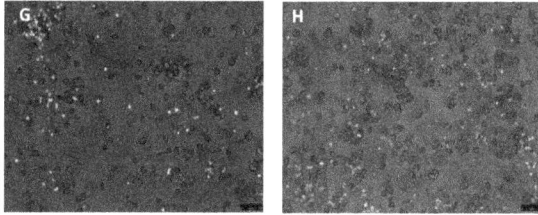

Figure 5. *Opuntia* extracts protect against APAP-induced necrotic cell death in primary cultures of rat hepatocytes. Cell toxicity was determined using the Sytox green fluorescent dye for necrotic cells. *Opuntia* extracts and NAC were added 30 min prior to APAP. Hepatocytes were exposed to 20 mmol/L APAP for 24 h, and subsequently, Sytox green was added. Micrographs were taken 15 min after addition of Sytox green. Different groups are explained in the lower-right panel. Magnification 100×. (**A**) Control; (**B**) APAP; (**C**) *O. robusta*; (**D**) *O. streptacantha*; (**E**) NAC; (**F**) *O. robusta* + APAP; (**G**) *O. streptacantha* + APAP; (**H**) NAC + APAP.

4. Discussion

Natural compounds have a huge structural diversity and many biological activities, thus offering ample opportunities to identify novel compounds for the treatment of different diseases [49,50]. The presence or absence of many bioactive compounds in leaves, fruits, roots, seeds and other natural subproducts depends on geographical and environmental factors, such as humidity, temperature, season, pollution, altitude, etc. Therefore, it is very difficult to standardize the composition of natural products, but it is acceptable to link their therapeutic benefits to the presence and concentration of specific compounds in the extracts used [51]. We studied two *Opuntia* species that are widely distributed in the central semi-arid regions of Mexico [52]. The fruits contained a large quantity of the most important phytochemical compounds with proven therapeutic activity as reported by Vinson et al. [53] and Coria Cayupán et al. [24]. A chemical characterization of the main bioactive compounds present in these two species of *Opuntia* fruits from different areas has been performed previously by different authors, and the results showed that the main components of them are mostly betalains, specifically betacyanins; flavonoids and phenolic compounds that apparently are responsible for their biologic activity [20,23].

Bioflavonoids are widely distributed in fruits and vegetables and have multiple biological effects, including free radical scavenging activity and chelation of metal ions [54]. It is well known that flavonoid effects are related to their chemical structure. This is especially true for flavonols, such as quercetin, which represents the most abundant dietary flavonoid. Mechanisms of antioxidant action include the suppression of reactive oxygen species (ROS) formation either by inhibition of ROS-generating enzymes; the chelation of trace elements that are involved in free radical generation; or by the induction of antioxidant defenses. These abilities are intimately related to the oxidation/reduction potential and the activation energy for electron transfer of the substance [55–57]. Several therapeutic effects of flavonoids have been linked to their antioxidant capacity, e.g., the inhibition of inflammation [58] and lipoperoxidation [59], as well as nephroprotective [60,61], neuroprotective [62] and hepatoprotective activities [63]. In addition, there is increasing evidence that polyphenols protect cellular constituents against oxidative damage and, therefore, limit the risk of chronic diseases associated with oxidative stress [64].

The fruit extracts of both *Opuntia* species investigated in this study contain high concentrations of betalains. The chemical structure of these pigments is derived from betalamic acid, and depending on the structures added to the main structure, they give rise to betacyanins and betaxanthins [65]. These bioactive compounds are natural antioxidants with a high radical scavenging potential [66]. The betanin molecule includes phenolic and cyclic amine groups, which are potent electron donors that endow betanin with an exceptionally high free radical scavenging ability [67]. Studies have investigated the capacity of betalains, mainly betanin, to scavenge free radicals in vitro, and this capacity is even higher than that of vitamin C [34,68]. Betanin has also been reported to inhibit cancer cell proliferation in vitro and in vivo [18], and it protects against acute lung injury and gastric lesions [30,69].

At high doses, the metabolism of APAP leads to the generation of the highly-reactive metabolite NAPQI, which leads to GSH depletion and the subsequent reaction of NAPQI with cellular proteins and lipids to form APAP adducts. Mitochondria are one of the most important targets of NAPQI, resulting in ATP depletion, oxidative stress and ultimately hepatocyte necrosis [7,8]. It has been reported that the hepatoprotective effect of some natural products is related to their antioxidant capacity to prevent liver cell damage or death, both prophylactically and therapeutically [70,71].

Our results suggest that the frequent consumption of *Opuntia robusta* and *Opuntia streptacantha* provides many bioactive compounds with antioxidant activity to counteract the cellular oxidative damage caused by APAP acute intoxication. Therapeutic treatment more closely resembles the clinical situation of APAP intoxication; however, the primary goal of this study was to demonstrate the protective effect of *Opuntia* extracts in APAP intoxication. Although we demonstrate in vitro the value of therapeutic treatment, this needs to be confirmed in vivo, as well. Animal studies have revealed the promising in vivo therapeutic value of antioxidants on liver diseases. Furthermore, APAP is a model of severe oxidative stress, and in many liver diseases, oxidative stress precedes or aggravates existing liver diseases (e.g., in non-alcoholic liver diseases). In fact, oxidative stress is considered as a common mechanism of liver injury in many (chronic) liver diseases, and the application of antioxidants is a rational strategy to prevent or ameliorate liver diseases involving oxidative stress [72]. Therefore, there is certainly value in the prophylactic use of *Opuntia* extracts as anti-oxidants, and we are currently testing *Opuntia* extracts in other models of (oxidative) liver damage.

The CYP2E1 enzyme is considered to be the main enzyme responsible for APAP biotransformation, and this enzyme is predominantly expressed in the centrilobular region [73]. In line with this, we observed the most prominent histological damage in the centrilobular area (Zones II/III of the hepatic acinus). Our histological data are also consistent with necrotic hepatocyte loss. This is confirmed by our in vitro data that clearly show that necrosis (Sytox green, LDH leakage) is the predominant mode of cell death in APAP intoxication. The *Opuntia* extracts are still protective when added up to 4 h after APAP intoxication, and in this respect, they are superior to NAC, the currently-used therapy for ALF induced by APAP. The reason for this might be that the *Opuntia* extracts contain a multitude of components that counteract oxidative damage via different mechanisms. Future studies should identify the components of *Opuntia* extracts that contribute to this protective effect.

In summary, we provide evidence that both *Opuntia* fruit extracts contain many bioactive compounds with antioxidant activity to counteract the oxidative damage caused by APAP. Our results also suggest that the daily ingestion of *Opuntia streptacantha* and *Opuntia robusta* fruit extracts at the indicated doses can increase liver detoxification and could be used as a dietary supplement to prevent APAP-induced acute liver failure. Finally, our results also suggest that the *Opuntia* extracts can be considered for other oxidative stress-related liver diseases like (non-)alcoholic fatty liver diseases.

Acknowledgments: Financial support for these studies was provided by the National Council of Science and Technology Mexico (CONACYT), Grant Number 336940, and the Abel Tasman Talent Program of the University Medical Center Groningen.

Author Contributions: H.A.G.-P., Ma.C.M.-S., A.R.R.-S. and F.J.-J. designed the in vivo experiments; H.A.G.-P., M.B.-H., K.N.F. and H.M. designed the in vitro experiments; H.A.G.-P. performed the in vivo and in vitro experiments; M.T.S.-M. contributed with reagents, materials and instruments for the chemical analysis of the extracts; H.A.G.-P., Ma.C.M.-S., M.T.S.-M., A.R.-R., M.B.-H., K.N.F., H.M. and F.J.-J. analyzed the data; H.A.G.-P. wrote the first draft of the paper; H.M. and F.J.-J. contributed to critical revisions of the text.

Conflicts of Interest: The authors declare no conflict of interest.

Abbreviations

AA	Ascorbic acid
ABTS	2,2'-Azino-bis(3-ethylbenzothiazoline-6-sulphonic acid)
ALF	Acute liver failure
ALP	Alkaline phosphatase
ALT	Alanine aminotransferase
ANOVA	Analysis of variance
APAP	Acetaminophen
AST	Aspartate aminotransferase
CAT	Catalase
Cu/Zn-SOD	Copper/zinc-superoxide dismutase
CYP450	Cytochrome P-450
CYP2E1	Cytochrome P-450 isoform 2E1
DNA	Deoxyribonucleic acid
DPPH	2,2-Diphenyl-1-picrylhydrazyl
EDTA	Ethylenediaminetetraacetic acid
FRAP	Ferric reducing antioxidant power
GPx	Glutathione peroxidase
GSH	Reduced glutathione
LDH	Lactate dehydrogenase
Mn-SOD	Manganese-superoxide dismutase
NAC	*N*-acetyl-L-cysteine
NAPQI	*N*-acetyl-*p*-benzoquinone imine
NSAID	Non-steroidal anti-inflammatory drugs
OPT	*o*-phtaldehyde
ORAC	Oxygen radical absorbance capacity
PAS	Periodic acid Schiff
PSF	Penicillin-streptomycin-fungizone
ROS	Reactive oxygen species
SEM	Standard error of the mean
SD	Standard deviation

References

1. Vonkeman, H.E.; van de Laar, M.A. Nonsteroidal Anti-Inflammatory Drugs: Adverse Effects and Their Prevention. *Semin. Arthritis Rheum.* **2010**, *39*, 294–312. [CrossRef] [PubMed]
2. Jones, R. Nonsteroidal anti-inflammatory drug prescribing: Past, present, and future. *Am. J. Med.* **2001**, *110*, S4–S7. [CrossRef]
3. Rumack, B.H. Acetaminophen misconceptions. *Hepatology* **2004**, *40*, 10–15. [CrossRef] [PubMed]
4. Jaeschke, H.; Bajt, M.L. Intracellular signaling mechanisms of acetaminophen-induced liver cell death. *Toxicol. Sci.* **2005**, *89*, 31–41. [CrossRef] [PubMed]
5. Craig, D.G.N.; Lee, A.; Hayes, P.C.; Simpson, K.J. The current management of acute liver failure. *Aliment. Pharmacol. Ther.* **2010**, *31*, 345–358. [CrossRef] [PubMed]
6. Jaeschke, H.; McGill, M.R.; Williams, C.D.; Ramachandran, A. Current issues with acetaminophen hepatotoxicity—A clinically relevant model to test the efficacy of natural products. *Life Sci.* **2011**, *88*, 737–745. [CrossRef] [PubMed]
7. McGill, M.R.; Jaeschke, H. Metabolism and disposition of acetaminophen: Recent advances in relation to hepatotoxicity and diagnosis. *Pharm. Res.* **2013**, *30*, 2174–2187. [CrossRef] [PubMed]
8. Jaeschke, H.; Knight, T.R.; Bajt, M.L. The role of oxidant stress and reactive nitrogen species in acetaminophen hepatotoxicity. *Toxicol. Lett.* **2003**, *144*, 279–288. [CrossRef]
9. Arai, T.; Koyama, M.; Kitamura, D.; Mizuta, R. Acrolein, a highly toxic aldehyde generated under oxidative stress in vivo, aggravates the mouse liver damage after acetaminophen overdose. *Biomed. Res.* **2014**, *35*, 389–395. [CrossRef] [PubMed]

10. Das, J.; Ghosh, J.; Manna, P.; Sil, P.C. Acetaminophen induced acute liver failure via oxidative stress and JNK activation: Protective role of taurine by the suppression of cytochrome P450 2E1. *Free Radic. Res.* **2010**, *44*, 340–355. [CrossRef] [PubMed]

11. Mahmoodi, M.; Soleimani Mehranjani, M.; Shariatzadeh, S.M.A.; Eimani, H.; Shahverdi, A. *N*-acetylcysteine improves function and follicular survival in mice ovarian grafts through inhibition of oxidative stress. *Reprod. Biomed. Online* **2015**, *30*, 101–110. [CrossRef] [PubMed]

12. Boeing, H.; Bechthold, A.; Bub, A.; Ellinger, S.; Haller, D.; Kroke, A.; Watzl, B. Critical review: Vegetables and fruit in the prevention of chronic diseases. *Eur. J. Nutr.* **2012**, *51*, 637–663. [CrossRef] [PubMed]

13. Poljsak, B.; Šuput, D.; Milisav, I. Achieving the Balance between ROS and Antioxidants: When to Use the Synthetic Antioxidants. *Oxid. Med. Cell. Longev.* **2013**, *2013*, 956792. [CrossRef] [PubMed]

14. Crozier, A.; Del Rio, D.; Clifford, M.N. Bioavailability of dietary flavonoids and phenolic compounds. *Mol. Asp. Med.* **2010**, *31*, 446–467. [CrossRef] [PubMed]

15. Heber, D. Vegetables, fruits and phytoestrogens in the prevention of diseases. *J. Postgrad. Med.* **2004**, *50*, 145–149. [PubMed]

16. Brahmi, D.; Bouaziz, C.; Ayed, Y.; Ben Mansour, H.; Zourgui, L.; Bacha, H. Chemopreventive effect of cactus *Opuntia ficus* indica on oxidative stress and genotoxicity of aflatoxin B1. *Nutr. Metab. (Lond.)* **2011**, *8*, 73. [CrossRef] [PubMed]

17. Illoldi-Rangel, P.; Ciarleglio, M.; Sheinvar, L.; Linaje, M.; Sánchez-Cordero, V.; Sarkar, S. Opuntia in México: Identifying Priority Areas for Conserving Biodiversity in a Multi-Use Landscape. *PLoS ONE* **2012**, *7*, e36650. [CrossRef] [PubMed]

18. Zou, D.; Brewer, M.; Garcia, F.; Feugang, J.M.; Wang, J.; Zang, R.; Zou, C. Cactus pear: A natural product in cancer chemoprevention. *Nutr. J.* **2005**, *4*, 25. [CrossRef] [PubMed]

19. Zorgui, L.; Ayed-Boussema, I.; Ayed, Y.; Bacha, H.; Hassen, W. The antigenotoxic activities of cactus (*Opuntia ficus-indica*) cladodes against the mycotoxin zearalenone in Balb/c mice: Prevention of micronuclei, chromosome aberrations and DNA fragmentation. *Food Chem. Toxicol.* **2009**, *47*, 662–667. [CrossRef] [PubMed]

20. Serra, A.T.; Poejo, J.; Matias, A.A.; Bronze, M.R.; Duarte, C.M.M. Evaluation of *Opuntia* spp. derived products as antiproliferative agents in human colon cancer cell line (HT29). *Food Res. Int.* **2013**, *54*, 892–901. [CrossRef]

21. Díaz Medina, E.M.; Rodríguez Rodríguez, E.M.; Díaz Romero, C. Chemical characterization of Opuntia dillenii and *Opuntia ficus indica* fruits. *Food Chem.* **2007**, *103*, 38–45. [CrossRef]

22. Moussa-Ayoub, T.E.; El-Samahy, S.K.; Rohn, S.; Kroh, L.W. Flavonols, betacyanins content and antioxidant activity of cactus *Opuntia macrorhiza* fruits. *Food Res. Int.* **2011**, *44*, 2169–2174. [CrossRef]

23. Yahia, E.M.; Mondragon-Jacobo, C. Nutritional components and anti-oxidant capacity of ten cultivars and lines of cactus pear fruit (*Opuntia* spp.). *Food Res. Int.* **2011**, *44*, 2311–2318. [CrossRef]

24. Coria Cayupán, Y.S.; Ochoa, M.J.; Nazareno, M.A. Health-promoting substances and antioxidant properties of *Opuntia* sp. fruits. Changes in bioactive-compound contents during ripening process. *Food Chem.* **2011**, *126*, 514–519. [CrossRef]

25. Kuti, J.O. Antioxidant compounds from four *Opuntia cactus* pear fruit varieties. *Food Chem.* **2004**, *85*, 527–533. [CrossRef]

26. Sumaya-Martínez, M.T.; Cruz-Jaime, S.; Madrigal-Santillán, E.; García-Paredes, J.D.; Cariño-Cortés, R.; Cruz-Cansino, N.; Alanís-García, E. Betalain, Acid Ascorbic, Phenolic Contents and Antioxidant Properties of Purple, Red, Yellow and White Cactus Pears. *Int. J. Mol. Sci.* **2011**, *12*, 6452–6468. [CrossRef] [PubMed]

27. Kaur, M. Pharmacological actions of *Opuntia ficus indica*: A Review. *J. App. Pharm. Sci.* **2012**, *2*, 15–18. [CrossRef]

28. Madrigal-Santillán, E.; García-Melo, F.; Morales-González, J.; Vázquez-Alvarado, P.; Muñoz-Juárez, S.; Zuñiga-Pérez, C.; Hernández-Ceruelos, A. Antioxidant and Anticlastogenic Capacity of Prickly Pear Juice. *Nutrients* **2013**, *5*, 4145–4158. [CrossRef] [PubMed]

29. Alimi, H.; Hfaeidh, N.; Bouoni, Z.; Sakly, M.; Ben Rhouma, K. Protective effect of *Opuntia ficus indica* f. inermis prickly pear juice upon ethanol-induced damages in rat erythrocytes. *Alcohol* **2012**, *46*, 235–243. [CrossRef] [PubMed]

30. Kim, S.H.; Jeon, B.J.; Kim, D.H.; Kim, T.I.; Lee, H.K.; Han, D.S.; Sung, S.H. Prickly Pear Cactus (*Opuntia ficus indica* var. saboten) Protects Against Stress-Induced Acute Gastric Lesions in Rats. *J. Med. Food* **2012**, *15*, 968–973. [CrossRef] [PubMed]

31. Wolfram, R.; Budinsky, A.; Efthimiou, Y.; Stomatopoulos, J.; Oguogho, A.; Sinzinger, H. Daily prickly pear consumption improves platelet function. *Prostaglandins Leukot. Essent. Fat. Acids* **2003**, *69*, 61–66. [CrossRef]

32. Jaeschke, H.; Williams, C.D.; McGill, M.R.; Xie, Y.; Ramachandran, A. Models of drug-induced liver injury for evaluation of phytotherapeutics and other natural products. *Food Chem. Toxicol.* **2013**, *55*, 279–289. [CrossRef] [PubMed]

33. Jia, Z.; Tang, M.; Wu, J. The determination of flavonoid contents in mulberry and their scavenging effects on superoxide radicals. *Food Chem.* **1999**, *64*, 555–559.

34. Stintzing, F.C.; Herbach, K.M.; Mosshammer, M.R.; Carle, R.; Yi, W.; Sellappan, S.; Akoh, C.C.; Bunch, R.; Felker, P. Color, Betalain Pattern, and Antioxidant Properties of Cactus Pear (*Opuntia* spp.) Clones. *J. Agric. Food Chem.* **2005**, *53*, 442–451. [CrossRef] [PubMed]

35. Dürüst, N.; Sümengen, D.; Dürüst, Y. Ascorbic acid and element contents of foods of Trabzon (Turkey). *J. Agric. Food Chem.* **1997**, *45*, 2085–2087. [CrossRef]

36. Georgé, S.; Brat, P.; Alter, P.; Amiot, M.J. Rapid Determination of Polyphenols and Vitamin C in Plant-Derived Products. *J. Agric. Food Chem.* **2005**, *53*, 1370–1373. [CrossRef] [PubMed]

37. Morales, F.J.; Jiménez-Pérez, S. Free radical scavenging capacity of Maillard reaction products as related to colour and fluorescence. *Food Chem.* **2001**, *72*, 119–125. [CrossRef]

38. Re, R.; Pellegrini, N.; Proteggente, A.; Pannala, A.; Yang, M.; Rice-Evans, C. Antioxidant activity applaying an improved ABTS radicalcation decolorization assay. *Free Radic. Biol. Med.* **1999**, *26*, 1231–1237. [CrossRef]

39. Kuskoski, E.M.; Asuero, A.G.; García-Parilla, M.C.; Troncoso, A.M.; Fett, R. Actividad antioxidante de pigmentos antociánicos. *Braz. J. Food Technol.* **2004**, *24*, 691–693. [CrossRef]

40. Hinneburg, I.; Damien Dorman, H.J.; Hiltunen, R. Antioxidant activities of extracts from selected culinary herbs and spices. *Food Chem.* **2006**, *97*, 122–129. [CrossRef]

41. Gulcin, İ.; Buyukokuroglu, M.E.; Kufrevioglu, O.I. Metal chelating and hydrogen peroxide scavenging effects of melatonin. *J. Pineal Res.* **2003**, *34*, 278–281. [CrossRef] [PubMed]

42. Huang, D.; Ou, B.; Hampsch-Woodill, M.; Flanagan, J.A.; Prior, R.L. High-Throughput Assay of Oxygen Radical Absorbance Capacity (ORAC) Using a Multichannel Liquid Handling System Coupled with a Microplate Fluorescence Reader in 96-Well Format. *J. Agric. Food Chem.* **2002**, *50*, 4437–4444. [CrossRef] [PubMed]

43. Conde de la Rosa, L.; Schoemaker, M.H.; Vrenken, T.E.; Buist-Homan, M.; Havinga, R.; Jansen, P.L.M.; Moshage, H. Superoxide anions and hydrogen peroxide induce hepatocyte death by different mechanisms: Involvement of JNK and ERK MAP kinases. *J. Hepatol.* **2006**, *44*, 918–929. [CrossRef] [PubMed]

44. Vrenken, T.E.; Buist-Homan, M.; Kalsbeek, A.J.; Faber, K.N.; Moshage, H. The active metabolite of leflunomide, A77 1726, protects rat hepatocytes against bile acid-induced apoptosis. *J. Hepatol.* **2008**, *49*, 799–809. [CrossRef] [PubMed]

45. Zhou, G.; Chen, Y.; Liu, S.; Yao, X.; Wang, Y. In vitro and in vivo hepatoprotective and antioxidant activity of ethanolic extract from *Meconopsis integrifolia* (Maxim.) Franch. *J. Ethnopharmacol.* **2013**, *148*, 664–670. [CrossRef] [PubMed]

46. Hissin, P.J.; Hilf, R. A fluorometric method for determination of oxidized and reduced glutathione in tissues. *Anal. Biochem.* **1976**, *74*, 214–226. [CrossRef]

47. Maeda, K.; Kimura, M.; Hayashi, S. Cellular mechanism of U78517F in the protection of porcine coronary artery endothelial cells from oxygen radical-induced damage. *Br. J. Pharmacol.* **1993**, *108*, 1077–1082. [CrossRef] [PubMed]

48. Woudenberg-Vrenken, T.E.; Buist-Homan, M.; Conde de la Rosa, L.; Faber, K.N.; Moshage, H. Anti-oxidants do not prevent bile acid-induced cell death in rat hepatocytes. *Liver Int.* **2010**, *30*, 1511–1521. [CrossRef] [PubMed]

49. Gu, J.; Gui, Y.; Chen, L.; Yuan, G.; Lu, H.-Z.; Xu, X. Use of Natural Products as Chemical Library for Drug Discovery and Network Pharmacology. *PLoS ONE* **2013**, *8*, e62839. [CrossRef] [PubMed]

50. Bankova, V. Chemical diversity of propolis and the problem of standardization. *J. Ethnopharmacol.* **2005**, *100*, 114–117. [CrossRef] [PubMed]

51. Kujumgiev, A.; Tsvetkova, I.; Serkedjieva, Y.; Bankova, V.; Christov, R.; Popov, S. Antibacterial, antifungal and antiviral activity of propolis of different geographic origin. *J. Ethnopharmacol.* **1999**, *64*, 235–240. [CrossRef]

52. Anderson, E.F. *The Cactus Family*; Timber Press: Portland, OR, USA, 2001; p. 776.

53. Vinson, J.A.; Su, X.; Zubik, L.; Bose, P. Phenol antioxidants quantity and quality in foods: Fruits. *J. Agric. Food Chem.* **2001**, *49*, 5315–5321. [CrossRef] [PubMed]

54. Van Acker, S.A.; de Groot, M.J.; van den Berg, D.-J.; Tromp, M.N.; Donné-Op den Kelder, G.; van der Vijgh, W.J.; Bast, A. A quantum chemical explanation of the antioxidant activity of flavonoids. *Chem. Res. Toxicol.* **1996**, *9*, 1305–1312. [CrossRef] [PubMed]

55. Nimse, S.B.; Pal, D. Free radicals, natural antioxidants, and their reaction mechanisms. *RSC Adv.* **2015**, *5*, 27986–28006. [CrossRef]

56. Russo, M.; Spagnuolo, C.; Tedesco, I.; Bilotto, S.; Russo, G.L. The flavonoid quercetin in disease prevention and therapy: Facts and fancies. *Biochem. Pharmacol.* **2012**, *83*, 6–15. [CrossRef] [PubMed]

57. Kumar, S.; Pandey, A.K. Chemistry and Biological Activities of Flavonoids: An Overview. *Sci. World J.* **2013**, *2013*, 162750. [CrossRef] [PubMed]

58. Pan, M.-H.; Lai, C.-S.; Ho, C.-T. Anti-inflammatory activity of natural dietary flavonoids. *Food Funct.* **2010**, *1*, 15–31. [CrossRef] [PubMed]

59. Frémont, L.; Gozzélino, M.T.; Franchi, M.P.; Linard, A. Dietary flavonoids reduce lipid peroxidation in rats fed polyunsaturated or monounsaturated fat diets. *J. Nutr.* **1998**, *128*, 1495–1502. [PubMed]

60. Fouad, A.A.; Albuali, W.H.; Zahran, A.; Gomaa, W. Protective effect of naringenin against gentamicin-induced nephrotoxicity in rats. *Environ. Toxicol. Pharmacol.* **2014**, *38*, 420–429. [CrossRef] [PubMed]

61. Yokozawa, T.; Dong, E.; Kawai, Y.; Gemba, M.; Shimizu, M. Protective effects of some flavonoids on the renal cellular membrane. *Exp. Toxicol. Pathol.* **1999**, *51*, 9–14. [CrossRef]

62. Nakayama, M.; Aihara, M.; Chen, Y.-N.; Araie, M.; Tomita-Yokotani, K.; Iwashina, T. Neuroprotective effects of flavonoids on hypoxia-, glutamate-, and oxidative stress-induced retinal ganglion cell death. *Mol. Vis.* **2011**, *17*, 1784. [PubMed]

63. Wu, Y.; Wang, F.; Zheng, Q.; Lu, L.; Yao, H.; Zhou, C.; Wu, X.; Zhao, Y. Hepatoprotective effect of total flavonoids from *Laggera alata* against carbon tetrachloride-induced injury in primary cultured neonatal rat hepatocytes and in rats with hepatic damage. *J. Biomed. Sci.* **2006**, *13*, 569–578. [CrossRef] [PubMed]

64. Pandey, K.B.; Rizvi, S.I. Plant polyphenols as dietary antioxidants in human health and disease. *Oxid. Med. Cell. Longev.* **2009**, *2*, 270–278. [CrossRef] [PubMed]

65. Castellar, R.; Obón, J.M.; Alacid, M.; Fernández-López, J.A. Color Properties and Stability of Betacyanins from *Opuntia* Fruits. *J. Agric. Food Chem.* **2003**, *51*, 2772–2776. [CrossRef] [PubMed]

66. Gandía-Herrero, F.; Escribano, J.; García-Carmona, F. Biological activities of plant pigments betalains. *Crit. Rev. Food Sci. Nutr.* **2016**, *56*, 937–945. [CrossRef] [PubMed]

67. Livrea, M.A.; Tesoriere, L. Lipoperoxyl Radical Scavenging and Antioxidative Effects of Red Beet Pigments. In *Red Beet Biotechnology: Food and Pharmaceutical Applications*; Neelwarne, B., Ed.; Springer: Boston, MA, USA, 2013; pp. 105–124.

68. Wu, L.; Hsu, H.-W.; Chen, Y.-C.; Chiu, C.-C.; Lin, Y.-I.; Ho, J.A. Antioxidant and antiproliferative activities of red pitaya. *Food Chem.* **2006**, *95*, 319–327. [CrossRef]

69. Han, J.; Ma, D.; Zhang, M.; Yang, X.; Tan, D. Natural antioxidant betanin protects rats from paraquat—induced acute lung injury interstitial pneumonia. *Biomed. Res. Int.* **2015**, *2015*, 608174. [CrossRef] [PubMed]

70. Madrigal-Bujaidar, E.; Álvarez-González, I.; Sumaya-Martínez, M.T.; Gutiérrez-Salinas, J.; Bautista, M.; Morales-González, Á.; González-Rubio, M.G.Y.; Aguilar-Faisal, J.L.; Morales-González, J.A. Review of natural products with hepatoprotective effects. *World J. Gastroenterol.* **2014**, *20*, 14787–14804. [CrossRef] [PubMed]

71. Kanner, J.; Harel, S.; Granit, R. Betalains, a new class of dietary cationized antioxidants. *J. Agric. Food Chem.* **2001**, *49*, 5178–5185. [CrossRef] [PubMed]

72. Li, S.; Tan, H.; Wang, N.; Zhang, Z.; Lao, L.; Wong, C.; Feng, Y. The role of oxidative stress and antioxidants in liver diseases. *Int. J. Mol. Sci.* **2015**, *16*, 26087–26124. [CrossRef] [PubMed]

73. Abdelmegeed, M.A.; Moon, K.-H.; Chen, C.; Gonzalez, F.J.; Song, B.-J. Role of cytochrome P450 2E1 in protein nitration and ubiquitin-mediated degradation during acetaminophen toxicity. *Biochem. Pharmacol.* **2010**, *79*, 57–66. [CrossRef] [PubMed]

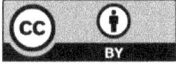

nutrients

MDPI

Article

Effect of Green Tea Extract on Systemic Metabolic Homeostasis in Diet-Induced Obese Mice Determined via RNA-Seq Transcriptome Profiles

Ji-Young Choi [1,2], Ye Jin Kim [1,2], Ri Ryu [1,2], Su-Jung Cho [1,2], Eun-Young Kwon [1,2] and Myung-Sook Choi [1,2,*]

[1] Department of Food Sciences and Nutrition, Kyungpook National University, 1370 Sankyuk Dong Puk-Ku, Daegu 702-701, Korea; jyjy31@hanmail.net (J.-Y.C.); freewilly59@hanmail.net (Y.J.K.); sangsang0119@gmail.com (R.R.); chocrystalhihi@hanmail.net (S.-J.C.); savage20@naver.com (E.-Y.K.)
[2] Center for Food and Nutritional Genomics Research, Kyungpook National University, 1370 Sankyuk Dong Puk-Ku, Daegu 702-701, Korea
* Correspondence: mschoi@knu.ac.kr; Tel.: +82-53-950-6232; Fax: +82-53-950-6229

Received: 13 July 2016; Accepted: 11 October 2016; Published: 14 October 2016

Abstract: Green tea (GT) has various health effects, including anti-obesity properties. However, the multiple molecular mechanisms of the effects have not been fully determined. The aim of this study was to elucidate the anti-obesity effects of GT via the analysis of its metabolic and transcriptional responses based on RNA-seq profiles. C57BL/6J mice were fed a normal, high-fat (60% energy as fat), or high-fat + 0.25% (w/w) GT diet for 12 weeks. The GT extract ameliorated obesity, hepatic steatosis, dyslipidemia, and insulin resistance in diet-induced obesity (DIO) mice. GT supplementation resulted in body weight gain reduction than mice fed high-fat through enhanced energy expenditure, and reduced adiposity. The transcriptome profiles of epididymal white adipose tissue (eWAT) suggested that GT augments transcriptional responses to the degradation of branched chain amino acids (BCAAs), as well as AMP-activated protein kinase (AMPK) signaling, which suggests enhanced energy homeostasis. Our findings provide some significant insights into the effects of GT for the prevention of obesity and its comorbidities. We demonstrated that the GT extract contributed to the regulation of systemic metabolic homeostasis via transcriptional responses to not only lipid and glucose metabolism, but also amino acid metabolism via BCAA degradation in the adipose tissue of DIO mice.

Keywords: energy expenditure; green tea extract; obesity; RNA-seq; transcriptome

1. Introduction

Obesity is a metabolic disorder characterized by excess fat accumulation in the body. It is associated with the development of hyperlipidemia, insulin resistance, type 2 diabetes mellitus, hypertension, and non-alcoholic fatty liver disease [1]. A major proportion of the excess body weight in obese subjects is attributable to the expansion of white adipose tissue (WAT). In obesity, WAT is more closely linked to metabolic complications than other tissues [2], while chronic inflammation in the WAT may play a vital role in the development of obesity related metabolic dysfunction [3]. Meanwhile, adipose tissue is considered as a regulator of energy homeostasis and a key endocrine organ secreting multiple adipokines. These adipokines may contribute to the whole-body homeostasis in normal conditions; however, in an obese state, enlarged adipose tissue leads to the dysregulated secretion of adipokines. The dysregulated production of adipokines in obesity may contribute not only to inflammation, but also to the development of various metabolic diseases via altered lipid and glucose homeostasis [4,5]. While the role of adipose tissue in glucose and lipid metabolism is relatively well known, its role in protein and amino acid metabolism is less well recognized. Several studies provide evidence that adipose tissue also contributes to amino acid metabolism, particularly that of branched chain amino acids (BCAAs) [6,7]. Metabolic diseases are characterized by higher levels of circulating BCAAs, which have recently been recognized as regulators of metabolic homeostasis [7–9]. Moreover, BCAA supplementation or BCAA deficiency is closely associated with the regulation of metabolic homeostasis [10,11].

Green tea (GT) has been widely studied for its health benefits in humans and animals. It contains caffeine and polyphenolic compounds known as catechins. The four major flavonoids in GT are the catechins such as epicatechin (EC), epigallocatechin (EGC), epicatechin gallate (ECG), and epigallocatechin gallate (EGCG). The efficacy of GT may be attributed to the presence of catechin polyphenols, and it has been suggested that EGCG could be responsible for the various health effects associated with GT [12,13]. GT has been reported to have various effects including anti-obesity, antioxidant, anti-hypertensive, anti-diabetic, and anti-inflammatory [13–17]. In particular, GT has been shown to increase energy expenditure [18] and enhance the metabolic rate and fat-burning ability [19,20]. Most recently, Rocha and colleagues [21] reported that GT extract activates AMP-activated protein kinase (AMPK) and ameliorates WAT metabolic dysfunction that is induced by obesity.

In the present study, we investigated the possible mechanisms of the anti-obesity effect of GT extract by focusing on its phenotypic and transcriptional responses in an obesogenic animal model. This is the first report on the efficacy of GT, with epididymal white adipose tissue (eWAT) and liver tissue transcriptomes obtained from RNA-seq.

2. Materials and Methods

2.1. Animals

Thirty 4-week-old male C57BL/6J mice were obtained from The Jackson Laboratory (Bar Harbor, ME, USA). All mice were individually housed at a constant temperature (24 °C) and with 12-h light/dark cycles. The mice were fed a normal chow diet for an acclimatization period of 1 week after their arrival. At 5 weeks of age, they were randomly divided into 3 groups of 10 mice per group, and fed either a normal diet (ND), high-fat diet (HFD), or HFD + 0.25% (*w*/*w*) GT extract for 12 weeks. The ND (AIN-93G, TD94045, Harlan, Madison, WI, USA) contained 17.2% kcal from fat, 18.8% kcal from protein, and 63.9% kcal from carbohydrate, while the HFD (TD06414, Harlan, Madison, WI, USA) contained 60.3% kcal from fat, 18.4% kcal from protein, and 21.3% kcal from carbohydrate. GT ethanol extract was obtained from Bioland (Ansan, Korea) and it was a functional food ingredient approved by the Ministry of Food and Drug Safety (MFDS, formerly known as the Korea Food & Drug Administration (KFDA)). The GT extract contained 40.5% catechins, which comprised 4.8% EC, 11.16% EGC, 3.16% ECG, and 21.33% EGCG, and 3.39% caffeine. The human dose of GT, determined based on the MFDS guidelines, is 500 mg/day for adults as catechin. The human GT dose was converted to a mouse dose using the body surface area normalization method [22]. The mice were provided free access to food and distilled water, while food intake, and body weight were measured daily and weekly, respectively. At the end of the diet period, all mice were anesthetized with isoflurane after a 12-h fast. Blood was taken from the inferior vena cava for determination of glucose, plasma lipid, and hormone concentrations. The liver and adipose tissue were removed, rinsed with physiological saline, weighed, immediately frozen in liquid nitrogen, and then stored at −70 °C until use. The animal study protocols were approved by the Ethics Committee of Kyungpook National University (KNU 2012-136).

2.2. Measurement of Energy Expenditures

Energy expenditure was measured using an indirect calorimeter (Oxylet; Panlab, Cornella, Spain) in five randomly selected mice per group during final week. The mice were placed into individual metabolic chambers at 25 °C, with free access to food and water. Oxygen and carbon dioxide analyzers were calibrated with high-purity gas. Oxygen consumption and carbon dioxide production were recorded at 3-min intervals, using a computer-assisted data acquisition program, (Chart 5.2; AD Instrument, Sydney, Australia) over a 24-h period, and the data were averaged for each mouse. Energy expenditure (EE) was calculated according to the following formula:

$$EE \ (kcal \cdot day^{-1} \cdot bodyweight^{-0.75}) = VO_2 \times 1.44 \times (3.815 + (1.232 \times VCO_2/VO_2)) \qquad (1)$$

2.3. Analysis of Plasma and Hepatic Lipids

Enzymatic assays to determine the plasma free fatty acid, total cholesterol and triglyceride levels were performed using kits purchased from Asan Pharm Co. (Seoul, Korea). Hepatic lipid was extracted according to the methods described by Folch [23]. This was followed by the determination of cholesterol and triglyceride levels using the same enzymatic kit used for the plasma analyses. The hepatic fatty acid level was measured using the Wako enzymatic kit (Wako Chemicals, Richmond, VA, USA). Plasma and hepatic lipids measurements were performed in triplicate.

2.4. Levels of Plasma Aspartate Aminotransferase (AST) and Alanine Aminotransferase (ALT)

AST and ALT activities were measured in triplicate using commercially available kits (Asan Pharm Co., Seoul, Korea).

2.5. Plasma Glucose and Insulin Resistance Index

The plasma glucose level was measured in triplicate using commercially available kit (Asan Pharm Co., Seoul, Korea). The homeostasis model assessment for insulin resistance (HOMA-IR) was calculated using the following formula:

$$HOMA\text{-}IR = (fasting\ insulin\ concentration\ (mU/L)) \times (fasting\ glucose\ concentration$$
$$(mg/dL) \times 0.05551)/22.5 \qquad (2)$$

2.6. Plasma Hormones, Adipokines, and Proinflammatory Cytokines

Plasma concentrations of hormones (insulin and glucagon) and adipokines (leptin, resistin, and plasminogen activator inhibitor 1 (PAI-1)) were quantified in triplicate using a multiplex detection kit (171-F7001M, Bio-Rad, Hercules, CA, USA) according to the manufacturer's protocol. Plasma concentrations of adiponectin and plasma cytokines (interferon γ (IFN-γ), monocyte chemoattractant protein 1 (MCP-1), and tumor necrosis factor α (TNF-α)) were quantified in triplicate using a detection kit (171-F7002M, Bio-Rad, Hercules, CA, USA) and multiplex detection kit (M60-009RDPD, Bio-Rad), respectively, according to the manufacturer's instructions.

2.7. Hepatic Enzyme Activities and Glycogen Concentration

Fatty acid β-oxidation and malic enzyme activities were measured in triplicate according to previously described protocols [24–26]. Microsomal HMG-CoA reductase (HMGCR) activity was measured in triplicate using [^{14}C]-HMG-CoA and [^{14}C]-Oleoyl CoA as substrates [27]. The hepatic glycogen concentration was determined in triplicate as previously described [28].

2.8. Histological Analysis of eWAT and the Liver

The liver and eWAT were excised from each mouse, fixed in 10% (v/v) paraformaldehyde in PBS, and embedded in paraffin for staining with hematoxylin and eosin (H & E), and Masson's trichrome (MT) dye. The stained slices were examined under an optical microscope (Zeiss Axioscope) at 200$\times$ magnification [29].

2.9. RNA Preparation, Library Preparation, and RNA-Seq

The eWAT and liver were collected from three randomly selected mice from each of the ND, HFD, and GT groups. Total RNA was extracted from the eWAT using TRIzol reagent (Invitrogen Life Technologies, NY, USA) according to the manufacturer's instructions. After synthesizing cDNA libraries, their quality was evaluated using an Agilent 2100 BioAnalyzer (Agilent, CA, USA). The cDNA libraries were quantified using the KAPA Library Quantification Kit (Kapa Biosystems, Boston, MA, USA). After cluster amplification of the denatured templates, samples in flow cells were sequenced as paired-end polymers (2 × 100 bp) using the Illumina HiSeq2500 (Illumina, San Diego, CA, USA).

2.10. Preprocessing of the RNA-Seq Data

Low-quality reads were filtered out according to the following criteria: reads containing >10% of skipped bases (marked as N's), reads containing >40% of bases whose quality scores were <20, and reads whose average quality score was <20. The filtering process was performed using in-house scripts. The remaining reads were mapped onto the mouse reference genome (Ensembl, release 72), using the aligner software STAR version 2.3.0e [30]. The gene expression levels were measured using Cufflinks version 2.1.1 [31], using the gene annotation database of Ensembl, release 72. The noncoding gene regions were removed by means of the mask option. To improve the accuracy of the measurement, "multiread correction" and "frag bias-correct" options were used. All other options were set to the default values.

2.11. Differential Transcriptome and Functional Analysis

For differential expression analysis, the data on gene level counts were generated using HTSeq-count version 0.5.4p3 [32]. Using the resulting read count data, differentially expressed genes (DEGs) were identified using the R software package, TCC (Bioconductor open source project) [33]. The TCC package uses robust normalization strategies to compare tag count data. Normalization factors were calculated using the iterative DEGES/edgeR method. The q-value was calculated from the p value using the p.adjust function in the R package and the default settings. DEGs were identified based on a q-value threshold of less than 0.05. K-means clustering was performed in the Bioinformatics Toolbox of MATLAB R2009a.

2.12. Molecular Pathway and Function Analysis

The DEG lists were analyzed using the Ingenuity Pathway Analysis (IPA) software (IPA, Ingenuity® systems, Qiagen, CA, USA). IPA allows for the identification of network interactions and pathway interactions between genes, based on an extensive manually curated database of published gene interactions. We uploaded the genes with a q-value threshold of less than 0.05, and a fold change in expression of more than 1.5, after HFD, with or without GT supplementation, and the associated expression value from the RNA-seq data into IPA.

2.13. Statistical Analysis

Results were expressed as the mean ± standard error of the mean (SEM). Differences among the ND, HFD, and GT groups were assessed for significance using one-way analysis of variance (one-way ANOVA), as calculated using the SPSS v18.0 software (SPSS Inc., Chicago, IL, USA). Any differences identified between groups at each time-point were analyzed further using Duncan's multiple-range post-hoc test. Results were considered statistically significant at $p < 0.05$.

3. Results

3.1. Supplementation with GT Ethanol Extract Reduced Body Weight Gain and Body Fat Mass with Enhanced Energy Expenditure and Plasma Lipid and Glucose Profiles in Diet-Induce Obesity (DIO) Mice

Body weight and body weight gain were significantly lower in the GT group than in the HFD group (Figure 1A,B). For this reason, the food efficiency ratio (FER) was significantly lower in the GT group than in the HFD group (Figure 1D). Similar to the trends observed in body weight, liver weight per 100 g of body weight was significantly lower in the GT-treated group than in the HFD group. The significant reductions in kidney and muscle weights observed in the HFD group were reversed upon treatment with GT (Figure 1E). Furthermore, treatment with GT resulted in significant decreases in the weights of perirenal, mesenteric, interscapular, and visceral tissue, in addition to total WAT when compared with the HFD group (Figure 1F).

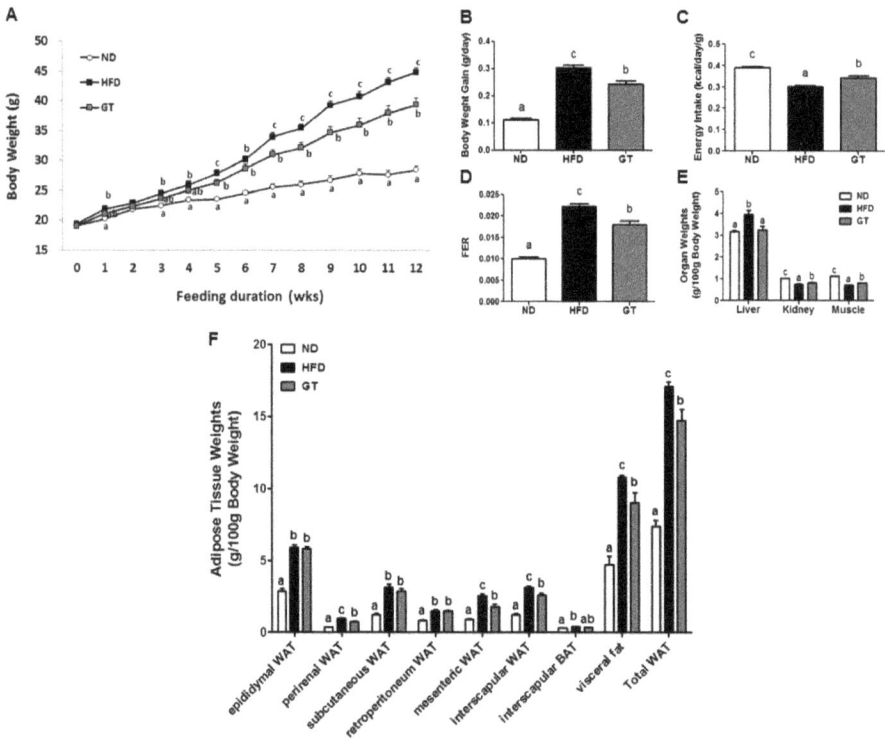

Figure 1. (**A**) Changes in body weight over 12 weeks; (**B**) body weight gain; (**C**) differences in energy intake; (**D**) food efficiency ratio; (**E**) organ weight; and (**F**) adipose tissue (AT) weights in diet-induced obese C57BL/6J mice treated with green tea extract for 12 weeks. The data are shown as mean ± standard error of the mean. [a-c] Mean values not sharing a common superscript were significantly different among the groups ($p < 0.05$). ND, normal diet, AIN-93G; HFD, high-fat diet, 60% kcal from fat; GT, green tea extract (0.25%, w/w). FER, Food efficiency ratio = body weight gain/energy intake per day. Energy intake (kcal/day/g) = food intake (g/day) × calories (kcal/g) × body weight (g). The energy intake was normalized by mouse body weight.

The energy expenditure decreased in the HFD group relative to the ND group during both light and dark phases, while GT supplementation significantly augmented the energy expenditure during the dark phase (Figure 2A,B). Furthermore, GT-treated mice exhibited higher oxygen consumption

(VO$_2$) than HFD-fed mice during the dark phase (Figure 2C). Plasma-free fatty acid and total-cholesterol levels were significantly lower in the GT group than in the HFD group (Figure 2D). Plasma glucose and insulin levels were also significantly reduced with GT supplementation after 12 weeks compared to that in the HFD group. Additionally, the HOMA-IR was significantly lower in the GT group than in the HFD group, which indicates decreased insulin resistance. The HFD-induced elevation in hepatic glycogen was attenuated by GT supplementation (Figure 2E).

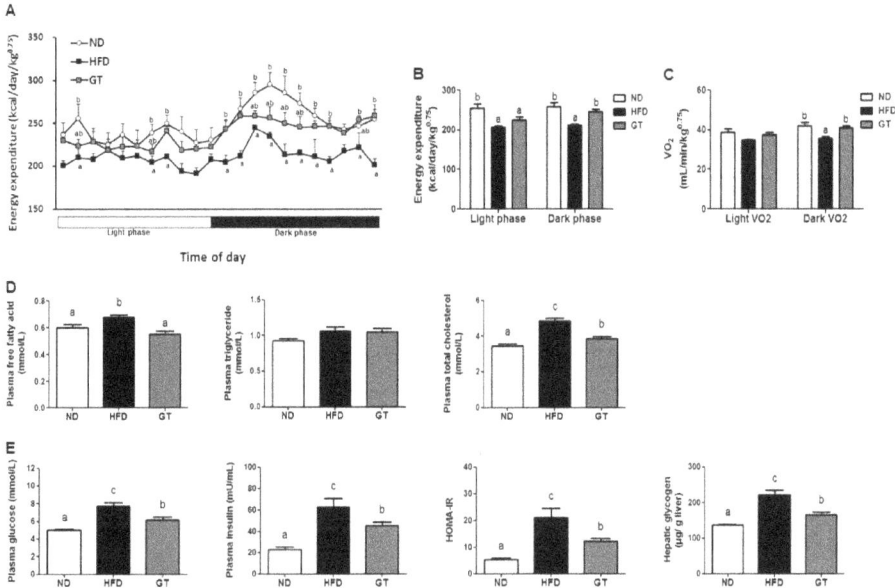

Figure 2. (**A,B**) Energy expenditure; (**C**) oxygen consumption (VO$_2$); (**D**) plasma lipid profiles; and (**E**) glucose metabolism-related markers in diet-induced obese C57BL/6J mice treated with green tea extract for 12 weeks. The data are shown as mean ± standard error of the mean. [a–c] Mean values not sharing a common superscript were significantly different among the groups ($p < 0.05$). ND, normal diet, AIN-93G; HFD, high-fat diet, 60% kcal from fat; GT, green tea extract (0.25%, w/w).

3.2. GT Ethanol Extract Attenuated the Level of Plasma Adipokines in DIO Mice and Modulated Transcriptional Responses to a HFD in eWAT

The epididymal adipocyte size in the HFD group was visibly larger than in the ND-fed mice. Treatment with GT reduced the epididymal adipocyte size when compared to the size in HFD-fed mice. According to the results of MT staining, HFD-fed mice exhibited visible morphological evidence of fibrosis when compared to the ND-fed mice, while no signs of fibrotic changes were identified in the GT group (Figure 3A). The plasma leptin and resistin levels were remarkably lower in GT-treated mice than in the HFD-fed mice. In contrast, plasma adiponectin levels were significantly elevated in the GT group (Figure 3B) than in the ND and HFD groups. Furthermore, GT supplementation resulted in a significant decrease in the plasma levels of tumor necrosis factor α (TNF-α), monocyte chemoattractant protein 1 (MCP-1), plasminogen activator inhibitor 1 (PAI-1), and interferon γ (IFN-γ) when compared to HFD group (Figure 3C).

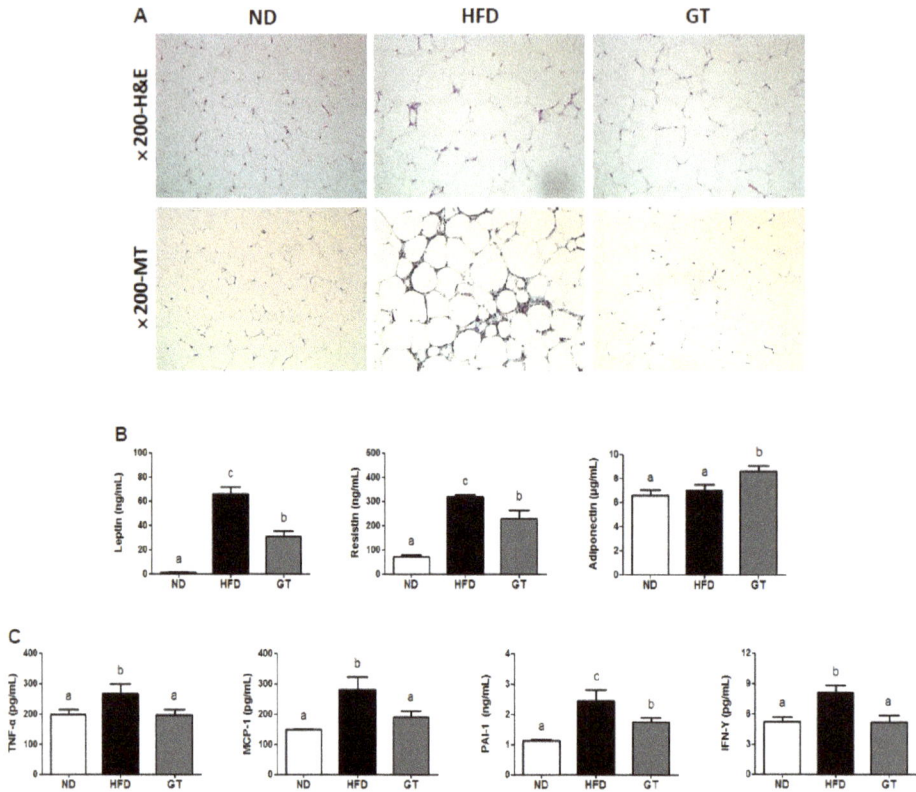

Figure 3. (**A**) Hematoxylin and eosin staining (H & E; upper panel) and Masson's trichrome staining (MT; lower panel) of epididymal adipocytes (magnification 200×); and (**B,C**) differences in plasma adipokines in diet-induced obese C57BL/6J mice treated with green tea extract for 12 weeks. The data are shown as mean ± standard error of the mean. [a–c] Mean values not sharing a common superscript were significantly different among the groups ($p < 0.05$). ND, normal diet, AIN-93G; HFD, high-fat diet, 60% kcal from fat; GT, green tea extract, 0.25% *w/w*.

To identify the global transcriptomic profiles associated with obesity and its comorbidities, we performed RNA-seq on eWAT and liver samples obtained from the ND, HFD, and GT groups and systematically analyzed the results. First, we identified differentially expressed genes (DEGs) between HFD-fed and GT-treated mice using the cutoff set to a fold change of ≥1.5 and a *q*-value of <0.05. In the eWAT, 1173 DEGs were identified between GT-treated and HFD-fed mice (703 upregulated and 470 downregulated). Next, we identified significant molecular pathways and functions when comparing GT to HFD groups using ingenuity pathway analysis (IPA). GT supplementation resulted in the up-regulation of AMPK signaling-related genes such as *Acacb*, *Adipoq*, *Adra1a*, *Adrb3*, *Akt2*, *Cpt2*, *Eef2k*, *Gys1*, *Insr*, *Irs2*, *Lipe*, *Mlycd*, *Nos3*, *Pfkfb3*, *Prkag2*, *Prkar2b*, and *Slc2a4* of adipose tissue in DIO mice (Figure 4A,B). Among the significant canonical pathways, triacylglycerol biosynthesis and degradation, and fatty acid β-oxidation pathway related genes, were up-regulated by GT supplementation (Figure 5A–C). Furthermore, GT supplementation increased the transcriptional response involved in thermogenesis (Figure 5D).

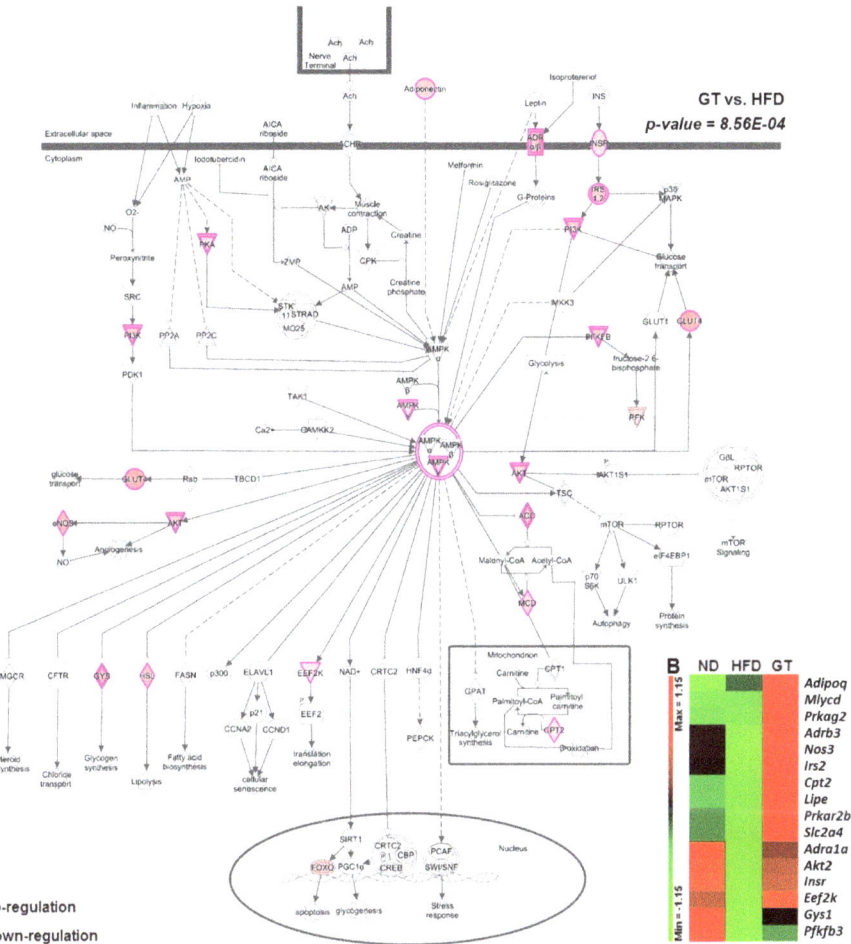

Figure 4. (**A**) Canonical pathway; and (**B**) heat map of the genes related to the AMP-activated protein kinase (AMPK) signaling pathway in epididymal white adipose tissue (eWAT) of diet-induced obese C57BL/6J mice treated with green tea extract for 12 weeks. ND, normal diet, AIN-93G; HFD, high-fat diet, 60% kcal from fat; GT, green tea extract, 0.25% *w/w*. The significant pathways and functions were obtained via Ingenuity Pathway Analysis (IPA).

Degradation pathways of amino acids, including valine, proline, alanine, histidine, leucine, tryptophan, tyrosine, and isoleucine, were also significantly altered by GT supplementation. It augmented the transcriptional response to the degradation of BCAA in the eWAT of DIO mice, and valine degradation was identified as the most significant canonical pathway among 298 canonical pathways based on IPA. The expression of genes related to the degradation of leucine and isoleucine was also up-regulated by GT supplementation (Figure 6A). In particular, mRNA expression of the branched-chain α-keto dehydrogenase (BCKD) complex components (*Bckdha*, *Bckdhb*, and *Dbt*) of the eWAT in DIO mice was significantly up-regulated by GT supplementation (Figure 6B).

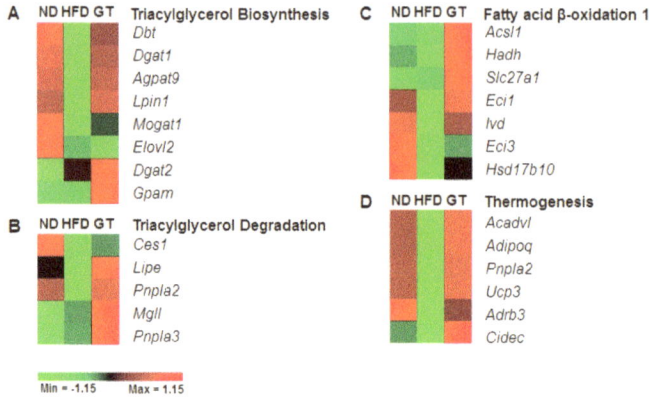

Figure 5. Expression profiles of lipid metabolism-related genes in epididymal white adipose tissue (eWAT) of diet-induced obese C57BL/6J mice treated with green tea extract for 12 weeks. ND, normal diet, AIN-93G; HFD, high-fat diet, 60% kcal from fat; GT, green tea extract, 0.25% w/w. The significant pathways and functions were obtained via Ingenuity Pathway Analysis (IPA).

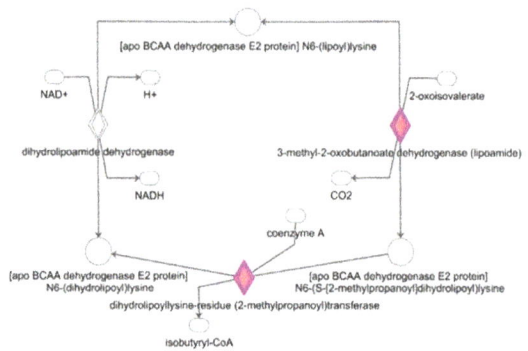

Figure 6. (**A**) A heat map of the genes involved in amino acid degradation; and (**B**) the transcriptional response related to branched-chain α-keto dehydrogenase (BCKD) in the epididymal white adipose tissue (eWAT) of diet-induced obese C57BL/6J mice treated with green tea extract for 12 weeks. The significant pathways were obtained via Ingenuity Pathway Analysis (IPA).

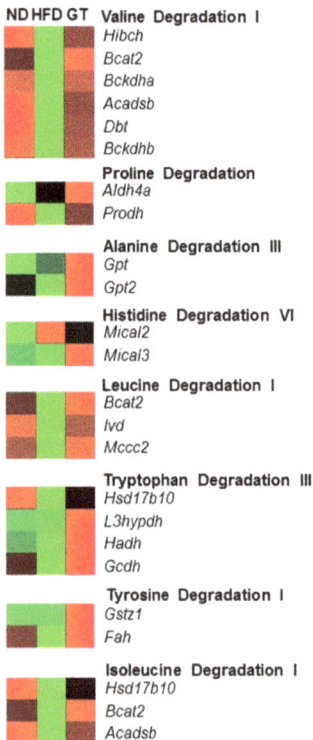

3.3. GT Extract Ameliorated Hepatic Steatosis via the Metabolic and Transcriptional Responses in the Livers of DIO Mice

The morphology of hepatic tissue revealed a decrease in the accumulation of hepatic lipid droplets in the GT group. MT staining of the liver also demonstrated no fibrotic changes in the ND and GT groups, whereas fibrosis was observed around the vessels in the HFD group (Figure 7A). Hepatic fatty acids, triglyceride, and cholesterol contents of the GT group were significantly lower when compared to the HFD group (Figure 7B). Although there was no significant difference in the activity of β-oxidation between GT and HFD groups, the activities of HMG-CoA reductase (HMGCR) and malic enzyme were markedly reduced in the GT group relative to the HFD group (Figure 7C). Furthermore, the levels of plasma aspartate aminotransferase (AST) and alanine aminotransferase (ALT), markers of hepatic toxicity, were significantly decreased by GT supplementation (Figure 7D).

The RNA-seq data revealed several adaptive molecular functions and pathways that partly explain why GT-treated mice were protected from the pathological conditions present in DIO mice. In the liver, 1561 DEGs were identified between the GT-treated and HFD-fed mice (1119 up-regulated and 442 down-regulated). The most significant identified pathway was the hepatic fibrosis/hepatic stellate cell activation of 289 canonical pathways obtained from IPA. The majority of hepatic fibrosis/hepatic stellate cell activation-associated genes were down-regulated in the liver upon GT-treatment (Figure 7E). Furthermore, GT attenuated transcriptional regulation such as the transport and synthesis of lipids in DIO mice (Figure 7F,G). It also reversed the transcriptional response associated with insulin resistance in the HFD (Figure 7H).

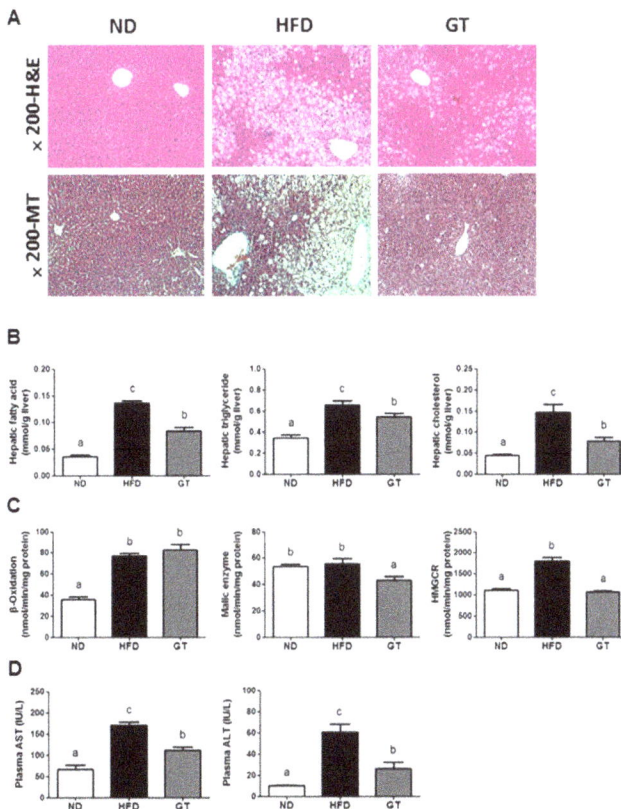

Figure 7. *Cont.*

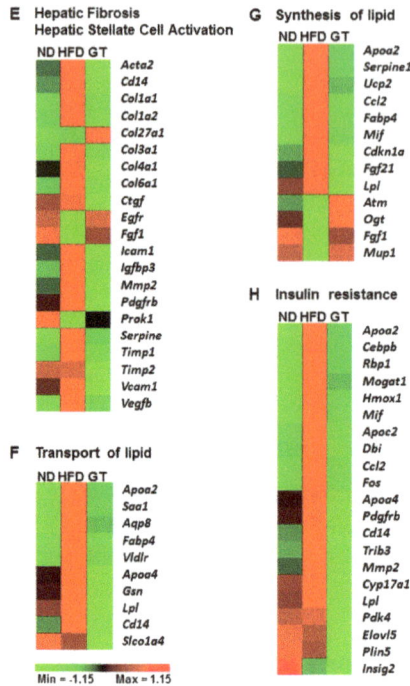

Figure 7. (**A**) Hematoxylin and eosin staining (H & E, upper panel) and Masson's trichrome (MT, lower panel) staining of the liver (magnification 200×); (**B**) hepatic lipid profiles; (**C**) hepatic activities of lipid-regulating enzymes; (**D**) plasma aspartate aminotransferase (AST) and alanine aminotransferase (ALT) levels; and (**E–H**) Heat map of the genes involved in hepatic fibrosis/hepatic stellate cell activation, transport of lipid, synthesis of lipid and insulin resistance in the liver of diet-induced obese C57BL/6J mice treated with green tea extract for 12 weeks. The data are shown as mean ± standard error of the mean. a–c Mean values not sharing a common superscript were significantly different among the groups ($p < 0.05$). ND, normal diet, AIN-93G; HFD, high-fat diet, 60% kcal from fat; GT, green tea extract, 0.25% *w/w*. The significant pathways and functions were obtained via Ingenuity Pathway Analysis (IPA).

4. Discussion

In this study, we have shown the multiple effects of GT extract that are involved in ameliorating metabolic disturbances in DIO mice. GT treatment attenuated HFD-induced obesity, dyslipidemia, hepatic steatosis, insulin resistance, and the inflammatory response. In the current study, we evaluated the effect of GT and the potential mechanisms underlying its metabolic regulation using RNA-seq transcriptomic profiles in a DIO model. The transcriptomic profiles based on RNA-seq revealed several adaptive mechanisms that may explain why GT-treated mice were protected from the pathological changes that occurred in HFD-fed mice.

We were able to find significant canonical pathways and molecular functions via IPA based on the DEGs between GT-treated and HFD-fed mice. In this study, GT supplementation resulted in the up-regulation of AMPK signaling-related genes in the eWAT of DIO mice. In particular, the expressions of *Adipoq* and *Adrb3*, considered to be AMPK activation factors, were significantly augmented and the expression of *Glut4* (also known as *Slc2a4*), a major glucose transporter, was also up-regulated because of GT supplementation. AMPK is a key regulator of cellular energy metabolism and the whole-body energy balance [34]. Previous studies reveal that EGCG, major catechin of green tea extract, and green tea extract activate AMPK in various cell lines and tissues. Several reports suggest that EGCG inhibits adipogenesis through activation of AMPK in 3T3-L1 cells [35,36] and EGCG anti-diabetic effects essentially depended on the AMPK activation in rat L6 muscle cells [37]. Moreover, EGCG prevents fatty liver by AMPK activation via liver kinase B1 inhibiting mediators responsible for the synthesis of fatty acid and de novo lipogenesis in mice fed a HFD [38]. In addition, similar effects of GT supplementation in the prevention of the deleterious effects of HFD have been supported by Rocha et al., whose results suggested that GT extract could improve WAT metabolic dysfunction induced via activation of AMPK [21]. Thus, GT supplementation contributed to the energy homeostasis of adipose tissue via the regulation of the AMPK signaling pathway in DIO mice. Furthermore, GT supplementation promoted the expression of genes involved in lipolysis, fatty acid oxidation, and thermogenesis in adipose tissue. Despite upregulating transcriptional pathways involved in triacylglycerol biosynthesis in adipose tissue, GT markedly reduced the WAT weights. It is plausible that GT restricts triglyceride availability by increasing lipolysis, oxidation, and thermogenesis prior to lipid droplet formation in adipose tissue. These transcriptional responses in the WAT suggest that although GT activates lipogenesis, it also simultaneously increases lipolysis, fatty acid oxidation, and thermogenesis, which may contribute to the reduction in adiposity.

Another possible explanation for the observed body fat reduction could be the increased transcriptional response of BCAA degradation upon treatment with GT when compared to the HFD group. Based on the IPA, the transcriptional profiles of the eWAT of GT-treated DIO mice were strongly linked with amino acid degradation, particularly BCAAs. The BCAAs, leucine, isoleucine, and valine, are three of the nine essential amino acids that have been recently recognized as regulators of metabolic homeostasis [8]. Several studies have reported that abnormal BCAA levels are associated with various metabolic diseases in both humans and rodents [6,9,39]. BCAA homeostasis is mainly controlled by BCKD, the rate-limiting enzyme in BCAA catabolism [40], the expression of which is reduced in an obese state [6]. While the role of adipose tissue in glucose and lipid metabolism is relatively well known, its role in protein and amino acid metabolism is less well recognized. Several studies have provided evidence of adipose tissue contributing to amino acid metabolism, particularly BCAAs [6,7]. In this study, GT supplementation augmented the mRNA expression of the BCKD complex components, *Bckdha*, *Bckdhb*, and *Dbt*, in the eWAT of DIO mice. A previous study reported that WAT BCKD protein was significantly reduced in various obesity models (fa/fa rats, *db/db* mice, and DIO mice), and that BCKD component transcripts were significantly lower in adipocytes from obese versus lean subjects [6]. Lian and colleagues [41] reported that impaired adiponectin signaling contributed to the disturbed catabolism of BCAA in diabetic mice. In the current study, both mRNA expression of *Adipoq* in the eWAT, and plasma adiponectin levels, were markedly up-regulated by GT supplementation in DIO mice. Therefore, it is thought that the GT extract contributes to whole-body homeostasis partly via increased transcriptional response to the degradation of BCAAs in the eWAT of DIO mice.

GT supplementation increased energy expenditure during the dark phase, without a difference in the energy intake of DIO mice. Accordingly, GT-treated mice were more metabolically active than HFD-fed mice, which was again reflected in their lower body weight and body fat mass. Consistent with the reduced adiposity, GT supplementation improved endocrine secretion, including a reduction in chemokines, cytokines, and hormone levels in mice fed an HFD. Plasma leptin and resistin levels were higher in HFD-fed mice than in ND-fed mice; however, this change was attenuated in GT-treated mice. In contrast, plasma adiponectin, a regulator of energy homeostasis, was significantly elevated by GT supplementation, with a concomitant increase in the mRNA expression of *Adipoq* in the eWAT. The accumulation of excess body fats was related to the augmentation of inflammatory markers including TNF-α, MCP-1, PAI-1, and IFN-γ. The down-regulation of these markers in GT-treated mice suggests that GT may suppress inflammation and improve immune responses.

HFD commonly induces metabolic alterations, which include dyslipidemia and hepatic steatosis. However, GT supplementation attenuated the plasma and hepatic lipid contents, with decreased hepatic lipogenic enzyme activities (malic enzyme and HMCGR). This suggests that GT may limit hepatic lipid availability by inhibiting lipogenesis, thereby, reducing hepatic lipotoxicity markers such as AST and ALT. A histological examination of liver tissue from GT-treated DIO mice revealed a reduction in lipid droplets when compared with the HFD group, indicating an amelioration of hepatic steatosis. In addition, notable hepatic fibrosis was observed around the vessels in the livers of HFD-fed mice, whereas the livers of mice in the GT group revealed no fibrotic changes. The alteration of these phenotype markers in GT-treated mice was underpinned by the transcriptomic profiles of the liver. Our present data obtained by IPA demonstrate that hepatic fibrosis/hepatic stellate cell activation is the most significant canonical pathway among the 289 canonical pathways. The hepatic stellate cell is the key cellular element involved in the development of hepatic fibrosis [42]. GT supplementation attenuated the expression of hepatic fibrosis/hepatic stellate cell activation-related genes, which was accompanied with the down-regulation of genes for lipid transport and synthesis. Accordingly, these transcriptional responses may contribute to the attenuation of hepatic steatosis as well as fibrosis.

There are limitations to this study. First, we only reported phenotype characteristics and transcriptomic profiles without direct evidence of each potential transcriptional pathway. In addition, it is difficult to distinguish the cause of increased energy expenditure that is product of increased movement, increased resting energy expenditure, or a combination, due to absence of physical activity data. Despite the aforementioned limitations, the present findings provide important insights into the mechanism by which the GT extract exerts its anti-obesity effects and ameliorates metabolic complications such as adiposity, dyslipidemia, hepatic steatosis, and insulin resistance. This modulation occurs partly through an increase in energy expenditure, and via metabolic and transcriptional regulation in the WAT and livers of DIO mice.

5. Conclusions

In conclusion, the overall metabolic and transcriptional responses to the GT extract in DIO proved to be desirable. GT contributes to systemic metabolic homeostasis via the transcriptional regulation of BCAA degradation, as well as lipid and glucose metabolism in adipose tissue.

Supplementary Materials: The following are available online at http://www.mdpi.com/2072-6643/8/10/640/s1, Table S1: Primer sequences used for RT-qPCR, Figure S1: Validation of RNA-seq data by RT-qPCR.

Acknowledgments: This work was supported by the Bio-Synergy Research Project (NRF-2012M3A9C4048818) and the Science Research Center Project (NRF-2015R1A5A6001906) of the Ministry of Science, ICT and Future Planning through the National Research Foundation of Korea.

Author Contributions: J.-Y.C. performed the experiments, analyzed the data and wrote/edited the manuscript. Y.J.K., R.R., S.-J.C. and E.-Y.K. performed the experiments and reviewed the manuscript. M.-S.C. supervised this work and had full access to all data and therefore takes full responsibility for the integrity of the results and accuracy of the data analysis.

Conflicts of Interest: The authors declare no conflict of interest.

Abbreviations

ALT	alanine aminotransferase
AMPK	AMP-activated protein kinase
AST	aspartate aminotransferase
BCAAs	branched chain amino acids
BCKD	branched-chain α-keto dehydrogenase
DEGs	differentially expressed genes
DIO	diet-induced obesity
EC	epicatechin
ECG	epicatechin gallate
EGC	epigallocatechin
EGCG	epigallocatechin gallate
eWAT	epididymal white adipose tissue
FER	food efficiency ratio

GT	green tea
HFD	high-fat diet
HMGCR	HMG-CoA reductase
HOMA-IR	homeostasis model assessment for insulin resistance
IFN-γ	interferon γ
IPA	ingenuity pathway analysis
MCP-1	monocyte chemoattractant protein 1
ND	normal diet
PAI-1	plasminogen activator inhibitor 1
TNF-α	tumor necrosis factor α

References

1. Kopelman, P.G. Obesity as a medical problem. *Nature* **2000**, *404*, 635–643. [PubMed]
2. Gesta, S.; Tseng, Y.H.; Kahn, R.C. Developmental origin of fat: Tracking obesity to its source. *Cell* **2007**, *131*, 242–256. [CrossRef] [PubMed]
3. Xu, H.; Barnes, G.T.; Yang, Q.; Tan, G.; Yang, D.; Chou, C.J.; Sole, J.; Nichols, A.; Ross, J.S.; Tartaglia, L.A.; et al. Chronic inflammation in fat plays a crucial role in the development of obesity-related insulin resistance. *J. Clin. Investig.* **2003**, *112*, 1821–1830. [CrossRef] [PubMed]
4. Kershaw, E.E.; Flier, J.S. Adipose tissue as an endocrine organ. *J. Clin. Endocrinol. Metab.* **2004**, *89*, 2548–2556. [CrossRef] [PubMed]
5. Hauner, H. Secretory factors from human adipose tissue and their functional role. *Proc. Nutr. Soc.* **2005**, *64*, 163–169. [CrossRef] [PubMed]
6. Lackey, D.E.; Lynch, C.J.; Olson, K.C.; Mostaedi, R.; Ali, M.; Smith, W.H.; Karpe, F.; Humphreys, S.; Bedinger, D.H.; Dunn, T.N.; et al. Regulation of adipose branched-chain amino acid catabolism enzyme expression and cross-adipose amino acid flux in human obesity. *Am. J. Physiol. Endocrinol. Metab.* **2013**, *304*, E1175–E1187. [CrossRef] [PubMed]
7. Herman, M.A.; She, P.; Peroni, O.D.; Lynch, C.J.; Kahn, B.B. Adipose Tissue Branched Chain Amino Acid (BCAA) Metabolism Modulates Circulating BCAA Levels. *J. Biol. Chem.* **2010**, *285*, 11348–11356. [CrossRef] [PubMed]
8. Lynch, C.J.; Adams, S.H.; Christopher, J.; Lynch, S.H.A. Branched-chain amino acids in metabolic signalling and insulin resistance. *Nat. Rev. Endocrinol.* **2014**, *10*, 723–736. [CrossRef] [PubMed]
9. McCormack, S.E.; Shaham, O.; McCarthy, M.A.; Deik, A.A.; Wang, T.J.; Gerszten, R.E.; Clish, C.B.; Mootha, V.K.; Grinspoon, S.K.; Fleischman, A. Circulating Branched-chain Amino Acid Concentrations Are Associated with Obesity and Future Insulin Resistance in Children and Adolescents. *Pediatr. Obes.* **2013**, *8*, 52–61. [CrossRef] [PubMed]
10. Freudenberg, A.; Petzke, K.J.; Klaus, S. Dietary L-leucine and L-alanine supplementation have similar acute effects in the prevention of high-fat diet-induced obesity. *Amino Acids* **2013**, *44*, 519–528. [CrossRef] [PubMed]
11. Guo, F.; Cavener, D.R. The GCN2 eIF2alpha kinase regulates fatty-acid homeostasis in the liver during deprivation of an essential amino acid. *Cell Metab.* **2007**, *5*, 103–114. [CrossRef] [PubMed]
12. Wolfram, S.; Wang, Y.; Thielecke, F. Anti-obesity effects of green tea: From bedside to bench. *Mol. Nutr. Food Res.* **2006**, *50*, 176–187. [CrossRef] [PubMed]
13. Bose, M.; Lambert, J.D.; Ju, J.; Reuhl, K.R.; Shapses, S.A.; Yang, C.S. The Major Green Tea Polyphenol, (−)-Epigallocatechin-3-Gallate, Inhibits Obesity, Metabolic Syndrome, and Fatty Liver Disease in High-Fat-Fed Mice. *J. Nutr.* **2008**, *138*, 1677–1683. [PubMed]
14. Park, H.J.; DiNatale, D.A.; Chung, M.Y.; Park, Y.K.; Lee, J.Y.; Koo, S.I.; O'Connor, M.; Manautou, J.E.; Bruno, R.S. Green tea extract attenuates hepatic steatosis by decreasing adipose lipogenesis and enhancing hepatic antioxidant defenses in *ob/ob* mice. *J. Nutr. Biochem.* **2011**, *22*, 393–400. [CrossRef] [PubMed]
15. Forester, S.C.; Lambert, J.D. The role of antioxidant versus pro-oxidant effects of green tea polyphenols in cancer prevention. *Mol. Nutr. Food Res.* **2011**, *55*, 844–854. [CrossRef] [PubMed]
16. Basu, A.; Betts, N.M.; Mulugeta, A.; Tong, C.; Newman, E.; Lyons, T.J. Green tea supplementation increases glutathione and plasma antioxidant capacity in adults with the metabolic syndrome. *Nutr. Res.* **2013**, *33*, 180–187. [CrossRef] [PubMed]

17. Peng, X.; Zhou, R.; Wang, B.; Yu, X.; Yang, X.; Liu, K.; Mi, M. Effect of green tea consumption on blood pressure: A meta-analysis of 13 randomized controlled trials. *Sci. Rep.* **2014**, *1*, 6251. [CrossRef] [PubMed]
18. Dulloo, A.G.; Duret, C.; Rohrer, D.; Girardier, L.; Mensi, N.; Fathi, M.; Chantre, P.; Vandermander, J. Efficacy of a green tea extract rich in catechin polyphenols and caffeine in increasing 24-h energy expenditure and fat oxidation in humans. *Am. J. Clin. Nutr.* **1999**, *70*, 1040–1045. [PubMed]
19. Diepvens, K.; Westerterp, K.R.; Westerterp-Plantenga, M.S. Obesity and thermogenesis related to the consumption of caffeine, ephedrine, capsaicin, and green tea. *Am. J. Physiol. Regul. Integr. Comp. Physiol.* **2007**, *292*, R77–R85. [CrossRef] [PubMed]
20. Bérubé-Parent, S.; Pelletier, C.; Doré, J.; Tremblay, A. Effects of encapsulated green tea and Guarana extracts containing a mixture of epigallocatechin-3-gallate and caffeine on 24 h energy expenditure and fat oxidation in men. *Br. J. Nutr.* **2005**, *94*, 432–436. [CrossRef] [PubMed]
21. Rocha, A.; Bolin, A.P.; Cardoso, C.A.; Otton, R. Green tea extract activates AMPK and ameliorates white adipose tissue metabolic dysfunction induced by obesity. *Eur. J. Nutr.* **2015**, *55*, 2231–2244. [CrossRef] [PubMed]
22. Reagan-Shaw, S.; Nihal, M.; Ahmad, N. Dose translation from animal to human studies revisited. *FASEB J.* **2008**, *22*, 659–661. [CrossRef] [PubMed]
23. Folch, J.; Lees, M.; Sloane-Stanley, G.H. A simple method for the isolation and purification of total lipides from animal tissues. *J. Biol. Chem.* **1957**, *226*, 497–509. [PubMed]
24. Lazarow, P.B. Assay of peroxisomal β-oxidation of fatty acids. *Methods Enzymol.* **1981**, *72*, 315–319. [PubMed]
25. Markwell, M.A.; McGroarty, E.J.; Bieber, L.L.; Tolbert, N.E. The Subcellular Distribution of Carnitine Acyltransferases in Mammalian Liver and Kidney A new peroxisomal enzyme. *J. Biol. Chem.* **1973**, *248*, 3426–3432. [PubMed]
26. Ochoa, S. Malic dehydrogenase from pig heart: L-Malate + DPN$^+$ ⇆ Oxalacetate + DPNH + H$^+$. *Methods Enzymol.* **1955**, *1*, 735–739.
27. Shapiro, D.J.; Nordstrom, J.L.; Mitschelen, J.J.; Rodwell, V.W.; Schimke, R.T. Micro assay for 3-hdyroxy-3-methylglutaryl-CoA reductase in rat liver and in L-cell fibroblasts. *Biochim. Biophys. Acta* **1974**, *70*, 369–377. [CrossRef]
28. Seifter, S.; Dayton, S.; Novic, B.; Muntwyler, E. The estimation of glycogen with the anthrone reagent. *Arch. Biochem.* **1950**, *25*, 191–200. [PubMed]
29. Do, G.M.; Jung, U.J.; Park, H.J.; Kwon, E.Y.; Jeon, S.M.; McGregor, R.A.; Choi, M.S. Resveratrol ameliorates diabetes-related metabolic changes via activation of AMP-activated protein kinase and its downstream targets in *db/db* mice. *Mol. Nutr. Food Res.* **2012**, *56*, 1282–1291. [CrossRef] [PubMed]
30. Dobin, A.; Davis, C.A.; Schlesinger, F.; Drenkow, J.; Zaleski, C.; Jha, S.; Batut, P.; Chaisson, M.; Gingeras, T.R. STAR: Ultrafast universal RNA-seq aligner. *Bioinformatics* **2013**, *29*, 15–21. [CrossRef] [PubMed]
31. Trapnell, C.; Williams, B.A.; Pertea, G.; Mortazavi, A.; Kwan, G.; van Baren, M.J.; Salzberg, S.L.; Wold, B.J.; Pachter, L. Transcript assembly and quantification by RNA-Seq reveals unannotated transcripts and isoform switching during cell differentiation. *Nat. Biotechnol.* **2010**, *8*, 511–515. [CrossRef] [PubMed]
32. Anders, S.; Pyl, P.T.; Huber, W. HTSeq-a Python framework to work with high-throughput sequencing data. *Bioinformatics* **2015**, *31*, 166–169. [CrossRef] [PubMed]
33. Sun, J.; Nishiyama, T.; Shimizu, K.; Kadota, K. TCC: An R package for comparing tag count data with robust normalization strategies. *BMC Bioinf.* **2013**, *14*, 219. [CrossRef] [PubMed]
34. Long, Y.C.; Zierath, J.R. AMP-activated protein kinase signaling in metabolic regulation. *J. Clin. Investig.* **2006**, *116*, 1776–1783. [CrossRef] [PubMed]
35. Hwang, J.T.; Park, I.J.; Shin, J.I.; Lee, Y.K.; Lee, S.K.; Baik, H.W.; Ha, J.; Park, O.J. Genistein, EGCG, and capsaicin inhibit adipocyte differentiation process via activating AMP-activated protein kinase. *Biochem. Biophys. Res. Commun.* **2005**, *338*, 694–699. [CrossRef] [PubMed]
36. Moon, H.S.; Chung, C.S.; Lee, H.G.; Kim, T.G.; Choi, Y.J.; Cho, C.S. Inhibitory effect of (−)-epigallocatechin-3-gallate on lipid accumulation of 3T3-L1 cells. *Obesity* **2007**, *15*, 2571–2582. [CrossRef] [PubMed]
37. Zhang, Z.F.; Li, Q.; Liang, J.; Dai, X.Q.; Ding, Y.; Wang, J.B.; Li, Y. Epigallocatechin-3-*O*-gallate (EGCG) protects the insulin sensitivity in rat L6 muscle cells exposed to dexamethasone condition. *Phytomedicine* **2010**, *17*, 14–18. [CrossRef] [PubMed]
38. Santamarina, A.B.; Oliveira, J.L.; Silva, F.P.; Carnier, J.; Mennitti, L.V.; Santana, A.A.; de Souza, G.H.; Ribeiro, E.B.; Oller do Nascimento, C.M.; Lira, F.S.; et al. Green Tea Extract Rich in Epigallocatechin-3-Gallate

Prevents Fatty Liver by AMPK Activation via LKB1 in Mice Fed a High-Fat Diet. *PLoS ONE* **2015**, *10*, e0141227. [CrossRef] [PubMed]

39. She, P.; Van Horn, C.; Reid, T.; Hutson, S.M.; Cooney, R.N.; Lynch, C.J. Obesity-related elevations in plasma leucine are associated with alterations in enzymes involved in branched-chain amino acid metabolism. *Am. J. Physiol. Endocrinol. Metab.* **2007**, *293*, E1552–E1563. [CrossRef] [PubMed]

40. Lu, G.; Sun, H.; She, P.; Youn, J.Y.; Warburton, S.; Ping, P.; Vondriska, T.M.; Cai, H.; Lynch, C.J.; Wang, Y. Protein phosphatase 2Cm is a critical regulator of branched-chain amino acid catabolism in mice and cultured cells. *J. Clin. Investig.* **2009**, *119*, 1678–1687. [CrossRef] [PubMed]

41. Lian, K.; Du, C.; Liu, Y.; Zhu, D.; Yan, W.; Zhang, H.; Hong, Z.; Liu, P.; Zhang, L.; Pei, H.; et al. Impaired adiponectin signaling contributes to disturbed catabolism of branched-chain amino acids in diabetic mice. *Diabetes* **2015**, *64*, 49–59. [CrossRef] [PubMed]

42. Mann, D.A.; Smart, D.E. Transcriptional regulation of hepatic stellate cell activation. *Gut* **2002**, *50*, 891–896. [CrossRef] [PubMed]

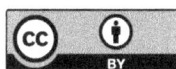

nutrients

MDPI

Review

The Role of Avocados in Maternal Diets during the Periconceptional Period, Pregnancy, and Lactation

Kevin B. Comerford [1,*], Keith T. Ayoob [2,†], Robert D. Murray [3,†] and Stephanie A. Atkinson [4,†]

1   Department of Nutrition, University of California at Davis, Davis, CA 95616, USA
2   Department of Pediatrics, Albert Einstein College of Medicine, Bronx, NY 10461, USA;
    keith.ayoob@einstein.yu.edu
3   Department of Human Sciences, The Ohio State University, Columbus, OH 43210, USA;
    murrayMD@live.com
4   Department of Pediatrics, McMaster University, Hamilton, ON L8S 4KI, Canada; satkins@mcmaster.ca
*   Correspondence: kbcomerford@ucdavis.edu; Tel.: +1-707-799-0699
†   These authors contributed equally to this work.

Received: 18 February 2016; Accepted: 13 May 2016; Published: 21 May 2016

Abstract: Maternal nutrition plays a crucial role in influencing fertility, fetal development, birth outcomes, and breast milk composition. During the critical window of time from conception through the initiation of complementary feeding, the nutrition of the mother is the nutrition of the offspring—and a mother's dietary choices can affect both the early health status and lifelong disease risk of the offspring. Most health expert recommendations and government-sponsored dietary guidelines agree that a healthy diet for children and adults (including those who are pregnant and/or lactating) should include an abundance of nutrient-rich foods such as fruits and vegetables. These foods should contain a variety of essential nutrients as well as other compounds that are associated with lower disease risk such as fiber and bioactives. However, the number and amounts of nutrients varies considerably among fruits and vegetables, and not all fruit and vegetable options are considered "nutrient-rich". Avocados are unique among fruits and vegetables in that, by weight, they contain much higher amounts of the key nutrients folate and potassium, which are normally under-consumed in maternal diets. Avocados also contain higher amounts of several non-essential compounds, such as fiber, monounsaturated fats, and lipid-soluble antioxidants, which have all been linked to improvements in maternal health, birth outcomes and/or breast milk quality. The objective of this report is to review the evidence that avocados may be a unique nutrition source for pregnant and lactating women and, thus, should be considered for inclusion in future dietary recommendations for expecting and new mothers.

Keywords: avocado; monounsaturated fat; oleic acid; fiber; carotenoids; fetal health; maternal diet; pregnancy; lactation

1. Introduction

The federal dietary recommendations in the U.S. only apply to Americans over the age of two years [1], yet one of the most critical times for proper nutrition is in the first two years of life when growth and development rates are at their peak. The development of federal dietary guidelines for maternal, infant, and toddler food patterns are due to be issued in 2020. Ideally, these guidelines should be based on foods and dietary patterns—not simply on nutrients—since the average American can understand and quantify food items much more accurately than individual nutrients. Furthermore, the federal recommendations for pregnant and lactating mothers, and for infants and toddlers, may be more practical and applicable if they included specific food items that are rich in multiple shortfall nutrients and low in empty calories. Doing so would help caregivers better understand what foods in each food group are actually recommended, instead of needing to interpret more complicated nutrient-based recommendations.

The basic cornerstones of a healthy diet for children and adults should include nutrient-rich foods such as fruits and vegetables, which contain a variety of essential nutrients and other health-promoting non-essential compounds such as fiber [2]. These foods should ideally be rich in shortfall nutrients identified in the 2015–2020 Dietary Guidelines for Americans (DGA)—calcium, vitamin D, potassium, and fiber [1]—as well as in key essential nutrients such as folate and iron, which have garnered global scientific support from the World Health Organization and the Food and Agriculture Organization (WHO/FAO) for their beneficial effects on mother-offspring health outcomes [1,3]. For example, breast milk is the ideal food for newborns and infants since it is rich in both essential and shortfall nutrients that are necessary for proper health and development, along with several bioactive compounds which can potentially modulate facets of immunity, digestion and nutrient uptake. Similarly, unsaturated oil-containing fruits such as avocados provide multiple shortfall nutrients without significantly contributing to any of the 2015 DGA nutrients of concern for overconsumption (*i.e.*, sodium and saturated fat), or to empty calories from added sugars (Table 1). Furthermore, the 2015 Dietary Guidelines for Americans Committee (DGAC) report indicates that several other vitamins found in avocados (*i.e.*, vitamin E, folate, and vitamin C) are currently under consumed relative to the estimated average requirement (EAR) for Americans above two years old [2]. Although these nutrients of concern have not yet been directly studied by the DGAC for infant/toddler populations, they are required in higher amounts by pregnant and lactating women compared to the general population [4]. In addition to containing multiple shortfall nutrients, avocados are a source of several promising non-essential compounds, such as monounsaturated fats (MUFA), lipid-soluble antioxidants, and various phytosterols that show promise for maternal, infant, and toddler health (Table 1).

Proper nutrition is never more critical for insuring the quality of human health and reducing the risk for disease than for mothers in the perinatal and neonatal periods, and for infants and toddlers in their first years of life [5]. However, these are difficult populations in whom to conduct clinical experiments due to ethical constraints. There is a need for review of dietary components that may influence health and development during these life stages. These concerns are being addressed by the Birth to 24 months and Pregnant Women Dietary Guidance Development Project expert work groups convened by the U.S. Department of Agriculture (USDA) and Department of Health and Human Services (HHS) [6].

Our paper, the first of a two-part series, covers a large body of epidemiological evidence, and a much smaller body of clinical research that has investigated the effects of dietary patterns, dietary components, and individual nutrients on maternal nutrition during the critical periods of conception, gestation, and lactation. The objective of this report is to review the evidence that dietary patterns which include avocados may provide both nutritive and bioactive components that are ideal for pregnant and lactating women, and thus additional research into the role of avocados should be performed in these populations. Throughout, where applicable, the paper addresses nutrition topic questions posed by the Birth to 24 months and Pregnant Women Dietary Guidance Development Project expert work groups. Two of the four areas of focus for the development project's working groups—Work Group 1—Infancy: Period of Sole Nutrient Source Feeding (0–6 months), and Work Group 4—Caregivers (Mothers and Others)—Factors Influencing Nutrient Needs, Infant Feeding Choice, Dietary Quality and Food Habits—are to investigate factors influencing maternal nutrient needs and infant nutrition extending from pregnancy until the first foods are introduced. While these sub-groups have each been tasked with answering dozens of questions on their respective topics, this report focuses on the following questions that are most closely related to food (especially fruits and vegetables) and nutrient intake, and their effects on birth outcomes and health outcomes:

- What is the influence of maternal dietary intake on micronutrients—including fat-soluble and water-soluble vitamins—and macronutrients—including total fat, *n*-3 polyunsaturated fatty acids (PUFA), *n*-6 PUFA, and *trans* fats—on human milk composition?

- What are the effects of dietary patterns—such as vegan, vegetarian, macrobiotic diets—on breast milk composition?
- What is the relationship between maternal dietary water-soluble vitamin intake and human milk water-soluble vitamin composition?
- What is the relationship between maternal dietary-fat intake and human milk-fat composition?
- What is the relationship between maternal dietary fat-soluble vitamin intake and human milk fat-soluble vitamin composition?

Table 1. California avocado composition (USDA 2015).

	1 Serving, 30 g (1 Ounce)	½ Fruit, 68 g (2.27 Ounces)	Per 100 g (3.33 Ounces)	1 Fruit, 136 g (4.53 Ounces)
Water (g)	22	49	72	98
Energy (kcal)	50	114	167	227
Protein (g)	0.6	1.3	2.0	2.7
Total Lipids (g)	4.6	10.5	15.4	21
Saturated Fat (g)	0.6	1.5	2.1	2.9
Monounsaturated Fat (g)	2.9	6.7	9.8	13.3
Polyunsaturated Fat (g)	0.5	1.2	1.8	2.5
Cholesterol (mg)	0	0	0	0
Stigmasterol (mg)	1.0	1.5	2.0	3
Campesterol (mg)	2.0	3.5	5.0	7
Beta-Sitosterol (mg)	23	51.5	76	103
Total Carbohydrate (g)	2.6	5.9	8.6	11.8
Insoluble Fiber (g)	1.4	3.2	4.8	6.4
Soluble Fiber (g)	0.6	1.4	2.0	2.8
Sugars (g)	0.1	0.2	0.3	0.4
Water-Soluble Vitamins				
Vitamin C (mg)	2.6	6.0	8.8	12
Thiamin (mg)	0	0.1	0.1	0.1
Riboflavin (mg)	0	0.1	0.1	0.2
Niacin (mg)	0.6	1.3	1.9	2.6
Pantothenic acid (mg)	0.4	1.0	1.5	2.0
Vitamin B-6 (mg)	0.1	0.2	0.3	0.4
Folate (μg)	27	60.5	89	121
Choline (mg)	4.3	9.7	14	19.3
Vitamin B-12 (μg)	0	0	0	0
Fat-Soluble Vitamins and Carotenoids				
Vitamin A (μg RAE)	2.0	5.0	7.0	10
Carotene, beta (μg)	19	43	63	86
Carotene, alpha (μg)	7	16.5	24	33
Cryptoxanthin, beta (μg)	8	18.5	27	37
Lutein + zeaxanthin (μg)	81	185	271	369
Vitamin E (α-tocopherol) (mg)	0.6	1.3	2.0	2.7
Vitamin D (μg)	0	0	0	0
Vitamin K1 (phylloquinone) (μg)	6.3	14.3	21	28.6
Minerals				
Calcium (mg)	4.0	9.0	13	18
Magnesium (mg)	9.0	19.5	29	39
Phosphorus (mg)	16	36.5	54	73
Potassium (mg)	152	345	507	690
Sodium (mg)	2	5.5	8	11
Iron (mg)	0.2	0.4	0.6	0.8
Zinc (mg)	0.2	0.5	0.7	0.9
Copper (mg)	0.1	0.1	0.2	0.2
Manganese (mg)	0.1	0.1	0.1	0.2
Selenium (ug)	0.1	0.3	0.4	0.5

Data sourced from: USDA Agricultural Research Service, National Nutrient Database for Standard Reference Release 27. Basic Report: 09038, Avocados, raw, California [7].

2. General Recommendations for Maternal Diet during the Preconceptional Period, Pregnancy, and Lactation

Maternal nutrient intake can affect every major aspect of reproduction from the early peri-conceptional period to the later post-natal stages. In essence, maternal nutrient status influences the entire range of maternal functions: the ability to conceive and maintain a healthy pregnancy [8], produce an effective placenta, assist the offspring's brain and body development, and manufacture adequate and nutritious breast milk [9]. Additionally, the maternal host environment during pregnancy influences gene expression and the health of the offspring for years after birth [10]. It remains unclear just how long before conception the importance of maternal nutrition—and even paternal nutrition [11]—is for the short-term and long-term health of the offspring. What is known is that proper maternal nutrition—especially for key nutrients and bioactives found in fruits and vegetables—is paramount for reducing the risk for congenital birth defects in the critical periods directly before and after conception occurs [12]. Optimal nutrition is a critical factor among all women of childbearing age, even before conception; however, many young mothers are not getting the foods and nutrients they need for themselves or their offspring [13].

The nutrients most commonly associated with prenatal and neonatal health are: iodine, iron, zinc, vitamin A and carotenoids, vitamin D, choline, folate, riboflavin, vitamin B-6 and vitamin B-12, protein, and several specific fatty acids [14–16]. Yet, pregnant women in the U.S. are known to have intakes of folate, potassium, fiber, and vitamins A, D, E, and C well below the EAR [2]. Thus, major deficits can occur especially for nutrients like iron and vitamin B6 which are required in nearly twice the normal recommended dietary allowance of the mother to promote a proper host environment and/or used to nourish the offspring by being passed along through the placenta or breast milk. The addition of healthy and nutrient-dense foods are ideal options for assisting expecting and lactating mothers in reaching their nutritional goals.

3. Adjusting and Improving the Federal Dietary Advice for Pregnancy and Lactation

Failure of women to meet the recommended guidelines during the perinatal period is well documented [17–20]. Whether this is due to unawareness, inability to adhere to, or simply an ambivalence towards the federal dietary recommendations is not clear. What is apparent is that the effects of suboptimal dietary choices in U.S. women are associated with increasing rates of maternal obesity [21] and gestational diabetes [22], both of which increase risks for birth defects [23] and affect lactation [24]. In this regard, the DGA may be too abstract for many expecting American mothers. For example, the federally run website ChooseMyPlate.gov specifically recommends fruits and vegetables that provide potassium and provitamin A for pregnant and breastfeeding mothers [25]. This is ambiguous advice, however, since many Americans do not know which fruits and vegetables best contain these nutrients and why they are important. This lack of understanding tends to lead to suboptimal dietary patterns and an unnecessary deference to supplements instead of food as a primary means of meeting their—and their offspring's—nutritional needs during pregnancy and lactation [26,27]. In order to address nutrition in a way that is more consumer-friendly and impactful, further efforts should be undertaken by the DGA to simplify the dietary recommendations for pregnant and lactating women. For example, providing examples of specific food items—not just nutrients or broad food groups—that are rich in multiple recommended nutrients—such as "eat more salmon, yogurt, walnuts or avocados"—will undoubtedly be better understood by those trying to figure out what to eat.

Currently, the federal dietary advice in the U.S. for pregnant mothers is largely based on what not to eat, such as recommendations to avoid alcohol and empty calories from added sugars and saturated fats [28]. This is valuable advice, but could be improved upon if it gave real-world examples on how to exchange a nutrient-poor food for a nutrient-rich one without losing flavor or textural properties. Recent research from the French Nutrition and Health Survey shows that food substitutions of this nature are a promising and effective dietary strategy for improving nutrient adequacy in the diet of adults [29]. For example, a simple substitution recommendation could be to choose fresh avocado over mayonnaise on a sandwich to reduce saturated fats while adding numerous other essential nutrients, potentially bioactive compounds (e.g., lipophilic antioxidants and phytosterols), and fiber. Another example would be to use an avocado- and yogurt-based dressing in place of many nutrient-poor commercial options in order to avoid added sugars and saturated fats while adding protein, fiber, and fat-soluble vitamins.

4. Maternal Diet: Effects on Fertility, Fetal Growth, and Birth Outcomes

Pregnant women have a higher requirement for many essential and non-essential nutrients during gestation. The most heavily researched nutrients for fetal health can be narrowed down to a few different groups: (1) micronutrients that regulate DNA synthesis, cell division, and growth (*i.e.*, folate, B-12, vitamin A, vitamin D, iron, and zinc); (2) nutrients that assist with brain development (*i.e.*, iodine and specific fatty acids); and (3) antioxidant nutrients which protect against free radical damage and DNA mutation (*i.e.*, vitamin A and carotenoids, vitamin C, and vitamin E). Another important class of nutrients for fetal health not currently recognized is regulatory nutrients—such as fiber and potassium—which may improve maternal health status (*i.e.*, reduce the risk of diseases such as hypertension, dyslipidemia, and gestational diabetes) [30–32], thereby potentially producing a more favorable host environment and reducing pregnancy and birth complications associated with maternal disease [31,33].

Infertility affects over 10% of U.S. women of reproductive age [34], or approximately one in six couples during their reproductive years [35]. While the current state of scientific knowledge on preconception diets is improving, there is still limited information available to date [11]. Studies that have investigated the effects of diet on fertility have shown that weight loss in overweight and obese women can improve insulin sensitivity, which is a key factor in improving fertility [8,36,37]. Studies have also shown that certain foods or diet plans can improve fertility [38]—in particular, diet plans involving increased fruit and vegetable intake, as well as increased intake of certain high-fat foods (e.g., dairy foods, foods like avocados that contain unsaturated plant oils, and fish oils) and reduced intake of other high-saturated fat foods (*i.e.*, red and processed meat, and foods that contain *trans* fats) [8].

4.1. Mediterranean-Style Diet and Fertility

The 2015 DGAC report recognized several dietary patterns (e.g., USDA-style, vegetarian-style, and Mediterranean-style) that can support beneficial health outcomes for the general population, including pregnant and breastfeeding mothers [2]. A particularly well-researched eating plan associated with general health and maternal health is a Mediterranean-style diet. A Mediterranean-style diet varies by region, but is traditionally based on regular intake of antioxidant- and fiber-rich fruits and vegetables, lean choices of protein, omega-3s in the form of fatty fish, whole grains, and MUFA from plant oils. A maternal Mediterranean-style diet has been associated with significantly improved health outcomes such as lower total and low-density cholesterol levels for the mother and up to a 90% lower risk for preterm delivery [39].

While avocados are not part of the "traditional" Mediterranean-style diet, according to the Mediterranean diet pyramid created by Oldways (a non-profit food and nutrition education organization), along with the Harvard School of Public Health and the WHO, avocados are Mediterranean-style foods because they are classified as an antioxidant- and fiber-rich fruit and have a fatty acid profile that is naturally rich in MUFA [40]. Two-thirds of the fatty acid content of avocados are MUFA. Several recent studies have shown that a greater adherence to a Mediterranean-style diet may enhance fertility rates by reducing the risk of obesity, hypertension [41], insulin resistance [42], and diabetes [43] in pregnant women. A Mediterranean-style diet has been associated with nearly a 70% lower risk of ovulatory disorders in infertile women [8] when compared to diets that are high in *trans* fats.

4.2. Low-Glycemic Diets: Effects on Fertility, Maternal Health, and Fetal Health Outcomes

The association between a low-glycemic maternal diet and birth outcomes begins in the pre-pregnancy period, with a lower intake of high-glycemic foods having been shown to increase the chances of fertility [44,45]. An analysis of the Nurses' Health Study population showed that higher intakes of MUFA, vegetable protein, fiber, and low-glycemic carbohydrates were associated with improved fertility outcomes in the Nurses' Health Study II population [35]. All of the dietary components listed above are also dietary components (or tenets) of a Mediterranean-style diet [46] and oil-containing fruits such as avocados (Figure 1). It should be noted that this research was gathered from women with no history of infertility [35] so it is still unknown how these findings apply to women with known fertility issues.

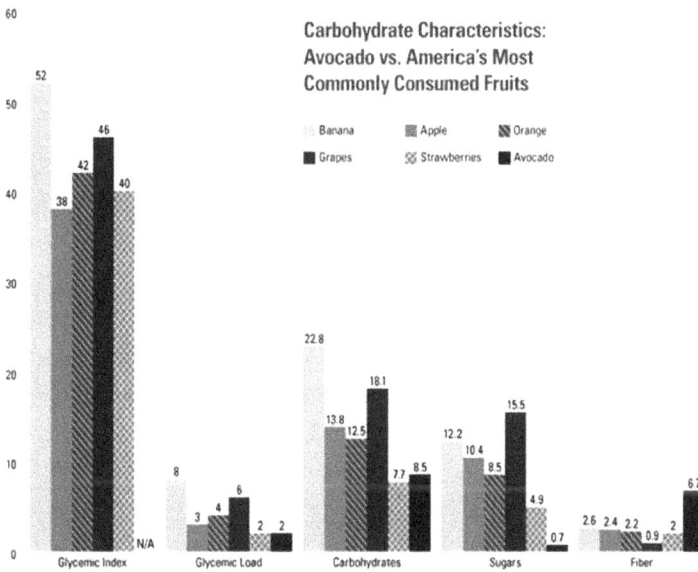

Figure 1. Carbohydrate Characteristics: Avocado vs. America's Most Commonly Consumed Fruits. Glycemic Index Scale: Glucose = 100. Carbohydrates, sugars, and fiber are all listed per 100 g serving. There are no glycemic index values given for avocados because they contain so few carbohydrates that it would be difficult for people to consume a large enough portion (50 g of available carbohydrates) to properly perform glycemic index testing. Data sources: Nutrients—USDA Nutrient Database for Standard Reference 27 [47,48]; Glycemic Load and Glycemic Index—International table of glycemic index and glycemic load values [49].

Randomized trials show that a low-glycemic index diet can be used in the management of gestational diabetes by reducing an expectant mother's need for insulin [50] and by improving maternal glycemia [51]—all while reducing the negative effects of maternal insulin resistance and hyperglycemia on the developing fetus. When compared to a high-glycemic diet, the effects of a low-glycemic diet are further seen (or more importantly not seen) throughout the offspring's early life in the form of a reduced rate for birth defects (*i.e.*, encephalocele, diaphragmatic hernia, small intestinal atresia/stenosis, and atrial septal defects) [23]. A low-glycemic maternal diet has also been associated with offspring birth weight, birth length, adiposity, and arterial wall thickness [52,53], and later life reductions in biomarkers for metabolic syndrome (*i.e.*, insulin levels, leptin levels, and homeostatic model assessment of insulin resistance [HOMA-IR]) [54]. Overall, dietary patterns that are based on nutrient-rich, low-glycemic foods, such as legumes, non-starchy vegetables, and oil-containing fruits, offer great building blocks for a nutritious dietary pattern for both a mother and her offspring.

4.3. Maternal Intake of Fruits and Vegetables

Fruits and vegetables are nutrient-dense foods and key components of all USDA recommended dietary patterns. Fruits and vegetables have been linked to reductions in numerous types of disease and deficiency states [55,56], largely because they contain essential nutrients and bioactive compounds [57], but also because consumption of fruits and vegetables generally displaces the consumption of other less nutrient-rich foods. Many of the essential nutrients in fruits and vegetables are the same nutrients that are recommended for mothers during the periconceptional and perinatal periods. [58]. Fruits and vegetables are also whole-food sources of fiber, magnesium, and vitamin C, as well as thousands of relatively unstudied bioactive compounds, including various antioxidants and phytosterols [59,60], which may also have modulatory effects on pregnancy outcomes. At present, the available evidence regarding maternal consumption of fruits and vegetables, especially those rich in multiple short-fall nutrients, supports their importance as part of a healthy and protective diet throughout pregnancy and early life [58,61,62]. In both highly developed and developing countries, however, fruit and vegetable intake levels for pregnant women are typically much lower than recommended and may contribute to increased risk of poor fetal development [58].

After conception occurs, fetal growth rate is one of the most useful indicators of an offspring's ability to survive and thrive later in life. Approximately 8% of infants in the U.S. are born with a low-birth-weight [63]. A suboptimal fetal growth rate—as well as an excessive fetal growth rate—has been associated with developmental issues in early life, childhood, and adolescence. Additional evidence even suggests that poor fetal nutrition increases the risk for poor health outcomes such as obesity, impaired bone health, immune dysfunction, impaired mental health, and cardiometabolic disease (e.g., cardiovascular disease and type 2 diabetes) many years later in life [63–65].

The growth and development of a fetus is dependent on several factors, some of which may occur before conception. Some data suggest fetal growth and development can be influenced by the nutritional status of the mother prior to and at the time of conception [66], but these findings have yet to be confirmed. What is currently known from epidemiological studies is that nutrient-poor maternal nutrition is associated with fetal disease [67] and below average fetal growth [63]. In regards to fetal health, the data suggest that an imbalance between dietary intake of macronutrients and micronutrients contributes to the pathogenesis of complex birth defects, and that specific dietary modifications, such as increased consumption of fruits and vegetables, may be able to help reduce the risk and severity of various defects.

In 2004, a case-control study of 206 mothers with a child that had a non-syndromic orofacial cleft and 203 control mother-child dyads, showed that a higher pre-conceptional intake of nutrients predominantly present in fruits and vegetables (*i.e.*, fiber, vegetable protein, beta-carotene, ascorbic acid, alpha-tocopherol, magnesium, and iron) was associated with a lowered risk for orofacial clefts in the offspring [68]. However, this study was limited in that all of the participants were Caucasian, and confounders such as body mass index (BMI) and physical activity were not adjusted for. Additionally, in 2004, a similar case-control study involving Caucasian women investigated the associations between maternal diet and risk for spina bifida in the offspring (106 cases and 181 controls). The researchers found that low pre-conceptional intakes of plant-based nutrients were associated with a two- to five-fold increase in spina bifida risk [69]. Taken together, these findings strengthen the advice that in order to lower the risk for orofacial and neural-tube defects in their children, women of child-bearing age should consume a balanced diet, with nutrient-rich fruits and vegetables before and after conception.

Fruit and vegetable intake is also associated with a reduced risk for preeclampsia (*i.e.*, maternal hypertension and proteinuria) [33,70] and insulin resistance [71]. When compared to the relatively low-calorie and low-protein options provided by most fruits and vegetables, it seems reasonable that birth weight is most strongly correlated with high-protein and high-calorie foods since those foods are associated with muscle and adipose tissue expansion in adults. Surprisingly, a 2006 prospective cohort study of 44,612 Danish women found that when pregnant mothers followed a high-calorie, high-protein Western-style diet (*i.e.*, higher amounts of red and processed meat, low fruit and vegetable intake, *etc.*), they tended to have an increased risk for low birth weight for gestational age compared to those who consumed fewer calories and greater quantities of plant foods [64]. A much smaller study of 2466 rural Indian mothers and their babies also showed similar results, where higher intakes of protein and calories by the mother were not associated with offspring birth weight, but green leafy vegetables and fruits were [72]. Therefore, it is unclear as to whether certain components of a high animal-protein and high-fat diet impair fetal growth, or if certain components in fruits and vegetables—such as key micronutrients—are uniquely responsible for proper fetal growth. It is most likely not simply one or the other, but rather that animal-based foods, fruits, and vegetables can all modulate fetal growth to varying degrees. The association found between fruit and vegetable intake and birth weight suggest the existence of potential micronutrient or phytochemical combinations present in plant-based foods that play an important role in optimal fetal development [62]. The types of nutrients from fruits and vegetables and their roles in fetal development deserve further investigation.

5. Maternal Intake of Key Avocado Compounds: Effects on Fertility, Fetal Health, and Birth Outcomes

5.1. MUFA—Oleic Acid

Among the classes of nutrients most frequently associated with fertility are lipids—especially fatty acids and fatty acid ratios—which appear to be key modulators of human fecundity [73]. The majority of research on fatty acid intake in pregnant mothers has focused on essential fatty acid intake—especially long-chain polyunsaturated fatty acids (LCPUFA) such as DHA. MUFA, however, also deserve attention for fetal health and birth outcomes.

The association between intake of MUFA in pregnant women and their offspring was demonstrated by Agostoni *et al.* who collected blood on 16 healthy women and their newborns to determine their whole blood-fatty acid profile. They found that MUFA made up approximately 29% of the blood fatty acids of pregnant mothers, 18% of the umbilical cord blood, and 23% of the blood of a newborn infant [74]. The MUFA oleic acid (18:1*n*-9) comprised approximately 75%–85% of the total MUFA in these blood compartments. Additional research by Agostoni *et al.* on 144 infants showed that MUFA levels were significantly lower in newborn infants who were small for gestational age when compared to those who were born appropriate for gestational age (23% *vs.* 25%, respectively) [75]. There were no differences in total PUFA or saturated fatty acids (SFA) in blood lipid profiles between groups. It is unclear from the report as to why this difference occurred, or as to whether increased MUFA consumption by the mother was responsible for the difference in size. Nonetheless, it is clear that MUFA (especially oleic acid) make up a large portion of an infant's blood fatty acid profile, and that the role of MUFA in gestational development should continue to be investigated. Furthermore, a recent case-control study of 11 cases of gastroschisis (a congenital birth defect where the baby's intestines and other internal organs can push out through a hole in the abdominal wall) and 34 controls, provided evidence that a peri-conceptional maternal diet rich in oleic acid may be able to significantly lower the odds of gastroschisis in the offspring [76]. In addition, mothers who had higher intake of vegetables had an even lower chance of having an infant with gastroschisis.

In their analysis of the Nurses' Health Study II, Chavarro and Willet analyzed the effects of lipid intake (cholesterol, fatty acids, and fatty acid ratios) on fertility in more than 18,500 women in the U.S. The researchers found that consuming just 2% of energy from unprocessed MUFA instead of hydrogenated *trans* fats was associated with less than half of the risk of ovulatory infertility [8]. A potential explanation for these findings is that certain unsaturated fatty acids, such as unprocessed MUFA from fruits or vegetables, can bind to the peroxisome proliferator-activated receptor γ (PPAR-γ), and thereby reduce inflammation and improve ovulatory function [77]. The researchers concluded that higher intake of unprocessed MUFA (commonly found in non-hydrogenated vegetable oils and oil-containing fruits) and lower intakes of *trans* fats may lead to lower incidences of ovulatory infertility [8]. A further study by Chavarro *et al.* investigated the effects of fat intake on preclinical and clinical outcomes in women undergoing *in vitro* fertilization (IVF) [78]. The researchers found that greater intakes of MUFA were related to nearly three and half times higher odds of live birth after embryo transfer, compared to lower intakes of MUFA. A recent critical review of the available literature on diet and fertility by Sinska *et al.* came to similar conclusions as Chavarro and Willet. After reviewing the current evidence, the Sinska group suggested that a larger intake of MUFA can help to improve a woman's fertility, while the intake of *trans* fats should be avoided [44]. Avocados are a well-tolerated food that can serve as an important source of lipids such as MUFA. An ounce of avocado provides 4.6 g total fat, 3 g of that is MUFA—primarily in the form of oleic acid [79].

5.2. Fiber

Fiber intake by Americans is low enough to be of public health concern [1]. According to the 2015 DGAC report, only 8% of women who were pregnant had adequate intake of fiber [2]. In 2012, Blumfield *et al.* performed a review of dietary intakes of pregnant women in developed countries and found that fiber intakes were consistently below the recommended levels [80]. Although fiber is generally not considered an essential nutrient—sometimes it is even referred to as an "anti-nutrient" since it can inhibit the absorption of certain nutrients [81]—it is still an important dietary component for maternal and fetal health [9,61]. Low fiber intake is associated with an increased risk for several maternal diseases (*i.e.*, chronic constipation, type 2 diabetes, and hypertension/preeclampsia) that can all dramatically affect the fetal environment [9,82]. Studies on fiber intake in pregnant women and the risk for preeclampsia and gestational diabetes consistently encourage greater maternal fiber intake for a reduced risk for both diseases [31,33,83].

Although there are different types and forms of dietary fiber, most of the observational research on fiber intake during pregnancy does not distinguish which type of fiber was consumed, and usually just aggregates all fibers into a general intake value. Many whole plant foods contain either predominantly soluble or insoluble fiber, but avocados contain a mix of both. Even a modest portion of avocado—30 g—contains 2 g of fiber, with a ratio of 70% insoluble to 30% soluble fiber [84]. Higher fiber intake in pregnant mothers has been shown to attenuate pregnancy-associated dyslipidemia, which along with hypertension, is an important clinical characteristic of preeclampsia [31]. Soluble and insoluble fiber intakes have both been shown to be associated with a lower relative risk for preeclampsia (soluble: RR = 0.30; 95% CI = 0.11–0.86 *vs.* insoluble: RR = 0.35; 95% CI = 0.14–0.87) [31]. Any compound that can reduce the risk for maternal disease during pregnancy should, in theory, also be beneficial for the developing fetus, which is heavily influenced by the mother's nutrient status and disease status.

5.3. Folate

Approximately 3% of U.S. babies are born with a birth defect [63]. The best known nutrient for reducing the risk for birth defects (*i.e.*, neural tube defects and some heart defects) is folate/folic acid. Folate is a cofactor for many essential cellular reactions, including DNA and nucleic acid synthesis. During pregnancy, the folate requirement for a mother increases due to new cell and tissue formation (*i.e.*, increase in red blood cell mass, enlargement of the uterus, development of the placenta, and growth of the fetus), and it is recommended that pregnant women consume 600 μg of dietary folate equivalents daily from all food sources [85]. Insufficient maternal folate intake has been linked to increased rates of low birth weight, preterm birth, cardiac defects and neural tube defects [14,15,86,87]; however, the risk for all of these outcomes can be significantly reduced with adequate intake. In addition, supplements and fortified foods, the highest food sources of folate tend to be beans, leafy green, and cruciferous vegetables. Avocados are also a source of this nutrient. A 30 g serving of avocado contains approximately 27 μg of folate [79], which is higher than a serving of most fruits, tree nuts, and seeds [79,88]. Based on a recent National Health and Nutrition Examination Survey (NHANES) survey, the average daily avocado consumption by persons who eat avocados is over twice that amount (70 g), at approximately one-half of a medium sized avocado [89]. At this level of average intake, avocado is a good source of folate providing approximately 62 µg (*i.e.*, 10%) of the recommended daily intake of folate per day for pregnant women.

5.4. Vitamin A and Carotenoids

Vitamin A and carotenoids are needed for proper health throughout a person's entire life span, but their effects are most critical during life stages when cells are rapidly proliferating and differentiating, such as during fetal development and infancy [90]. Some carotenoids have vitamin A activity (e.g., beta-carotene, alpha-carotene and beta-cryptoxanthin) while others do not (e.g., lutein, lycopene, and zeaxanthin). All of these compounds have antioxidant properties, and they exhibit a range of functions involving eye health, immune function, and neurological development [90]. A deficiency in vitamin A, especially at critical times in development, can cause a host of severe health issues such as blindness and immunodeficiency complications [91], whereas intakes of various carotenoids, whether they have vitamin A activity or not, are associated with immune health [92,93], eye health, and brain development [94].

Henriksen *et al.* have suggested that levels of carotenoids are depleted through placental transfer to the fetus during pregnancy, thereby the dietary need increases for carotenoid intake by pregnant mothers in order to avoid deficiencies in both the mother and the offspring [95]. Lutein and zeaxanthin are critical for proper eye development *in utero*, making them key carotenoids for fetal development especially in the third trimester [95]. These particular carotenoids are either not present in, or not well absorbed from, most fruits and vegetables; however, they are both present in avocados and well-absorbed due to the fatty acid content of avocado. For example, carotenoid absorption has been shown to be improved by 5–15 times when avocado is present in a salad, when compared to an avocado free salad [96]. The fetal demand for these nutrients suggest that maternal intake of carotenoids should be monitored closely, with emphasis on beta-carotene, lutein, and zeaxanthin [95]; and adequate dietary fat to encourage their absorption. The fatty acid and fat-soluble carotenoid (especially lutein and zeaxanthin) composition of avocados make them an ideal food for assisting pregnant mothers in attaining the nutrients necessary for proper early brain, eye, and immune development of their offspring. One ounce of avocado contains approximately 3.2 RE (20 µg) of beta-carotene, and 80 µg of lutein + zeaxanthin [79], which is absorbed in considerably higher quantities than a serving of most fruits and vegetables [97].

5.5. Potassium

Potassium is considered a shortfall nutrient by the 2015 DGA report [1], thus intakes are low enough to be a public health concern. On one hand, according to the What We Eat in America (WWEIA) data from 2007 to 2010, the usual intake distributions for pregnant and non-pregnant women in the U.S. ages 19–50 years show that only 3% of women had intakes above the adequate intakes (AI) for potassium [2]. On the other hand, most Americans tend to get too much sodium from their diets. An imbalance between high levels of dietary sodium and low levels of dietary potassium is associated with hypertension; and hypertension can increase the risk for stroke, cardiovascular disease, and insulin resistance [98,99]. Pregnant woman without a history of hypertension are only at a 3%–5% higher risk for developing preeclampsia, while 17%–25% of women with chronic hypertension will develop preeclampsia [100]. Both hypertension and preeclampsia can be harmful to fetal health, resulting in higher congenital malformations, particularly cardiac defects [101]. Higher potassium intake than sodium intake has been shown to blunt the effects of sodium on blood pressure in populations with hypertension [102], further supporting the importance of obtaining adequate dietary potassium for maternal health.

The influence of dietary potassium on blood pressure was demonstrated by, Kazemian *et al.* who performed a study on women with gestational hypertension that showed the odds of getting gestational hypertension decreased significantly with roughly 250–300 mg higher intakes of potassium per day [103]. This is less than the amount of potassium found in one-half of a medium-sized avocado, but more than in one-half of a medium sized banana or a large apple. Frederick *et al.* independently arrived at similar conclusions when investigating the effects of diet on preeclampsia [33]. Their results showed diets high in potassium (>4.1 g/day) are associated with an odds ratio of 0.49 for preeclampsia compared to lower potassium diets (<2.4 g/day). Pregnant mothers and their offspring can likely benefit from increasing their potassium intake while maintaining or lowering their sodium intake. A multicenter longitudinal study on teenage girls has also shown that even when sodium intakes are above recommended levels, higher potassium intakes were associated with lower systolic and diastolic blood pressure [104]. Avocados have more potassium by weight than most other common fruits and vegetables [105]; they contain roughly 152 mg potassium per ounce, and only 2 mg sodium [79], which can help pregnant women meet recommendations.

6. Maternal Intake of Fruits, Vegetables, and Key Avocado Compounds: Effects on Milk Production and Composition

Breast milk is recommended as the only necessary source of nutrition for the first months of life [106]; and human milk is often used as the basis from which to derive nutrient requirements for infants during the first year of life. While the influence of fruit and vegetable intake on breast milk production and composition is unknown, maternal consumption of fruits and vegetables is associated with specific flavor preferences in breastfed infants from the variety of food flavors received through the milk [107,108]. These early flavor experiences may help explain why infants who are breastfed tend to be more willing to try new foods, which may contribute to greater fruit and vegetable consumption later in life [109–111].

Maternal intake of some but not all nutrients can be reflected in the nutrient composition of breast milk [112,113]. For example, maternal folate intake does not significantly alter breast milk folate despite being a proven critical nutrient for fetal development [113]. In contrast, maternal intake of vitamin A, vitamin B6, and vitamin B12), as well as iodine and fatty acids directly influence the composition of breast milk [112–114]. Few fruits or vegetables are rich in both vitamins and fatty acids, with the exception of oil-containing fruits such as avocados, which contain MUFA.

6.1. MUFA—Oleic Acid

Human breast milk provides more than 50% of its energy from fat. The fatty acids in breast milk can be taken up directly from circulation (*i.e.*, from food or from mobilized fat stores) into the mammary glands and used in milk production, or they can be synthesized in the liver or mammary glands as needed [115]. Breast milk supplies SFA, PUFA, and MUFA [116], and the specific fatty acid profile is heavily implicated in infant health and development [112]. The primary fatty acids in breast milk are palmitic acid (16:0), linoleic acid (18:2*n*-6), and oleic acid (18:1*n*-9). These three fatty acids account for roughly three-fourths of the fatty acids in human milk [117]; with the MUFA oleic acid being the most abundant fatty acid of the three. Oleic acid is also the same fatty acid that is most abundant in oil-containing fruits such as avocados and olives, but the sodium content of ready-to-eat olives, ranging up to 1000 mg per serving, make them less than ideal as a daily food for pregnant and lactating mothers.

The quantity of total fat in the milk is fairly stable even with changes to the maternal diet [118]; however, the ratio of specific fatty acids in breast milk show extreme sensitivity to maternal nutrition. Several researchers have shown that the mother's dietary habits can impact specific short-, medium, -and long-chain fatty acids in their milk, but the SFA content of the milk is generally unaffected by maternal dietary patterns [116,119]. Early researchers discovered that maternal dietary fatty acids are rapidly transferred into breast milk and within a few days the quality of human milk fat can be significantly influenced by dietary fat [120]. Therefore, the consumption of higher quantities of unsaturated fatty acids such as oleic acid by a nursing mother can be used to increase the oleic acid ratio in her milk, while a higher maternal intake of SFA does not get passed along in the breast milk in the same manner—possibly as a protection mechanism to maintain the fluidity of the breast milk, and/or to protect the infant from high levels of SFA in its early developmental stages.

Maternal lipid intake is the single most influential factor contributing to breast milk fatty acid composition [112], while carbohydrate intake has lesser influence [106]. A study in Brazilian mothers who consumed fruits four to six times per week, and whose primary fat source was soybean oil, showed that approximately 40%–42% of the fat calories in their milk came from SFA and another 20%–30% from PUFA [116]. On one hand, these values did not change much with variations in what the mother consumed. On the other hand, approximately 30%–35% of the fat calories in their milk came from MUFA, and this value was shown to change significantly depending on eating habits. Studies on European and Israeli mothers have shown that MUFA levels in their breast milk account for roughly 30%–45% of the total fatty acids, with oleic acid accounting for over 90% of the MUFA [117,121]. Furthermore, studies on Western women show that they have several-fold more *trans* oleic acid isomers in their milk than their non-Western counterparts because they ingest a higher percentage of partially hydrogenated oils in their diets [122]. The *trans* oleic acid isomers can be transferred to the fetus via cord blood and to the infant through milk. These *trans* isomers may have deleterious effects on milk liquidity and the health of the mother and offspring [122]. Experts consistently recommend replacing most forms of *trans* fatty acids with the *cis* forms [122,123]. Food manufacturers have been removing *trans* fats from their formulations for several years and the FDA is considering banning trans fats entirely. Until such time, and due to a history of higher amounts of *trans* oleic acid in the breast milk of American mothers, and lower overall MUFA ingestion in the American diet compared to a European or Mediterranean-style diet, it may be beneficial for the health of pregnant and lactating American mothers and their infants to continue to actively seek out and consume sources of *cis* MUFA—such as those found in oil-containing fruits like avocados and olives.

According to the Continuing Survey of Food Intakes by Individuals (CSFII), the most common sources of MUFA, not including breast milk, in children ages zero to two years old are cow's milk, peanut butter, white potato/French fries, hot dogs, eggs, chicken nuggets, corn puffs, and macaroni with cheese [124]. All of these sources, except peanut butter, have higher levels of SFA and/or starchy carbohydrates, than they do MUFA. In comparison, oil-containing fruits such as avocados have much higher levels of MUFA than any other fatty acids, and they also contain more fiber than starch, making them an optimal source of MUFA with likely no nutritional components associated with high cholesterol levels and insulin resistance (Figure 2). Rather, they have multiple nutritional components that research shows are inversely associated with the risk factors involved in the development of cardiovascular disease and metabolic syndrome [124–126].

In sum, MUFA in the form of oleic acid are critical to breast milk quality beyond nutritive role because it reduces the melting point of triglycerides, thus providing the proper liquidity required for the breast milk formation [122]. MUFA, along with PUFA, are also necessary for the proper development of the human nervous system [118], and substantial structural and functional brain development in the first year of life [112]. Maternal and infant MUFA intakes are clearly an area of lactation research that deserves more attention. The future research should focus on how maternal nutrition and early infant nutrition can affect health outcomes in later life stages, especially in regards to the targets of obesity, hypertension, and diabetes—all of which can negatively impact pregnant mothers and the health of their offspring.

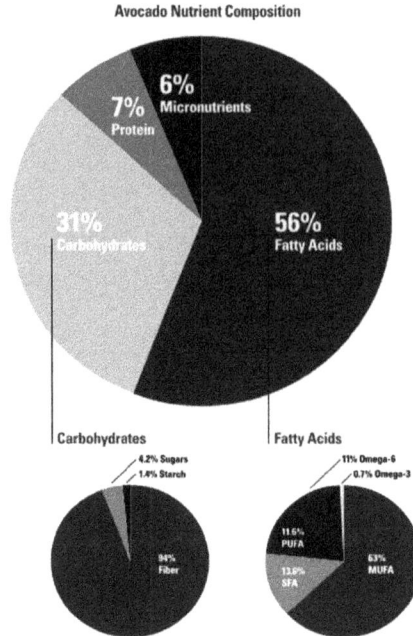

Figure 2. Avocado nutrient composition. Data sourced from: USDA Agricultural Research Service, National Nutrient Database for Standard Reference Release 27. Basic Report: 09038, Avocados, raw, California [7].

6.2. Carotenoids

Breast milk carotenoids decrease in concentration over the period of lactation. However, lutein is a carotenoid of particular interest because lutein in breast milk rises with maternal intake [119], represents roughly 25% of the carotenoid in breast milk in the first few days of breastfeeding and actually increases to nearly 50% by the end of the first month [127]. In addition to proper infant eye development, improved cognitive function, and various neuroprotective effects [128–130], plasma lutein has also been inversely correlated with oxidative DNA damage [79,131]. Lutein is the most abundant carotenoid in avocados [132]; and it is absorbed in greater quantities from avocados relative to other fruits and vegetables with low or no lipid content [96]. There is growing evidence suggesting that maternal antioxidant intake is an important factor in reducing the risk for abnormal pregnancies and birth defects [133]. Therefore, the intake of foods such as avocados—which have the highest recorded lipophilic antioxidant capacity among fruits and vegetables [134]—may also assist fetal and infant health in ways which have yet to be discovered.

7. Conclusions

Maternal nutrition plays a crucial role in influencing fetal growth and birth outcomes. Maternal nutrition also influences breast milk composition of some nutrients (*i.e.*, fatty acids and some vitamins). Avocados are a unique nutrient-rich plant-based food that contain many of the critical nutrients for fetal and infant health and development. They fit within the guidelines for a Mediterranean-style diet (*i.e.*, they contain MUFA, fiber, antioxidants, and are low-glycemic), which is known to be beneficial for disease reduction in most populations including pregnant and lactating populations. Based on this review, avocados offer a range of beneficial nutrients that can make a substantial contribution to a nutrient-rich diet when offered as a staple food for the periconceptional period, as well as during pregnancy and lactation. While they are not currently listed on the ChooseMyPlate.gov website as a recommended fruit or vegetable, they do precisely fit the description of a federally recommended food for a pregnant or lactating population. Avocados contain several recommended nutrients for reproductive health such as folate, potassium, carotenoids, and other key compounds for general health such as fiber, MUFA, and antioxidants. They do not contain empty calories from added sugars, saturated fats, or alcohol, and they are also sodium-free. Future research is required to directly study the effects of inclusion of avocados in the diet on maternal health during each of the key periods from pre-conception to the end of breastfeeding, with an emphasis on both the short-term and long-term health of the mother and offspring.

Acknowledgments: All authors have read and approved the final manuscript. This research was funded by the Hass Avocado Board.

Author Contributions: K.B.C. drafted the manuscript. K.T.A., R.D.M., and S.A.A. provided expert guidance, review and feedback throughout the manuscript development process.

Conflicts of Interest: All authors received consulting fees from the Hass Avocado Board. All conclusions are those of the authors.

References

1. U.S. Department of Health; Human Services and U.S. Department of Agriculture. 2015–2020 Dietary Guidelines for Americans. Available online: http://www.cnpp.usda.gov/2015-2020-dietary-guidelines-americans (accessed on 26 January 2016).
2. U.S. Department of Agriculture; U.S. Department of Health and Human Services. Scientific Report of the 2015 Dietary Guidelines Advisory Committee—Advisory Report to the Secretary of Health and Human Services and the Secretary of Agriculture. Available online: http://health.gov/dietaryguidelines/2015-scientific-report/pdfs/scientific-report-of-the-2015-dietary-guidelines-advisory-committee.pdf (accessed on 13 January 2016).
3. WHO/FAO. *Vitamin and Mineral Requirements in Human Nutrition: Report of a Joint FAO/WHO Expert Consultation*, 2nd ed.; World Health Organization: Geneva, Switzerland, 2004.
4. Otten, J.J.; Hellwig, J.P.; Meyers, L.D. *Dietary Reference Intakes: The Essential Guide to Nutrient Requirements*; The National Academies Press: Washington, DC, USA, 2006.
5. Christian, P.; Mullany, L.C.; Hurley, K.M.; Katz, J.; Black, R.E. Nutrition and maternal, neonatal, and child health. *Semin. Perinatol.* **2015**, *39*, 361–372. [CrossRef] [PubMed]
6. Raiten, D.J.; Raghavan, R.; Porter, A.; Obbagy, J.E.; Spahn, J.M. Executive summary: Evaluating the evidence base to support the inclusion of infants and children from birth to 24 months of age in the Dietary Guidelines for Americans—"The B-24 Project". *Am. J. Clin. Nutr.* **2014**, *99*, 663S–691S. [CrossRef] [PubMed]
7. USDA. National Nutrient Database for Standard Reference Release 27, Basic Report: 09038, Avocados, Raw, California. Available online: http://www.ars.usda.gov/Services/docs.htm?docid=25706 (accessed on 23 August 2015).
8. Chavarro, J.E.; Rich-Edwards, J.W.; Rosner, B.A.; Willett, W.C. Dietary fatty acid intakes and the risk of ovulatory infertility. *Am. J. Clin. Nutr.* **2007**, *85*, 231–237. [PubMed]
9. Champ, M.; Hoebler, C. Functional food for pregnant, lactating women and in perinatal nutrition: A role for dietary fibres? *Curr. Opin. Clin. Nutr. Metab. Care* **2009**, *12*, 565–574. [CrossRef] [PubMed]
10. Vanhees, K.; Vonhogen, I.G.; van Schooten, F.J.; Godschalk, R.W. You are what you eat, and so are your children: The impact of micronutrients on the epigenetic programming of offspring. *Cell. Mol. Life Sci.* **2014**, *71*, 271–285. [CrossRef] [PubMed]
11. Twigt, J.M.; Bolhuis, M.E.; Steegers, E.A.; Hammiche, F.; van Inzen, W.G.; Laven, J.S.; Steegers-Theunissen, R.P. The preconception diet is associated with the chance of ongoing pregnancy in women undergoing IVF/ICSI treatment. *Hum. Reprod.* **2012**, *27*, 2526–2531. [CrossRef] [PubMed]
12. Abu-Saad, K.; Fraser, D. Maternal nutrition and birth outcomes. *Epidemiol. Rev.* **2010**, *32*, 5–25. [CrossRef] [PubMed]
13. Mason, J.B.; Saldanha, L.S.; Martorell, R. The importance of maternal undernutrition for maternal, neonatal, and child health outcomes: An editorial. *Food Nutr. Bull.* **2012**, *33*, S3–S5. [CrossRef] [PubMed]

14. Ramakrishnan, U.; Grant, F.; Goldenberg, T.; Zongrone, A.; Martorell, R. Effect of women's nutrition before and during early pregnancy on maternal and infant outcomes: A systematic review. *Paediatr. Perinat. Epidemiol.* **2012**, *26*, 285–301. [CrossRef] [PubMed]
15. Cetin, I.; Berti, C.; Calabrese, S. Role of micronutrients in the periconceptional period. *Hum. Reprod. Update* **2010**, *16*, 80–95. [CrossRef] [PubMed]
16. Cox, J.T.; Phelan, S.T. Prenatal nutrition: Special considerations. *Minerva Ginecol.* **2009**, *61*, 373–400. [PubMed]
17. Fowler, J.K.; Evers, S.E.; Campbell, M.K. Inadequate dietary intakes among pregnant women. *Can. J. Diet Pract. Res.* **2012**, *73*, 72–77. [CrossRef] [PubMed]
18. Schatzer, M.; Rust, P.; Elmadfa, I. Fruit and vegetable intake in Austrian adults: Intake frequency, serving sizes, reasons for and barriers to consumption, and potential for increasing consumption. *Public Health Nutr.* **2010**, *13*, 480–487. [CrossRef] [PubMed]
19. De Weerd, S.; Steegers, E.A.; Heinen, M.M.; van den Eertwegh, S.; Vehof, R.M.; Steegers-Theunissen, R.P. Preconception nutritional intake and lifestyle factors: First results of an explorative study. *Eur. J. Obstet. Gynecol. Reprod. Biol.* **2003**, *111*, 167–172. [CrossRef]
20. American Dietetic Association; American Society of Nutrition; Siega-Riz, A.M.; King, J.C. Position of the American Dietetic Association and American Society for Nutrition: Obesity, reproduction, and pregnancy outcomes. *J. Am. Diet Assoc.* **2009**, *109*, 918–927.
21. Heslehurst, N.; Ells, L.J.; Simpson, H.; Batterham, A.; Wilkinson, J.; Summerbell, C.D. Trends in maternal obesity incidence rates, demographic predictors, and health inequalities in 36,821 women over a 15-year period. *BJOG* **2007**, *114*, 187–194. [CrossRef] [PubMed]
22. Ferrara, A. Increasing prevalence of gestational diabetes mellitus: A public health perspective. *Diabetes Care* **2007**, *30*, S141–S146. [CrossRef] [PubMed]
23. Parker, S.E.; Werler, M.M.; Shaw, G.M.; Anderka, M.; Yazdy, M.M.; National Birth Defects Prevention Study. Dietary Glycemic Index and the risk of birth defects. *Am. J. Epidemiol.* **2012**, *176*, 1110–1120. [CrossRef] [PubMed]
24. Matias, S.L.; Dewey, K.G.; Quesenberry, C.P., Jr.; Gunderson, E.P. Maternal prepregnancy obesity and insulin treatment during pregnancy are independently associated with delayed lactogenesis in women with recent gestational diabetes mellitus. *Am. J. Clin. Nutr.* **2014**, *99*, 115–121. [CrossRef] [PubMed]
25. ChooseMyPlate.gov. Health and Nutrition Information for Pregnant and Breastfeeding Women: Making Healthy Choices in Each Food Group. Available online: http://www.choosemyplate.gov/pregnancy-breastfeeding/making-healthy-food-choices.html (accessed on 17 November 2014).
26. Lundqvist, A.; Johansson, I.; Wennberg, A.; Hultdin, J.; Hogberg, U.; Hamberg, K.; Sandstrom, H. Reported dietary intake in early pregnant compared to non-pregnant women inverted question mark a cross-sectional study. *BMC Pregnancy Childbirth* **2014**, *14*, 373. [CrossRef] [PubMed]
27. Picciano, M.F.; McGuire, M.K. Use of dietary supplements by pregnant and lactating women in North America. *Am. J. Clin. Nutr.* **2009**, *89*, 663S–667S. [CrossRef] [PubMed]
28. ChooseMyPlate.gov. Health and Nutrition Information for Pregnant and Breastfeeding Women: Nutritional Needs during Pregnancy. Available online: http://www.choosemyplate.gov/pregnancy-breastfeeding/pregnancy-nutritional-needs.html (accessed on 17 November 2014).
29. Verger, E.O.; Holmes, B.A.; Huneau, J.F.; Mariotti, F. Simple changes within dietary subgroups can rapidly improve the nutrient adequacy of the diet of French adults. *J. Nutr.* **2014**, *144*, 929–936. [CrossRef] [PubMed]
30. Kelly, T.N.; Gu, D.; Rao, D.C.; Chen, J.; Chen, J.; Cao, J.; Li, J.; Lu, F.; Ma, J.; Mu, J.; et al. Maternal history of hypertension and blood pressure response to potassium intake: The gensalt study. *Am. J. Epidemiol.* **2012**, *176*, S55–S63. [CrossRef] [PubMed]
31. Qiu, C.; Coughlin, K.B.; Frederick, I.O.; Sorensen, T.K.; Williams, M.A. Dietary fiber intake in early pregnancy and risk of subsequent preeclampsia. *Am. J. Hypertens.* **2008**, *21*, 903–909. [CrossRef] [PubMed]
32. Hernandez, T.L.; Anderson, M.A.; Chartier-Logan, C.; Friedman, J.E.; Barbour, L.A. Strategies in the nutritional management of gestational diabetes. *Clin. Obstet. Gynecol.* **2013**, *56*, 803–815. [CrossRef] [PubMed]
33. Frederick, I.O.; Williams, M.A.; Dashow, E.; Kestin, M.; Zhang, C.; Leisenring, W.M. Dietary fiber, potassium, magnesium and calcium in relation to the risk of preeclampsia. *J. Reprod. Med.* **2005**, *50*, 332–344. [PubMed]
34. Centers for Disease Control and Prevention (CDC). Faststats: Infertility. Available online: http://www.cdc.gov/nchs/fastats/infertility.htm25706 (accessed on 17 November 2014).

35. Chavarro, J.; Willett, W.; Skerrett, P.J. *The Fertility Diet: Groundbreaking Research Reveals Natural Ways to Boost Ovulation & Improve Your Chances of Getting Pregnant*; McGraw-Hill: New York, NY, USA, 2008.

36. Kulak, D.; Polotsky, A.J. Should the ketogenic diet be considered for enhancing fertility? *Maturitas* **2013**, *74*, 10–13. [CrossRef] [PubMed]

37. Crosignani, P.G.; Vegetti, W.; Colombo, M.; Ragni, G. Resumption of fertility with diet in overweight women. *Reprod. Biomed. Online* **2002**, *5*, 60–64. [CrossRef]

38. Santangelo, C.; Vari, R.; Scazzocchio, B.; Filesi, C.; Masella, R. Management of reproduction and pregnancy complications in maternal obesity: Which role for dietary polyphenols? *Biofactors* **2014**, *40*, 79–102. [CrossRef] [PubMed]

39. Khoury, J.; Henriksen, T.; Christophersen, B.; Tonstad, S. Effect of a cholesterol-lowering diet on maternal, cord, and neonatal lipids, and pregnancy outcome: A randomized clinical trial. *Am. J. Obstet. Gynecol.* **2005**, *193*, 1292–1301. [CrossRef] [PubMed]

40. Mediterranean Diet Pyramid Poster. Available online: http://www.californiaavocado.com/mediterranean-diet/ (accessed on 7 January 2015).

41. Timmermans, S.; Steegers-Theunissen, R.P.; Vujkovic, M.; Bakker, R.; den Breeijen, H.; Raat, H.; Russcher, H.; Lindemans, J.; Hofman, A.; Jaddoe, V.W.; *et al.* Major dietary patterns and blood pressure patterns during pregnancy: The generation R study. *Am. J. Obstet. Gynecol.* **2011**, *205*. [CrossRef] [PubMed]

42. Toledo, E.; Lopez-del Burgo, C.; Ruiz-Zambrana, A.; Donazar, M.; Navarro-Blasco, I.; Martinez-Gonzalez, M.A.; de Irala, J. Dietary patterns and difficulty conceiving: A nested case-control study. *Fertil. Steril.* **2011**, *96*, 1149–1153. [CrossRef] [PubMed]

43. Hirai, S.; Takahashi, N.; Goto, T.; Lin, S.; Uemura, T.; Yu, R.; Kawada, T. Functional food targeting the regulation of obesity-induced inflammatory responses and pathologies. *Mediat. Inflamm.* **2010**, *2010*, 367838. [CrossRef] [PubMed]

44. Sinska, B.; Kucharska, A.; Dmoch-Gajzlerska, E. The Diet in improving fertility in women. *Pol. Merkur. Lekarski.* **2014**, *36*, 400–402. [PubMed]

45. Becker, G.F.; Passos, E.P.; Moulin, C.C. Short-term effects of a hypocaloric diet with low glycemic index and low glycemic load on body adiposity, metabolic variables, ghrelin, leptin, and pregnancy rate in overweight and obese infertile women: A randomized controlled trial. *Am. J. Clin. Nutr.* **2015**, *102*, 1365–1372. [CrossRef] [PubMed]

46. De Lorgeril, M.; Salen, P.; Paillard, F.; Laporte, F.; Boucher, F.; de Leiris, J. Mediterranean diet and the French paradox: Two distinct biogeographic concepts for one consolidated scientific theory on the role of nutrition in coronary heart disease. *Cardiovasc. Res.* **2002**, *54*, 503–515. [CrossRef]

47. USDA. National Nutrient Database for Standard Reference Release 27: Sugars, Total (G): "Compared to Fruits and Fruit Juices". Available online: https://ndb.nal.usda.gov/ (accessed on 23 August 2015).

48. USDA. National Nutrient Database for Standard Reference Release 27: Fiber, Total Dietary (G): "Compared to Fruits and Fruit Juices". Available online: https://ndb.nal.usda.gov/ (accessed on 23 August 2015).

49. Foster-Powell, K.; Holt, S.H.; Brand-Miller, J.C. International table of glycemic index and glycemic load values: 2002. *Am. J. Clin. Nutr.* **2002**, *76*, 5–56. [PubMed]

50. Moses, R.G.; Barker, M.; Winter, M.; Petocz, P.; Brand-Miller, J.C. Can a low-glycemic index diet reduce the need for insulin in gestational diabetes mellitus? A randomized trial. *Diabetes Care* **2009**, *32*, 996–1000. [CrossRef] [PubMed]

51. McGowan, C.A.; Walsh, J.M.; Byrne, J.; Curran, S.; McAuliffe, F.M. The influence of a low glycemic index dietary intervention on maternal dietary intake, glycemic index and gestational weight gain during pregnancy: A randomized controlled trial. *Nutr. J.* **2013**, *12*, 140. [CrossRef] [PubMed]

52. Kizirian, N.V.; Kong, Y.; Muirhead, R.; Brodie, S.; Garnett, S.P.; Petocz, P.; Sim, K.A.; Celermajer, D.S.; Louie, J.C.; Markovic, T.P.; *et al.* Effects of a low-glycemic index diet during pregnancy on offspring growth, body composition, and vascular health: A pilot randomized controlled trial. *Am. J. Clin. Nutr.* **2016**, *103*, 1073–1082. [CrossRef] [PubMed]

53. Horan, M.K.; McGowan, C.A.; Gibney, E.R.; Byrne, J.; Donnelly, J.M.; McAuliffe, F.M. Maternal nutrition and glycaemic index during pregnancy impacts on offspring adiposity at 6 months of age-analysis from the rolo randomised controlled trial. *Nutrients* **2016**, *8*. [CrossRef] [PubMed]

54. Danielsen, I.; Granstrom, C.; Haldorsson, T.; Rytter, D.; Hammer Bech, B.; Henriksen, T.B.; Vaag, A.A.; Olsen, S.F. Dietary glycemic index during pregnancy is associated with biomarkers of the metabolic syndrome in offspring at age 20 years. *PLoS ONE* **2013**, *8*, e64887. [CrossRef]

55. Hung, H.C.; Joshipura, K.J.; Jiang, R.; Hu, F.B.; Hunter, D.; Smith-Warner, S.A.; Colditz, G.A.; Rosner, B.; Spiegelman, D.; Willett, W.C. Fruit and vegetable intake and risk of major chronic disease. *J. Natl. Cancer Inst.* **2004**, *96*, 1577–1584. [CrossRef] [PubMed]

56. Tobias, M.; Turley, M.; Stefanogiannis, N.; Vander Hoorn, S.; Lawes, C.; Mhurchu, C.N.; Rodgers, A. Vegetable and fruit intake and mortality from chronic disease in New Zealand. *Aust. N. Z. J. Public Health* **2006**, *30*, 26–31. [CrossRef] [PubMed]

57. Liu, R.H. Health-promoting components of fruits and vegetables in the diet. *Adv. Nutr.* **2013**, *4*, 384S–392S. [CrossRef] [PubMed]

58. Murphy, M.M.; Stettler, N.; Smith, K.M.; Reiss, R. Associations of consumption of fruits and vegetables during pregnancy with infant birth weight or small for gestational age births: A systematic review of the literature. *Int. J. Womens Health* **2014**, *6*, 899–912. [CrossRef] [PubMed]

59. Wojdylo, A.; Oszmianski, J. Bioactive compounds of selected fruit juices. *Nat. Prod. Commun.* **2009**, *4*, 671–676. [PubMed]

60. Stoewsand, G.S. Bioactive organosulfur phytochemicals in Brassica oleracea vegetables—A review. *Food Chem. Toxicol.* **1995**, *33*, 537–543. [CrossRef]

61. Grieger, J.A.; Clifton, V.L. A review of the impact of dietary intakes in human pregnancy on infant birthweight. *Nutrients* **2015**, *7*, 153–178. [CrossRef] [PubMed]

62. Loy, S.L.; Marhazlina, M.; Azwany, Y.N.; Hamid Jan, J.M. Higher intake of fruits and vegetables in pregnancy is associated with birth size. *Southeast Asian J. Trop. Med. Public Health* **2011**, *42*, 1214–1223. [PubMed]

63. Procter, S.B.; Campbell, C.G. Position of the academy of nutrition and dietetics: Nutrition and lifestyle for a healthy pregnancy outcome. *J. Acad. Nutr. Diet* **2014**, *114*, 1099–1103. [CrossRef] [PubMed]

64. Knudsen, V.K.; Orozova-Bekkevold, I.M.; Mikkelsen, T.B.; Wolff, S.; Olsen, S.F. Major dietary patterns in pregnancy and fetal growth. *Eur. J. Clin. Nutr.* **2008**, *62*, 463–470. [CrossRef] [PubMed]

65. Hanley, B.; Dijane, J.; Fewtrell, M.; Grynberg, A.; Hummel, S.; Junien, C.; Koletzko, B.; Lewis, S.; Renz, H.; Symonds, M.; *et al.* Metabolic imprinting, programming and epigenetics—A review of present priorities and future opportunities. *Br. J. Nutr.* **2010**, *104*, S1–S25. [CrossRef] [PubMed]

66. Organization, W.H. *Promoting Optimal Fetal Development: Report of a Technical Consultation*; World Health Organization: Geneva, Switzerland, 2006.

67. Gesteiro, E.; Rodriguez Bernal, B.; Bastida, S.; Sanchez-Muniz, F.J. Maternal diets with low healthy eating index or mediterranean diet adherence scores are associated with high cord-blood insulin levels and insulin resistance markers at birth. *Eur. J. Clin. Nutr.* **2012**, *66*, 1008–1015. [CrossRef] [PubMed]

68. Krapels, I.P.; van Rooij, I.A.; Ocke, M.C.; West, C.E.; van der Horst, C.M.; Steegers-Theunissen, R.P. Maternal nutritional status and the risk for orofacial cleft offspring in humans. *J. Nutr.* **2004**, *134*, 3106–3113. [PubMed]

69. Groenen, P.M.; van Rooij, I.A.; Peer, P.G.; Ocke, M.C.; Zielhuis, G.A.; Steegers-Theunissen, R.P. Low maternal dietary intakes of iron, magnesium, and niacin are associated with spina bifida in the offspring. *J. Nutr.* **2004**, *134*, 1516–1522. [PubMed]

70. Brantsaeter, A.L.; Haugen, M.; Samuelsen, S.O.; Torjusen, H.; Trogstad, L.; Alexander, J.; Magnus, P.; Meltzer, H.M. A dietary pattern characterized by high intake of vegetables, fruits, and vegetable oils is associated with reduced risk of preeclampsia in nulliparous pregnant norwegian women. *J. Nutr.* **2009**, *139*, 1162–1168. [CrossRef] [PubMed]

71. Ley, S.H.; Hanley, A.J.; Retnakaran, R.; Sermer, M.; Zinman, B.; O'Connor, D.L. Effect of macronutrient intake during the second trimester on glucose metabolism later in pregnancy. *Am. J. Clin. Nutr.* **2011**, *94*, 1232–1240. [CrossRef] [PubMed]

72. Rao, S.; Yajnik, C.S.; Kanade, A.; Fall, C.H.; Margetts, B.M.; Jackson, A.A.; Shier, R.; Joshi, S.; Rege, S.; Lubree, H.; *et al.* Intake of micronutrient-rich foods in rural indian mothers is associated with the size of their babies at birth: Pune maternal nutrition study. *J. Nutr.* **2001**, *131*, 1217–1224. [PubMed]

73. Schisterman, E.F.; Mumford, S.L.; Browne, R.W.; Barr, D.B.; Chen, Z.; Louis, G.M. Lipid concentrations and couple fecundity: The life study. *J. Clin. Endocrinol. Metab.* **2014**, *99*, 2786–2794. [CrossRef] [PubMed]

74. Agostoni, C.; Galli, C.; Riva, E.; Rise, P.; Colombo, C.; Giovannini, M.; Marangoni, F. Whole blood fatty acid composition at birth: From the maternal compartment to the infant. *Clin. Nutr.* **2011**, *30*, 503–505. [CrossRef] [PubMed]

75. Agostoni, C.; Marangoni, F.; Stival, G.; Gatelli, I.; Pinto, F.; Rise, P.; Giovannini, M.; Galli, C.; Riva, E. Whole blood fatty acid composition differs in term versus mildly preterm infants: Small versus matched appropriate for gestational age. *Pediatr. Res.* **2008**, *64*, 298–302. [CrossRef] [PubMed]

76. Canovas-Conesa, A.; Gomariz-Penalver, V.; Sanchez-Sauco, M.F.; Jaimes Vega, D.C.; Ortega-Garcia, J.A.; Aranda Garcia, M.J.; Delgado Marin, J.L.; Trujillo Ascanio, A.; Lopez Hernandez, F.; Ruiz Jimenez, J.I.; *et al.* The Association of adherence to a mediterranean diet during early pregnancy and the risk of gastroschisis in the offspring. *Cir. Pediatr.* **2013**, *26*, 37–43. [PubMed]

77. Yamashita, D.; Shimizu, M.; Osumi, T. Mechanism for the action of PPARs. *Nihon Rinsho* **2005**, *63*, 536–537. [PubMed]

78. Chavarro, J.E.; Colaci, D.S.; Afeiche, M.; Gaskins, A.J.; Wright, D.; Toth, T.L.; Hauser, R. Dietary Fat Intake and *in-vitro* Fertilization Outcomes: Saturated Fat Intake is Associated with Fewer Metaphase 2 Oocytes. Available online: http://humrep.oxfordjournals.org/content/27/suppl_2/ii78.abstract (accessed on 17 August 2015).

79. Dreher, M.L.; Davenport, A.J. Hass avocado composition and potential health effects. *Crit. Rev. Food Sci. Nutr.* **2013**, *53*, 738–750. [CrossRef] [PubMed]

80. Blumfield, M.L.; Hure, A.J.; Macdonald-Wicks, L.; Smith, R.; Collins, C.E. Systematic review and meta-analysis of energy and macronutrient intakes during pregnancy in developed countries. *Nutr. Rev.* **2012**, *70*, 322–336. [CrossRef] [PubMed]

81. Gibson, R.S.; Ferguson, E.L.; Lehrfeld, J. Complementary foods for infant feeding in developing countries: Their nutrient adequacy and improvement. *Eur. J. Clin. Nutr.* **1998**, *52*, 764–770. [CrossRef] [PubMed]

82. Quinn, M. Sustained constipation and subsequent reproductive outcomes: Is there a link? *J. Obstet. Gynaecol.* **2006**, *26*, 366–367. [CrossRef] [PubMed]

83. Zhang, C.; Liu, S.; Solomon, C.G.; Hu, F.B. Dietary fiber intake, dietary glycemic load, and the risk for gestational diabetes mellitus. *Diabetes Care* **2006**, *29*, 2223–2230. [CrossRef] [PubMed]

84. Marlett, J.A.; Cheung, T.F. Database and quick methods of assessing typical dietary fiber intakes using data for 228 commonly consumed foods. *J. Am. Diet Assoc.* **1997**, *97*, 1139–1151. [CrossRef]

85. U.S. Department of Agriculture; U.S. Department of Health and Human Services. *Dietary Guidelines for Americans*, 7th ed.; U.S. Government Printing Office: Washington, DC, USA, 2010.

86. Ionescu-Ittu, R.; Marelli, A.J.; Mackie, A.S.; Pilote, L. Prevalence of severe congenital heart disease after folic acid fortification of grain products: Time trend analysis in Quebec, Canada. *BMJ* **2009**, *338*. [CrossRef] [PubMed]

87. Scholl, T.O.; Hediger, M.L.; Schall, J.I.; Khoo, C.S.; Fischer, R.L. Dietary and serum folate: Their influence on the outcome of pregnancy. *Am. J. Clin. Nutr.* **1996**, *63*, 520–525. [PubMed]

88. USDA. National Nutrient Database for Standard Reference Release 27: Folate, Food (µg): "Compared to Fruits and Fruit Juices, and Vegetables and Vegetable Products". Available online: https://ndb.nal.usda.gov/ (accessed on 23 August 2015).

89. Fulgoni, V.L., III; Dreher, M.; Davenport, A.J. Avocado consumption is associated with better diet quality and nutrient intake, and lower metabolic syndrome risk in US adults: Results from the National Health and Nutrition Examination Survey (NHANES) 2001–2008. *Nutr. J.* **2013**, *12*. [CrossRef] [PubMed]

90. Azais-Braesco, V.; Pascal, G. Vitamin a in pregnancy: Requirements and safety limits. *Am. J. Clin Nutr.* **2000**, *71*, 1325S–1333S. [PubMed]

91. Elmadfa, I.; Meyer, A.L. Vitamins for the first 1000 days: Preparing for life. *Int. J. Vitam. Nutr. Res.* **2012**, *82*, 342–347. [CrossRef] [PubMed]

92. Ruhl, R. Non-pro-vitamin a and pro-vitamin a carotenoids in atopy development. *Int. Arch. Allergy Immunol.* **2013**, *161*, 99–115. [CrossRef] [PubMed]

93. Ruhl, R. Effects of dietary retinoids and carotenoids on immune development. *Proc. Nutr. Soc.* **2007**, *66*, 458–469. [CrossRef] [PubMed]

94. Henriksen, B.S.; Chan, G.M. Importance of carotenoids in optimizing eye and brain development. *J. Pediatr. Gastroenterol. Nutr.* **2014**, *59*, 552. [CrossRef] [PubMed]

95. Henriksen, B.S.; Chan, G.; Hoffman, R.O.; Sharifzadeh, M.; Ermakov, I.V.; Gellermann, W.; Bernstein, P.S. Interrelationships between maternal carotenoid status and newborn infant macular pigment optical density and carotenoid status. *Investig. Ophthalmol. Vis. Sci.* **2013**, *54*, 5568–5578. [CrossRef] [PubMed]

96. Unlu, N.Z.; Bohn, T.; Clinton, S.K.; Schwartz, S.J. Carotenoid absorption from salad and salsa by humans is enhanced by the addition of avocado or avocado oil. *J. Nutr.* **2005**, *135*, 431–436. [PubMed]

97. Sommerburg, O.; Keunen, J.E.; Bird, A.C.; van Kuijk, F.J. Fruits and vegetables that are sources for lutein and zeaxanthin: The macular pigment in human eyes. *Br. J. Ophthalmol.* **1998**, *82*, 907–910. [CrossRef] [PubMed]

98. Lima, N.K.; Abbasi, F.; Lamendola, C.; Reaven, G.M. Prevalence of insulin resistance and related risk factors for cardiovascular disease in patients with essential hypertension. *Am. J. Hypertens.* **2009**, *22*, 106–111. [CrossRef] [PubMed]

99. Maillot, M.; Monsivais, P.; Drewnowski, A. Food pattern modeling shows that the 2010 dietary guidelines for sodium and potassium cannot be met simultaneously. *Nutr. Res.* **2013**, *33*, 188–194. [CrossRef] [PubMed]

100. Seely, E.W.; Ecker, J. Chronic hypertension in pregnancy. *Circulation* **2014**, *129*, 1254–1261. [CrossRef] [PubMed]

101. Bateman, B.T.; Huybrechts, K.F.; Fischer, M.A.; Seely, E.W.; Ecker, J.L.; Oberg, A.S.; Franklin, J.M.; Mogun, H.; Hernandez-Diaz, S. Chronic hypertension in pregnancy and the risk of congenital malformations: A cohort study. *Am. J. Obstet. Gynecol.* **2015**, *212*, 337.e1–337.e14. [CrossRef] [PubMed]

102. Rodrigues, S.L.; Baldo, M.P.; Machado, R.C.; Forechi, L.; Molina Mdel, C.; Mill, J.G. High potassium intake blunts the effect of elevated sodium intake on blood pressure levels. *J. Am. Soc. Hypertens.* **2014**, *8*, 232–238. [CrossRef] [PubMed]

103. Kazemian, E.; Dorosty-Motlagh, A.R.; Sotoudeh, G.; Eshraghian, M.R.; Ansary, S.; Omidian, M. Nutritional status of women with gestational hypertension compared with normal pregnant women. *Hypertens. Pregnancy* **2013**, *32*, 146–156. [CrossRef] [PubMed]

104. Buendia, J.R.; Bradlee, M.L.; Daniels, S.R.; Singer, M.R.; Moore, L.L. Longitudinal effects of dietary sodium and potassium on blood pressure in adolescent girls. *JAMA Pediatr.* **2015**, *169*, 560–568. [CrossRef] [PubMed]

105. USDA. National Nutrient Database for Standard Reference Release 27: Potassium, Food (Mg): "Compared to Fruits and Fruit Juices, and Vegetables and Vegetable Products". Available online: https://ndb.nal.usda.gov/ (accessed on 23 August 2015).

106. Rocquelin, G.; Tapsoba, S.; Dop, M.C.; Mbemba, F.; Traissac, P.; Martin-Prevel, Y. Lipid content and essential fatty acid (EFA) composition of mature congolese breast milk are influenced by mothers' nutritional status: Impact on infants' EFA supply. *Eur. J. Clin. Nutr.* **1998**, *52*, 164–171. [CrossRef] [PubMed]

107. Mennella, J.A.; Beauchamp, G.K. Maternal diet alters the sensory qualities of human milk and the nursling's behavior. *Pediatrics* **1991**, *88*, 737–744. [PubMed]

108. Mennella, J.A. *The Chemical Senses and the Development of Flavor Preferences in Humans*; Hale Publishing: Amarillo, TX, USA, 2007.

109. Nicklaus, S.; Boggio, V.; Chabanet, C.; Issanchou, S. A prospective study of food variety seeking in childhood, adolescence and early adult life. *Appetite* **2005**, *44*, 289–297. [CrossRef] [PubMed]

110. Cooke, L.J.; Wardle, J.; Gibson, E.L.; Sapochnik, M.; Sheiham, A.; Lawson, M. Demographic, familial and trait predictors of fruit and vegetable consumption by pre-school children. *Public Health Nutr.* **2004**, *7*, 295–302. [CrossRef] [PubMed]

111. Skinner, J.D.; Carruth, B.R.; Bounds, W.; Ziegler, P.; Reidy, K. Do food-related experiences in the first 2 years of life predict dietary variety in school-aged children? *J. Nutr. Educ. Behav.* **2002**, *34*, 310–315. [CrossRef]

112. Innis, S.M. Impact of maternal diet on human milk composition and neurological development of infants. *Am. J. Clin. Nutr.* **2014**, *99*, 734S–741S. [CrossRef] [PubMed]

113. Allen, L.H. B vitamins in breast milk: Relative importance of maternal status and intake, and effects on infant status and function. *Adv. Nutr.* **2012**, *3*, 362–369. [CrossRef] [PubMed]

114. Innis, S.M. Human milk: Maternal dietary lipids and infant development. *Proc. Nutr. Soc.* **2007**, *66*, 397–404. [CrossRef] [PubMed]

115. Jensen, R.G. The lipids in human milk. *Prog. Lipid Res.* **1996**, *35*, 53–92. [CrossRef]

116. Da Cunha, J.; Macedo da Costa, T.H.; Ito, M.K. Influences of maternal dietary intake and suckling on breast milk lipid and fatty acid composition in low-income women from Brasilia, Brazil. *Early Hum. Dev.* **2005**, *81*, 303–311. [CrossRef] [PubMed]

117. Saphier, O.; Blumenfeld, J.; Silberstein, T.; Tzor, T.; Burg, A. Fatty acid composition of breastmilk of Israeli mothers. *Indian Pediatr.* **2013**, *50*, 1044–1046. [CrossRef] [PubMed]
118. Martysiak-Zurowska, D.; Zoralska, K.; Zagierski, M.; Szlagtys-Sidorkiewicz, A. Fatty acid composition in breast milk of women from Gdansk and the surrounding district in the course of lactation. *Med. Wieku Rozwoj.* **2011**, *15*, 167–177. [PubMed]
119. Del Prado, M.; Villalpando, S.; Elizondo, A.; Rodriguez, M.; Demmelmair, H.; Koletzko, B. Contribution of dietary and newly formed arachidonic acid to human milk lipids in women eating a low-fat diet. *Am. J. Clin. Nutr.* **2001**, *74*, 242–247. [PubMed]
120. Insull, W., Jr.; Hirsch, J.; James, T.; Ahrens, E.H., Jr. The fatty acids of human milk. II. Alterations produced by manipulation of caloric balance and exchange of dietary fats. *J. Clin. Investig.* **1959**, *38*, 443–450. [CrossRef] [PubMed]
121. Lopez-Lopez, A.; Lopez-Sabater, M.C.; Campoy-Folgoso, C.; Rivero-Urgell, M.; Castellote-Bargallo, A.I. Fatty acid and sn-2 fatty acid composition in human milk from Granada (Spain) and in infant formulas. *Eur. J. Clin. Nutr.* **2002**, *56*, 1242–1254. [CrossRef] [PubMed]
122. Jensen, R.G. Lipids in human milk. *Lipids* **1999**, *34*, 1243–1271. [CrossRef] [PubMed]
123. Ascherio, A.; Willett, W.C. Health effects of *trans* fatty acids. *Am. J. Clin. Nutr.* **1997**, *66*, 1006S–1010S. [PubMed]
124. Nicklas, T.A.; Hampl, J.S.; Taylor, C.A.; Thompson, V.J.; Heird, W.C. Monounsaturated fatty acid intake by children and adults: Temporal trends and demographic differences. *Nutr. Rev.* **2004**, *62*, 132–141. [CrossRef] [PubMed]
125. Root, M.M.; Dawson, H.R. Dash-like diets high in protein or monounsaturated fats improve metabolic syndrome and calculated vascular risk. *Int. J. Vitam. Nutr. Res.* **2013**, *83*, 224–231. [CrossRef] [PubMed]
126. Gillingham, L.G.; Harris-Janz, S.; Jones, P.J. Dietary monounsaturated fatty acids are protective against metabolic syndrome and cardiovascular disease risk factors. *Lipids* **2011**, *46*, 209–228. [CrossRef] [PubMed]
127. Cena, H.; Castellazzi, A.M.; Pietri, A.; Roggi, C.; Turconi, G. Lutein concentration in human milk during early lactation and its relationship with dietary lutein intake. *Public Health Nutr.* **2009**, *12*, 1878–1884. [CrossRef] [PubMed]
128. Johnson, E.J. Role of lutein and zeaxanthin in visual and cognitive function throughout the lifespan. *Nutr. Rev.* **2014**, *72*, 605–612. [CrossRef] [PubMed]
129. Ozawa, Y.; Sasaki, M.; Takahashi, N.; Kamoshita, M.; Miyake, S.; Tsubota, K. Neuroprotective effects of lutein in the retina. *Curr. Pharm. Des.* **2012**, *18*, 51–56. [CrossRef] [PubMed]
130. Vishwanathan, R.; Kuchan, M.J.; Sen, S.; Johnson, E.J. Lutein and preterm infants with decreased concentrations of brain carotenoids. *J. Pediatr. Gastroenterol. Nutr.* **2014**, *59*, 659–665. [CrossRef] [PubMed]
131. Haegele, A.D.; Gillette, C.; O'Neill, C.; Wolfe, P.; Heimendinger, J.; Sedlacek, S.; Thompson, H.J. Plasma xanthophyll carotenoids correlate inversely with indices of oxidative dna damage and lipid peroxidation. *Cancer Epidemiol. Biomark. Prev.* **2000**, *9*, 421–425.
132. Ashton, O.B.; Wong, M.; McGhie, T.K.; Vather, R.; Wang, Y.; Requejo-Jackman, C.; Ramankutty, P.; Woolf, A.B. Pigments in avocado tissue and oil. *J. Agric. Food Chem.* **2006**, *54*, 10151–10158. [CrossRef] [PubMed]
133. Allen, L.H. Multiple micronutrients in pregnancy and lactation: An overview. *Am. J. Clin. Nutr.* **2005**, *81*, 1206S–1212S. [PubMed]
134. Wu, X.; Beecher, G.R.; Holden, J.M.; Haytowitz, D.B.; Gebhardt, S.E.; Prior, R.L. Lipophilic and hydrophilic antioxidant capacities of common foods in the United States. *J. Agric. Food Chem.* **2004**, *52*, 4026–4037. [CrossRef] [PubMed]

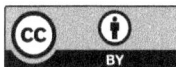

nutrients

MDPI

Review

The Role of Avocados in Complementary and Transitional Feeding

Kevin B. Comerford [1,*], Keith T. Ayoob [2,†], Robert D. Murray [3,†] and Stephanie A. Atkinson [4,†]

[1] Department of Nutrition, University of California at Davis, Davis, CA 95616, USA
[2] Department of Pediatrics, Albert Einstein College of Medicine, Bronx, NY 10461, USA; keith.ayoob@einstein.yu.edu
[3] Department of Human Sciences, The Ohio State University, Columbus, OH 43210, USA; murrayMD@live.com
[4] Department of Pediatrics, McMaster University, Hamilton, ON L8S 4KI, Canada; satkins@mcmaster.ca
* Correspondence: kbcomerford@ucdavis.edu; Tel.: +1-707-799-0699
† These authors contributed equally to this work.

Received: 18 February 2016; Accepted: 29 March 2016; Published: 21 May 2016

Abstract: Infant dietary patterns tend to be insufficient sources of fruits, vegetables, and fiber, as well as excessive in salt, added sugars, and overall energy. Despite the serious long-term health risks associated with suboptimal fruit and vegetable intake, a large percentage of infants and toddlers in the U.S. do not consume any fruits or vegetables on a daily basis. Since not all fruits and vegetables are nutritionally similar, guidance on the optimal selection of fruits and vegetables should emphasize those with the greatest potential for nutrition and health benefits. A challenge is that the most popularly consumed fruits for this age group (*i.e.*, apples, pears, bananas, grapes, strawberries) do not closely fit the current general recommendations since they tend to be overly sweet and/or high in sugar. Unsaturated oil-containing fruits such as avocados are nutritionally unique among fruits in that they are lower in sugar and higher in fiber and monounsaturated fatty acids than most other fruits, and they also have the proper consistency and texture for first foods with a neutral flavor spectrum. Taken together, avocados show promise for helping to meet the dietary needs of infants and toddlers, and should be considered for inclusion in future dietary recommendations for complementary and transitional feeding.

Keywords: avocado; monounsaturated fat; fiber; infant; toddler complementary feeding; transitional feeding

1. Introduction

Proper nutrition is one of the most influential factors for insuring normal growth and development during a child's first years of life, yet there are currently very few research-based dietary recommendations for parents and caregivers regarding this critical time period [1]. Currently, U.S. dietary guidelines do not differentiate between age groups of children under two years old even though the nutritional requirements of infants and toddlers differ from each other, and from the nutritional requirements of older children, adolescents, and adults. Without age-appropriate dietary guidelines from birth to 24 months of age, the diets of infants and toddlers often reflect the dietary preferences and nutrient composition of their parents' and caregivers' diets, which tend to lack adequate sources of fiber-rich and nutrient-dense fruits and vegetables and contain excessive sodium and sugar [1].

Nutrition delivery to infants is influenced by physiological development, growth demands, and to some extent by family dietary practices. During the first six months after birth, breast milk is recommended as the exclusive source of nutrition necessary for early infant health and development [2], especially because during the early stages of development, a baby's swallowing and digestive systems are not yet fully developed for the intake and processing of non-liquid food sources [3]. As an infant grows and develops, it experiences physiological shifts in nutrient and energy requirements that can no longer be supported by breast milk alone [2]. Additionally, as an infant transitions from a strictly maternal-sourced food supply to a varied diet and familial table foods, the emphasis on energy and nutrient requirements is placed on a whole new set of dietary options—many of which are not ideal for young children.

Although the timeframes for complementary and transitional feeding are not officially defined, for this review, the complementary feeding period is considered to start when the first foods (other than breast milk or formula) are consumed and continues throughout the infant's first year of life (approximately six to 12 months), while the transitional feeding period covers a toddler's dietary pattern during their second year of life (13–24 months). Nutrient and energy deficiencies during the early developmental stages can have lasting effects on the health of the offspring [4–6]. Therefore, nutrient-rich foods that are also moderately energy-dense (while being low in sugar content) are ideal early foods for infants [7,8]. The first food exposures should meet the infant's/toddler's high nutritional requirements for energy, certain fatty acids, and key vitamins and minerals, such as vitamin A/provitamin A carotenoids, several B vitamins, iodine, iron, and zinc [9,10]. Deficiencies in any of these nutrients during the critical times of development can have both immediate and long-lasting effects on the health of the offspring.

Fruits and vegetables are some of the most consistently recommended early food options, but few of the most popular fruit options such as apples, bananas and grapes have the characteristics of being both moderate in energy-density and low in sugar content. Avocados—technically classified as fleshy, single-seeded berries—differ from most other fruits, however, in that they are a source of several promising non-essential compounds, such as fat-soluble antioxidants and monounsaturated fatty acids (MUFA). The sugar content is less than 1 g per serving, which is the lowest amount compared to all other fresh fruits. A 1-ounce (30 g) serving of avocado is higher in key developmental nutrients such as folate, vitamin E, and lutein compared to a Nutrition Labeling and Education Act (NLEA) serving size of the most popular complementary and transitional feeding fruits (*i.e.*, apples, pears, bananas, grapes, strawberries, and peaches) (Table 1) [11–13]. A standard serving of avocados is also less than one fourth the weight of any of the other commonly consumed fruits, making them a very efficient vehicle food for delivering essential nutrition in a portion size that an infant or toddler would more likely be able to consume in one sitting. Avocado is also higher in unsaturated fatty acids compared to most fruits and vegetables [14] (Table 1). The fatty acids in avocados allow for greater absorption of fat-soluble nutrients, either inherent in the fruit or from other foods eaten with avocado, when compared to other fruits and vegetables that are low in fat (or fat-free) [15,16].

This paper is the second of a two-part series on ideal food and nutrient intake and related health outcomes covering the first 1000 days of life (*i.e.*, from the time of conception to the end of a toddler's second year). The first paper in the series provides evidence for the regular inclusion of key nutrients as well as low-glycemic fruits and vegetables, such as avocados, in a maternal diet for improving birth outcomes and various aspects of maternal health extending from the pre-conceptional period through pregnancy and lactation [17]. This report provides further evidence regarding the regular inclusion of such key nutrients and their food sources, including avocados, on many potential early- and later-life health benefits, as well as explore the potential beneficial effects of monounsaturated fatty acids and bioactive compounds during the complementary and transitional feeding periods. The paper also addresses nutrition topic questions posed by the U.S. Department of Agriculture (USDA) and U.S. Department of Health and Human Services (HHS) expert work groups that comprise the Birth to 24 months and Pregnant Women Dietary Guidance Development Project—specifically Work Group 2–Infancy: Period of Complementary Feeding (6–12 months) and Work Group 3–Period of Transitional Feeding (12–24 months):

- What types and amounts of complementary foods are necessary for infants fed human milk, formula, or mixed feedings to promote favorable health outcomes, such as (1) growth and physical development; (2) cognitive, behavioral or neuromotor development?
- What strategies can be used to improve dietary quality and micronutrient intake in infants six to 12 months of age?
- What are the evidence-based strategies to enhance acceptance of nutrient-dense foods like fruits and vegetables?
- Does exposure (timing, quantity, frequency) to nutrient-dense foods in weaned infants increase acceptance of nutrient-dense foods?
- Does increased acceptance/preference for nutrient-dense foods in the first year of life persist? Does it improve dietary intake of nutrient-dense foods at 12–24 months?
- Does the intake of foods with added salt and sugar in infancy influence the preference and analgesic appeal of dietary salt and sweet in infants, young children, and adults?
- What are the energy requirements for toddlers, ages 12–24 months, to promote optimal growth and physical development?
- What is the relationship between observed intakes of fiber, vitamin A, and folate and the estimated average requirement (EAR) and upper limits (UL) for toddlers 12–24 months of age?
- What food characteristics (e.g., taste/flavor characteristics, portion size, energy, nutrient-density, novel or familiar) impact the development of food preferences and dietary intake?

Table 1. Meeting the developmental needs of infants and toddlers. Comparison of a serving (30 g) of avocado *versus* a Nutrition Labeling and Education Act (NLEA) serving (Range: 126–242 g) of the most popular complementary and transitional fruits.

Per NLEA Serving	Apples (242 g)	Avocados (30 g)	Bananas (126 g)	Grapes (126 g)	Peaches (147 g)	Pears (166 g)	Strawberries (147 g)
>150 mg potassium/serving	√	√	√	√	√	√	√
>25 µg folate/serving		√	√				√
>0.50 mg α-tocopherol/serving		√			√		
>80 µg Lutein + zeaxanthin/serving		√		√	√		
>40 IU vitamin A/serving	√	√	√	√	√	√	
>6 µg vitamin K/serving		√		√		√	
>2.5 g MUFA/serving		√					
≥2 g fiber/serving	√	√	√		√	√	√

Data sourced from: USDA Agricultural Research Service, National Nutrient Database for Standard Reference Release 27 [18]. Basic Report: 09003, apples, raw, with skin; 09038, avocados, raw, California; 09040, bananas, raw; 09131, grapes, American type (slip skin) raw; 09236, peaches, yellow, raw; 09252, pears, raw; 09316, strawberries, raw.

2. Background Information and General Recommendations for Complementary Feeding (6 to 12 Months)

Current guidance from the World Health Organization (WHO) and other leading developed countries is consistent in the recommendations that complementary feedings should begin at about six months of age to support sufficient infant growth and development [19–22], and should last through the end of the first year of life. During this period breastfeeding should still remain a primary source of nutrition [23]. Therefore, breastfeeding mothers should pay careful attention to the quality of their own diets, since for some nutrients (especially vitamins and fatty acids), the foods mothers eat directly influence the nutrient profile of the milk consumed by their infants [24]. When introducing new foods to an infant, experts recommend that parents and caregivers offer a variety of nutrient-dense, soft- and mixed-textured fruits, vegetables, cereals, and meats that contain little or no added sugar or salt [3,7,25]. The WHO recommends that infants start receiving complementary foods in addition to breast milk two to three times a day from six to eight months of age, and three to four times a day from nine months of age through the end of the complementary feeding period [26].

A consensus statement from the American Heart Association (AHA) on dietary recommendations for children acknowledged that only a small percentage of infants in the U.S. remain exclusively breastfed after four months of age [27]. Corroborating the AHA findings, a recent Hass Avocado Board (HAB) funded survey (HAB Caregiver Survey) conducted among 338 caregivers of infants between the ages of four and 24 months also shows nearly half of the respondents introduced fruits and vegetables between four and six months of age, while approximately one-third introduced protein foods (meat, beans, eggs, peanut butter), grains or dairy in that same time period [28].

Infants will usually triple their body weight between birth and the end of their first year, and much of this growth occurs in the complementary feeding period [29]. In order to accomplish the high rate of growth and development, infants must consume both adequate amounts of energy and essential nutrients. Foods consumed throughout the complementary feeding stage should balance the nutrients from milk or formula, without imposing excess intakes of energy or nutrients [30]. Since complementary foods are initially consumed in very small quantities, caregivers should offer moderately energy-dense foods, rich in multiple nutrients that are key for proper infant health and development (*i.e.*, iron, zinc, calcium, provitamin A/carotenoids, vitamin C, and folate) [8].

3. Background Information and General Recommendations for Transitional Feeding (13 to 24 Months)

Similarly to complementary feeding, transitional feeding (13 to 24 months) is defined as all solid and liquid foods consumed other than breast milk and infant formula. The main differences between complementary foods and transitional foods are: (1) the timeframe in which they are consumed (*i.e.*, first year *versus* second year of life); (2) the texture and consistency of foods recommended, which require more developed mastication and digestive abilities; and (3) the portions consumed, based on individual appetite, breast milk and/or formula consumption, and nutritional needs. Toddlers typically consume an increasingly complex diet, moving further away from milk and/or formula towards a diet more focused on a variety of table foods, especially those consumed by other family members [31]. On average, approximately two-thirds of a toddler's energy intake from 12 to 24 months comes from transitional foods [20,23], more than double the energy intake from table foods when compared to the last months of the complementary period [32].

Currently, little research exists on nutrition and health in the toddler age group (13–24 months). The existing evidence is further complicated by datasets that do not distinguish between age groups and combine one- and two-year-olds together without teasing out the differences between these age groups [1]. This gap in scientific knowledge is reflected in the DRI for toddlers, which were generally derived by extrapolating data from studies involving infants or adults [33]. Toddlers' nutrition needs are different however. They are less dependent on breast milk for their nutrients and need more fiber, while experiencing greater growth velocity than older children [1]. Therefore ideal toddler foods should contain adequate energy, as well as fiber and key nutrients not found in sufficient amounts in breast milk or other popular family foods [23,34].

4. Ideal Complementary and Transitional Foods: Recommendations *versus* Reality

Many of the nutrient-rich foods recommended by the *2015 Dietary Guidelines for Americans* (DGA) [35] for child and adult health have been linked to allergy development and are thought to be contraindicated in the complementary feeding period for infants. These foods include seafood, nuts, and eggs [36,37], although recent evidence has challenged the early exposure hypothesis linking these foods to the development of allergies [38,39]. Other nutrient-dense food options contain too much saturated fat, added salt, sugar, spices, preservatives, additives or artificial ingredients [8,20]. Furthermore, in addition to their nutritional properties, ideal complementary and transitional foods should also have specific physical and chemical attributes such as a proper texture and consistency, along with natural and relatively neutral flavors, to encourage toddlers to develop familiarity and taste preferences for them [20,31].

Data from the landmark Feeding Infants and Toddlers Studies (FITS I and FITS II) along with recent National Health and Nutrition Examination Survey (NHANES) data (from children over two years old) show that young children consume nearly 40% of their total energy from foods like refined grains, sugar-sweetened beverages, and fruit juice. [40,41]. The findings also showed a general decline in fruit and vegetable intake, especially fiber-rich fruits and vegetables as children age from infancy into toddlerhood [27]. The data also showed that infants and toddlers were much more likely to consume sweets, such as cookies or candies rather than nutrient-rich options such as fruits or vegetables [5]. This trend continued through the end of the transitional feeding period, when approximately one-third of U.S. toddlers consumed no fruit on a daily basis [42] and deep yellow vegetable intake went from being consumed by nearly 40% of infants during the middle of the complementary feeding period down to 13% by the time they reached the end of the transitional feeding period [31]. Nutrient- and antioxidant-dense dietary options were consistently replaced by lower-nutrient and higher-energy options such as candies, desserts, and sugar-sweetened beverages [31,43].

The most popular fruits consumed by infants were apples, bananas, peaches, and pears [42], and often times these were in forms that contained added sugars. Apples, bananas, grapes, peaches, and strawberries ranked as the most popular in a child's second year of life [41,42]. Apples and bananas were also the most popular fruits among infants [28]. In summary, despite the popularity of these fruits, only avocados, actually meet almost all of the expert recommendations (*i.e.*, nutrient-rich, colorful, naturally soft texture, low in sugar/not overly sweet, low-glycemic). This positions avocados as both a unique and ideal food for infants and toddlers.

5. Fruits and Vegetables: Early Exposure Can Lead to Life Long Benefits

Fruits and vegetables are vital to a healthy eating pattern as they contain essential nutrients, various forms of fiber, and potentially beneficial bioactive components such as antioxidants and phytosterols [44,45]. Yet, increasing fruit and vegetable exposure and intake among infants/toddlers remains a challenge for both caregivers and dietetic professionals [46,47]. Both fruit and vegetable intake in children of all ages remains below recommendations in most countries worldwide [48], and a large percentage of U.S. infants from six to 12 months of age do not consume any fruits or vegetables on a daily basis [42,49]. A practical goal would be simple dietary changes focused on exchanging empty-calorie foods and beverages for nutrient-rich, high-fiber fruits and vegetables containing no added sugar.

Experts suggest that vegetables and low-sugar fruits, such as avocados, should be introduced in the early stages in order to avoid invoking an early preference for sweet foods, which may influence early childhood and later life eating behaviors [7,8]. The dietary patterns of infants and young children have been shown to correlate to patterns in later childhood [50,51] and even to adulthood [52]; adult health factors, such as cholesterol metabolism, may be programmed from the lipids consumed in infancy [53].

Observational studies have demonstrated later health benefits of healthful early nutrition choices. Better body weights in later years were observed in infants who consumed higher amounts of fruits and/or vegetables and thus less total energy in their diets [5]. Infants given home-prepared fruits or vegetables more frequently at six months of age were more likely to eat more fruits and vegetables several years later compared to infants who were given similar foods less often [54]. Furthermore, frequent fruit and vegetable consumption by younger children was associated with lower blood pressure and a lower risk of stroke in their adult years [55,56], and a lower risk for some cancers [6]. While these studies showed associations between early and later life dietary patterns and health outcomes, very little research has addressed the introduction of specific fruits and vegetables in the complementary and transitional feeding periods, or how consumption of specific "ideal" or popular complementary foods or specific nutrients in those foods (e.g., iron-fortified cereal grains, bananas, apples, avocados, potatoes) may promote long-term health, help build good dietary habits, or assist in reducing health risks. Avocados, and other foods that fit the description of an "ideal complementary food" deserve more clinical research attention, especially since the health status of an infant in its first year of life affects its risk for certain chronic diseases in later years [57].

6. Macronutrients: Amount and Specific Structural/Functional Characteristics are Key for Infant and Toddler Health

6.1. Dietary Fat: Quantity and Quality Both Matter for Growth and Development

In infancy, fat should comprise about 50% of energy intake in order to provide adequate energy for rapid growth and the essential fatty acids for brain development [58]. With the introduction of complementary foods, energy intake may become inadequate as foods such as fruits, vegetables and cereal grains are generally very low in fat. Complementary foods that are a good source of both fat and energy are important to maintain energy intake. Once in the toddler period, the percentage of fat in the diet may be reduced; however, the total energy and nutrients, including essential fatty acids, must increase to cover the energy cost of activity and growth. Achieving adequate fat intake may be a challenge since in the FITS II data, total fat intakes were below the acceptable macronutrient distribution range in one in four toddlers from the U.S. [59]. Diets of infants and toddlers that are low fat are associated with lower vitamin and mineral intakes [58], and lower fat-soluble vitamin absorption [60]. A Joint Food and Agriculture Organization (FAO)/WHO Expert Consultation report underlined the importance of not only the quantity, but also the quality of fat for proper infant health and development [60].

A joint statement from Health Canada, the Canadian Pediatric Society, Dietitians of Canada, and Breastfeeding Committee for Canada suggests that parents and caregivers should provide adequate amounts of healthy fats in addition to breast milk, and specifically includes avocados as an example of a nutritious fat-containing food for infant health [20]. Avocados are unique among the commonly recommended complementary and transitional fruits and vegetables in that they contain 3.5 g of unsaturated fats per 1-ounce (30 g) serving, accounting for more than 75% of their fat content. The unsaturated fatty acids are primarily in the form of the MUFA oleic acid (C18:1; $n = 9$), while a lesser amount comes from other MUFA, polyunsaturated fatty acids (PUFA), and saturated fatty acids (SFA). Although oleic acid is not considered an essential fatty acid because the human body can synthesize it from other fatty acids, it is the most abundant fatty acid in breast milk [61]. MUFA, such as oleic acid, has also been shown to be important for the normal growth and development of the central nervous system and brain [62], as well as being beneficial for fat-soluble nutrient absorption [15,16]. A 30 g serving of avocado contains approximately 0.5 g of the PUFA linoleic acid (18:2*n*-6) [14], which comprises roughly 10%–15% of the fatty acid content in avocados [63]. Evidence exists showing that as little as 3%–4.5% of total energy intake from linoleic acid is associated with optimal growth and development for infants and toddlers [60].

Since avocados provide energy, MUFA, and PUFA, they would contribute to achieving nutrient balance in infant diets, as well as aiding in absorption of fat-soluble nutrients, providing a source of antioxidants, and thereby potentially contributing to health benefits [16,64,65].

6.2. Fiber: Balancing Intake for Optimal Health

Breast milk contains various non-digestible oligosaccharides, which are small-chain prebiotic fiber compounds that are important for infant gut health and immune development [66,67]. While other infant foods are not rich sources of non-digestible oligosaccharides, many fruits and vegetables are rich sources of both soluble and insoluble fibers (e.g., non-digestible carbohydrates and lignin), which may have health benefits even in young children [68]. Currently, there is no infant adequate intake (AI) established for fiber, but it has been suggested by the American Academy of Pediatrics that the amount be gradually increased to provide roughly 5 g per day by the end of the first year of life [69,70].

Neither the appropriate amount nor type of fiber for infants is as yet determined, with both too little and too much dietary fiber posing their own unique set of problems. Too little fiber can lead to constipation [71], and excessive fiber intake has the potential to negatively impact energy and nutrient intake by increasing fecal energy losses, extending satiety (therefore leading to lower energy and nutrient intakes), and binding up minerals through fiber-associated phytates and oxalates [71–73]. However, fiber intakes of about 4 g/day in infants at 8 months and 7 g/day in infants at 13 months of age have been positively associated with energy intake and weight gain [74]. Additionally, higher dietary fiber intake in infancy was associated with higher intakes of vitamins and minerals compared to lower fiber intakes [74]. In the FITS I data, infants in the highest quartile of fiber intake were also in the highest quartile of energy and macronutrient intake from table foods, providing further evidence that higher fiber intakes in infancy are not associated with under eating [32].

Concern is expressed by practitioners and researchers about both too much fiber intake in the early feeding periods, and inadequate fiber consumption throughout every life stage thereafter [20,68,69,75]. A decline in fiber intake from the complementary period to transitional period was demonstrated in Finnish infants in which 55%–70% of the fiber in an infant's diet was from fruits and vegetables, while only 40%–45% of fiber in a toddler's diet comes from fruits and vegetables [76]. In American infants in FITS I the top sources of dietary fiber for toddlers were primarily refined grains such as non-infant cereals and breads, rolls, biscuits, bagels, and tortillas, along with carbohydrate-rich fruits and vegetables such as bananas and white potatoes [76].

Avocados could contribute to infant fiber intake as they have approximately 2 g of fiber in a 30 g serving [14], which is equal to or greater than nearly all other commonly consumed complementary or transitional foods or fruits by weight [11]. Of the total fiber in avocados, 30%–40% is soluble while 60%–70% is insoluble [14]. When the fiber content of more than 30 fruits and vegetables were compared, avocados stood out as the only food source with relatively high amounts of both soluble fiber (2.1% by weight) and insoluble fiber (2.7% by weight). Additionally, avocados also contain lower levels of phytates and oxalates compared to the most popular fiber sources such as cereal fibers, vegetables, and legumes, thus minimizing loss of calcium and other key essential minerals due to binding by such substances [77].

The higher soluble fiber content of avocados compared to other fruits may be of benefit to the development of an infant's/toddler's gut microflora as it is fermented by the colonic microflora to a greater extent. While fermentable soluble fibers (*i.e.*, prebiotics such as oligosaccharides) from breast milk are known to have potent beneficial effects on infant health [78], the dose response and potential effects of plant-based soluble fiber sources on infant health requires further research. The soluble fiber in avocados may also contribute an energy source for infants since the fermentable nature of soluble fiber allows the colonic microflora to metabolize undigested polysaccharides and produce various short-chain fatty acids (e.g., acetic acid, butyric acid and propionic acid), which are then able to be absorbed [79–81].

7. Micronutrients: Avoiding Deficiencies during the Complementary and Transitional Feeding Periods

7.1. Nutrients for Building the Blood

The selection of complementary foods to meet the micronutrient needs of infants is challenging as essential nutrients like iron are present in low concentrations in typical infant foods, even in breast milk [82]. Avocados, while low in iron, contain folate, vitamin C, riboflavin, and vitamin B6 that are all essential to various aspects of iron absorption, red blood cell formation and/or hemoglobin function. Vitamin C enhances non-heme iron absorption and is a key factor in its bioavailability [83–85]. Folate is critical for the proper synthesis of red blood cells; and is therefore important for prevention of megaloblastic anemia [86]. Vitamin B6 plays a role in the synthesis of hemoglobin and in oxygen transport, and a deficiency in vitamin B6 can lead to microcytic hypochromic anemia. Riboflavin is required for the enzymatic activation of folate and vitamin B6 as well as for red blood cell production, and a deficiency in riboflavin can lead to normocytic anemia. Foods such as avocados, should be considered as providing a unique combination of several blood-building nutrients that can act as iron-absorption enhancers and/or function in red blood cell synthesis.

7.2. Potassium

As infants and toddlers begin to consume less electrolyte-rich breast milk, complementary food sources must provide a balance of electrolytes necessary to maintain proper fluid balance and bone turnover. However, it is observed that about 45%–80% of toddlers exceed the recommended sodium intake levels, and only 5% of toddlers meet the recommended intake levels for potassium [59,87]. To reduce sodium and provide potassium, complementary foods like avocados offer not only a sodium-free, complementary food, but they are also rich in potassium (Table 1) [14].

7.3. Enhanced Fat-Soluble Nutrient Absorption

Natural food sources of lipid-soluble vitamins and antioxidant compounds are important to identify as it is known that toddlers receive a substantial amount of nutrients, such as vitamin A, from supplements and fortified foods instead of from unprocessed whole foods [76]. More than 60% of toddlers in the U.S. consume less vitamin E than the EAR [59]. Avocados contribute three of the four fat-soluble vitamins such that a 1-ounce serving of avocado provides more provitamin A in the form of carotenoids than almost all other fruits, as well as small amounts of vitamin E and vitamin K (Table 1). Absorption of fat-soluble vitamins is enhanced in the presence of adequate fat intake, which is known to be less than adequate in the toddler age group [58]. The MUFA content of avocados is unique among other fruits and vegetables as fatty acids help fat-soluble vitamins and carotenoids (e.g., lutein, lycopene, alpha-carotene, and beta-carotene) be more effectively absorbed from other foods [15,16]. Avocado consumption can also enhance the efficiency of conversion of carotenoids to vitamin A by two to six fold [16].

8. Avocado Dietary Bioactive Components: Playing an Important Role in Infant Health

Breast milk is known to have numerous bioactive properties (*i.e.*, properties above and beyond their nutritive roles) that are associated with infant health and development [88–90]. Complementary and transitional foods contain bioactive components such as fiber, antioxidants, electrolytes, carotenoids, and flavonoids [14,91]. Avocados also contain many lipophilic phytochemicals and bioactive compounds that may confer health benefits (e.g., sterols, polyhydroxylated fatty alcohols (PFA), alkaloids, acetogenins, and volatile oils) [91–93]. While understanding of the interplay of antioxidant, prebiotic and sterol components in foods and food combinations is just emerging, it has been suggested that a wide variety of bioactive compounds are responsible for the health benefits of fruits and vegetables through additive and synergistic interactions by targeting multiple signal transduction pathways [94].

For early infant foods, such as fruits and vegetables, the health effects are attributed to different bioactive compounds such as vitamin C, carotenoids, and various phenolic compounds [95]. The antioxidant potential of components like carotenoids (beta-carotene, lutein and zeaxanthin) in fruits and vegetables not only provide the precursors for vitamin A (which is essential for proper growth, development, vision, immunity, hair and skin health, and mucous membrane formation) [25], but may also act as free-radical scavenging antioxidants [96]. Additionally, these carotenoids have functional roles in the tissues of the infant brain [97].

Lutein accounts for the majority of infant brain carotenoids, representing approximately 60% of total carotenoids [98]. Recent metabolomics studies on post-mortem infants showed correlations between brain lutein concentrations and energy metabolite pathways, lipid metabolite pathways, and amino acid neurotransmission pathways [99]. Further, formula-fed infants compared to breast-fed infants had significantly lower lutein concentrations in their blood [100]. Lutein was approved by the FDA for use in infant formulas, despite it not being officially classified as an essential nutrient.

As complementary foods begin to displace breast milk or formula in the diet, adequate sources of lutein from complementary foods may be important in infant health [99]. Avocados contain some of the highest levels of lutein and dietary fat of any fruit or vegetable (Table 1), along with the added benefit of a dietary MUFA fat source to aid absorption of the fat-soluble lutein [15,16].

Phytosterols and PFA are two other lipid-soluble compounds that account for a large portion of the lipid content of avocados but their potential benefits have not been studied in infants or toddlers [25]. In adults, both phytosterols and PFA have been shown to support a healthy inflammatory response [25]. Lipophilic acetogenins in avocados [92] are a group of antioxidants that are synthesized from fatty acid precursors that have promise for their anti-proliferative and apoptotic effects on cancer cells [101–103]. The amino-acid based antioxidant glutathione, also in avocados in higher concentration (8.4 mg/30 g) that any other fruit [104], is involved in immune function, lipid metabolism, detoxification, and several aspects of cellular defense and replication [105]. Since heating and processing reduces glutathione levels in foods, foods which are commonly consumed raw, such as avocados, contain higher levels of this antioxidant compound. Future research is required to identify the types of foods with fat-soluble nutrient absorption-enhancing properties that may optimize infant and toddler health, as well as provide protection against free-radical damage and future chronic disease risk [95].

9. Food Preferences: Early Exposure to Flavor and Texture Can Influence Acceptability

Beyond choosing the most ideal nutrient-rich foods to feed their infants and toddlers, parents and caregivers should also understand the roles that the flavors and textures of foods play in transitional and complementary feeding. Food learning and flavor preferences start in utero and are heavily influenced by breastfeeding and the infant's complementary diet in the first year of life [106]. The early taste preferences appear to be biologically driven with certain flavors, such as sweetness indicating available calories, and bitter flavors indicating potentially dangerous compounds present in the food [106]. These preferences have been shown to be somewhat malleable and dependent on environmental factors such as repeated exposures to flavors [1,107]. Once established, many of the early dietary preferences and habits tend to have a long-lasting influence [47], even into adulthood where there is a tendency to favor foods the way they were initially introduced [8]. Therefore, proper early food exposure is important for laying the foundation of a long-term varied diet. Beyond taste and texture, early exposure to a myriad of food taste and texture profiles also teaches societal and familial ideals, attitudes, and beliefs about food and eating behaviors [108].

In order to establish a varied eating pattern—which includes neutral, sour, and bitter taste acceptance—the ideal initial foods should be those that are both nutritious and have a low to moderate sweet and salty flavor profile [8]. Such presentation takes advantage of the plasticity of early flavor learning [106]. Additionally, infants who have positive early experiences with fruits and vegetables are significantly more likely to choose and consume those foods later in life [109–111]. Unfortunately, findings from the HAB Caregiver Survey indicate that this approach is not being readily followed. Nearly 60% of infants and toddlers were described as picky eaters, and the most common foods offered and consumed early in life were sweet fruits and starchy vegetables [28]. Further, the caregivers' overarching goal was to give "foods that the infant/toddler really enjoyed eating", while the actual nutritional value of the food provided ranked lower on their agendas [28]. In order to combat the overly sweet and salty flavors of the standard American diet without offending the child's innate dislikes for bitter and sour, some pediatricians recommend introducing mild foods (*i.e.*, neither sweet, salty, sour, or bitter) with a neutral flavor profile in the early complementary period [7]. Avocados can provide children with the types of nutrients and phytochemicals found in many sweet-tasting, sugar-rich fruits and bitter-tasting vegetables.

In addition to flavor preferences, infants also have texture preferences due to their developing abilities to chew and swallow. When foods are being introduced to infants it is important that caregivers provide a variety of soft textures—such as creamy, lumpy, tender, pureed, mashed or ground—in order to properly develop oro-sensory functions and the swallowing mechanism [20]. Different textures are necessary to gradually introduce the baby to solid foods while reducing the risk of choking or swallowing large chunks of food that are difficult to digest. Soft fruit and vegetable consumption—such as from peaches, bananas, and avocados—is consistent with several recommendations from the federal feeding assistance program Special Supplemental Nutrition Program for Women, Infants, and Children (WIC) for infant feeding (although peaches and bananas do not have an ideal sweetness/sugar factor). Soft, neutral-flavored, and nutrient-dense avocado—which does not need to be cooked and can easily be stored—appears to be one of the most ideal complementary and transitional foods available. In essence, the avocado's natural characteristics match what health professionals and caregivers are most likely to consider important for an infant's first food offerings [28].

10. Future Guidelines for Complementary and Transitional Feeding: Importance of Clear and Specific Recommendations

A consistent message from recent literature is that fruit and vegetable intake needs to be increased in infant and toddler dietary patterns; selection of those foods that are lower in sugar and higher in fiber should be recommended above varieties that are higher in sugar and overly sweet. Most specific recommendations for parents and caregivers suggest offering a wide variety of fruits and vegetables on a daily basis, with an emphasis on colorful fruits and dark green, leafy, and deep yellow vegetables [31]. For fruit, recommendations could be clearer to ensure caregivers are making the best choices by specifically calling out: "colorful fruits that are a good source of fiber and low in sugar". Further, naming of specific examples of these types of fruits would limit confusion and clearly point caregivers to the best options for infants and toddlers.

Avocados are a good example of a fruit that could be specifically recommended as an optimal transitional food. Beyond its texture, flavor and nutrient profile, avocado consumption among infants and toddlers may be able to displace empty calorie offerings more effectively than other nutrient-rich complementary and transitional foods due to their higher amount of appetite suppressing fatty acids and fiber [112,113]. According to the American Dietetic Association (now the Academy of Nutrition and Dietetics), "foods that are rich in energy and nutrients such as avocado should be used when the infant is being weaned [34]". Therefore, the avocado with its fiber-content, MUFA, moderate energy-density, more than 20 vitamins and minerals, and array of phytonutrients appears to one of the most ideal fruits—and possibly foods—for complementary and transitional feeding [114].

11. Conclusions

Major transitions occur in the dietary patterns of infants and toddlers over the first two years of life. Exposure to certain foods and nutrients during the first two years may impact their future health through metabolic programming or development of specific tastes [115]. The most ideal complementary and transitional foods—nutritionally and physiochemically—should be offered regularly to infants and toddlers in order to ensure their optimal health, as well to expand their range of flavor preferences and acceptance for nutrient-rich dietary options. As detailed in this paper, avocados are unique among complementary and transitional foods in that they:

- Contain a spectrum of essential and non-essential nutrients with potential health benefits that minimize undesirable components such as sodium, empty calories, and unhealthy fats.
- Provide an ideal source of energy (high in healthy unsaturated fats and low in sugar) to meet the increasing energy and growth demands of weaning infants and toddlers.
- By weight and serving size, contain some of the highest levels of the antioxidants lutein, zeaxanthin, and glutathione among complementary and transitional foods.
- Are rich in unsaturated fatty acids, which significantly enhance the absorption of lipid-soluble compounds.

- Contain more total fiber and soluble fiber per gram than almost all other complementary and transitional foods, and at the same time contain less mineral-binding phytates and oxalates than other popular high-fiber foods.
- Have a neutral flavor and smooth consistency that is ideal for early infant foods.

At present, the current infant feeding recommendations tend to be based on anecdotal and observational findings, which are largely dependent on an infant's learned preference for sweet foods. Future development of complementary and transitional feeding recommendations should utilize evidence from controlled studies that investigate the critical nutrient needs of infants and toddlers, and should progress toward identifying the most ideal foods (*i.e.*, those that meet the majority of recommended guidelines). Future research on ideal infant and toddler foods, including avocados, is warranted to further explore their potential in both early life and later life health outcomes.

Acknowledgments: This research was funded by the Hass Avocado Board.

Author Contributions: K.B.C. drafted the manuscript. K.T.A., R.D.M., and S.A.A. provided expert guidance, review and feedback throughout the manuscript development process.

Conflicts of Interest: All authors received consulting fees from the Hass Avocado Board. All conclusions are those of the authors.

References

1. Birch, L.L.; Doub, A.E. Learning to eat: Birth to age 2 years. *Am. J. Clin. Nutr.* **2014**, *99*, 723S–728S. [CrossRef] [PubMed]
2. Solomons, N.W.; Vossenaar, M. Nutrient Density in Complementary Feeding of Infants and Toddlers. *Eur. J. Clin. Nutr.* **2013**, *67*, 501–506. [CrossRef] [PubMed]
3. USDA. *Food and Nutrition Service: Feeding Infants: A Guide for Use in Child Nutrition Programs*; USDA: Alexandria, VA, USA, 2002.
4. Gale, C.R.; Martyn, C.N.; Marriott, L.D.; Limond, J.; Crozier, S.; Inskip, H.M.; Godfrey, K.M.; Law, C.M.; Cooper, C.; Robinson, S.M.; *et al.* Dietary Patterns in Infancy and Cognitive and Neuropsychological Function in Childhood. *J. Child Psychol. Psychiatry* **2009**, *50*, 816–823. [CrossRef] [PubMed]
5. Saavedra, J.M.; Deming, D.; Dattilo, A.; Reidy, K. Lessons from the Feeding Infants and Toddlers Study in North America: What Children Eat, and Implications for Obesity Prevention. *Ann. Nutr. Metab.* **2013**, *62* (Suppl. 3), 27–36. [CrossRef] [PubMed]
6. Maynard, M.; Gunnell, D.; Emmett, P.; Frankel, S.; Davey Smith, G. Fruit, Vegetables, and Antioxidants in Childhood and Risk of Adult Cancer: The Boyd Orr Cohort. *J. Epidemiol. Community Health* **2003**, *57*, 218–225. [CrossRef] [PubMed]
7. Stettler, N.; Bhatia, J.; Parish, A.; Stallings, V.A. Feeding Healthy Infants, Children, and Adolescents. In *Nelson Textbook of Pediatrics*, 19th ed.; Kliegman, R.M., Stanton, B.M.D., Geme, J.S., Schor, N.F., Behrman, R.E., Eds.; Elsevier & Saunders: Philadelphia, PA, USA, 2011; Chapter 42.
8. Monte, C.M.; Giugliani, E.R. Recommendations for the Complementary Feeding of the Breastfed Child. *J. Pediatr. (Rio J.)* **2004**, *80*, S131–S141. [CrossRef]
9. Ramakrishnan, U.; Grant, F.; Goldenberg, T.; Zongrone, A.; Martorell, R. Effect of Women's Nutrition before and During Early Pregnancy on Maternal and Infant Outcomes: A Systematic Review. *Paediatr. Perinat. Epidemiol.* **2012**, *26* (Suppl. 1), 285–301. [CrossRef] [PubMed]
10. Cetin, I.; Berti, C.; Calabrese, S. Role of Micronutrients in the Periconceptional Period. *Hum. Reprod. Update* **2010**, *16*, 80–95. [CrossRef] [PubMed]
11. USDA. National Nutrient Database for Standard Reference Release 27: Fiber, Total Dietary (G): "Compared to Fruits and Fruit Juices". 2014. Available online: https://ndb.nal.usda.gov/ (accessed on 23 August 2015).
12. USDA. National Nutrient Database for Standard Reference Release 27: Sugars, Total (G): "Compared to Fruits and Fruit Juices". 2014. Available online: https://ndb.nal.usda.gov/ (accessed on 23 August 2015).
13. USDA. National Nutrient Database for Standard Reference Release 27: Fatty Acids, Total Monounsaturated (G): "Compared to Fruits and Fruit Juices". 2014. Available online: https://ndb.nal.usda.gov/ (accessed on 23 August 2015).

14. Dreher, M.L.; Davenport, A.J. Hass Avocado Composition and Potential Health Effects. *Crit. Rev. Food Sci. Nutr.* **2013**, *53*, 738–750. [CrossRef] [PubMed]

15. Unlu, N.Z.; Bohn, T.; Clinton, S.K.; Schwartz, S.J. Carotenoid Absorption from Salad and Salsa by Humans Is Enhanced by the Addition of Avocado or Avocado Oil. *J. Nutr.* **2005**, *135*, 431–436. [PubMed]

16. Kopec, R.E.; Cooperstone, J.L.; Schweiggert, R.M.; Young, G.S.; Harrison, E.H.; Francis, D.M.; Clinton, S.K.; Schwartz, S.J. Avocado Consumption Enhances Human Postprandial Provitamin a Absorption and Conversion from a Novel High-Beta-Carotene Tomato Sauce and from Carrots. *J. Nutr.* **2014**, *144*, 1158–1166. [CrossRef] [PubMed]

17. Comerford, K.B.; Ayoob, K.T.; Murray, R.D.; Atkinson, S.A. The Role of Avocados in Maternal Diets During the Periconceptional Period, Pregnancy, and Lactation. *Nutrients* **2016**. [CrossRef]

18. US Department of Agriculture, Agricultural Research Service, Nutrient Data Laboratory. USDA National Nutrient Database for Standard Reference, Release 27. 2014. Available online: http://www.ars.usda.gov/nea/bhnrc/ndl (accessed on 23 August 2015).

19. Michaelsen, K.F.; Larnkjaer, A.; Lauritzen, L.; Molgaard, C. Science Base of Complementary Feeding Practice in Infancy. *Curr. Opin. Clin. Nutr. Metab. Care* **2010**, *13*, 277–283. [CrossRef] [PubMed]

20. Health Canada: Infant Feeding Joint Working Group. Nutrition for Healthy Term Infants: Recommendations from Six to 24 months, 2014. Available online: http://www.Hc-Sc.Gc.Ca/Fn-an/Nutrition/Infant-Nourisson/Recom/Recom-6-24-Months-6-24-Mois-Eng.Php#A3 (accessed on 21 August 2015).

21. Australia National Health and Medical Research Council. Infant Feeding Guidelines Information for Health Workers. 2012. Available online: http://www.Eatforhealth.Gov.Au/Sites/Default/Files/Files/the_Guidelines/N56_Infant_Feeding_Guidelines.Pdf (accessed on 21 August 2015).

22. National Health Service: Pregnancy and Baby. 2015. Available online: http://www.Nhs.Uk/Conditions/Pregnancy-and-Baby/Pages/Solid-Foods-Weaning.Aspx#Close (accessed on 21 August 2015).

23. WHO. *Infant and Young Child Feeding: Model Chapter for Textbooks for Medical Students and Allied Health Professionals*; WHO: Geneva, Switzerland, 2009.

24. Champ, M.; Hoebler, C. Functional Food for Pregnant, Lactating Women and in Perinatal Nutrition: A Role for Dietary Fibres? *Curr. Opin. Clin. Nutr. Metab. Care* **2009**, *12*, 565–574. [CrossRef] [PubMed]

25. USDA. Food and Nutrition Service: Woman, Infants and Children (Wic). Infant Nutrition and Feeding: A Guide for Use in the Wic and Csf Programs. 2009. Available online: http://www.Nal.Usda.Gov/Wicworks/Topics/Fg/Completeifg.Pdf (accessed on 23 August 2015).

26. WHO. Nutrition: Complementary Feeding. 2014. Available online: http://www.Who.Int/Nutrition/Topics/Complementary_Feeding/En/ (accessed on 23 August 2015).

27. Gidding, S.S.; Dennison, B.A.; Birch, L.L.; Daniels, S.R.; Gillman, M.W.; Lichtenstein, A.H.; Rattay, K.T.; Steinberger, J.; Stettler, N.; Van Horn, L.; *et al.* Dietary Recommendations for Children and Adolescents: A Guide for Practitioners: Consensus Statement from the American Heart Association. *Circulation* **2005**, *112*, 2061–2075. [CrossRef] [PubMed]

28. Hass Avocado Board: Infant & Toddler Caregiver Survey. 2014. Available online: http://www.Hassavocadoboard.Com (accessed on 6 June 2015).

29. Kathy, C. Complementary Feeding for Infants 6 to 12 months. *J. Fam. Health Care* **2010**, *20*, 20–23. [PubMed]

30. Kuo, A.A.; Inkelas, M.; Slusser, W.M.; Maidenberg, M.; Halfon, N. Introduction of Solid Food to Young Infants. *Mater. Child Health J.* **2011**, *15*, 1185–1194. [CrossRef] [PubMed]

31. Fox, M.K.; Pac, S.; Devaney, B.; Jankowski, L. Feeding Infants and Toddlers Study: What Foods Are Infants and Toddlers Eating? *J. Am. Diet. Assoc.* **2004**, *104*, s22–s30. [CrossRef] [PubMed]

32. Briefel, R.R.; Reidy, K.; Karwe, V.; Jankowski, L.; Hendricks, K. Toddlers' Transition to Table Foods: Impact on Nutrient Intakes and Food Patterns. *J. Am. Diet. Assoc.* **2004**, *104*, s38–s44. [CrossRef] [PubMed]

33. Otten, J.J.; Hellwig, J.P.; Meyers, L.D. *Dietary Reference Intakes: The Essential Guide to Nutrient Requirements*; Medicine, I.O., Ed.; National Academies Press: Washington, DC, USA, 2006.

34. Craig, W.J.; Mangels, A.R.; American Dietetic, A. Position of the American Dietetic Association: Vegetarian Diets. *J. Am. Diet. Assoc.* **2009**, *109*, 1266–1282. [PubMed]

35. U.S. Department of Health, Human Services, U.S. Department of Agriculture. 2015–2020 Dietary Guidelines for Americans, 8th ed. Available online: http://www.cnpp.usda.gov/2015-2020-dietary-guidelines-americans (accessed on 26 January 2016).

36. Fiocchi, A.; Assa'ad, A.; Bahna, S. Food Allergy and the Introduction of Solid Foods to Infants: A Consensus Document. Adverse Reactions to Foods Committee, American College of Allergy, Asthma and Immunology. *Ann. Allergy Asthma Immunol.* **2006**, *97*, 10–21. [CrossRef]

37. Chin, B.; Chan, E.S.; Goldman, R.D. Early Exposure to Food and Food Allergy in Children. *Can. Fam. Phys.* **2014**, *60*, 338–339.

38. Pham-Thi, N.; Bidat, E. Solid Food Introduction and Allergic Risk. *Arch. Pediatr.* **2014**, *21*, 1392–1395. [CrossRef] [PubMed]

39. Abrams, E.M.; Becker, A.B. Food Introduction and Allergy Prevention in Infants. *CMAJ* **2015**, *187*, 1297–1301. [CrossRef] [PubMed]

40. Reedy, J.; Krebs-Smith, S.M. Dietary Sources of Energy, Solid Fats, and Added Sugars among Children and Adolescents in the United States. *J. Am. Diet. Assoc.* **2010**, *110*, 1477–1484. [CrossRef] [PubMed]

41. Fox, M.K.; Condon, E.; Briefel, R.R.; Reidy, K.C.; Deming, D.M. Food Consumption Patterns of Young Preschoolers: Are They Starting off on the Right Path? *J. Am. Diet. Assoc.* **2010**, *110*, S52–S59. [CrossRef] [PubMed]

42. Siega-Riz, A.M.; Deming, D.M.; Reidy, K.C.; Fox, M.K.; Condon, E.; Briefel, R.R. Food Consumption Patterns of Infants and Toddlers: Where Are We Now? *J. Am. Diet. Assoc.* **2010**, *110*, S38–S51. [CrossRef] [PubMed]

43. Mennella, J.A.; Ziegler, P.; Briefel, R.; Novak, T. Feeding Infants and Toddlers Study: The Types of Foods Fed to Hispanic Infants and Toddlers. *J. Am. Diet. Assoc.* **2006**, *106*, S96–S106. [CrossRef] [PubMed]

44. Slavin, J.L.; Lloyd, B. Health Benefits of Fruits and Vegetables. *Adv. Nutr.* **2012**, *3*, 506–516. [CrossRef] [PubMed]

45. Poiroux-Gonord, F.; Bidel, L.P.; Fanciullino, A.L.; Gautier, H.; Lauri-Lopez, F.; Urban, L. Health Benefits of Vitamins and Secondary Metabolites of Fruits and Vegetables and Prospects to Increase Their Concentrations by Agronomic Approaches. *J. Agric. Food Chem.* **2010**, *58*, 12065–12082. [CrossRef] [PubMed]

46. Ashman, A.M.; Collins, C.E.; Hure, A.J.; Jensen, M.; Oldmeadow, C. Maternal Diet During Early Childhood, but Not Pregnancy, Predicts Diet Quality and Fruit and Vegetable Acceptance in Offspring. *Mater. Child Nutr.* **2014**. [CrossRef] [PubMed]

47. Hetherington, M.M.; Schwartz, C.; Madrelle, J.; Croden, F.; Nekitsing, C.; Vereijken, C.M.; Weenen, H. A Step-by-Step Introduction to Vegetables at the Beginning of Complementary Feeding. The Effects of Early and Repeated Exposure. *Appetite* **2015**, *84*, 280–290. [CrossRef] [PubMed]

48. de Lauzon-Guillain, B.; Jones, L.; Oliveira, A.; Moschonis, G.; Betoko, A.; Lopes, C.; Moreira, P.; Manios, Y.; Papadopoulos, N.G.; Emmett, P.; *et al.* The Influence of Early Feeding Practices on Fruit and Vegetable Intake among Preschool Children in 4 European Birth Cohorts. *Am. J. Clin. Nutr.* **2013**, *98*, 804–812. [CrossRef] [PubMed]

49. Young, B.E.; Krebs, N.F. Complementary Feeding: Critical Considerations to Optimize Growth, Nutrition, and Feeding Behavior. *Curr. Pediatr. Rep.* **2013**, *1*, 247–256. [CrossRef] [PubMed]

50. Northstone, K.; Emmett, P.M. Are Dietary Patterns Stable Throughout Early and Mid-Childhood? A Birth Cohort Study. *Br. J. Nutr.* **2008**, *100*, 1069–1076. [CrossRef] [PubMed]

51. Golley, R.K.; Smithers, L.G.; Mittinty, M.N.; Emmett, P.; Northstone, K.; Lynch, J.W. Diet Quality of U.K. Infants Is Associated with Dietary, Adiposity, Cardiovascular, and Cognitive Outcomes Measured at 7–8 years of Age. *J. Nutr.* **2013**, *143*, 1611–1617. [CrossRef] [PubMed]

52. Mikkila, V.; Rasanen, L.; Raitakari, O.T.; Pietinen, P.; Viikari, J. Consistent Dietary Patterns Identified from Childhood to Adulthood: The Cardiovascular Risk in Young Finns Study. *Br. J. Nutr.* **2005**, *93*, 923–931. [CrossRef] [PubMed]

53. Owen, C.G.; Whincup, P.H.; Kaye, S.J.; Martin, R.M.; Davey Smith, G.; Cook, D.G.; Bergstrom, E.; Black, S.; Wadsworth, M.E.; Fall, C.H.; *et al.* Does Initial Breastfeeding Lead to Lower Blood Cholesterol in Adult Life? A Quantitative Review of the Evidence. *Am. J. Clin. Nutr.* **2008**, *88*, 305–314. [PubMed]

54. Coulthard, H.; Harris, G.; Emmett, P. Long-Term Consequences of Early Fruit and Vegetable Feeding Practices in the United Kingdom. *Public Health Nutr.* **2010**, *13*, 2044–2051. [CrossRef] [PubMed]

55. Moore, L.L.; Singer, M.R.; Bradlee, M.L.; Djousse, L.; Proctor, M.H.; Cupples, L.A.; Ellison, R.C. Intake of Fruits, Vegetables, and Dairy Products in Early Childhood and Subsequent Blood Pressure Change. *Epidemiology* **2005**, *16*, 4–11. [CrossRef] [PubMed]

56. Ness, A.R.; Maynard, M.; Frankel, S.; Smith, G.D.; Frobisher, C.; Leary, S.D.; Emmett, P.M.; Gunnell, D. Diet in Childhood and Adult Cardiovascular and All Cause Mortality: The Boyd Orr Cohort. *Heart* **2005**, *91*, 894–898. [CrossRef] [PubMed]

57. U.S. Department of Agriculture; U.S. Department of Health and Human Services. *Dietary Guidelines for Americans*, 7th ed.; U.S. Government Printing Office: Washington, DC, USA, 2010.

58. Picciano, M.F.; Smiciklas-Wright, H.; Birch, L.L.; Mitchell, D.C.; Murray-Kolb, L.; McConahy, K.L. Nutritional Guidance Is Needed During Dietary Transition in Early Childhood. *Pediatrics* **2000**, *106*, 109–114. [CrossRef] [PubMed]

59. Butte, N.F.; Fox, M.K.; Briefel, R.R.; Siega-Riz, A.M.; Dwyer, J.T.; Deming, D.M.; Reidy, K.C. Nutrient Intakes of Us Infants, Toddlers, and Preschoolers Meet or Exceed Dietary Reference Intakes. *J. Am. Diet. Assoc.* **2010**, *110*, S27–S37. [CrossRef] [PubMed]

60. Fats and Fatty Acids in Human Nutrition. Proceedings of the Joint Fao/Who Expert Consultation. 10–14 November 2008. Geneva, Switzerland. *Ann. Nutr. Metab.* **2009**, *55*, 5–300.

61. Saphier, O.; Blumenfeld, J.; Silberstein, T.; Tzor, T.; Burg, A. Fatty Acid Composition of Breastmilk of Israeli Mothers. *Indian Pediatr.* **2013**, *50*, 1044–1046. [CrossRef] [PubMed]

62. Martysiak-Zurowska, D.; Zoralska, K.; Zagierski, M.; Szlagtys-Sidorkiewicz, A. Fatty Acid Composition in Breast Milk of Women from Gdansk and the Surrounding District in the Course of Lactation. *Med. Wieku Rozwoj.* **2011**, *15*, 167–177. [PubMed]

63. Lu, Q.Y.; Zhang, Y.; Wang, Y.; Wang, D.; Lee, R.P.; Gao, K.; Byrns, R.; Heber, D. California Hass Avocado: Profiling of Carotenoids, Tocopherol, Fatty Acid, and Fat Content During Maturation and from Different Growing Areas. *J. Agric. Food Chem.* **2009**, *57*, 10408–10413. [CrossRef] [PubMed]

64. Stunkard, A.J.; Berkowitz, R.I.; Schoeller, D.; Maislin, G.; Stallings, V.A. Predictors of Body Size in the First 2 years of Life: A High-Risk Study of Human Obesity. *Int. J. Obes. Relat. Metab. Disord.* **2004**, *28*, 503–513. [CrossRef] [PubMed]

65. Heppe, D.H.; Kiefte-de Jong, J.C.; Durmus, B.; Moll, H.A.; Raat, H.; Hofman, A.; Jaddoe, V.W. Parental, Fetal, and Infant Risk Factors for Preschool Overweight: The Generation R Study. *Pediatr. Res.* **2013**, *73*, 120–127. [CrossRef] [PubMed]

66. Kapiki, A.; Costalos, C.; Oikonomidou, C.; Triantafyllidou, A.; Loukatou, E.; Pertrohilou, V. The Effect of a Fructo-Oligosaccharide Supplemented Formula on Gut Flora of Preterm Infants. *Early Hum. Dev.* **2007**, *83*, 335–339. [CrossRef] [PubMed]

67. Euler, A.R.; Mitchell, D.K.; Kline, R.; Pickering, L.K. Prebiotic Effect of Fructo-Oligosaccharide Supplemented Term Infant Formula at Two Concentrations Compared with Unsupplemented Formula and Human Milk. *J. Pediatr. Gastroenterol. Nutr.* **2005**, *40*, 157–164. [CrossRef] [PubMed]

68. Kranz, S.; Brauchla, M.; Slavin, J.L.; Miller, K.B. What Do We Know About Dietary Fiber Intake in Children and Health? The Effects of Fiber Intake on Constipation, Obesity, and Diabetes in Children. *Adv. Nutr.* **2012**, *3*, 47–53. [CrossRef] [PubMed]

69. Agostoni, C.; Riva, E.; Giovannini, M. Dietary Fiber in Weaning Foods of Young Children. *Pediatrics* **1995**, *96*, 1002–1005. [PubMed]

70. Committee on Nutrition, American Academy of Pediatrics. *Pediatric Nutrition Handbook*, 4th ed.; American Academy of Pediatrics: Elk Grove Village, IL, USA, 1998.

71. Stewart, M.L.; Schroeder, N.M. Dietary Treatments for Childhood Constipation: Efficacy of Dietary Fiber and Whole Grains. *Nutr. Rev.* **2013**, *71*, 98–109. [CrossRef] [PubMed]

72. Hambidge, K.M. Micronutrient Bioavailability: Dietary Reference Intakes and a Future Perspective. *Am. J. Clin. Nutr.* **2010**, *91*, 1430S–1432S. [CrossRef] [PubMed]

73. Moilanen, B.C. Vegan Diets in Infants, Children, and Adolescents. *Pediatr. Rev.* **2004**, *25*, 174–176. [CrossRef] [PubMed]

74. Ruottinen, S.; Lagstrom, H.K.; Niinikoski, H.; Ronnemaa, T.; Saarinen, M.; Pahkala, K.A.; Hakanen, M.; Viikari, J.S.; Simell, O. Dietary Fiber Does Not Displace Energy but Is Associated with Decreased Serum Cholesterol Concentrations in Healthy Children. *Am. J. Clin. Nutr.* **2010**, *91*, 651–661. [CrossRef] [PubMed]

75. Donini, L.M.; Savina, C.; Cannella, C. Nutrition in the Elderly: Role of Fiber. *Arch. Gerontol. Geriatr.* **2009**, *49* (Suppl. 1), 61–69. [CrossRef] [PubMed]

76. Fox, M.K.; Reidy, K.; Novak, T.; Ziegler, P. Sources of Energy and Nutrients in the Diets of Infants and Toddlers. *J. Am. Diet. Assoc.* **2006**, *106*, S28–S42. [CrossRef] [PubMed]

77. Kasidas, G.P.; Rose, G.A. Oxalate Content of Some Common Foods: Determination by an Enzymatic Method. *J. Hum. Nutr.* **1980**, *34*, 255–266. [CrossRef] [PubMed]

78. Bode, L. Human Milk Oligosaccharides: Every Baby Needs a Sugar Mama. *Glycobiology* **2012**, *22*, 1147–1162. [CrossRef] [PubMed]

79. Cummings, J.H.; Englyst, H.N. Fermentation in the Human Large Intestine and the Available Substrates. *Am. J. Clin. Nutr.* **1987**, *45*, 1243–1255. [PubMed]

80. Kaji, I.; Karaki, S.; Kuwahara, A. Short-Chain Fatty Acid Receptor and Its Contribution to Glucagon-Like Peptide-1 Release. *Digestion* **2014**, *89*, 31–36. [CrossRef] [PubMed]

81. den Besten, G.; van Eunen, K.; Groen, A.K.; Venema, K.; Reijngoud, D.J.; Bakker, B.M. The Role of Short-Chain Fatty Acids in the Interplay between Diet, Gut Microbiota, and Host Energy Metabolism. *J. Lipid Res.* **2013**, *54*, 2325–2340. [CrossRef] [PubMed]

82. Dewey, K.G. The Challenge of Meeting Nutrient Needs of Infants and Young Children During the Period of Complementary Feeding: An Evolutionary Perspective. *J. Nutr.* **2013**, *143*, 2050–2054. [CrossRef] [PubMed]

83. Vitolo, M.R.; Bortolini, G.A. Iron Bioavailability as a Protective Factor against Anemia among Children Aged 12 to 16 months. *J. Pediatr. (Rio J.)* **2007**, *83*, 33–38. [CrossRef]

84. Hazell, T. Vitamin C Has a Key Physiological Role in Facilitating the Absorption of Non-Heme Iron from the Diet. *Hum. Nutr. Appl. Nutr.* **1987**, *41*, 286–287. [PubMed]

85. Cook, J.D.; Reddy, M.B. Effect of Ascorbic Acid Intake on Nonheme-Iron Absorption from a Complete Diet. *Am. J. Clin. Nutr.* **2001**, *73*, 93–98. [PubMed]

86. Pacheco, M.M.; Gomez, R.L.; Garciglia, R.S.; Calderon, M.R.; Muñoz, R.E.M. Folates and *Persea americana* Mill (Avocado). *Emir. J. Food Agric.* **2011**, *23*, 204–213.

87. Tian, N.; Zhang, Z.; Loustalot, F.; Yang, Q.; Cogswell, M.E. Sodium and Potassium Intakes among US Infants and Preschool Children, 2003–2010. *Am. J. Clin. Nutr.* **2013**, *98*, 1113–1122. [CrossRef] [PubMed]

88. Casazza, K.; Hanks, L.J.; Fields, D.A. The Relationship between Bioactive Components in Breast Milk and Bone Mass in Infants. *Bonekey Rep.* **2014**, *3*, 577. [CrossRef] [PubMed]

89. Lonnerdal, B. Bioactive Proteins in Breast Milk. *J. Paediatr. Child Health* **2013**, *49* (Suppl. 1), 1–7. [CrossRef] [PubMed]

90. McEvoy, B. Transfer of Bioactive Substances in Breast Milk. *Med. J. Aust.* **1984**, *141*, 196. [PubMed]

91. Yasir, M.; Das, S.; Kharya, M.D. The Phytochemical and Pharmacological Profile of Persea Americana Mill. *Pharmacogn. Rev.* **2010**, *4*, 77–84. [CrossRef] [PubMed]

92. Rodriguez-Sanchez, D.; Silva-Platas, C.; Rojo, R.P.; Garcia, N.; Cisneros-Zevallos, L.; Garcia-Rivas, G.; Hernandez-Brenes, C. Activity-Guided Identification of Acetogenins as Novel Lipophilic Antioxidants Present in Avocado Pulp (*Persea Americana*). *J. Chromatogr. B Anal. Technol. Biomed. Life Sci.* **2013**, *942–943*, 37–45. [CrossRef] [PubMed]

93. Rodriguez-Sanchez, D.G.; Flores-Garcia, M.; Silva-Platas, C.; Rizzo, S.; Torre-Amione, G.; De la Pena-Diaz, A.; Hernandez-Brenes, C.; Garcia-Rivas, G. Isolation and Chemical Identification of Lipid Derivatives from Avocado (Persea Americana) Pulp with Antiplatelet and Antithrombotic Activities. *Food Funct.* **2014**, *6*, 193–203. [CrossRef] [PubMed]

94. Liu, R.H. Dietary Bioactive Compounds and Their Health Implications. *J. Food Sci.* **2013**, *78* (Suppl. 1), A18–A25. [CrossRef] [PubMed]

95. Carbonell-Capella, J.M.; Barba, F.J.; Esteve, M.J.; Frigola, A. Quality Parameters, Bioactive Compounds and Their Correlation with Antioxidant Capacity of Commercial Fruit-Based Baby Foods. *Food Sci. Technol. Int.* **2014**, *20*, 479–487. [CrossRef] [PubMed]

96. Lee, J.; Koo, N.; Min, D.B. Reactive Oxygen Species, Aging, and Antioxidative Nutraceuticals. *Compr. Rev. Food Sci. Food Saf.* **2004**, *3*, 21–33. [CrossRef]

97. Moukarzel, A.A.; Bejjani, R.A.; Fares, F.N. Xanthophylls and Eye Health of Infants and Adults. *J. Med. Liban.* **2009**, *57*, 261–267. [PubMed]

98. Vishwanathan, R.; Kuchan, M.J.; Sen, S.; Johnson, E.J. Lutein and Preterm Infants with Decreased Concentrations of Brain Carotenoids. *J. Pediatr. Gastroenterol. Nutr.* **2014**, *59*, 659–665. [CrossRef] [PubMed]

99. Lieblein-Boff, J.C.; Johnson, E.J.; Kennedy, A.D.; Lai, C.S.; Kuchan, M.J. Exploratory Metabolomic Analyses Reveal Compounds Correlated with Lutein Concentration in Frontal Cortex, Hippocampus, and Occipital Cortex of Human Infant Brain. *PLoS ONE* **2015**, *10*, e0136904.

100. Bettler, J.; Zimmer, J.P.; Neuringer, M.; DeRusso, P.A. Serum Lutein Concentrations in Healthy Term Infants Fed Human Milk or Infant Formula with Lutein. *Eur. J. Nutr.* **2010**, *49*, 45–51. [CrossRef] [PubMed]

101. Silva-Platas, C.; Garcia, N.; Fernandez-Sada, E.; Davila, D.; Hernandez-Brenes, C.; Rodriguez, D.; Garcia-Rivas, G. Cardiotoxicity of Acetogenins from Persea Americana Occurs through the Mitochondrial Permeability Transition Pore and Caspase-Dependent Apoptosis Pathways. *J. Bioenerg. Biomembr.* **2012**, *44*, 461–471. [CrossRef] [PubMed]

102. Kojima, N.; Fushimi, T.; Tatsukawa, T.; Yoshimitsu, T.; Tanaka, T.; Yamori, T.; Dan, S.; Iwasaki, H.; Yamashita, M. Structure-Activity Relationships of Hybrid Annonaceous Acetogenins: Powerful Growth Inhibitory Effects of Their Connecting Groups between Heterocycle and Hydrophobic Carbon Chain Bearing Thf Ring on Human Cancer Cell Lines. *Eur. J. Med. Chem.* **2013**, *63*, 833–839. [CrossRef] [PubMed]

103. Matsui, Y.; Takeuchi, T.; Kumamoto-Yonezawa, Y.; Takemura, M.; Sugawara, F.; Yoshida, H.; Mizushina, Y. The Relationship between the Molecular Structure of Natural Acetogenins and Their Inhibitory Activities Which Affect DNA Polymerase, DNA Topoisomerase and Human Cancer Cell Growth. *Exp. Ther. Med.* **2010**, *1*, 19–26. [PubMed]

104. Jones, D.P.; Coates, R.J.; Flagg, E.W.; Eley, J.W.; Block, G.; Greenberg, R.S.; Gunter, E.W.; Jackson, B. Glutathione in Foods Listed in the National Cancer Institute's Health Habits and History Food Frequency Questionnaire. *Nutr. Cancer* **1992**, *17*, 57–75. [CrossRef] [PubMed]

105. Michel, S.H.; Maqbool, A.; Hanna, M.D.; Mascarenhas, M. Nutrition Management of Pediatric Patients Who Have Cystic Fibrosis. *Pediatr. Clin. N. Am.* **2009**, *56*, 1123–1141. [CrossRef] [PubMed]

106. Ventura, A.K.; Worobey, J. Early Influences on the Development of Food Preferences. *Curr. Biol.* **2013**, *23*, R401–R408. [CrossRef] [PubMed]

107. Beauchamp, G.K.; Mennella, J.A. Early Flavor Learning and Its Impact on Later Feeding Behavior. *J. Pediatr. Gastroenterol. Nutr.* **2009**, *48* (Suppl. 1), S25–S30. [CrossRef] [PubMed]

108. Thompson, A.L.; Bentley, M.E. The Critical Period of Infant Feeding for the Development of Early Disparities in Obesity. *Soc. Sci. Med.* **2013**, *97*, 288–296. [CrossRef] [PubMed]

109. Ahern, S.M.; Caton, S.J.; Bouhlal, S.; Hausner, H.; Olsen, A.; Nicklaus, S.; Moller, P.; Hetherington, M.M. Eating a Rainbow. Introducing Vegetables in the First Years of Life in 3 European Countries. *Appetite* **2013**, *71*, 48–56. [CrossRef] [PubMed]

110. Anzman, S.L.; Rollins, B.Y.; Birch, L.L. Parental Influence on Children's Early Eating Environments and Obesity Risk: Implications for Prevention. *Int. J. Obes. (Lond.)* **2010**, *34*, 1116–1124. [CrossRef] [PubMed]

111. Mennella, J.A.; Nicklaus, S.; Jagolino, A.L.; Yourshaw, L.M. Variety Is the Spice of Life: Strategies for Promoting Fruit and Vegetable Acceptance During Infancy. *Physiol. Behav.* **2008**, *94*, 29–38. [CrossRef] [PubMed]

112. Karhunen, L.J.; Juvonen, K.R.; Huotari, A.; Purhonen, A.K.; Herzig, K.H. Effect of Protein, Fat, Carbohydrate and Fibre on Gastrointestinal Peptide Release in Humans. *Regul. Pept.* **2008**, *149*, 70–78. [CrossRef] [PubMed]

113. Paniagua, J.A.; de la Sacristana, A.G.; Sanchez, E.; Romero, I.; Vidal-Puig, A.; Berral, F.J.; Escribano, A.; Moyano, M.J.; Perez-Martinez, P.; Lopez-Miranda, J.; *et al.* A Mufa-Rich Diet Improves Posprandial Glucose, Lipid and Glp-1 Responses in Insulin-Resistant Subjects. *J. Am. Coll. Nutr.* **2007**, *26*, 434–444. [CrossRef] [PubMed]

114. Chang, K.T.; Lampe, J.W.; Schwarz, Y.; Breymeyer, K.L.; Noar, K.A.; Song, X.; Neuhouser, M.L. Low Glycemic Load Experimental Diet More Satiating Than High Glycemic Load Diet. *Nutr. Cancer* **2012**, *64*, 666–673. [CrossRef] [PubMed]

115. Zalewski, B.M.; Patro, B.; Veldhorst, M.; Kouwenhoven, S.; Escobar, P.C.; Lerma, J.C.; Koletzko, B.; Van Goudoever, J.B.; Szajewska, H. Nutrition of Infants and Young Children (1–3 years) and Its Effect on Later Health: A Systematic Review of Current Recommendations (Earlynutrition Project). *Crit. Rev. Food Sci. Nutr.* **2015**. in presss. [CrossRef] [PubMed]

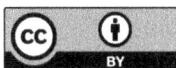

![nutrients](nutrients logo) *nutrients*

MDPI

Article

Avenanthramides Prevent Osteoblast and Osteocyte Apoptosis and Induce Osteoclast Apoptosis in Vitro in an Nrf2-Independent Manner

Gretel G. Pellegrini [1,2,]*, Cynthya C. Morales [1], Taylor C. Wallace [3,4,5], Lilian I. Plotkin [1,2] and Teresita Bellido [1,2,6,]*

[1] Department of Anatomy & Cell Biology, School of Medicine, Indiana University, Indianapolis, IN 46202, USA; moralecy@iupui.edu (C.C.M.); lplotkin@iupui.edu (L.I.P.)
[2] Roudebush Veterans Administration Medical Center, Indianapolis, IN 46202, USA
[3] Department of Nutrition and Food Studies, George Mason University, Fairfax, VA 22030, USA; taylor.wallace@nof.org
[4] Think Healthy Group, LLC, Washington, DC 20001, USA
[5] National Osteoporosis Foundation, Arlington, VA 22202, USA
[6] Department of Medicine, Division of Endocrinology, School of Medicine, Indiana University, Indianapolis, IN 46202, USA
* Correspondence: gpellegr@iupui.edu (G.G.P.); tbellido@iupui.edu (T.B.); Tel.: +1-317-274-2323 (G.G.P.); +1-317-274-7410 (T.B.)

Received: 23 May 2016; Accepted: 6 July 2016; Published: 11 July 2016

Abstract: Oats contain unique bioactive compounds known as avenanthramides (AVAs) with antioxidant properties. AVAs might enhance the endogenous antioxidant cellular response by activation of the transcription factor Nrf2. Accumulation of reactive oxygen species plays a critical role in many chronic and degenerative diseases, including osteoporosis. In this disease, there is an imbalance between bone formation by osteoblasts and bone resorption by osteoclasts, which is accompanied by increased osteoblast/osteocyte apoptosis and decreased osteoclast apoptosis. We investigated the ability of the synthethic AVAs 2c, 2f and 2p, to 1-regulate gene expression in bone cells, 2-affect the viability of osteoblasts, osteocytes and osteoclasts, and the generation of osteoclasts from their precursors, and 3-examine the potential involvement of the transcription factor Nrf2 in these actions. All doses of AVA 2c and 1 and 5 µM dose of 2p up-regulated collagen 1A expression. Lower doses of AVAs up-regulated OPG (osteoprotegerin) in OB-6 osteoblastic cells, whereas 100 µM dose of 2f and all concentrations of 2c down-regulated RANKL gene expression in MLO-Y4 osteocytic cells. AVAs did not affect apoptosis of OB-6 osteoblastic cells or MLO-Y4 osteocytic cells; however, they prevented apoptosis induced by the DNA topoisomerase inhibitor etoposide, the glucocorticoid dexamethasone, and hydrogen peroxide. AVAs prevented apoptosis of both wild type (WT) and Nrf2 Knockout (KO) osteoblasts, demonstrating that AVAs-induced survival does not require Nrf2 expression. Further, KO osteoclast precursors produced more mature osteoclasts than WT; and KO cultures exhibited less apoptotic osteoclasts than WT cultures. Although AVAs did not affect WT osteoclasts, AVA 2p reversed the low apoptosis of KO osteoclasts. These in vitro results demonstrate that AVAs regulate, in part, the function of osteoblasts and osteocytes and prevent osteoblast/osteocyte apoptosis and increase osteoclast apoptosis; further, these regulatory actions are independent of Nrf2.

Keywords: avenanthramides; oxidative stress; apoptosis; gene expression; bone cells

1. Introduction

Oxidative stress is caused by the imbalance between free radical generation and the scavenging activities of intracellular antioxidants and plays a critical role in many chronic and degenerative diseases, including osteoporosis, cancer, and neurodegenerative diseases [1–3]. High levels of reactive oxygen species (ROS), especially hydrogen peroxide (H_2O_2), in the bone/bone marrow microenvironment play a pathogenic role in osteoporosis due to estrogen deficiency with menopause, androgen deficiency during aging in both women and men [4], and/or glucocorticoid therapy used in treating many inflammatory and autoimmune diseases [5]. ROS accumulation increases the number of osteoclasts (the cells that resorb bone) by enhancing the expression by osteoblastic cells of the pro-osteoclastogenic cytokines RANKL (Receptor Activator for Nuclear Factor κB Ligand) and TNFα (Tumor Necrosis Factor alpha) [6–8]. ROS increase osteoclast differentiation directly by activating the transcription factor NFATc1, which in turn increases transcription of osteoclast-specific genes [6]. ROS also promotes osteoclast survival. On the other hand, ROS accumulation decreases the number of osteoblasts (the cells that form bone) by inhibiting their proliferation and differentiation; and induces premature osteoblast apoptosis [9–12]. In addition, ROS induces apoptosis of osteocytes, the most abundant cells in the bone that orchestrate osteoclast and osteoblast function [13,14].

Two main therapeutic approaches have been developed for the management of osteoporosis: (1) Anti-resorptive medications including bisphosphonates, estrogen replacement, and anti-RANKL antibodies; and (2) Anabolic treatments such as daily injections of parathyroid hormone (PTH) [15]. The first approach seeks to block osteoclast formation and/or function and the second stimulates osteoblast production and function. Although therapies for treating osteoporosis have been shown to be effective, prevention strategies through optimal lifestyle patterns (e.g., nutrition and physical activity) are actively being sought to help decrease the overall burden of osteoporosis and high bone fracture risk. There is an increase in the prevalence of degenerative diseases that affect bone and involve increased oxidative stress. Therefore, alternative therapeutic interventions that counteract ROS effects in bone without causing harmful effects in other tissues are needed.

Nuclear factor erythroid derived 2-related factor-2 (Nrf2) plays an important role in the cellular defense against oxidative stress by inducing enzymes that regulate oxidative stress [16,17]. Recent studies have demonstrated that Nrf2 is an important regulator of bone homeostasis in bone cells, since activation of Nrf2 can enhance the endogenous antioxidant response against ROS [1,16,18,19].

Increasing evidence, including epidemiological, clinical, and animal experimentation, suggests that consumption of plant foods, containing polyphenols helps to protect against the development of oxidative stress pathologies, including cancer, cardiovascular diseases, diabetes, neurodegenerative diseases, and osteoporosis [20–23]. Oat is a commonly consumed whole-grain cereal that is gaining scientific and public interest for their health benefits beyond basic nutrition [24,25]. Oats contain phytochemicals with high antioxidant properties, among them tocopherols, tocotrienols, phenolic compounds, phytic acid, avenanthramides (AVAs), and flavonoids and sterols in a lesser amount [24,26,27]. AVAs are a group of alkaloid phenols uniquely found in oats [28]. These compounds consist of an anthranilic acid derivate and a hydroxycinnamic acid derivate linked by a pseudo-peptide bond [29], and exhibit strong antioxidant activity and anti-inflammatory and anti-proliferative properties both in vitro and in vivo [25,30–32]. AVAs inhibit the expression of adhesion molecules and inflammatory cytokines, such as IL-6, IL-8, and monocyte chemoattractant protein 1 in human aortic endothelial cell cultures [33]; and inhibit the growth of human colon cancer cells in vitro [28]. Further, dietary intake of AVAs by postmenopausal women decreased the inflammatory response induced by physical exercise and increased the total antioxidant capacity of plasma and the superoxide dismutase (SOD) activity of red blood cells [34]. Addition of AVAs extracts to mouse diets enhanced the hepatic mRNA expression of Cu-Zn SOD1, Mn SOD2, and glutathione peroxidase (GPx) [35]. AVAs also increase hemeoxygenase (HO) 1 expression in human kidney cells in a dose- and time-dependent manner and induce the nuclear translocation of the transcription factor Nrf2 [36].

To date, there are no studies addressing the effect of AVAs on bone cells in vitro. The aims of this study, were to investigate the ability of the three major synthetic AVAs (2c, 2f and 2p), which differ in the type of hydroxylcinnamic acid component (ferulic, caffeic or p-coumaric acid), to 1-regulate gene expression in bone cells, 2-affect the viability of osteoblasts, osteocytes and osteoclasts, and the generation of osteoclasts from their precursors, and 3-examine the potential involvement of the transcription factor Nrf2 in these actions.

2. Material and Methods

2.1. AVAs Preparation and Cell Treatment

The synthethic AVA 2f, 2c and 2p were provided by Quaker Oats Center of Excellence (Barrington, IL, USA). Purity was controlled by HPLC measurements (2f > 95.1%; 2c > 94.9%; 2p > 96%). AVAs were dissolved in dimethylsulfoxide (DMSO) and added to the cell culture medium with a maximum final DMSO concentration of 0.1%, which showed no cytotoxicity [37]. AVAs were kept as 0.05 M stock solutions and stored at $-80\ ^\circ$C until used. Osteoblastic and osteocytic cells were treated with doses ranging from 1 to 100 µM of the AVAs. The dose range was chosen based on previous studies using AVAs in other cell systems [32,36].

2.2. Cell Culture

Adherent primary osteoblastic C57BL/6 wild type (WT) and Nrf2 knock-out (KO) cells were seeded at a density of $1.5 \times 10^4/cm^2$ before being prepared as previously described in the scientific literature [38–40]. The cells were cultured in growth medium consisting of α-Minimum Essential Medium Eagle (α-MEM) supplemented with 10% fetal bovine serum (FBS), (Invitrogen, Carlsbad, CA, USA), 1% penicillin/streptomycin (Invitrogen) and 50 mg/mL normocin (Invivogen, San Diego, CA, USA).

Adherent OB-6 osteoblastic cells were seeded at a density of 5000 cells/cm^2 in α-MEM supplemented with 10% FBS and MLO-Y4 cells were seeded at a density of 1×10^4 to 2×10^4 cells/cm^2 on collagen type I—coated plates in α-MEM supplemented with 2.5% FBS and 2.5% bovine calf serum (BCS, Invitrogen), as previously published [41–43].

WT or KO bone marrow precursors were seeded at a density of $4 \times 10^5/cm^2$ and cultured for 48 h in α-MEM supplemented with 15% FBS, and 1% penicillin/streptomycin and 50 mg/mL normocin. Next, "non adherent cells", were collected and seeded at a density of $6 \times 10^5/cm^2$ and cultured with α-MEM with 10% FBS and 1% penicillin/streptomycin, and 80 ng/mL of recombinant murine soluble Receptor Activator for Nuclear Factor κB Ligand (sRANKL) (PreproTech, Rocky Hill, NJ, USA) and 20 ng/mL recombinant murine Macrofage Colony Stimulating Factor (M-CSF) (PreproTech). Medium was changed every 2 days for 5 days, as previously reported [44].

2.3. RNA Extraction and Quantitative RT-PCR (qPCR)

To determine the effects of AVAs on gene expression, total RNA was purified from cell preparations using Trizol reagent (Invitrogen) according to the manufacturer's instructions. RNA was reverse-transcribed using a High Capacity cDNA Archive Kit (Applied Biosystems, Foster City, CA, USA). Gene expression was analyzed by quantitative PCR using the ΔCt method as previously described with Mrps2 (mitochondrial ribosomal protein S2) or GAPDH (Glyceraldehyde-3-phosphate dehydrogenase) as housekeeping genes [45,46]. The following primer probe sets were purchased from Applied Biosystems: Collagen 1A (COL1A) (Mm00801666 g1); Osteocalcin (OCN) (AIT97T5); Osteoprotegerin (OPG) (Mm01205928 m1); RANKL (Mm00441906 m1); Cathepsin K (Cat K) (Mm00484036 m1); Tartrate-resistant acid phosphate (TRAPase) (Mm00475698 m1); Nrf2 (Mm00477784 m1); Mps2 (Mm00475529 m1); GAPDH (Mm99999915 g1). For the other genes, primer probe sets were designed using the Assay Design Center of Roche Applied Science (Indianapolis, IN, USA), and were as follows. For OSTERIX: probe 106, forward primer:

gggaagggtgggtagtcatt, reverse primer: ctcctgcaggcagtcctc; Runt-related transcription factor 2 (RUNX2): probe 34, forward primer: tgcctggctcttcttactgag, reverse primer: gcccaggcgtatttcaga; Calcitonin receptor (CAL R): probe 15, forward primer: agaactggagttgggctcac, reverse primer: ggttccttctcgtgaacaggt; NAD(P)H dehydrogenase, quinone 1 (NQO1): probe 50, forward primer: agtacaatcagggctcttctcg, reverse primer: agcgttcggtattacgatcc; HO-1: probe 17, forward primer: tgtgttcctctgtcagcatca, reverse primer: aggctaagaccgccttcct; SOD1: probe 49, forward primer: tgcccaggtctccaacat, reverse primer: caggacctcattttaatcctcac. Glutathione S-transferase 1 (GSTP1): probe 105, forward primer: ggacagcagggtctcaaaag, reverse primer: tgtcaccctcatctacaccaac.

2.4. TRAPase Staining and Osteoclast Counting

After 24 h-treatment with AVAs 2f, 2c or 2p at 1 μM or vehicle (DMSO), mature osteoclasts differentiated from WT or KO bone marrow precursors, were examined for the activity of the osteoclast-specific enzyme TRAPase [47]. Briefly, cells were washed with PBS and fixed in 10% formaldehyde for 10 min. Next, cells were stained using a commercial TRAPase staining kit (Sigma-Aldrich, St. Louis, MO, USA) and counterstained with hematoxylin according to the manufacturer's instructions. TRAPase + cells were considered osteoclasts if having more than 3 nuclei. Osteoclast apoptosis was assessed by quantifying the percentage of osteoclasts that presented at least 50% condensed chromatin and dark nuclei.

Results are expressed as number of osteoclast/well or as percentage of apoptotic osteoclasts. Images were acquired using a Zeiss Axiovert 35 microscope equipped with a digital camera.

2.5. Quantification of Osteoblastic Cell Viability

Osteoblastic cells (OB-6 and WT and KO primary cells) and osteocytic cells were seeded in a 48-well plate at a density of 1×10^4 cells/well in αMEM + PSG + 10% FBS and cultured for 20 h. Next, the medium was changed to αMEM + PSG + 2% FBS + each AVA 2c, 2f, 2p at 1, 10, or 100 μM or the vehicle (DMSO) for 1 h. Cells were then exposed to the pro-apoptotic agents dexamethasone (10^{-6} M), etoposide (50 μM), or H_2O_2, (50 μM) or vehicle (DMSO) for an additional 6 h. Non-adherent cells were combined with adherent cells released from the culture dish using trypsin—Ethylenediaminetetraacetic acid (EDTA), re-suspended in medium containing serum, and collected by centrifugation. Subsequently, 0.04% trypan blue was added and the percentage of cells exhibiting both nuclear and cytoplasmic staining was determined using a hemocytometer. Cells that excluded the dye were considered alive, and cells stained were considered dead. Data is reported as the percentage of dead cells [48].

2.6. Statistical Analysis

Statistical analysis was performed using SigmaPlot (Systat Software Inc., Version 12.0, San Jose, CA, USA). All the results are presented as mean ± standard deviation of multiple cultures. At least 3 experiments per cell type with 5 independent replicates per experiment were performed for gene expression and apoptosis of osteoblastic and osteocytic cells. Three independent replicates were performed for osteoclast quantification and apoptosis. Sample differences were determined by one or two-way ANOVA, followed by pairwise multiple comparisons using Holm-Sidak or Tukey method, depending on the number of variables. Means were considered significantly different at $p < 0.05$.

3. Results

3.1. AVAs Regulate OPG and RANKL Gene Expression in OB-6 Osteoblastic and MLO-Y4 Osteocytic Cells

Gene expression analysis in OB-6 cells did not show significant changes on the expression of the osteoblast markers OCN, RUNX2 or osterix (Figure 1A), whereas RANKL was not detected in these cells (not shown). On the other hand, AVA 2c and 2p (1, 5 and 10 μM and 1 and 5 μM, respectively) increased COL1A expression. Further, lower doses of the three compounds upregulated

OPG expression with more potency than higher doses in OB-6 cells, showing an inverse dose-effect relationship. The reason behind this unexpected biological response is not known and could be due to the involvement of two different mechanisms or molecular mediators, one operating at lower doses and another at higher doses of the compounds. In MLO-Y4 cells, AVAs 2f (100 μM) and 2c (at all concentrations) downregulated the expression of RANKL, whereas AVA 2p (at 1 μM) increased it (Figure 1B). No statistical differences were found for OPG in MLO-Y4 cells. These results suggest that AVAs regulate in part the function of osteoblasts and osteocytes.

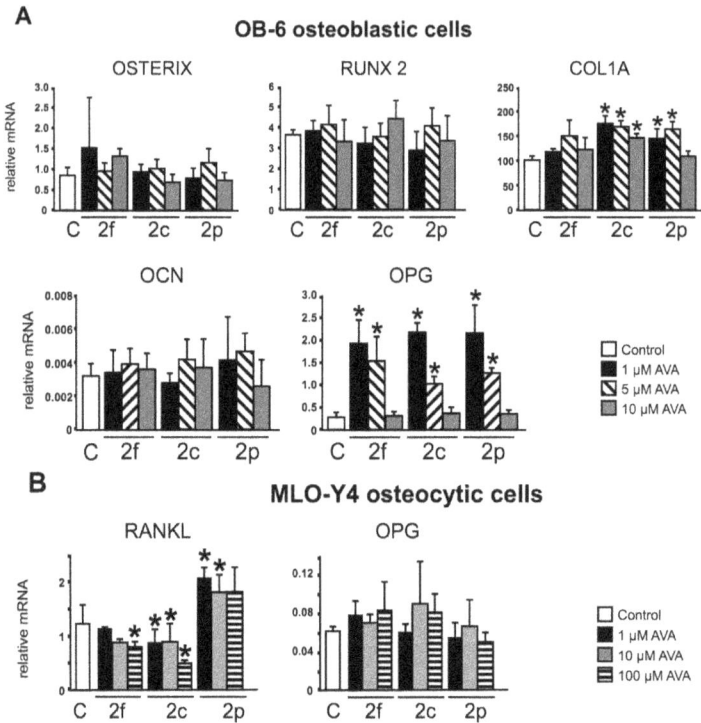

Figure 1. AVAs (Avenanthramides) regulate Collagen 1A (COL1A), osteoprotegerin (OPG) and Receptor Activator for Nuclear Factor κB Ligand (RANKL) in osteoblastic and osteocytic cells, respectively. 24-h gene expression of OB-6 osteoblastic (**A**), and MLO-Y4 cells (**B**); treated with vehicle (**C**) or AVA 2f, 2c or 2p. mRNA levels were measured by qPCR and corrected by Mrps2. The bars represent means ± SD, $n = 5$ replicates/treatment. * $p < 0.05$ vs. control, by One-Way ANOVA, followed by pairwise multiple comparisons using Holm-Sidak method.

3.2. AVAs Do Not Affect Cell Death in the Absence of Pro-Apoptotic Agents but Prevent the Effect Induced by Pro-Apoptotic Agents in Ob-6 Osteoblastic and Mlo-Y4 Osteocytic Cells

AVAs were further investigated for their effects on osteoblast and osteocyte survival in the absence or in the presence of pro-apoptotic agents. One h pre-treatment with AVA 2f, 2c or 2p at the concentrations tested (1, 10 and 100 μM) did not affect the survival of osteoblastic cells in the absence of pro-apoptotic agents (Figure 2A). As previously reported, the pro-apoptotic agent etoposide, increases the percentage of cells with increased membrane permeability [49]. However, the three AVA compounds, at the same doses, prevented etoposide induced-apoptosis. Since the lowest concentration of AVAs (1 μM) effectively blocked apoptosis of osteblastic cells, this dose was used for the next set of experiments, aiming to examine whether AVAs regulate survival in the presence of the pro-apoptotic agents dexamethasone or H_2O_2. Six h-treatment with dexamethasone or H_2O_2 increased significantly the percentage of cells exhibiting trypan blue uptake; however 1-h pre-treatment with AVAs prevented dexamethasone or H_2O_2-induced OB-6 and MLO-Y4 cell death (Figure 2B,C). These findings demonstrate that AVAs 2f, 2c and 2p preserve the viability of osteoblastic and osteocytic cells in vitro.

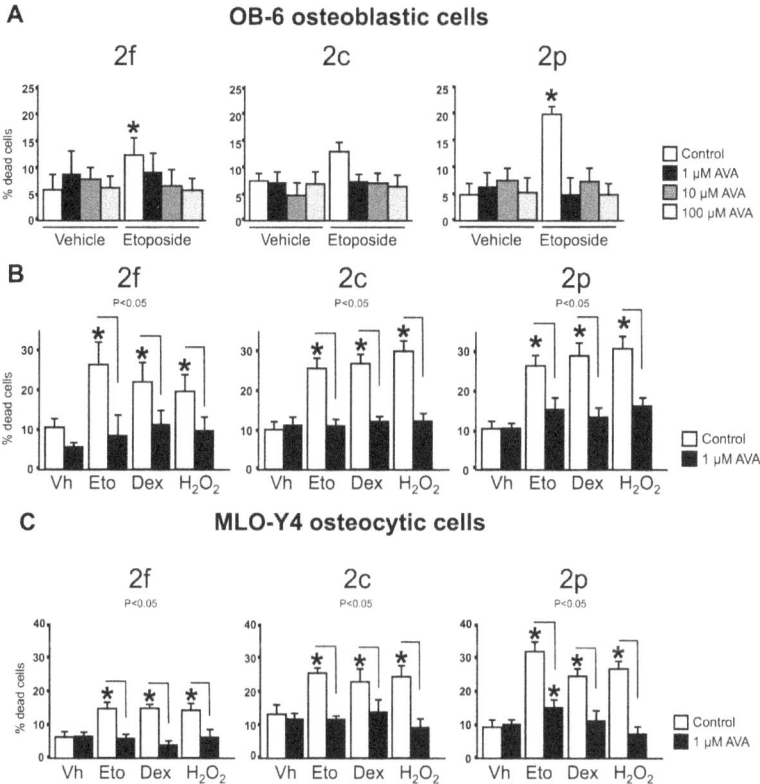

Figure 2. AVAs do not induce apoptosis and prevent cell death induced by proapototic agents in osteoblastic and osteocytic cells. (**A**) Cell death was examined in osteoblastic cells pretreated for 1-h with vehicle (control) or 3 different doses of AVA 2f, 2c and 2p, followed by exposure to vehicle (Vh, dimethylsulfoxide (DMSO)) or etoposide for 6-h; (**B,C**) Cells were treated with vehicle (control) or 1 μM AVAs for 1 h, followed by 6 h-treatment with the indicated compounds. Vh, vehicle; Eto, etoposide; Dex, dexamethasone or H_2O_2. Cell death was assessed by trypan blue uptake. Bars represent the means $\pm$ SD of n = 6 independent wells/treatment. * $p < 0.05$ vs. Vh control, and lines connect conditions with significant differences by One-Way ANOVA, followed by Tukey method.

3.3. The Survival Effect of Avas in Osteoblastic Cells Does Not Require Nrf2 Expression

We examined whether activation of the Nrf2 pathway, a key component of the antioxidant cellular defense mechanism, was involved in the protective effects of AVAs on osteoblastic cells, by comparing the effects of AVAs in WT or Nrf2 KO osteoblastic cells. Pre-treatment with AVA 2f, 2c or 2p prevented cell death induced by etoposide, dexamethasone or H_2O_2 in WT primary osteoblastic cells (Figure 3A). Surprisingly, AVAs were also effective in promoting survival in primary KO osteoblastic cells (Figure 3B). Moreover, AVA 2f was more effective to decrease cell death in the absence or in the presence of pro-apoptotic agents, in primary KO osteoblastic cells compared to WT cells. These findings demonstrate that the survival effect of AVAs on osteoblastic cells does not require Nrf2 expression. Consistent with this conclusion, the mRNA expression of the Nrf2 target genes, cytoprotective enzymes SOD1, HO-1 or GSTP1 were not affected by treatment with AVAs in MLO-Y4 osteocytic cells (Figure 3C).

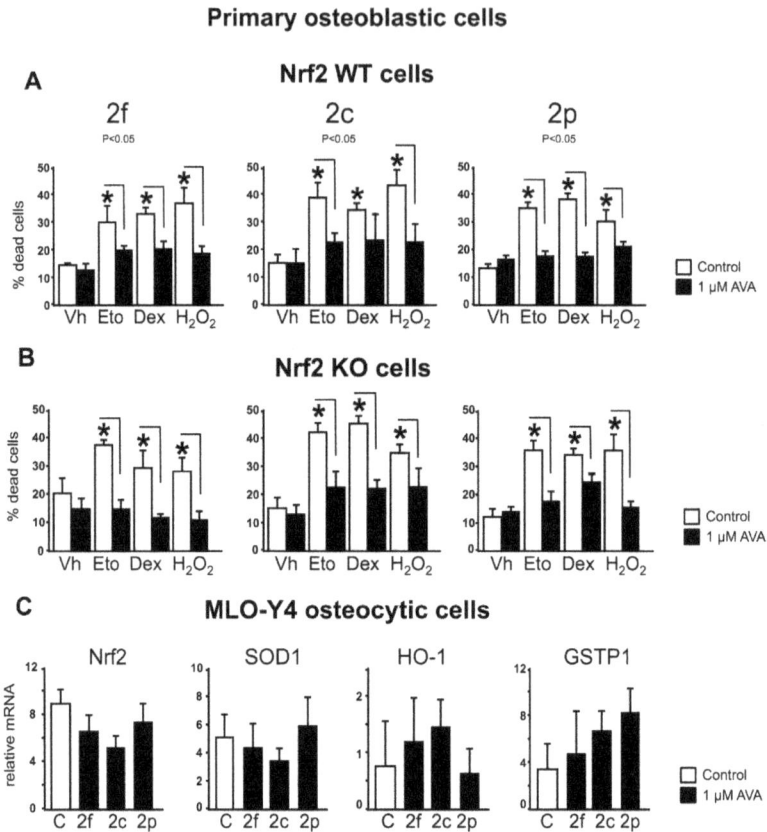

Figure 3. The survival effect of AVAs in osteoblastic cells does not require the expression of Nrf2. (**A**,**B**) Cell death was quantify by trypan blue uptake. Bars represent means $\pm$ SD of $n = 6$ samples per treatment. * $p < 0.05$ vs. cells treated with vehicle, by One-Way ANOVA, followed by Tukey method; (**C**) MLO-Y4 osteocytic cells mRNA levels were measured by qPCR and corrected by Mrps2. The bars represent means $\pm$ SD, $n = 5$ replicates/treatment. * $p < 0.05$ vs. control, and lines connect conditions with significant differences by One-Way ANOVA, followed by pairwise multiple comparisons using Holm-Sidak method.

3.4. Nrf2 Is Not Required for the Regulation of Gene Expression and Survival of Osteoclasts by AVAs

We next examined the effect of AVAs on osteoclasts and the potential requirement of Nrf2. Bone marrow osteoclast precursors lacking Nrf2 (KO cultures) treated with vehicle (control) produced 30% $\pm$ 2% more osteoclasts than WT control cultures (Figure 4A,B). In addition, KO control cultures exhibited lower number of apoptotic osteoclasts compared to WT control cultures (13% $\pm$ 2% vs. 23% $\pm$ 2% for KO and WT, respectively). Although AVAs did not affect the number or the percentage of dead osteoclasts in WT cultures (Figure 4A,B), AVAs 2f and 2p increased the percentage of apoptotic osteoclasts in KO cultures to reach levels found in WT cultures. Consistent with the increased osteoclast number observed in KO cultures, the expression of genes that characterize mature osteoclasts, including Cat K, CAL R and TRAPase, were higher in these preparations compared to WT cultures (Figure 4C). AVA 2f did not affect osteoclastic gene expression either in WT control or KO cultures. AVA 2c increased CAL R expression in WT cultures. Further, AVA 2p increased the expression of CAL R and TRAPase in WT cultures, whereas it decreased CAL R in KO cultures. This latter effect is consistent with the pro-apoptotic effect of AVA 2p on KO cultures (Figure 4A).

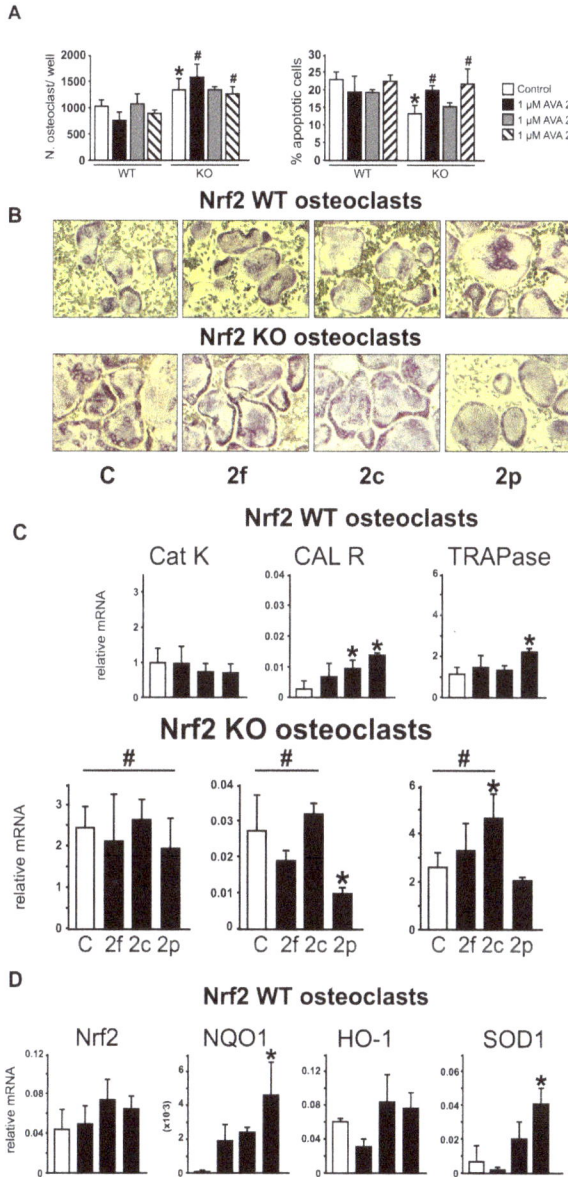

Figure 4. *Cont.*

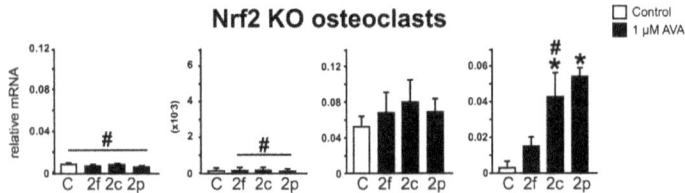

Figure 4. AVAs effect on the regulation of osteoclast gene expression and survival does not require Nrf2 expression. Non adherent cells were differentiated into osteoclasts by treatment with Macrofage Colony Stimulating Factor (M-CSF) and Receptor Activator for Nuclear Factor κB Ligand (sRANKL) for 5 days and treated for 24-h with AVAs. (**A**) Osteoclast number and percentage of dead osteoclasts were quantified by TRAPase-Hematoxylin staining $n = 3$ replicates/treatment; (**B**) Representative images of osteoclasts stained for TRAP are shown; (**C,D**) Gene expression in Nrf2 WT and KO cells. mRNA levels were measured by qPCR and corrected by GAPDH. Bars represent means $\pm$ SD, $n = 5$ replicates/treatment. * $p < 0.05$ versus cells treated with vehicle by One-Way ANOVA, followed by pairwise multiple comparisons using Holm-Sidak method. # $p < 0.05$ versus the corresponding WT treatment by Two-Way ANOVA, followed by pairwise multiple comparisons using Student-Newman-Keuls method.

As expected, KO cultures exhibit minimal expression of Nrf2 mRNA compared to WT cultures (Figure 4D). AVAs did not change Nrf2 expression in cultures of either genotype. In addition, NQO1 was the only antioxidant enzyme whose expression was dependent on Nrf2, as mRNA NQO1 transcripts were markedly reduced in KO compared to WT cultures (Figure 4D). In contrast, HO-1 and SOD1 expressions were similar in cultures of both genotypes. AVA 2p increased NQO1 expression in WT, but not in KO cultures. Similar results were obtained with AVA 2f and 2c, although the increase in NQO1 expression did not reach significance in WT cultures. AVAs did not alter HO-1 in cells of either genotype. In contrast, AVAs increased SOD1 expression in both WT and KO cultures, with AVA 2p exhibiting the strongest effect. Taken together, these results show a differential effect of AVAs on the expression of antioxidant enzymes that depends on the enzyme and of the presence or absence of Nrf2.

4. Discussion

The results of this study demonstrate that AVAs, compounds found uniquely in oats, regulate the expression of some genes in osteoblastic cells and affect the life span of the bone cells, osteoblasts, osteocytes and osteoclasts. Remarkably, AVAs were similarly effective in WT or Nrf2 KO cells to exert their anti-apoptotic effects on osteoblastic cells and their pro-apoptotic effects on osteoclasts. Although previous studies have shown that AVAs exert cytoprotective effects on other cell types in vitro [50,51], to our knowledge, this is the first study that evaluates the effects of AVAs on bone cell survival.

Osteoblasts express extracellular matrix proteins such as alkaline phosphatase, OCN and COL1A during the cell proliferation, matrix maturation, and mineralization phases [52]. The levels of mRNA expression of these osteoblast markers allows distinguishing the stages of differentiation and maturation of osteoblasts. COL1A among others, is secreted during the early stage of osteogenic differentiation, whereas OCN is a marker of a mature osteoblasts [53–55]. Our results revealed that AVA 2c and 2p potentially enhanced osteogenic differentiation by increasing the expression levels of COL1A. Cells of the osteoblastic lineage, osteoblasts, osteocytes and stromal/osteoblastic cells, play an important role in bone remodeling by expressing pro- and anti-osteoclastogenic cytokines [56–59]. These cells express the master osteoclast differentiation factor RANKL in response to osteoclast-stimulating hormones and cytokines, including PTH, tumor necrosis factor and interleukin-1; and they also express the RANKL decoy receptor OPG that inhibits osteoclastogenesis [45,58,60–62]. OPG protects bone from excessive resorption by preventing RANKL from binding to its receptor

(RANK) [63]. In our study, the lowest doses of all three AVAs increased OPG in OB-6 cells, suggesting a beneficial effect of AVAs by inhibiting osteoclast differentiation. Furthermore, we found that AVAs 2f and 2c decrease RANKL expression in MLO-Y4 osteocytic cells. Taken together these findings suggest that AVAs could modulate osteoclastogenesis by altering the expression of RANKL and OPG. Future studies are required to examine the relevance of our in vitro findings for the potential beneficial effects of AVAs on the skeleton in vivo; and the mechanistic basis of the differential effects of individual AVAs on bone cell gene expression.

Apoptosis plays a central role in the maintenance of skeletal mass and strength and several molecular mechanisms are involved in apoptosis regulation in bone cells [64,65]. Changes in the prevalence of osteoblast apoptosis have a significant impact in the number of osteoblasts present at sites of bone formation and their function [66]. Hence, increased osteoblast apoptosis is at least partially responsible for the decreased bone formation associated with the osteopenia induced by glucocorticoid excess [67], and conversely, inhibition of osteoblast apoptosis might contribute to the anabolic effect of intermittent administration of PTH [40,68]. Several studies have emphasized the importance of osteocyte viability for the maintenance of bone structure and strength [69]. Accumulation of apoptotic osteocytes preceded the increase in osteoclasts, suggesting a cause-effect relationship between dead osteocytes and bone resorption [70,71]. Thus, the increased bone fragility that occurs as consequence of glucocorticoid excess, sex steroid deficiency, immobilization and aging, is associated with increased osteoblast and osteocyte apoptosis [72]. It is known that osteoclasts die by apoptosis after completing a bone resorption cycle and that the majority of osteoblasts also die, whereas the remainders become lining cells or osteocytes. Osteocytes also can die prematurely with devastating consequences for bone fragility. Furthermore, it is recognized that systemic hormones, local growth factors, cytokines and pharmacological agents, as well as physical stimuli such as mechanical forces regulate the rate of bone cell apoptosis [66]. The data presented in this report indicate that AVAs do not induce apoptosis of osteoblastic or osteocytic cells. However, AVAs inhibit the effect of several pro-apoptotic stimuli. Moreover, AVA 2p induced apoptosis of KO osteoclasts. Similar to our findings with osteoclasts, AVA 2p induced apoptosis of the human cervical cancer cell line HeLa [73]. Because exaggerated ROS induces apoptosis of osteoblasts and osteocytes whereas it preserves osteoclast viability, it is possible that AVA actions are mediated by their antioxidant properties.

The Nrf2 pathway constitutes one of the major cellular defense mechanisms against oxidative stress, as evidenced by the fact that mice lacking Nrf2 are prone to the damaging effects of oxidative stress in different tissues [18,74]. The Nrf2 signaling pathway is emerging as a critical factor in the regulation of bone metabolism [75]. Deletion of Nrf2 suppresses antioxidant enzymes and elevates the intracellular ROS level in osteoclasts, increasing osteoclast number and stimulating osteoclast activity [76,77]. Consistent with this previous evidence, we found that bone marrow precursors in KO cultures presented higher number of osteoclasts and that the lack of Nrf2 also enhances osteoclast survival. Furthermore, we showed that AVAs induce osteoclast apoptosis in KO cultures. These findings are consistent with the fact that ROS is required for osteoclast generation and survival. On the other hand, WT, as well as KO primary osteoblastic cells treated with AVAs, were protected from apoptosis. This finding suggests that the pro-survival effect of AVAs on osteoblastic cells as well as the pro-apoptotic effect on osteoclasts does not require Nrf2 expression. Collectively, these outcomes demonstrate that AVAs, at the concentrations and exposure times tested, act by mechanisms independent of Nrf2 in bone cells of both osteoblastic and osteoclastic lineage. Future experiments are needed to determine whether the effective concentrations of AVAs in the current study are found in the bone tissue after dietary intakes of these compounds.

We also found that NQO1 was the only antioxidant enzyme which expression is strictly dependent on Nrf2; and that the expression of other antioxidant enzymes, including HO-1 and SOD1 was still high in KO cultures, strongly suggesting that they are controlled by alternative factors. AVAs did not have a major effect on the expression of these enzymes, recognized as Nrf2 target genes. However, AVA 2p increased NQO1 in WT cultures and SOD1 in both WT and KO cultures, suggesting that it activates the endogenous antioxidant defense by a mechanism that does not involve Nrf2.

Our results demonstrating actions of AVA independent of Nrf2 appear to be inconsistent with findings demonstrating that the increase in the expression of the antioxidant enzyme HO-1 induced by AVAs is associated with Nrf2 nuclear translocation in human kidney cells [36]. This difference could be due to the cell type, as well as the dose and time of treatment.

5. Conclusions

In conclusion, although further studies are needed to examine the mechanism(s) by which AVAs regulate bone cell survival, our findings demonstrate that AVAs affect gene expression in bone cells in vitro, as well as cell viability, preventing osteoblastic and osteocytic cell apoptosis and increasing osteoclast apoptosis; and that these effects of AVAs in the studied cells are not mediated by Nrf2.

Acknowledgments: The authors thank, Marta Maycas and Hannah Marie Davis for their technical support. This research was supported by an unrestricted educational grant from the National Osteoporosis Foundation through the generous support of PepsiCo, Inc.

Author Contributions: T.B. and G.G.P. conceived experimental design; G.G.P. and C.C.M. performed the experiments; G.G.P. and T.B. analyzed and interpreted the data; G.G.P., L.I.P., and T.B. wrote the paper. T.C.W. reviewed the manuscript.

Conflicts of Interest: The authors declare no conflict of interest.

References

1. Lin, H.; Gao, X.; Chen, G.; Sun, J.; Chu, J.; Jing, K.; Li, P.; Zeng, R.; Wei, B. Indole-3-carbinol as inhibitors of glucocorticoid-induced apoptosis in osteoblastic cells through blocking ROS-mediated Nrf2 pathway. *Biochem. Biophys. Res. Commun.* **2015**, *460*, 422–427. [CrossRef] [PubMed]

2. Benz, C.C.; Yau, C. Ageing, oxidative stress and cancer: Paradigms in parallax. *Nat. Rev. Cancer* **2008**, *8*, 875–879. [CrossRef] [PubMed]

3. Tarozzi, A.; Angeloni, C.; Malaguti, M.; Morroni, F.; Hrelia, S.; Hrelia, P. Sulforaphane as a potential protective phytochemical against neurodegenerative diseases. *Oxid. Med. Cell. Longev.* **2013**. [CrossRef] [PubMed]

4. Almeida, M. Aging mechanisms in bone. *Bonekey Rep.* **2012**. [CrossRef] [PubMed]

5. Almeida, M.; Han, L.; Ambrogini, E.; Weinstein, R.S.; Manolagas, S.C. Glucocorticoids and tumor necrosis factor (TNF) alpha increase oxidative stress and suppress WNT signaling in osteoblasts. *J. Biol. Chem.* **2011**, *286*, 44326–44335. [CrossRef] [PubMed]

6. Callaway, D.A.; Jiang, J.X. Reactive oxygen species and oxidative stress in osteoclastogenesis, skeletal aging and bone diseases. *J. Bone Miner. Metab.* **2015**, *33*, 359–370. [CrossRef] [PubMed]

7. Bai, X.C.; Lu, D.; Liu, A.L.; Zhang, Z.M.; Li, X.M.; Zou, Z.P.; Zeng, W.S.; Cheng, B.L.; Luo, S.Q. Reactive oxygen species stimulates receptor activator of NF-kappaB ligand expression in osteoblast. *J. Biol. Chem.* **2005**, *280*, 17497–17506. [CrossRef] [PubMed]

8. Lean, J.M.; Jagger, C.J.; Kirstein, B.; Fuller, K.; Chambers, T.J. Hydrogen peroxide is essential for estrogen-deficiency bone loss and osteoclast formation. *Endocrinology* **2005**, *146*, 728–735. [CrossRef] [PubMed]

9. Xu, Z.S.; Wang, X.Y.; Xiao, D.M.; Hu, L.F.; Lu, M.; Wu, Z.Y.; Bian, J.S. Hydrogen sulfide protects MC3T3-E1 osteoblastic cells against H_2O_2-induced oxidative damage-implications for the treatment of osteoporosis. *Free Radic. Biol. Med.* **2011**, *50*, 1314–1323. [CrossRef] [PubMed]

10. Mody, N.; Parhami, F.; Sarafian, T.A.; Demer, L.L. Oxidative stress modulates osteoblastic differentiation of vascular and bone cells. *Free Radic. Biol. Med.* **2001**, *31*, 509–519. [CrossRef]

11. Bai, X.; Lu, D.; Bai, J.; Zheng, H.; Ke, Z.; Li, X.; Luo, S. Oxidative stress inhibits osteoblastic differentiation of bone cells by ERK and NF-kappaB. *Biochem. Biophys. Res. Commun.* **2004**, *314*, 197–207. [CrossRef] [PubMed]

12. Arai, M.; Shibata, Y.; Pugdee, K.; Abiko, Y.; Ogata, Y. Effects of reactive oxygen species (ROS) on antioxidant system and osteoblastic differentiation in MC3T3-E1 cells. *IUBMB Life* **2007**, *59*, 27–33. [CrossRef] [PubMed]

13. Almeida, M.; Han, L.; Martin-Millan, M.; Plotkin, L.I.; Stewart, S.A.; Roberson, P.K.; Kousteni, S.; O'Brien, C.A.; Bellido, T.; Parfitt, A.M.; et al. Skeletal involution by age-associated oxidative stress and its acceleration by loss of sex steroids. *J. Biol. Chem.* **2007**, *282*, 27285–27297. [CrossRef] [PubMed]

14. Almeida, M.; Han, L.; Ambrogini, E.; Bartell, S.M.; Manolagas, S.C. Oxidative stress stimulates apoptosis and activates NF-κB in osteoblastic cells via a PKCβ/p66shc signaling cascade: Counter regulation by estrogens or androgens. *Mol. Endocrinol.* **2010**, *24*, 2030–2037. [CrossRef] [PubMed]

15. Mazziotti, G.; Bilezikian, J.; Canalis, E.; Cocchi, D.; Giustina, A. New understanding and treatments for osteoporosis. *Endocrine* **2012**, *41*, 58–69. [CrossRef] [PubMed]

16. Ibanez, L.; Ferrandiz, M.L.; Brines, R.; Guede, D.; Cuadrado, A.; Alcaraz, M.J. Effects of Nrf2 deficiency on bone microarchitecture in an experimental model of osteoporosis. *Oxid. Med. Cell. Longev.* **2014**. [CrossRef]

17. Jung, K.A.; Kwak, M.K. The Nrf2 system as a potential target for the development of indirect antioxidants. *Molecules* **2010**, *15*, 7266–7291. [CrossRef] [PubMed]

18. Sun, Y.X.; Xu, A.H.; Yang, Y.; Li, J. Role of Nrf2 in bone metabolism. *J. Biomed. Sci.* **2015**. [CrossRef] [PubMed]

19. Park, C.K.; Lee, Y.; Kim, K.H.; Lee, Z.H.; Joo, M.; Kim, H.H. Nrf2 is a novel regulator of bone acquisition. *Bone* **2014**, *63*, 36–46. [CrossRef] [PubMed]

20. Pandey, K.B.; Rizvi, S.I. Plant polyphenols as dietary antioxidants in human health and disease. *Oxid. Med. Cell. Longev.* **2009**, *2*, 270–278. [CrossRef] [PubMed]

21. Arts, I.C.; Hollman, P.C. Polyphenols and disease risk in epidemiologic studies. *Am. J. Clin. Nutr.* **2005**, *81*, 317S–325S. [PubMed]

22. Scalbert, A.; Holvoet, S.; Mercenier, A. Dietary polyphenols and the prevention of diseases. *Crit. Rev. Food Sci. Nutr.* **2005**, *41*, 287–306. [CrossRef] [PubMed]

23. Pawlowski, J.W.; Martin, B.R.; McCabe, G.P.; Ferruzzi, M.G.; Weaver, C.M. Plum and soy aglycon extracts superior at increasing bone calcium retention in ovariectomized sprague dawley rats. *J. Agric. Food Chem.* **2014**, *62*, 6108–6117. [CrossRef] [PubMed]

24. Boz, H. Phenolic amides (avenanthramides) in Oats—A review. *Czech J. Food Sci.* **2015**, *34*, 399–404. [CrossRef]

25. Meydani, M. Potential health benefits of avenanthramides of oats. *Nutr. Rev.* **2009**, *67*, 731–735. [CrossRef] [PubMed]

26. Emmons, C.L.; Peterson, D.M.; Paul, G.L. Antioxidant capacity of oat (*Avena sativa* L.) extracts. 2. In vitro antioxidant activity and contents of phenolic and tocol antioxidants. *J. Agric. Food Chem.* **1999**, *47*, 4894–4898. [CrossRef] [PubMed]

27. Mourikis, P.; Sambasivan, R.; Castel, D.; Rocheteau, P.; Bizzarro, V.; Tajbakhsh, S. A critical requirement for notch signaling in maintenance of the quiescent skeletal muscle stem cell state. *Stem Cells* **2012**, *30*, 243–252. [CrossRef] [PubMed]

28. Lee-Manion, A.M.; Price, R.K.; Strain, J.J.; Dimberg, L.H.; Sunnerheim, K.; Welch, R.W. In vitro antioxidant activity and antigenotoxic effects of avenanthramides and related compounds. *J. Agric. Food Chem.* **2009**, *57*, 10619–10624. [CrossRef] [PubMed]

29. Collins, F.W. Oat phenolics: Avenanthramides, novel substituted N-cinnamoylanthranilate alkaloids from oat groats and hulls. *J. Agric. Food Chem.* **1989**, *37*, 60–66. [CrossRef]

30. Bryngelsson, S.; Dimberg, L.H.; Kamal-Eldin, A. Effects of commercial processing on levels of antioxidants in oats (*Avena sativa* L.). *J. Agric. Food Chem.* **2002**, *50*, 1890–1896. [CrossRef] [PubMed]

31. Chen, C.Y.; Milbury, P.E.; Kwak, H.K.; Collins, F.W.; Samuel, P.; Blumberg, J.B. Avenanthramides and phenolic acids from oats are bioavailable and act synergistically with vitamin C to enhance hamster and human LDL resistance to oxidation. *J. Nutr.* **2004**, *134*, 1459–1466. [PubMed]

32. Wang, P.; Chen, H.; Zhu, Y.; McBride, J.; Fu, J.; Sang, S. Oat avenanthramide-C (2c) is biotransformed by mice and the human microbiota into bioactive metabolites. *J. Nutr.* **2015**, *145*, 239–245. [CrossRef] [PubMed]

33. Liu, L.; Zubik, L.; Collins, F.W.; Marko, M.; Meydani, M. The antiatherogenic potential of oat phenolic compounds. *Atherosclerosis* **2004**, *175*, 39–49. [CrossRef] [PubMed]

34. Koenig, R.; Dickman, J.R.; Kang, C.; Zhang, T.; Chu, Y.F.; Ji, L.L. Avenanthramide supplementation attenuates exercise-induced inflammation in postmenopausal women. *Nutr. J.* **2014**. [CrossRef] [PubMed]

35. Ren, Y.; Yang, X.; Niu, X.; Liu, S.; Ren, G. Chemical characterization of the avenanthramide-rich extract from oat and its effect on D-galactose-induced oxidative stress in mice. *J. Agric. Food Chem.* **2011**, *59*, 206–211. [CrossRef] [PubMed]

36. Fu, J.; Zhu, Y.; Yerke, A.; Wise, M.L.; Johnson, J.; Chu, Y.; Sang, S. Oat avenanthramides induce heme oxygenase-1 expression via Nrf2-mediated signaling in HK-2 cells. *Mol. Nutr. Food Res.* **2015**, *59*, 2471–2479. [CrossRef] [PubMed]

37. Nie, L.; Wise, M.; Peterson, D.; Meydani, M. Mechanism by which avenanthramide-c, a polyphenol of oats, blocks cell cycle progression in vascular smooth muscle cells. *Free Radic. Biol. Med.* **2006**, *41*, 702–708. [CrossRef] [PubMed]

38. Lezcano, V.; Bellido, T.; Plotkin, L.I.; Boland, R.; Morelli, S. Role of connexin 43 in the mechanism of action of alendronate: Dissociation of anti-apoptotic and proliferative signaling pathways. *Arch. Biochem. Biophys.* **2012**, *518*, 95–102. [CrossRef] [PubMed]

39. Lecanda, F.; Warlow, P.M.; Sheikh, S.; Furlan, F.; Steinberg, T.H.; Civitelli, R. Connexin43 deficiency causes delayed ossification, craniofacial abnormalities, and osteoblast dysfunction. *J. Cell Biol.* **2000**, *151*, 931–944. [CrossRef] [PubMed]

40. Bellido, T.; Ali, A.A.; Plotkin, L.I.; Fu, Q.; Gubrij, I.; Roberson, P.K.; Weinstein, R.S.; O'Brien, C.A.; Manolagas, S.C.; Jilka, R.L. Proteasomal degradation of Runx2 shortens parathyroid hormone-induced anti-apoptotic signaling in osteoblasts. A putative explanation for why intermittent administration is needed for bone anabolism. *J. Biol. Chem.* **2003**, *278*, 50259–50272. [CrossRef] [PubMed]

41. Lecka-Czernik, B.; Gubrij, I.; Moerman, E.A.; Kajkenova, O.; Lipschitz, D.A.; Manolagas, S.C.; Jilka, R.L. Inhibition of Osf2/Cbfa1 expression and terminal osteoblast differentiation by PPAR-gamma 2. *J. Cell. Biochem.* **1999**, *74*, 357–371. [CrossRef]

42. Plotkin, L.I.; Weinstein, R.S.; Parfitt, A.M.; Roberson, P.K.; Manolagas, S.C.; Bellido, T. Prevention of osteocyte and osteoblast apoptosis by bisphosphonates and calcitonin. *J. Clin. Investig.* **1999**, *104*, 1363–1374. [CrossRef] [PubMed]

43. Kato, Y.; Windle, J.J.; Koop, B.A.; Mundy, G.R.; Bonewald, L.F. Establishment of an osteocyte-like cell line, MLO-Y4. *J. Bone Miner. Res.* **1997**, *12*, 2014–2023. [CrossRef] [PubMed]

44. Pacheco-Costa, R.; Hassan, I.; Reginato, R.D.; Davis, H.M.; Bruzzaniti, A.; Allen, M.R.; Plotkin, L.I. High bone mass in mice lacking Cx37 due to defective osteoclast differentiation. *J. Biol. Chem.* **2014**, *289*, 8508–8520. [CrossRef] [PubMed]

45. Ben-Awadh, A.; Delgado-Calle, J.; Tu, X.; Kuhlenschmidt, K.; Allen, M.R.; Plotkin, L.I.; Bellido, T. Parathyroid hormone receptor signaling induces bone resorption in the adult skeleton by directly regulating the RANKL gene in osteocytes. *Endocrinology* **2014**, *155*, 2797–2809. [CrossRef] [PubMed]

46. O'Brien, C.A.; Plotkin, L.I.; Galli, C.; Goellner, J.; Gortazar, A.R.; Allen, M.R.; Robling, A.G.; Bouxsein, M.; Schipani, E.; Turner, C.H.; et al. Control of bone mass and remodeling by PTH receptor signaling in osteocytes. *PLoS ONE* **2008**, *3*, e2942.

47. Bellido, T.; Plotkin, L.I.; Bruzzaniti, A. Bone cells. In *Basic and Applied Bone Biology*, 1st ed.; Burr, D., Allen, M., Eds.; Elsevier: Oxford, UK, 2014; pp. 27–45.

48. Bellido, T.; Plotkin, L.I. Detection of apoptosis of bone cells in vitro. In *Osteoporosis*; Westendorf, J.J., Ed.; Humana Press: Totowa, NJ, USA, 2007; pp. 51–75.

49. Plotkin, L.I.; Mathov, I.; Aguirre, J.I.; Parfitt, A.M.; Manolagas, S.C.; Bellido, T. Mechanical stimulation prevents osteocyte apoptosis: Requirement of integrins, Src kinases and ERKs. *Am. J. Physiol. Cell Physiol.* **2005**, *289*, C633–C643. [CrossRef] [PubMed]

50. Guo, W.; Wise, M.L.; Collins, F.W.; Meydani, M. Avenanthramides, polyphenols from oats, inhibit IL-1beta-induced NF-kappaB activation in endothelial cells. *Free Radic. Biol. Med.* **2008**, *44*, 415–429. [CrossRef] [PubMed]

51. Lv, N.; Song, M.Y.; Lee, Y.R.; Choi, H.N.; Kwon, K.B.; Park, J.W.; Park, B.H. Dihydroavenanthramide D protects pancreatic beta-cells from cytokine and streptozotocin toxicity. *Biochem. Biophys. Res. Commun.* **2009**, *387*, 97–102. [CrossRef] [PubMed]

52. Hu, Y.; Tang, X.X.; He, H.Y. Gene expression during induced differentiation of sheep bone marrow mesenchymal stem cells into osteoblasts. *Genet. Mol. Res.* **2013**, *12*, 6527–6534. [CrossRef] [PubMed]

53. Balcerzak, M.; Hamade, E.; Zhang, L.; Pikula, S.; Azzar, G.; Radisson, J.; Bandorowicz-Pikula, J.; Buchet, R. The roles of annexins and alkaline phosphatase in mineralization process. *Acta Biochim. Pol.* **2003**, *50*, 1019–1038. [PubMed]

54. Janssens, K.; Ten, D.P.; Janssens, S.; Van, H.W. Transforming growth factor-beta1 to the bone. *Endocr. Rev.* **2005**, *26*, 743–774. [CrossRef] [PubMed]

55. Osyczka, A.M.; Leboy, P.S. Bone morphogenetic protein regulation of early osteoblast genes in human marrow stromal cells is mediated by extracellular signal-regulated kinase and phosphatidylinositol 3-kinase signaling. *Endocrinology* **2005**, *146*, 3428–3437. [CrossRef] [PubMed]

56. Jimi, E.; Nakamura, I.; Amano, H.; Taguchi, Y.; Tsurkai, T.; Tamura, M.; Takahasi, N.; Suda, T. Osteoclast function is activated by osteoblastic cells through a mechanism involving cell-to-cell contact. *Endocrinology* **1996**, *137*, 2187–2190. [PubMed]

57. Udagawa, N.; Takahashi, N.; Jimi, E.; Matsuzaki, K.; Tsurukai, T.; Itoh, K.; Nakagawa, N.; Yasuda, H.; Goto, M.; Tsuda, E.; et al. Osteoblasts/stromal cells stimulate osteoclast activation through expression of osteoclast differentiation factor/RANKL but not macrophage colony-stimulating factor: Receptor activator of NF-kappa B ligand. *Bone* **1999**, *25*, 517–523. [CrossRef]

58. Nakashima, T.; Hayashi, M.; Fukunaga, T.; Kurata, K.; Oh-hora, M.; Feng, J.Q.; Bonewald, L.F.; Kodama, T.; Wutz, A.; Wagner, E.F.; et al. Evidence for osteocyte regulation of bone homeostasis through RANKL expression. *Nat. Med.* **2011**, *17*, 1231–1234. [CrossRef] [PubMed]

59. Xiong, J.; Onal, M.; Jilka, R.L.; Weinstein, R.S.; Manolagas, S.C.; O'Brien, C.A. Matrix-embedded cells control osteoclast formation. *Nat. Med.* **2011**, *17*, 1235–1241. [CrossRef] [PubMed]

60. Simonet, W.S.; Lacey, D.L.; Dunstan, C.R.; Kelley, M.; Chang, M.S.; Luthy, R.; Nguyen, H.Q.; Wooden, S.; Bennett, L.; Boone, T.; et al. Osteoprotegerin: A novel secreted protein involved in the regulation of bone density. *Cell* **1997**, *89*, 309–319. [CrossRef]

61. Kramer, I.; Halleux, C.; Keller, H.; Pegurri, M.; Gooi, J.H.; Weber, P.B.; Feng, J.Q.; Bonewald, L.F.; Kneissel, M. Osteocyte Wnt/beta-catenin signaling is required for normal bone homeostasis. *Mol. Cell Biol.* **2010**, *30*, 3071–3085. [CrossRef] [PubMed]

62. Zhao, S.; Zhang, Y.K.; Harris, S.; Ahuja, S.S.; Bonewald, L.F. MLO-Y4 osteocyte-like cells support osteoclast formation and activation. *J. Bone Miner. Res.* **2002**, *17*, 2068–2079. [CrossRef] [PubMed]

63. Theoleyre, S.; Wittrant, Y.; Tat, S.K.; Fortun, Y.; Redini, F.; Heymann, D. The molecular triad OPG/RANK/RANKL: Involvement in the orchestration of pathophysiological bone remodeling. *Cytokine Growth Factor Rev.* **2004**, *15*, 457–475. [CrossRef] [PubMed]

64. Jilka, R.L.; Bellido, T.; Almeida, M.; Plotkin, L.I.; O'Brien, C.A.; Weinstein, R.S.; Manolagas, S.C. Apoptosis in bone cells. In *Principles of Bone Biology*, 3rd ed.; Bilezikian, J.P., Raisz, L.G., Martin, T.J., Eds.; Academic Press: San Diego/San Francisco, CA, USA; New York, NY, USA; London, UK; Sydney, Australia; Tokyo, Japan, 2008; pp. 237–261.

65. Bilezikian, J.P.; Raisz, L.G.; Rodan, G.A. *Principles of Bone Biology*; Academic Press: San Diego, CA, USA, 1996.

66. Bellido, T.; Plotkin, L.I. Novel actions of bisphosphonates in bone: Preservation of osteoblast and osteocyte viability. *Bone* **2011**, *49*, 50–55. [CrossRef] [PubMed]

67. Weinstein, R.S.; Jilka, R.L.; Parfitt, A.M.; Manolagas, S.C. Inhibition of osteoblastogenesis and promotion of apoptosis of osteoblasts and osteocytes by glucocorticoids: Potential mechanisms of their deleterious effects on bone. *J. Clin. Investig.* **1998**, *102*, 274–282. [CrossRef] [PubMed]

68. Jilka, R.L.; Weinstein, R.S.; Bellido, T.; Roberson, P.; Parfitt, A.M.; Manolagas, S.C. Increased bone formation by prevention of osteoblast apoptosis with parathyroid hormone. *J. Clin. Investig.* **1999**, *104*, 439–446. [CrossRef] [PubMed]

69. Plotkin, L.I. Apoptotic osteocytes and the control of targeted bone resorption. *Curr. Osteoporos. Rep.* **2014**, *12*, 121–126. [CrossRef] [PubMed]

70. Aguirre, J.I.; Plotkin, L.I.; Stewart, S.A.; Weinstein, R.S.; Parfitt, A.M.; Manolagas, S.C.; Bellido, T. Osteocyte apoptosis is induced by weightlessness in mice and precedes osteoclast recruitment and bone loss. *J. Bone Miner. Res.* **2006**, *21*, 605–615. [CrossRef] [PubMed]

71. Verborgt, O.; Gibson, G.; Schaffler, M.B. Loss of osteocyte integrity in association with microdamage and bone remodeling after fatigue in vivo. *J. Bone Miner. Res.* **2000**, *15*, 60–67. [CrossRef] [PubMed]

72. Plotkin, L.I.; Bivi, N.; Bellido, T. A bisphosphonate that does not affect osteoclasts prevents osteoblast and osteocyte apoptosis and the loss of bone strength induced by glucocorticoids in mice. *Bone* **2011**, *49*, 122–127. [CrossRef] [PubMed]

73. Wang, D.; Wise, M.L.; Li, F.; Dey, M. Phytochemicals attenuating aberrant activation of beta-catenin in cancer cells. *PLoS ONE* **2012**, *7*, e50508.

74. Motohashi, H.; Yamamoto, M. Nrf2-Keap1 defines a physiologically important stress response mechanism. *Trends Mol. Med.* **2004**, *10*, 549–557. [CrossRef] [PubMed]

75. Sun, Y.X.; Li, L.; Corry, K.A.; Zhang, P.; Yang, Y.; Himes, E.; Mihuti, C.L.; Nelson, C.; Dai, G.; Li, J. Deletion of Nrf2 reduces skeletal mechanical properties and decreases load-driven bone formation. *Bone* **2015**, *74*, 1–9. [CrossRef] [PubMed]

76. Hyeon, S.; Lee, H.; Yang, Y.; Jeong, W. Nrf2 deficiency induces oxidative stress and promotes RANKL-induced osteoclast differentiation. *Free Radic. Biol. Med.* **2013**, *65*, 789–799. [CrossRef] [PubMed]

77. Kanzaki, H.; Shinohara, F.; Kajiya, M.; Kodama, T. The Keap1/Nrf2 protein axis plays a role in osteoclast differentiation by regulating intracellular reactive oxygen species signaling. *J. Biol. Chem.* **2013**, *288*, 23009–23020. [CrossRef] [PubMed]

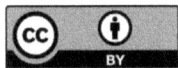

nutrients

MDPI

Review

Yacon (*Smallanthus sonchifolius*) as a Food Supplement: Health-Promoting Benefits of Fructooligosaccharides

Brunno F. R. Caetano [1], Nelci A. de Moura [1], Ana P. S. Almeida [2], Marcos C. Dias [3], Kátia Sivieri [2] and Luís F. Barbisan [1,*]

[1] Department of Morphology, Institute of Biosciences, Sao Paulo State University, Botucatu 18618-689, Brazil; brnncaetano@gmail.com (B.F.R.C.); nelcimoura@gmail.com (N.A.d.M.)

[2] Departament of Food and Nutrition, Faculty of Pharmaceutical Sciences, Sao Paulo State University, Araraquara 14800-903, Brazil; anap.almeida@terra.com.br (A.P.S.A.); katiasiv@hotmail.com (K.S.)

[3] Institute of Health Sciences, Federal University of Mato Grosso, Sinop 78550-000, Mato Grosso, Brazil; marcosdias16@gmail.com

* Correspondence: barbisan@ibb.unesp.br; Tel.: +55-14-3880-0469; Fax: +55-14-3880-0479

Received: 13 May 2016; Accepted: 16 June 2016; Published: 21 July 2016

Abstract: Yacon (*Smallanthus sonchifolius*), a perennial plant of the family Asteraceae native to the Andean regions of South America, is an abundant source of fructooligosaccharides (FOS). This comprehensive review of the literature addressed the role of yacon supplementation in promoting health and reducing the risk of chronic diseases. According to several preclinical and clinical trials, FOS intake favors the growth of health-promoting bacteria while reducing pathogenic bacteria populations. Moreover, the endproducts of FOS fermentation by the intestinal microbiota, short chain fatty acids (SCFA), act as substrates or signaling molecules in the regulation of the immune response, glucose homeostasis and lipid metabolism. As a result, glycemic levels, body weight and colon cancer risk can be reduced. Based on these findings, most studies reviewed concluded that due to their functional properties, yacon roots may be effectively used as a dietary supplement to prevent and treat chronic diseases.

Keywords: yacon; prebiotics; fructooligosacharides; functional food; chronic diseases

1. Introduction

Yacon (*Smallanthus sonchifolius*) is a perennial herbaceous plant of the family Asteraceae, native to the Andean regions of South America [1,2]. This plant has a branching system that gives rise to aerial stems about 2 to 2.5 m high. Yacon yields starchy, fruit-like roots of different shapes and sizes that are usually consumed raw and taste sweet. Their crunchy texture very much resembles that of an apple. One plant is estimated to produce more than 10 kilos of roots [3,4]. The fact that the yacon plant adapts to different climatic regions, altitudes and soils explains its expansion outside the Andean region. Yacon is currently cultivated in Argentina, Bolívia, Brazil, the Czech Republic, Ecuador, Italy, Japan, Korea, New Zealand, Peru and the United States [4].

There is a variety of common names for yacon around the world. These include aricoma and aricuma in Bolivia, jicama, chicama and shicama in Ecuador, and arboloco in Colombia. However, the Spanish term yacon, derived from the Quéchua word "yaku" which means "watery", is the most used worldwide. Interestingly, water is the most abundant component of the yacon root [2,4].

Yacon roots' water content usually exceeds 70% of the fresh weight while the major portion of the dry matter consists of fructooligosacharides (FOS) [5]. FOS content ranges from 6.4% to 70% of the dry matter (0.7% to 13.2% of the fresh weight) depending upon the specific crop and location. In yacon roots, the antioxidant capacity varies between 23 and 136 µmol/g trolox equivalent of the dry matter, and total phenolic compounds represent 0.79% to 3.08% of the dry matter [6–8]. Figure 1 summarizes the physicochemical and functional characteristics of yacon roots.

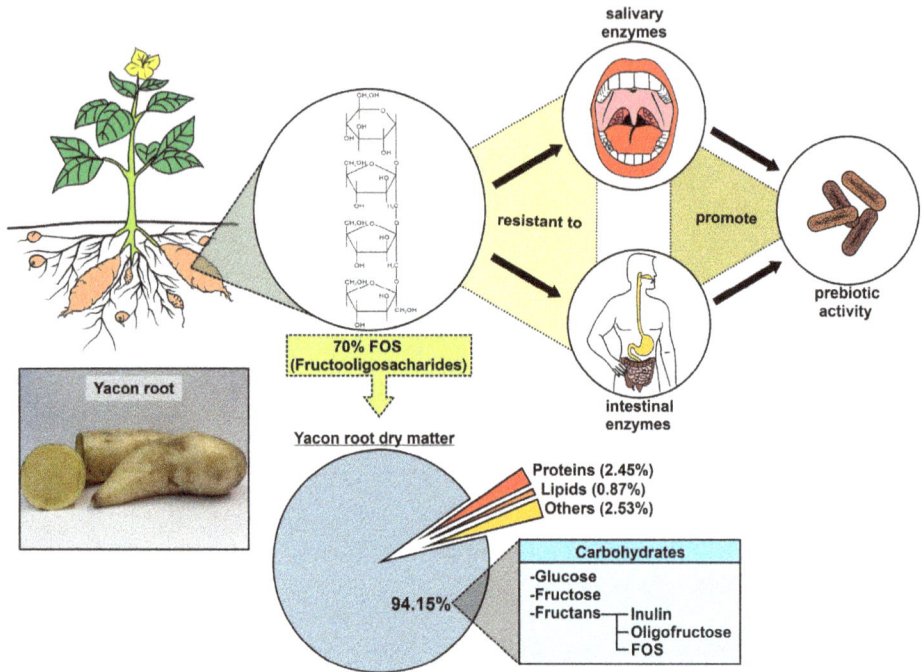

Figure 1. Chemical composition and functional properties of yacon roots.

The high content of FOS in yacon roots is considered to offer health benefits, as it can reduce glycemic index, body weight and the risk of colon cancer [9]. Yacon functional properties, long recognized by folk medicine, have been the subject of a number of research projects and clinical trials [10]. Thus, the nutraceutical potential of yacon roots has garnered great public interest as a dietary supplement. In this comprehensive review, we focused on yacon FOS health-promoting benefits regarding human chronic diseases.

2. Fructooligosacharides: Bioactivity and Potential Health Benefits

Fructooligosacharides (FOS) are fructans consisting of linear short chains of fructose molecules. Fructans are synthesized from sucrose in the cell vacuoles of plant leaves, stems and roots. They help protect against drying out and are carbohydrate reserves in a wide number of plant families [11,12]. FOS are natural food components that can be found in garlic, onion, asparagus, artichoke, banana, wheat and yacon. However, the highest concentrations of FOS are found in yacon [13].

FOS are able to escape enzymatic digestion in the upper gastrointestinal tract, reaching the colon intact before undergoing microbial fermentation. FOS intake elicits a bifidogenic effect by selectively stimulating the proliferation of bifidobacteria, a group of beneficial bacteria naturally found in the human colon (Figure 2) [14–16]. Short chain fatty acids (SCFA), the endproducts of FOS fermentation by the intestinal microbiota, can also favor the growth of health-promoting bacteria such as *Bifidobacterium* spp. and *Lactobacillus* spp., while reducing or maintaining pathogenic populations (e.g., *Clostridium* spp. and *Escherichia coli*) at low levels [17–19]. Thus, FOS are small soluble dietary fibers that exhibit prebiotic activity.

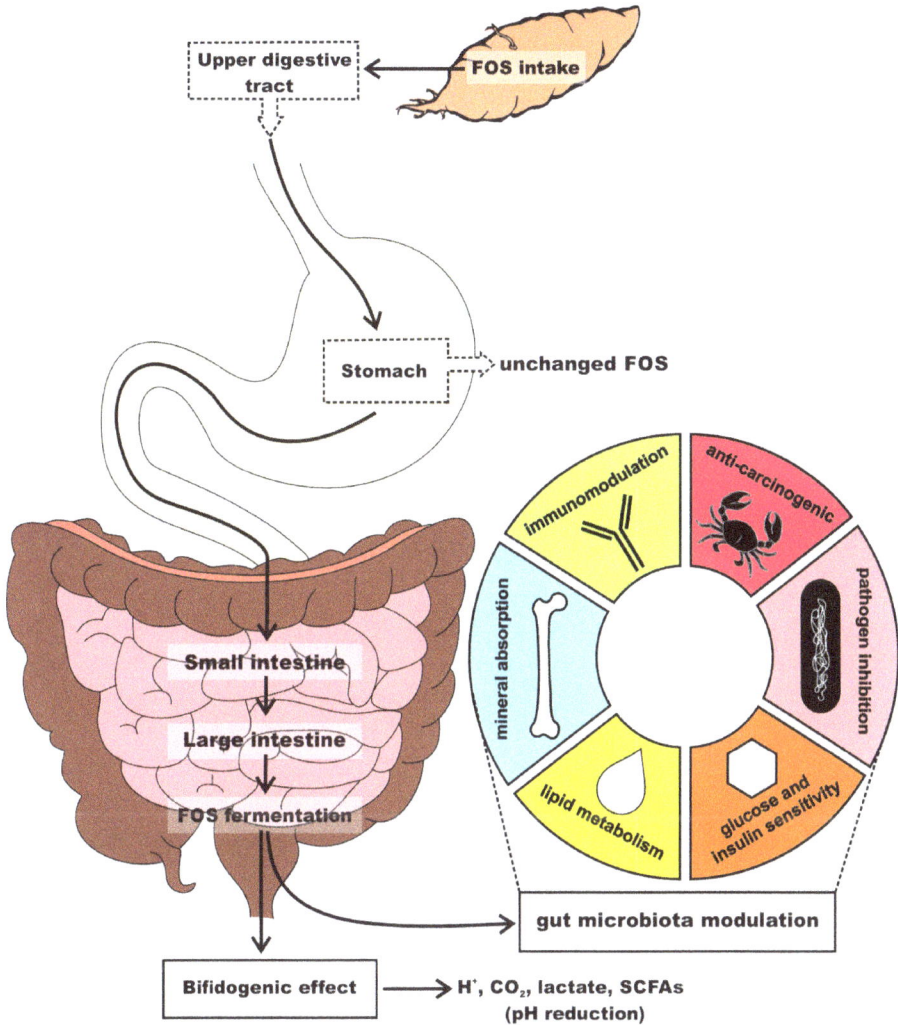

Figure 2. Yacon root consumption and health-promoting benefits of FOS.

The term prebiotic was coined by Gibson and Roberfroid in 1995 to describe a "non-digestible food ingredient that beneficially affects the host by selectively stimulating the growth and/or activity of one or a limited number of bacteria in the colon, thus improving host health" [20]. This concept was later revised by Roberfroid who redefined a prebiotic as "a selectively fermented ingredient that allows specific changes, both in the composition and/or activity in the gastrointestinal microflora that confers benefits upon host well-being and health" [21].

Several other concepts have been proposed since then, but they all describe a prebiotic as a non-digestible compound able to selectively stimulate the growth of gut bacteria. According to the criteria proposed by FAO at the technical meeting on prebiotics [22], to be classified as a prebiotic, a compound must present the following qualifications: (a) component: a compound or substance that can be chemically characterized—not an organism or drug normally presented as a food-grade component; (b) health benefit: a compound or substance must resist digestion and absorption in the small intestine, over-riding any adverse effects; and (c) modulation: a compound or substance must promote health-related changes in the composition and/or activities of the colonic microbiota in the target host.

There is sufficient evidence to support the categorization of FOS as prebiotics. FOS offers physiological benefits that justify its use as a food supplement, particularly in cases of chronic diseases [14,23,24]. Since yacon has long been used in folk medicine for treating diabetes, constipation and various other human diseases, the present study aimed at reviewing the mechanisms underlying yacon FOS health benefits in colon cancer, diabetes, and obesity.

3. FOS Effects on Colorectal Cancer

Colorectal Cancer (CRC) is the third most commonly diagnosed type of cancer and a leading cause of death in the Western world. Although family history is an important risk factor for CRC development, only 15% of new cases have been linked to hereditary causes. In fact, the majority of CRCs (80%) occur sporadically and are associated with acquired risk factors, such as lifestyle and diet [25,26]. Dietary factors that potentially increase the risk of CRC include a high intake of red and processed meat, saturated fats and refined starches [27,28]. Diabetes and obesity are also associated with a higher risk of developing CRC [29].

Little is known about the feasibility, safety and efficacy of using dietary yacon to modulate or suppress CRC. Our research group was the first to report the chemopreventive effects of yacon root intake on dimethylhydrazine (DMH)-induced colon cancer in male rats. We showed a reduction in cell proliferation, number and multiplicity of preneoplastic lesions and invasive adenocarcinomas in a group receiving 1% of yacon powder [30]. In a more recent study evaluating the effects of yacon aqueous extract on the initiation step of CRC carcinogenesis, we found that yacon aqueous extract alone or that associated with *Lactobacillus acidophilus* (synbiotic formulation) reduced DMH-induced DNA damage in leukocytes. Moreover, we observed a reduction in cell proliferation indexes and a decrease in apoptosis levels in the group supplemented with the synbiotic formulation [31].

There is growing evidence that human intestinal microbiota plays an essential role in CRC carcinogenesis. The interplay between the intestinal microbiota, the intestinal epithelium and the host innate immune system is associated with several human diseases, including colitis and CRC [32,33]. Dysbiosis is a condition in which an imbalance in the microbial community favors the growth of specific pathogens that are potentially pro-carcinogenic. Intestinal microbiota disruption also exerts a great impact on colon metabolic profiles under the influence of the microbial community [34].

The influence of dietary habits on the composition of the microbiota has been widely accepted in the scientific community, supporting the hypothesis that diet patterns can induce dysbiosis [35]. Hence, the yacon root is thought to be a good dietary supplement, since its high content of FOS can selectively modulate the composition and function of the intestinal microbiota. FOS promote the growth of bifidobacteria, a genus of Gram-positive pleomorphic rods that play a regulatory role in the colon by inhibiting the growth of putrefactive bacteria. Bifidobacteria have been suggested to decrease the expression of xenobiotic-metabolizing enzymes and stimulate the immune system in the colonic mucosa [36–38].

FOS consumption also leads to increased SCFA production, primarily acetate, propionate and butyrate. Recent findings suggest that SCFA can suppress inflammation and cancer by increasing local immune response, decreasing colon pH and promoting ammonia and amine excretion [36,38]. During carcinogenesis, SCFA production in the colon by beneficial bacteria decreases cellular proliferation and induces apoptosis, especially in colon tumor cells. In fact, increasing butyrate production has also been shown to decrease the development of preneoplastic aberrant crypt foci lesions and delay tumor progression in rats [30,39,40].

FOS can indirectly influence immune activity via SCFA production that modifies the intestinal microbiota composition. SCFA promote a state of immune tolerance and modulate interleukin (IL) production and natural killer (NK) cell activity [41]. Vaz-Tostes et al. [42] reported that the consumption of yacon flour (0.14 g FOS kg body weight) over 18 weeks increased serum IL-4 and fecal secretory IgA in overweight preschool children with an inadequate dietary intake of zinc and fiber [42]. However, the role of prebiotic-induced immunomodulation in CRC is still unclear.

Increasing evidence suggests that FOS can also directly modulate the immune system through the gut-associated lymphoid tissue (GALT) rather than the gut microbiota [43]. Natural plant compounds such as fructans and polysaccharides may activate specialized immune cells (macrophages, dendritic cells, lymphocytes and neutrophils) by mimicking pathogen-associated molecular patterns (PAMPs) that bind to toll-like receptors (TLR), causing immunomodulatory effects [44]. For instance, TLR-mediated activation of NK cells can promote IFN-γ production and thus increase anti-tumor cytotoxicity. Furthermore, direct and indirect immunomodulation mechanisms can synergistically induce robust regulatory cellular immune responses [45]. Indeed, yacon treatment increased cytokine production (i.e., IL-10, IFN-α and IL-4) and the expression of toll-like receptor 4 (TLR4) and CD206 in cells in infant mice [46,47]. The increase in the expression of these receptors in gut-associated immune cells results in an enhanced status of the innate immune response with remarkable macrophage activity. The increased phagocytic activity of macrophages, mediated by the CD206 receptor and TLR4, is able to maintain colonic homeostasis without inducing inflammatory responses, reinforcing the intestinal barrier against pathogens and improving anti-tumor defense [47,48].

Table 1 shows that the effects of yacon consumption on colorectal cancer include: (a) suppressed cell proliferation; (b) reduced preneoplastic lesions; (c) significantly changed composition of the colonic microbiota; and (d) modulated immune response in CRC.

Table 1. Effects of yacon consumption on colorectal cancer.

Yacon Source	Research, Subject Randomized, Dose and Duration	Health Properties	References
Dried extract of yacon root	Mouse (BALB/c) Dose: 340 mg/kg day in diet, for 75 days	Growth of *Bifidobacteria* and *Lactobacilli*	Bonet et al. [16]
Dried extract of yacon root	Rats (Wistar) Dose: 0.5%, 1.0% (20.4% FOS) in diet for 13 weeks	Reduce tumor multiplicity, preneoplastic lesions and cell proliferation	De Moura et al. [27]
Aqueous extract of yacon root	Rats (Wistar) Dose: 2.2 mL (1% FOS) for 8 months	Reduce DNA damage and cell proliferation	Almeida et al. [28]
Dried extract of yacon root	Mouse (BALB/c) Dose: 3.0%, 5% FOS in diet for 30 days	Improves the immune parameters	Delgado et al. [46]

4. FOS Effects on Diabetes

Diabetes is the most common chronic disorder in developed countries, and a leading cause of death worldwide, with the global prevalence being 8.4% among adults (>18 years) in 2014 [49]. Obesity and physical inactivity have been related to increased risk of developing diabetes. Diabetes mellitus is a group of metabolic diseases characterized by hyperglycemia resulting from defects in insulin secretion and/or insulin action. Untreated chronic hyperglycemia can cause long-term tissue damage and dysfunction that might lead to adverse outcomes such as skin ulcers and amputations. Type 2 diabetes mellitus, characterized by insulin resistance and pancreatic β-cell dysfunction, is the most common form of diabetes [50,51].

The current standard care for diabetes type 2 prevention and management is dietary intervention [52]. Hence, antidiabetic nutraceuticals, such as yacon, with reduced or no side effects have been high in demand. Due to their hypoglycemic properties, yacon roots have long been recognized by folk medicine as an effective alternative for diabetes treatment. Moreover, yacon roots, either crude or refined, can be used as low-calorie sweeteners by dieters as well as people suffering from diabetes [53].

Several preclinical and clinical trials have shown that yacon root FOS have a notable hypoglycemic effect. In an experiment using streptozotocin-induced diabetic rats, the number of insulin-positive pancreatic cells and glucagon-like peptide-1 (GLP-1) significantly increased, while visceral abdominal fat was reduced and fasting insulin serum levels were slightly increased in diabetic rats supplemented with yacon flour (340 or 6800 mg FOS/kg body weight (bw).) for 90 days [54]. In another study using Zucker fa/fa male rats, yacon at 6.5% in chow reduced blood glucose levels and improved hepatic insulin sensitivity. In this case, dietary yacon significantly reduced Trb3 hepatic expression and increased Akt expression, improving insulin sensitivity in the liver [55].

In a trial evaluating the daily intake of freeze-dried yacon among elderly individuals, FOS content (7.4 g) was positively correlated with decreasing serum glucose levels [56]. Among obese and slightly dyslipidemic pre-menopausal women, Genta et al. observed that yacon syrup at 0.14 g/kg bw reduced fasting serum insulin and was significantly associated with decreased beta-cell function and insulin resistance in a homeostasis model assessment (HOMA), suggesting that yacon syrup FOS promote glucose absorption in peripheral tissues and improve insulin sensitivity via SCFA production [57].

Plasma glucose homeostasis is achieved through a tightly controlled balance between glucose input (food intake and liver production) and glucose uptake by multiple organs [58]. FOS putative effects on glucose disposal and insulin tolerance are mediated via multiple mechanisms. These mechanisms are part of the milieu of interactions that take place between the intestinal microflora and the host metabolism, and converge to a similar outcome—the production of SCFA by FOS fermentation. SCFA produced by the intestinal microbiota are promptly absorbed in the colon and conveyed into blood, where they play their physiological roles as substrates or signaling molecules [59–61].

Several studies have been conducted to elucidate the underlying mechanisms of SCFA on glucose homeostasis. For instance, acetate has been shown to reduce free fatty acids (FFA) plasma levels, which are known to cause peripheral insulin resistance in obese individuals, inhibiting glucose uptake and glycogen synthesis [62]. The oral administration of propionate to both diabetic hyperglycemic and normal rats has been shown to decrease gluconeogenesis by increasing AMPK expression in the liver [63]. SCFA have also been reported to affect glycemic levels through the gut hormones peptide YY (PYY) and GLP-1 by directly activating colonic free fatty acid receptors 2 and 3 (Ffar2 and Ffar3). PYY and GLP-1 have also been proposed to improve plasma glucose levels after a meal in a dependent manner, stimulating insulin and inhibiting glucagon secretion in the pancreas [64,65].

Table 2 shows that the effects of yacon consumption on diabetes include: (a) increased glucose absorption in peripheral tissues; (b) decreased gluconeogenesis; (c) improved insulin tolerance in the liver; and (d) increased insulin secretion in the pancreas.

Table 2. Effects of yacon consumption on diabetes.

Yacon Source	Research, Subject Randomized, Dose and Duration	Health Properties	References
Yacon flour	Rats (Wistar) Dose: Yacon flour (340 mg FOS/kg/day) for 90 days	Increase insulin-positive pancreatic cell	Habib et al. [54]
Dried extract of yacon root	Rats (Zucker fa/fa) Dose: 6.5% yacon for 5 weeks	Improve insulin sensitivity in the insulin-resistant state	Satoh et al. [55]
Dried extract of yacon root	Elderly man and woman Dose: Yacon powder (7.4 g of FOS) for 9 weeks	Decrease in serum glucose levels	Scheid et al. [56]
Yacon syrup	Obese and slightly dyslipidemic pre-menopausal women Dose: Yacon syrup (0.29 g and 0.14 g FOS/kg/day), for 120 days	Improve insulin-resistance state	Genta et al. [57]

5. FOS Effects on Obesity

Overweight and obesity comprises one of the main public health challenges worldwide because of the associated increased risk of developing type 2 diabetes, heart disease, hypertension, cancer and a number of other diseases [66]. Over the past few decades, the increasing number of overweight and obese people has been claimed as a pandemic. According to the World Health Organization (WHO), the prevalence of overweight was estimated to be 39% among adults aged 18 years and over, while obesity represented 13% of the overall world's adult population in 2014 [67]. Overweight and obesity are defined as a condition of abnormal or excessive accumulation of adipose tissue in the body. This condition may impair health and lead, for instance, to the development of chronic inflammation and metabolic syndrome [68]. The main causes of overweight and obesity are related to energy imbalance (i.e., energy intake exceeds energy expenditure) modulated by metabolic factors, diet and physical activity. Hence, there has been a global trend to an increasing intake of energy-dense foods that are rich in saturated fat and refined starches, as well as increasing rates of physical inactivity and a sedentary lifestyle [69].

Metabolic syndrome is a cluster of cardiometabolic risk factors that arises from insulin resistance accompanying abnormal visceral adiposity, glucose intolerance, dyslipidemia and hypertension [70]. As a consequence, metabolic syndrome leads to a state of chronic inflammation produced by a complex interaction between genetic and environmental factors. At the moment, there is no consensus on what is the most appropriate nutritional intervention for treating metabolic syndrome related to obesity [71]. However, certain dietary bioactive compounds found in over 800 plants can help to prevent or ameliorate multiple facets of metabolic syndrome. In this regard, yacon has been hypothesized to exert anti-obesity and hypolipidemic effects by improving biochemical parameters and satiety [72]. Though there is a popular claim that yacon syrup can aid in weight loss, scientific evidence is nevertheless scarce. These properties, however, are thought to be directly related to the high content of FOS found in yacon root.

In a sub-chronic four-month oral toxicity study, dried yacon root (340 mg and 6800 mg FOS/kg bw) was given as a diet supplement to healthy, non-obese Wistar rats. During the feeding trial, yacon administration was well tolerated and did not produce any toxic effect. Furthermore, yacon consumption at both doses significantly reduced post-prandial serum triacylglycerol (TAG) levels [73]. Similar findings were reported when yacon flour (340 or 6800 mg FOS/kg bw) was administered to streptozotocin-induced diabetic rats. The oral consumption of yacon flour decreased fasting plasma TAG, very low-density lipoprotein (VLDL) and the postprandial peak of plasma TAG [54]. In another study using synbiotic formulations, a positive effect on TAG and high-density lipoprotein (HDL) cholesterol levels was reported in diabetic rats that received an aqueous extract of yacon roots and soybean, in association or not with *Enterococcus faecium* CRL 183 and *Lactobacillus helveticus* ssp jugurti [74].

Although the hypolipidemic effects of yacon roots have been demonstrated in pre-clinical studies, evidence from well-designed human trials is still scarce. As cited before, in a study with premenopausal, obese and slightly dyslipidemic women, yacon syrup intake (0.14 g FOS/kg bw) over 120 days showed improvements in fasting low density lipoproteins (LDL) and visceral fat [57]. Otherwise, no such effect was reported in a study conducted in elderly who consumed a daily intake of freeze-dried powdered yacon [56]. Moreover, yacon administered to healthy individuals (6.4 g FOS/day) over two weeks markedly accelerated colonic transit in a placebo-controlled, double-blind study design [75].

The beneficial effects of FOS on lipid metabolism are well recognized, although the underlying mechanisms are still unclear. FOS exert hypolipidemic effects through SCFA production by the intestinal microbiota, resulting in the modulation of biochemical and cellular pathways related to lipid metabolism, satiety and intestinal transit [76]. Indeed, SCFA have been shown to positively regulate the lipid homeostasis by inhibiting lipolysis, increasing triglyceride mobilization and adipogenic differentiation [60,77]. In vitro studies also reported that SCFA were able to reduce cholesterol synthesis by decreasing hepatic activity of the 3-hydroxy-3-methylglutaryl-CoA synthase (HMGCS) and 3-hydroxy-3-methylglutaryl-CoA reductase (HMGCR) enzymes [68]. AMPK activation by SFCAs has also been suggested to inhibit HMGCS and HMGCR activation in an independent manner [60].

It has also been shown that dietary FOS are able to increase the secretion of peptides by the gastrointestinal diffuse neuroendocrine system via SCFA production, acting as modulators of appetite and increasing satiety [78]. The physiological control of satiety is partly regulated by intestinal peptide secretion including cholecystokinin (CCK), PYY and GLP-1. It is noteworthy that this regulation is complex and involves a range of mechanisms and multiple control systems [79]. Nevertheless, SCFA can directly increase PYY and GLP-1 secretion by Ffar1 and Ffar2 activation in the colon [80]. Conversely, long-term studies have suggested that a long exposure time is needed for the intestinal microbiota to adapt and produce the amounts of SCFA to elicit the physiological effect of satiety. Increased gut motility may also be affected by intestinal peptide secretion [81]. However, SCFA such as butyrate are able to exert direct effects on myenteric neurons and increase the intestinal motility, supporting the hypothesis by which a high fiber intake accelerates the colonic transit [82].

Although there have been several studies reporting the beneficial effects of yacon intake on obesity, much needs to be understood about the mechanisms and processes that underlie such effects. Table 3 shows that the effects of yacon consumption on obesity include: (a) modulated biochemical and cellular pathways related to lipid homeostasis; (b) increased satiety; and (c) increased gut motility.

Table 3. Effects of yacon consumption on obesity.

Yacon Source	Research, Subject Randomized, Dose and Duration	Health properties	References
Yacon flour	Rats (Wistar) Dose: Yacon flour (340 mg FOS/kg/day) for 90 days	Hypolipidemic effect	Habib et al. [54]
Yacon syrup	Obese and slightly dyslipidemic pre-menopausal women Dose: Yacon syrup (0.29/g and 0.14/g FOS/kg/day) for 120 days.	Increased defecation frequency and satiety sensation	Genta et al. [57]
Dried extract of yacon root	Rats (wistar) Dose: Dried yacon root (340 mg and 6800 mg FOS/bw) for 4 months	Reduced post-prandial serum TAG levels	Genta et al. [73]
Aqueous extract of yacon root	Rats (wistar) Dose: 1 mL/kg body weight/day, 4.30 g/100 g of frutans, for 7 weeks	Positive effect on TAG and HDL	Roselino et al. [74]
Yacon syrup	Healthy individuals Dose: 6.4 g FOS/day	Accelerates the colonic transit	Geyer et al. [75]

6. Yacon Consumption Adverse Effects

Although yacon consumption is safe at recommended dosages, overdosing may be uncomfortable, but not life-threatening. Symptoms of yacon overdose include abdominal pain, bloating, flatulence and diarrhea [57]. In addition, yacon consumption markedly accelerates colonic transit, increasing stool frequency [75]. The only report of adverse effects found in the literature describes the case of a 55-year-old woman who developed anaphylaxis after yacon ingestion [83].

A side effect that should be taken into account when evaluating the proportion of oligofructans/fructose within yacon roots is the partial hydrolysis of yacon oligofructans to fructose that starts shortly after harvest and may accelerate during food processing [84]. This can seriously affect yacon's health-promoting benefits because high-fructose administration correlates with the induction of insulin resistance by modifying the early steps of insulin signal transduction [85]. Therefore, cold storage and temperature-controlled environments are highly recommended to keep the functional properties of the yacon roots [84].

7. Conclusions

Experimental and clinical studies have reported that yacon consumption is important to regulate several pathways related to colon cancer, diabetes, and obesity. The FOS content found in yacon roots can modulate the human intestinal microbiota, increase glucose absorption in peripheral tissues, stimulate insulin secretion in the pancreas and modulate cellular pathways related to lipid homeostasis. Therefore, based on these findings, most studies reviewed concluded that due to their functional properties, yacon roots may be effectively used as a dietary supplement to prevent and treat chronic diseases.

Acknowledgments: This review is based upon research projects supported by the Sao Paulo Research Foundation (FAPESP) under grants 09/12239-2, 11/01126-2 and 16/12800-0. The authors acknowledge the support of PROPe-PROINTER/UNESP.

Author Contributions: All authors contributed equally to this work.

Conflicts of Interest: The authors declare no conflict of interest.

Abbreviations

The following abbreviations are used in this manuscript:

BW	body weight
CRC	colorectal cancer
CCK	cholecystokinin
DMH	1,2-dimethylhydrazine
GLP-1	glucagon-like peptide 1
SCFA	short chain fatty acids
FFA	free fatty acids
FFAR	free fatty acid receptor
FOS	fructooligosaccharides
HDL	high density lipoprotein
LDL	low density lipoprotein
PAMPs	pathogen-associated molecular patterns
PYY	peptide YY
TAG	tryacylglycerol
TLR	toll-like receptors
VLDL	very low density lipoprotein

References

1. Lachman, J.; Fernández, E.C.; Orsák, M. Yacon (Smallanthus sonchifolia (Poepp. et Endl.) H. Robinson) chemical composition and use-a review. *Plant Soil Environ.* **2003**, *49*, 283–290.
2. Zardini, E. Ethnobotanical notes of yacon, Polymnia sonchifolia (Asteraceae). *Econ Bot.* **1991**, *45*, 72–85. [CrossRef]
3. Grau, A.; Rea, J. Yacon. Smallanthus sonchifolius (Poepp. & Endl.) H. Robinson. In *Andean Roots and Tuberous Roots: Ahipa, Arracacha, Maca and Yacon*; Gatersleben/IPGRI: Rome, Italy, 1997; pp. 199–256.
4. Ojansivua, I.; Ferreira, C.L.; Salminena, S. Yacon, a new source of prebiotic oligosaccharides with a history of safe use. *Trends Food Sci. Tech.* **2011**, *22*, 40–46. [CrossRef]
5. Campos, D.; Betalleluz-Pallardel, I.; Chirinos, R.; Aguilar-Galvez, A.; Noratto, G. Prebiotic effects of yacon (*Smallanthus sonchifolius* Poepp. & Endl), a source of fructooligosaccharides and phenolic compounds with antioxidant activity. *Food Chem.* **2012**, *135*, 1592–1599. [CrossRef] [PubMed]
6. Castro, A.; Céspedes, G.; Carballo, S.; Bergenståhl, B.; Tornberg, E. Dietary fiber, fructooligosaccharides, and physicochemical properties of homogenized aqueous suspensions of yacon (*Smallanthus sonchifolius*). *Food Res. Int.* **2013**, *50*, 392–400. [CrossRef]

7. Jiménez, M.E.; Sammán, N. Chemical characterization and quantification of fructooligosaccharides, phenolic compounds and antiradical activity of Andean roots and tubers grown in Northwest of Argentina. *Arch. Latinoam Nutr.* **2014**, *64*, 131–138. [PubMed]
8. Pereira, J.A.R.; Barcelos, M.F.P.; Pereira, M.C.A.; Ferreira, E.B. Studies of chemical and enzymatic characteristics of Yacon (*Smallanthus sonchifolius*) and its flour. *Food Sci. Technol.* **2013**, *33*. [CrossRef]
9. Delgado, G.T.; Tamashiro, W.M.; Maróstica-Junior, M.R.; Pastore, G.M. Yacon (*Smallanthus sonchifolius*): A functional food. *Plant Foods Hum. Nutr.* **2013**, *68*, 222–228. [CrossRef] [PubMed]
10. De Almeida, P.H.A.; Abranches, M.V.; de Luces Fortes Ferreira, C.L. Yacon (*Smallanthus sonchifolius*): A food with multiple functions. *Crit. Rev. Food Sci. Nutr.* **2015**, *55*, 32–40. [CrossRef] [PubMed]
11. Apolinário, A.C.; de Lima Damasceno, B.P.; de Macêdo Beltrão, N.E; Pessoa, A.; Converti, A.; da Silva, J.A. Inulin-type fructans: A review on different aspects of biochemical and pharmaceutical technology. *Carbohydr Polym.* **2014**, *30*, 368–378. [CrossRef] [PubMed]
12. Fujishima, M.; Furuyama, K.; Ishihiro, Y.; Onodera, S.; Fukushi, E.; Benkeblia, N.; Shiomi, N. Isolation and Structural Analysis In Vivo of Newly Synthesized Fructooligosaccharides in Onion Bulbs Tissues (*Allium cepa* L.) during storage. *Int. J. Carbohydr.* **2009**. [CrossRef]
13. Santana, I.; Cardoso, M.H. Yacon tuberous root (*Smallanthus sonchifolius*): Cultivation potentialities, technological and nutritional aspects. *Ciência Rural* **2008**, *38*, 898–905. [CrossRef]
14. Sabater-Molina, M.; Larqué, E.; Torrella, F.; Zamora, S. Dietary fructooligosaccharides and potential benefits on health. *J. Physiol. Biochem.* **2009**, *65*, 315–328. [CrossRef] [PubMed]
15. Sivieri, K.; Morales, M.V.; Saad, S.M.I.; Adorno, M.A.; Sakamoto, I.K.; Rossi, E.A. Prebiotic effect of fructooligosaccharide in the Simulator of the Human Intestinal Microbial Ecosystem (SHIME Model). *J. Med. Food.* **2014**, *17*, 1–8. [CrossRef] [PubMed]
16. Bibas Bonet, M.E.; Meson, O.; de Moreno de LeBlanc, A.; Dogib, C.A.; Chaves, S.; Kortsarz, A.; Grau, A.; Perdigón, G. Prebiotic effect of yacon (*Smallanthus sonchifolius*) on intestinal mucosa using a mouse model. *Food Agric. Immunol.* **2010**. [CrossRef]
17. Gibson, G.R. Dietary modulation of the human gut microflora using prebiotics. *Br. J. Nutr.* **1998**, *4*, 209–212.
18. Whelan, K. Mechanisms and effectiveness of prebiotics in modifying the gastrointestinal microbiota for the management of digestive disorders. *Proc. Nutr. Soc.* **2013**, *72*, 288–298. [CrossRef] [PubMed]
19. Sun, Y.; O'Riordan, M.X.D. Regulation of Bacterial Pathogenesis by Intestinal Short-Chain Fatty Acids. *Adv. Appl. Microbiol.* **2013**, *85*, 93–118. [CrossRef] [PubMed]
20. Gibson, G.R.; Roberfroid, M.B. Dietary modulation of the human colonic microbiota: Introducing the concept of prebiotics. *J. Nutr.* **1995**, *125*, 1401–1412. [PubMed]
21. Roberfroid, M. Prebiotics: The concept revisited. *J. Nutr.* **2007**, *137*, 830S–837S. [PubMed]
22. Pineiro, M.; Asp, N.G.; Reid, G.; Macfarlane, S.; Morelli, L.; Brunser, O.; Tuohy, K. FAO Technical meeting on prebiotics. *J. Clin. Gastroenterol.* **2008**. [CrossRef] [PubMed]
23. Valentová, K.; Ulrichová, J. *Smallanthus sonchifolius* and *Lepidium meyenii*—Prospective andean crops for the prevention of chronic diseases. *Biomed. Papers* **2003**, *147*, 119–130. [CrossRef]
24. Slavin, J. Fiber and prebiotics: Mechanisms and health benefits. *Nutrients* **2013**, *22*, 1417–1435. [CrossRef] [PubMed]
25. Siegel, R.L.; Miller, K.D.; Jemal, A. Cancer statistics, 2016. *CA Cancer J. Clin.* **2016**, *66*. [CrossRef] [PubMed]
26. Jasperson, K.W.; Tuohy, T.M.; Neklason, D.W.; Burt, R.W. Hereditary and familial colon cancer. *Gastroenterology* **2010**, *138*, 2044–2058. [CrossRef] [PubMed]
27. Baena, R.; Show, S. Diet and colorectal cancer. *Maturitas* **2015**, *80*, 258–264. [CrossRef] [PubMed]
28. Steck, S.E.; Guinter, M.; Zheng, J.; Thomson, C.A. Index-based dietary patterns and colorectal cancer risk: A systematic review. *Adv. Nutr.* **2015**, *6*, 763–773. [CrossRef] [PubMed]
29. Peeters, P.J.; Bazelier, M.T.; Leufkens, H.G.; de Vries, F.; De Bruin, M.L. The risk of colorectal cancer in patients with type 2 diabetes: Associations with treatment stage and obesity. *Diabetes Care* **2015**, *38*, 495–502. [CrossRef] [PubMed]
30. De Moura, N.A.; Caetano, B.F.R.; Sivieri, K.; Urbano, L.H.; Cabello, C.; Rodrigues, M.A.; Barbisan, L.F. Protective effects of yacon (*Smallanthus sonchifolius*) intake on experimental colon carcinogenesis. *Food Chem. Toxicol.* **2012**, *50*, 2902–2910. [CrossRef] [PubMed]

31. Almeida, A.P.S.; Avia, C.M.; Barbisan, L.F.; de Moura, N.A.; Caetano, B.F.R.; Romualdo, G.R.; Sivieri, K. Yacon (*Smallanthus sonchifolius*) and Lactobacillus acidophilus CRL 1014 reduce the early phases of colon carcinogenesis in male Wistar rats. *Food Res. Int.* **2015**, *74*, 48–54. [CrossRef]

32. Vipperla, K.; O'Keefe, S. Diet, microbiota, and dysbiosis: A "recipe" for colorectal cancer. *Food Funct.* **2016**, *20*, 1731–1740. [CrossRef] [PubMed]

33. Louis, P.; Hold, G.L.; Flint, H.J. The gut microbiota, bacterial metabolites and colorectal cancer. *Nat. Rev. Microbiol.* **2009**, *12*, 661–672. [CrossRef] [PubMed]

34. Mondot, S.; Lepage, P. The human gut microbiome and its dysfunctions through the meta-omics prism. *Ann NY Acad. Sci.* **2016**. [CrossRef] [PubMed]

35. Brown, K.; DeCoffe, D.; Molcan, E.; Gibson, D.L. Diet-Induced Dysbiosis of the Intestinal Microbiota and the Effects on Immunity and Disease. *Nutrients* **2012**, *4*, 1095–1119. [CrossRef] [PubMed]

36. Rolim, P.M. Development of prebiotic food products and health benefits. *Food Sci. Technol.* **2015**, *35*. [CrossRef]

37. Respondek, F.; Gerard, P.; Bossis, M.; Boschat, L.; Bruneau, A.; Rabot, S.; Wagner, A.; Martin, J.C. Short-chain fructo-oligosaccharides modulate intestinal microbiota and metabolic parameters of humanized gnotobiotic diet induced obesity mice. *PLoS ONE* **2013**, *8*, e71026. [CrossRef] [PubMed]

38. Raman, M.; Ambalam, P.; Kondepudi, K.K; Pithva, S.; Kothari, C.; Patel, A.T.; Purama, R.K.; Dave, J.M.; Vyas, B.R. Potential of probiotics, prebiotics and synbiotics for management of colorectal cancer. *Gut. Microbes* **2013**, *4*, 181–192. [CrossRef] [PubMed]

39. Wong, J.M.; de Souza, R.; Kendall, C.W.; Emam, A.; Jenkins, D. Colonic health: Fermentation and short chain fatty acids. *J. Clin. Gastroenterol.* **2006**, *40*, 235–243. [CrossRef] [PubMed]

40. Tang, Y.; Chen, Y.; Jiang, H.; Nie, D. The role of short-chain fatty acids in orchestrating two types of programmed cell death in colon cancer. *Autophagy* **2011**, *7*, 235–237. [CrossRef] [PubMed]

41. Kim, H.C.; Park, J.; Kim, M. Gut Microbiota-Derived Short-Chain Fatty Acids, T Cells, and Inflammation. *Immune Netw.* **2014**, *14*, 277–288. [CrossRef] [PubMed]

42. Vaz-Tostes, M.; Viana, M.L.; Grancieri, M.; Luz, T.C.; Paula, H.; Pedrosa, R.G.; Costa, N.M. Yacon effects in immune response and nutritional status of iron and zinc in preschool children. *Nutrition* **2014**, *30*, 666–672. [CrossRef] [PubMed]

43. Peshev, D.; Van den Ende, W. Fructans: Prebiotics and immunomodulators. *J. Funct. Foods.* **2014**, *8*, 348–357. [CrossRef]

44. Liu, X.; Zheng, J.; Zhou, H. TLRs as pharmacological targets for plant-derived compounds in infectious and inflammatory diseases. *Int. Immunopharmacol.* **2011**, *10*, 1451–1456. [CrossRef] [PubMed]

45. Vogt, L.; Ramasamy, U.; Meyer, D.; Pullens, G.; Venema, K.; Faas, M.M.; Schols, H.A.; de Vos, P. Immune modulation by different types of β2→1-fructans is toll-like receptor dependent. *PLoS ONE* **2013**, *5*, e68367. [CrossRef] [PubMed]

46. Delgado, G.T.; Thomé, R.; Gabriel, D.L.; Tamashiro, W.M.; Pastore, G.M. Yacon (*Smallanthus sonchifolius*)-derived fructooligosaccharides improves the immune parameters in the mouse. *Nutr. Res.* **2012**, *32*, 884–892. [CrossRef] [PubMed]

47. Velez, E.; Castillo, N.; Mesón, O.; Grau, A.; Bonet, M.E.B.; Perdigón, G. Study of the effect exerted by fructo-oligosaccharides from yacon (*Smallanthus sonchifolius*) root flour in an intestinal infection model with Salmonella Typhimurium. *Br. J. Nutr.* **2013**, *109*, 1971–1979. [CrossRef] [PubMed]

48. Nakamura, Y.; Nosaka, S.; Suzuki, M.; Nagafuchi, S.; Takahashi, T.; Yajima, T.; Takenouchi-Ohkubo, N.; Iwase, T.; Moro, I. Dietary fructooligosaccharides up-regulate immunoglobulin A res-ponse and polymeric immunoglobulin receptor expression in intestines of infant mice. *Clin. Exp. Immunol.* **2004**, *137*, 52–58. [CrossRef] [PubMed]

49. World Health Organization (WHO)—Diabetes Fact Sheet. Available online: http://www.who.int/mediacentre/factsheets/fs312/en/ (accessed on 9 May 2016).

50. Qin, L.; Mirjam, J.; Knol, S.; Corpeleijn, E.; Ronald, P. Does physical activity modify the risk of obesity for type 2 diabetes: A review of epidemiological data. *Eur. J. Epidemiol.* **2010**, *25*, 5–12. [CrossRef] [PubMed]

51. Tunaiji, H.A.; Davis, J.C.; Mackey, D.C.; Khan, K.M. Population attributable fraction of type 2 diabetes due to physical inactivity in adults: A systematic review. *BMC Public Health* **2014**, *14*, 469. [CrossRef] [PubMed]

52. Franz, M.J.; Boucher, J.L.; Evert, A.B. Evidence-based diabetes nutrition therapy recommendations are effective: The key is individualization. *Diabetes Metab. Syndr. Obes.* **2014**, *7*, 65–72. [CrossRef] [PubMed]

53. Russo, D.; Valentão, P.; Andrade, P.B.; Fernandez, E.C.; Milellal, L. Evaluation of Antioxidant, Antidiabetic and Anticholinesterase Activities of Smallanthus sonchifolius Landraces and Correlation with Their Phytochemical Profiles. *Int. J. Mol. Sci.* **2015**, *16*, 17696–17718. [CrossRef] [PubMed]
54. Habib, N.C.; Honoré, S.M.; Genta, S.B.; Sánchez, S.S. Hypolipidemic effect of *Smallanthus sonchifolius* (yacon) roots on diabetic rats: Biochemical approach. *Chem. Biol. Interact.* **2011**, *194*, 31–39. [CrossRef] [PubMed]
55. Satoh, H.; Nguyen, M.T.A.; Kudoh, A.; Watanabe, T. Yacon diet (*Smallanthus sonchifolius*, Asteraceae) improves hepatic insulin resistance via reducing Trb3 expression in Zucker fa/fa rats. *Nutr. Diabetes.* **2013**. [CrossRef] [PubMed]
56. Scheid, M.M.; Genaro, P.S.; Moreno, Y.M.; Pastore, G.M. Freeze-dried powdered yacon: Effects of FOS on serum glucose, lipids and intestinal transit in the elderly. *Eur. J. Nutr.* **2014**, *53*, 1457–1464. [CrossRef] [PubMed]
57. Genta, S.; Cabrera, W.; Habib, N.; Pons, J.; Carillo, I.M.; Grau, A.; Sara, S. Yacon syrup: Beneficial effects on obesity and insulin resistance in humans. *Clin. Nutr.* **2009**, *28*, 182–187. [CrossRef] [PubMed]
58. Triplitt, C.L. Examining the mechanisms of glucose regulation. *Am. J. Manag. Care* **2012**, *18*, S4–10. [PubMed]
59. López, V.L.; Medina, J.A.L.; Gutiérrez, M.V.; Soto, M.L.F. Carbohydrate: Current role in diabetes mellitus and metabolic disease. *Nutr. Hosp.* **2014**, *30*, 1020–1031. [CrossRef]
60. Den Besten, G.; van Eunen, K.; Groen, A.K.; Venema, K.; Reijngoud, D.J.; Bakker, B.M. The role of short-chain fatty acids in the interplay between diet, gut microbiota, and host energy metabolism. *J. Lipid Res.* **2013**, *54*, 2325–2340. [CrossRef] [PubMed]
61. Canfora, E.E.; Jocken, J.W.; Blaak, E.E. Short-chain fatty acids in control of body weight and insulin sensitivity. *Nat. Rev. Endocrinol.* **2014**, *11*, 577–591. [CrossRef] [PubMed]
62. Fernandes, J.; Vogt, J.; Wolever, T.M. Intravenous acetate elicits a greater free fatty acid rebound in normal than hyperinsulinaemic humans. *Eur. J. Clin. Nutr.* **2012**, *66*, 1029–1034. [CrossRef] [PubMed]
63. Boillot, J.; Alamowitch, C.; Berger, A.M.; Luo, J.; Bruzzo, F.; Bornet, F.R.; Slama, G. Effects of dietary propionate on hepatic glucose production, whole-body glucose utilization, carbohydrate and lipid metabolism in normal rats. *Br. J. Nutr.* **1995**, *73*, 241–251. [CrossRef] [PubMed]
64. Tolhurst, G.; Heffron, H.; Lam, Y.S.; Parker, H.E.; Habib, A.M; Diakogiannaki, E.; Cameron, J.; Grosse, J.; Reimann, F.; Gribble, F.M. Short-chain fatty acids stimulate glucagon-like peptide-1 secretion via the G-protein-coupled receptor FFAR2. *Diabetes* **2012**, *61*, 364–371. [CrossRef] [PubMed]
65. Psichas, A.; Sleeth, M.L.; Murphy, K.G.; Brooks, L.; Bewick, G.A.; Hanyaloglu, A.C.; Ghatei, M.A.; Bloom, S.R.; Frost, G. The short chain fatty acid propionate stimulates GLP-1 and PYY secretion via free fatty acid receptor 2 in rodents. *Int. J. Obes.* **2015**, *39*, 424–429. [CrossRef] [PubMed]
66. Ahima, R.S.; Lazar, M.A. The Health Risk of Obesity—Better Metrics Imperative. *Science* **2013**, *341*, 6148. [CrossRef] [PubMed]
67. World Health Organization (WHO)—Obesity and overweight Fact Sheet. Available online: http://www.who.int/mediacentre/factsheets/fs311/en/ (accessed on 9 May 2016).
68. Lehnert, T.; Sonntag, D.; Konnopka, A.; Riedel-Heller, S.; König, H.H. Economic costs of overweight and obesity. *Best Pract. Res. Clin. Endocrinol. Metab.* **2013**, *27*, 105–115. [CrossRef] [PubMed]
69. Lifshitz, F.; Lifshitz, J.Z. Globesity: The root causes of the obesity epidemic in the USA and now worldwide. *Pediatr. Endocrinol. Rev.* **2014**, *12*, 17–34. [PubMed]
70. Kaur, J. A Comprehensive Review on Metabolic Syndrome. *Cardiol. Res. Pract.* **2014**. [CrossRef] [PubMed]
71. Leão, L.S.; de Moraes, M.M.; de Carvalho, G.X.; Koifman, R.J. Nutritional interventions in metabolic syndrome: A systematic review. *Arq. Bras. Cardiol.* **2011**, *97*, 260–265. [CrossRef] [PubMed]
72. Mohamed, S. Functional foods against metabolic syndrome (obesity, diabetes, hypertension and dyslipidemia) and cardio vascular disease. *Trends Food Sci. Technol.* **2014**, *35*, 114–128. [CrossRef]
73. Genta, S.B.; Cabrera, W.M.; Grau, A.; Sánchez, S.S. Subchronic 4-month oral toxicity study of dried *Smallanthus sonchifolius* (yacon) roots as a diet supplement in rats. *Food Chem. Toxicol.* **2005**, *43*, 1657–1665. [CrossRef] [PubMed]
74. Roselino, M.N.; Pauly-Silveira, N.D.; Cavallini, D.C.; Celiberto, L.S.; Pinto, R.A.; Vendramini, R.C.; Rossi, E.A. A potential synbiotic product improves the lipid profile of diabetic rats. *Lipids Health Dis.* **2012**. [CrossRef] [PubMed]
75. Geyer, M.; Manrique, I.; Degen, L.; Beglinger, C. Effect of yacon (*Smallanthus sonchifolius*) on colonic transit time in healthy volunteers. *Digestion* **2008**, *78*, 30–33. [CrossRef] [PubMed]

76. Mora, S.; Fullerton, R. Effects of Short Chain Fatty Acids on Glucose and Lipid metabolism in Adipocytes. *FASEB J.* **2015**, *29*, 627–625.
77. Hara, H.; Haga, S.; Aoyama, Y.; Kiriyama, S. Short-chain fatty acids suppress cholesterol synthesis in rat liver and intestine. *J. Nutr.* **1999**, *129*, 942–948. [PubMed]
78. Byrne, S.; Chambers, E.S.; Morrison, D.J.; Frost, G. The role of short chain fatty acids in appetite regulation and energy homeostasis. *Int. J. Obes.* **2015**, *39*, 1331–1338. [CrossRef] [PubMed]
79. D'Alessio, D. Intestinal hormones and regulation of satiety: The case for CCK, GLP-1, PYY, and Apo A-IV. *JPEN J. Parenter Enteral Nutr.* **2008**, *32*, 567–568. [CrossRef] [PubMed]
80. Ichimura, A.; Hasegawa, S.; Kasubuchi, M.; Kimura, I. Free fatty acid receptors as therapeutic targets for the treatment of diabetes. *Front Pharmacol.* **2014**, *5*, 236. [CrossRef] [PubMed]
81. Isken, F.; Klaus, S.; Osterhoff, M.; Pfeiffer, A.F.; Weickert, M.O. Effects of long-term soluble vs. insoluble dietary fiber intake on high-fat diet-induced obesity in C57BL/6J mice. *J. Nutr. Biochem.* **2010**, *21*, 278–284. [CrossRef] [PubMed]
82. Eswaran, S.; Muir, J.; Chey, W.D. Fiber and functional gastrointestinal disorders. *Am. J. Gastroenterol.* **2013**, *108*, 718–727. [CrossRef] [PubMed]
83. Yun, E.Y.; Kim, H.S.; Kim, Y.E.; Kang, M.K.; Ma, J.E.; Lee, G.D.; Cho, Y.J.; Kim, H.C.; Lee, J.D.; Hwang, Y.S.; et al. A case of anaphylaxis after the ingestion of yacon. *Allergy Asthma. Immunol. Res.* **2010**, *2*, 149–152. [CrossRef] [PubMed]
84. Graefea, S.; Hermann, M.; Manrique, I.; Golombeka, S.; Buerkerta, A. Effects of post-harvest treatments on the carbohydrate composition of yacon roots in the Peruvian Andes. *F. Cr. Res.* **2004**, *86*, 157–165. [CrossRef]
85. Di Bartolomeo, F.; Van den Ende, W. Fructose and Fructans: Opposite Effects on Health. *Plant Foods Hum. Nutr.* **2015**, *70*, 227–237. [CrossRef] [PubMed]

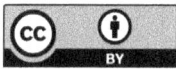

nutrients

Article

Reaching Low-Income Mothers to Improve Family Fruit and Vegetable Intake: Food Hero Social Marketing Campaign—Research Steps, Development and Testing

Lauren N. Tobey [1,*], Harold F. Koenig [2], Nicole A. Brown [2] and Melinda M. Manore [3]

1   Extension Family and Community Health, College of Public Health and Human Sciences,
    Oregon State University, 106 Ballard Hall, Corvallis, OR 97331, USA
2   College of Business, Oregon State University, 474 Austin Hall, Corvallis, OR 97331, USA;
    koenig@bus.oregonstate.edu (H.F.K.); nicole.brown@bus.oregonstate.edu (N.A.B.)
3   School of Biological and Population Health Sciences, College of Public Health and Human Sciences,
    Oregon State University, 103 Milam Hall, Corvallis, OR 97331, USA; melinda.manore@oregonstate.edu
*   Correspondence: lauren.tobey@oregonstate.edu; Tel.: +1-541-737-1017

Received: 6 June 2016; Accepted: 31 August 2016; Published: 13 September 2016

Abstract: The objective of this study was to create/test a social marketing campaign to increase fruit/vegetable (FV) intake within Oregon Supplemental Nutrition Assistance Program (SNAP) eligible families. Focus groups ($n = 2$) and pre/post campaign phone surveys ($n = 2082$) were conducted in intervention counties (IC) and one control county. Participants were female (86%–100%) with 1–2 children at home. Mean FV intake/without juice was 3.1 servings/day; >50% preferred the Internet for delivery of healthy eating information. Participants reported time/financial burdens, low household FV variety and desirability of frozen/canned FV, and acceptance of positive messages. A Food Hero (FH) campaign was created/delivered daily August–October 2009 to mothers through multiple channels (e.g., grocery stores, online, educators). Results showed that the IC had better FH name recall (12%) and interpretation of intended messages (60%) vs. control (3%, 23%, respectively). Compared to controls, the IC were less likely to report healthy food preparation as time consuming or a FV rich diet expensive, and it was easier to get their family to eat fruit. Results did not vary based on county/household characteristics. The FH campaign increased FH awareness and positive FV beliefs. A longer campaign with FV assessments will increase understanding of the target audience, and allow for campaign refinement.

Keywords: low-income women; focus group; survey; nutrition; social media; Supplemental Nutrition Assistance Program (SNAP); audience-centered positive messaging; health behavior messages; canned; frozen

1. Introduction

Between 2000 and 2013 Oregon experienced increases in Supplemental Nutrition Assistance Program (SNAP) participation (246%) and food insecurity (3%–4%) [1,2]. Only 2009 data from Oregon Behavioral Risk Factor Surveillance System (BRFSS) provide obesity rates based on income. For Oregon households with income <$15,000 the obesity rate was 28.6%, and for those with incomes between $15,000–$24,999 the rate was 31.8% [3]. These obesity rates are higher than those reported across all income categories ≥$25,000 (20.6%–25.7%). Currently, the prevalence of obesity among all adult Oregonians is 27.9% [4]. Low fruit and vegetable (FV) consumption may be one factor linked to increases in obesity. National research shows that higher quality diets that include FVs are more prevalent in populations with higher socioeconomic status, while rates of obesity and chronic disease are lower [5,6]. In addition, the 2015 Dietary Guidelines for Americans Advisory Committee Scientific Report states that FVs are the only diet characteristic consistently identified with positive health outcomes in every conclusion of the report [7]. Unfortunately, individual and community level barriers limit access to FV by low-income families. Barriers at the individual level include cost, inadequate time for preparation, poor nutrition knowledge, and limited cooking skills, while community barriers include cost, transportation, quality, variety, changing food environment, and societal norms on food [8]. Thus, low FV intake may be an important determinant of obesity and chronic disease risk.

Consistent with the nationwide trend, Oregonians continue to show low intakes of FVs [9]. Although the Center for Disease Control and Prevention reported that Oregon adults eat more FVs compared to other states, intake levels are still below the recommendations of 4–5 cups and 5–6.5 cups of FVs/day for adult (19–50 years) women and men, respectively [9,10]. Using the most recent BRFSS data (2013) only 21% of Oregon adults reported consuming FVs $\geq$5 times per day [11]. Finally, 2013 BRFSS data show that healthy weight adults in Oregon consume more FVs compared to adults who are obese, 24% versus 17%, respectively [11,12].

Social marketing (SM) can increase healthful eating behaviors, including FV intake [13–15]. By definition, SM is "a process that applies marketing principles and techniques to create, communicate, and deliver value in order to influence target audience behaviors that benefit society (public health, safety, the environment and communities) and the target audience" [16]. Based on research supported by the United Kingdom's National Social Marketing Center, SM effectiveness increases if eight SM benchmark criteria are followed: behavior, customer orientation, theory, insight, exchange, competition, segmentation and methods mix [13,14,17]. These benchmark criteria focus on the target audience in all project phases, including dividing the target audience into subgroups with common characteristics, called segments, to improve targeting.

Behavioral interventions aimed at promoting FV consumption are often grounded in the social cognitive theory (SCT) [18]. Although not all SM campaigns are theory based, those that are frequently use the SCT [19]. The SCT recognizes that people influence their environments just as their environments influence them, thus, this theory focuses on reciprocal determinism or associations between behavior, personal factors, and environment. Important components of the SCT include self-efficacy or the personal belief in one's ability to do something, observational learning, and a person's expectancies about the consequences of an action(s) [20].

To address Oregon's rising obesity rates and low FV intake, Oregon State University (OSU) Extension Service received funds to improve FV intake within low-income Oregon families using SM as part of Oregon SNAP-Education (SNAP-Ed), the nutrition promotion and obesity-prevention component of SNAP. Materials and messages from out-of-state SNAP-Ed funded SM campaigns were tested (described in Section 3.1), but none were a "good fit" for the Oregon target audience. Thus, in 2009 OSU began developing a new pilot SM campaign that now reaches Oregonians millions of times each year through indirect/direct education, SM, and policy, systems and environmental (PSE) change efforts. The PSE efforts focus on local policy changes, using local food systems and improving school food environments. The campaign goal was to increase FV consumption within the Oregon SNAP-eligible population, which is at risk for poverty, food insecurity, low intake of FVs, chronic disease, and obesity.

To our knowledge there are no published studies outlining the formative development steps, implementation, and testing of a SM campaign aimed at increasing low-income families FV intake by targeting mothers with children in the home. Thus, this article describes the steps used to develop, implement, and test the Food Hero SM campaign with SNAP participants, and presents the findings from this process. One of the first steps was to determine our target audience within SNAP that was ultimately identified as mothers with their children living in their home. The campaign development strategy was to identify how best to empower and support SNAP-eligible Oregonian's to overcome perceived and actual barriers to FV consumption and reinforce existing positive behaviors. Our campaign development objectives were to (1) define a target audience and develop a robust understanding of them; (2) identify barriers and what "moves and motivates" them regarding FV intake; and (3) use data gathered to create and test a pilot SM campaign (2-months) that could eventually result in positive behavior change. We hypothesized that a multi-channel, targeted and segmented short pilot SM campaign would increase awareness of the campaign and positive beliefs about FV intakes. We did not expect changes in FV behaviors in 2 months, since the goal was to further refine the campaign through formative/process evaluation and then assess changes in FV intake.

2. Materials and Methods

2.1. Study Overview

Two contractors were hired to add expertise to the campaign development team, a business research firm and a SM firm. The research firm (*Close to the Customer Project*, OSU's School of Business) assisted with writing research phone surveys (PS) and focus group (FG) questions, managed all phases of participant recruitment, lead the FGs, produced verbatim transcripts of FG discussions and analyzed FG data for common themes, conducted PSs, analyzed the data, and created data summary reports. The SM firm (*EnviroMedia*, Portland, OR, USA) assisted with brand creation, campaign message development, project management, and gave input into PS and FG questions. The campaign development included the eight elements of the SM benchmark criteria [17]. OSU's nutrition researchers gave input on all steps of the project (Figure 1).

Campaign Development Steps		Major Goal	Dates
STEP 1	Focus Groups 1 (n=25)	Learn more about the target audience and guide development of Phone Survey 1.	September 2008
STEP 2	Phone Survey 1 (n=1244)	Learn more about the target audience.	January-February 2009
STEP 3	Pilot Campaign Development	Develop draft campaign components with input from the results of Steps 1 and 2.	February-May 2009
STEP 4	Focus Groups 2 (n=11)	Test campaign components drafted in Step 3.	June 2009
STEP 5	Pilot Campaign Finalized	Create final campaign components.	June-July 2009
STEP 6	Pilot Campaign	Implement the campaign.	August-October 2009
STEP 7	Phone Survey 2 (n=802)	Gain insights for future campaign development.	September 2009

Figure 1. Food Hero development steps, goals and timeline.

All research was conducted with SNAP participants in select Oregon counties. The timeline and steps of the research and campaign development are outlined in Figure 1. Pre-campaign research included conducting FGs (Step 1: FG-1; n = 25 participants), which were used to help design a pre-campaign PS, including FV belief and barrier questions (Step 2: PS-1; n = 1244 participants). The PS's also included the validated BRFSS FV questions to assess FV intake [21]. In addition, the FGs provided information related to health priorities, beliefs and experiences. Using the results from FG-1 and PS-1, Step 3 developed the campaign, including creating draft campaign names, logos, messages and delivery channels (Figure 2 and Table 1). Key components of the SCT aligned with the FG-1 and PS-1 results; thus, the SCT was used to inform campaign development/implementation (Steps 3–6). As second set of FGs (Step 4: FG-2, n = 11) were used to test messages and components of the developed campaign. In Step 5, final campaign materials and delivery channels were determined/created and then implemented in Step 6. The campaign was delivered through multiple channels, including a web site, direct mail, billboards, web banner ads, grocery store demonstrations, grocery cart ads, and county

SNAP-Ed educators delivering the campaign using Food Hero Community Kits [22]. The community kits were designed to provide locally adaptable campaign tools and materials for OSU's Extension county educators and their partners. The goal of the community kit was to assure that comprehensive educator/partner Food Hero promotion occurred concurrently with other campaign communication channels. Public relations efforts throughout the campaign included television and radio interviews, a family video makeover contest, and social media postings (i.e., YouTube and Facebook). The Food Hero social media project is described elsewhere [23]. Due to the time left in the project funding cycle, the campaign could only run for 2-months. Near the end of the campaign, a second PS was conducted to test for campaign awareness and FV beliefs, and to gain further insights for future campaign development (Step 7: PS-2; *n* = 802).

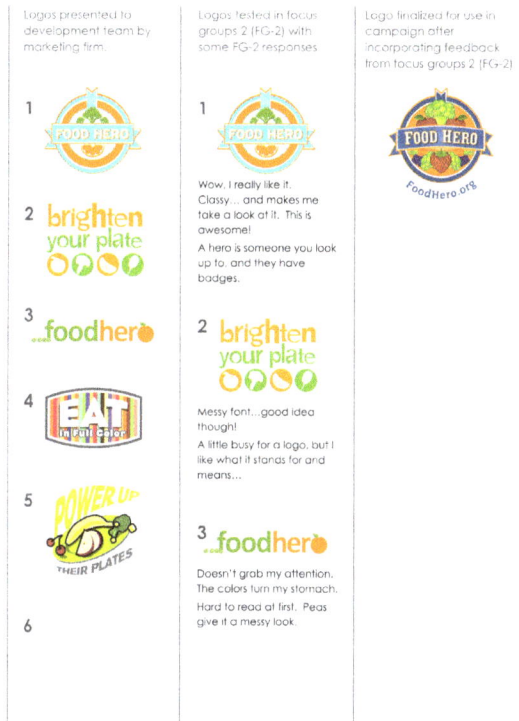

Figure 2. Process for the Design and Testing of Food Hero Logos (Focus Groups 2).

Table 1. Food Hero Messages: Tested and Used in Pilot Campaign.

	Message Priority Given by Participants from Highest (1) to Lowest (7) Preference
Messages Tested in Focus Groups 2 (FG-2)	1. Canned, frozen, or fresh they all start out the same. 2. Kids would pick candy for every meal, good thing you're in charge. 3. Canned and frozen fruits and vegetables make your money go further. 4. Buying canned and frozen helps you get more for less. 5. An apple a day is not that far away. 6. Fruits and vegetables are within reach. 7. In these tough economic times get more of a good thing.
Messages Used in Campaign and then Tested in Phone Survey 2 (PS-2)	1. Give them more of the good stuff (direct mail and billboards). 2. Brighten your plate (website banners, refrigerator magnet grocery store reinforcement).

2.2. Study Design

From Oregon's 36 counties, four (rural = 2; metropolitan = 2) were selected for data collection and to receive the Food Hero campaign (Figure 3). Inclusion criteria for all groups included current SNAP-Ed series of adult/family classes at multiple sites, availability of multiple media buy options, adequate population base for data collection, and SNAP staff available for assistance. Due to cost constraints, only one control county (Benton) was selected for PS-2 data collection because it had qualities of Oregon's rural and metropolitan counties (i.e., mid-sized population, ethnic diversity, away from a major highway). Benton county residents were also less likely to see Food Hero campaign billboards because it is located off Oregon's only major highway.

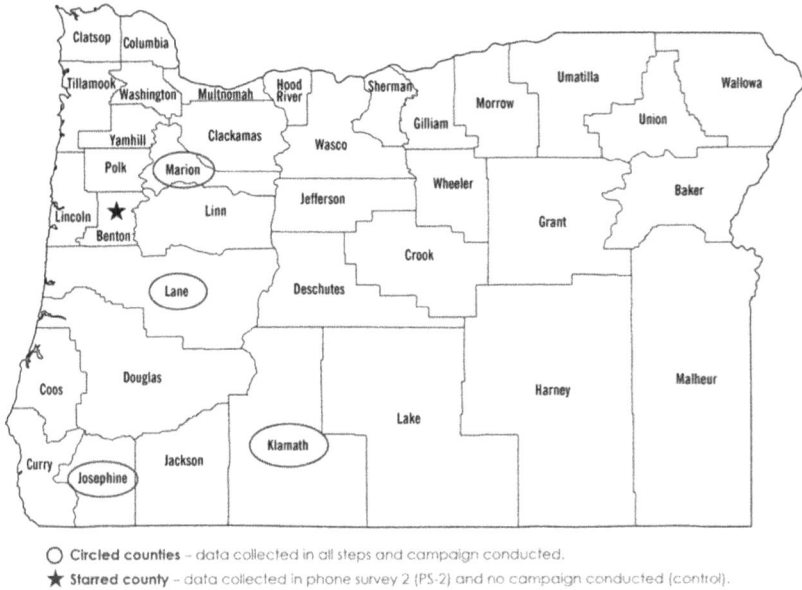

○ **Circled counties** – data collected in all steps and campaign conducted.
★ **Starred county** – data collected in phone survey 2 (PS-2) and no campaign conducted (control).

Figure 3. Oregon counties where formative research and pilot campaign were conducted (circled names).

2.3. Participants and Recruitment

All FG and PS participants were randomly selected from a list of all English speaking SNAP families living in the targeted counties. The Oregon Department of Human Services (DHS) provided the names and phone numbers, either landlines or cell. For PS-1 it was determined that 250 responses were needed per county, which allowed for counties to be analyzed by themselves with a margin of error ±5% on dichotomous questions (Table 2). Oversampling was done to assure adequate sample size. Calls were made and consenting participants self-verified that they met the following inclusion criteria; SNAP enrollment, county residency, being the primary household food preparer, and having one or more children <18 years living in their home.

Table 2. Mean responses across all counties to belief statements about fruit and vegetable intake from Phone Survey I (PS-1, *n* = 1244) and Phone Survey 2 (PS-2, *n* = 802) [1].

Belief Statement		PS-1 Mean ± SD	PS-2 Mean ± SD	*p* Value (PS-1 vs. PS-2)	PS-2 Control Mean ± SD	*p* Value (PS-2 vs. Control)
1.	I know how to prepare many different vegetables.	4.25 ± 1.06	4.25 ± 1.08	*p* = 0.50	4.23 ± 1.16	*p* = 0.44
2.	I want to serve more balanced meals to my family.	4.33 ± 1.03	4.35 ± 1.09	*p* = 0.35	4.13 ± 1.14	*p* = 0.03 [2]
3.	Canned fruit is just as healthy as fresh fruit.	2.17 ± 1.17	2.21 ± 1.25	*p* = 0.30	1.93 ± 0.96	*p* = 0.01 [2]
4.	Frozen vegetables are just as healthy as fresh.	2.90 ± 1.37	3.00 ± 1.30	*p* = 0.065	2.91 ± 1.25	*p* = 0.24
5.	It is easy to get my family to eat vegetables.	3.73 ± 1.30	3.82 ± 1.26	*p* = 0.055	3.79 ± 1.22	*p* = 0.38
6.	It is easy to get my family to eat fruit.	4.37 ± 1.00	4.49 ± 0.90	*p* = 0.005 [2]	4.43 ± 1.06	*p* = 0.27
7.	Eating a diet that includes a lot of fruits and vegetables is expensive.	3.42 ± 1.39	3.17 ± 1.45	*p* = 0.0005 [2]	3.06 ± 1.30	*p* = 0.21
8.	It is time consuming to prepare healthy food.	2.45 ± 1.31	2.29 ± 1.27	*p* = 0.005 [2]	2.45 ± 1.28	*p* = 0.09

[1] Responses were recorded on a five point scale where 1 = Strongly Disagree and 5 = Strongly Agree; [2] One sided *t*-test used to test changes after the Food Hero campaign; *p* < 0.05 was considered significant.

Rural versus urban responses from FG-1 and PS-1 were similar, thus, FG-2 was conducted in only one county (Marion) (Figure 3). Participants in FG-1 and PS-1 were 86%–92% female, thus, only females were recruited for FG-2. Due to DHS privacy requirements we do not know if participants overlap between or within the FG and PS samples, but FG participants represented less than 2% of the total study sample. Rural and urban responses on PS-1 were similar; therefore, the sample size for PS-2 was decreased. The research was approved by the Oregon State University Institutional Review Board and participants gave informed consent.

2.4. Instruments and Procedures

2.4.1. Focus Groups

For each FG 10-12 participants were recruited via phone calls, then mailed information packets, and received a reminder called prior to the meeting. Compensation was given for the 2-h FG meetings (FG-1: meal +$50; FG-2: meal +$25). *Close to the Customer Project* provided trained facilitators who lead participants through a series of pre-determined questions designed to elicit information regarding FV intake by the family, beliefs regarding FV intake, and barriers to FV intake. Questions for FG-1 focused on campaign development, while questions for FG-2 focused on testing potential campaign messages and components. Follow-up and probing questions were used as necessary, and participants engaged in writing responses and small group discussion.

2.4.2. Phone Surveys

PS-1 data were collected early in the pre-campaign, while PS-2 was conducted the last 2-weeks of the campaign (Figure 1). Both PSs used identical recruitment procedures. Due to DHS privacy requirements, all potential participants received a letter from DHS with the following information: (1) the purpose and time commitment of the survey; (2) that DHS had given their phone number to OSU;

and (3) they might receive a phone call asking them to participate in the survey. Trained PS interviewers conducted the surveys, which included moving systematically through a series of questions (PS-1: 70 questions, 24% response rate, interview time ~10 min; PS-2: 32 questions, 11% response rate, interview time was ~5.5 min). If the call resulted in no answer/answering machine, four more call attempts were made before discarding the telephone number. Participants received no compensation. Using mock phone interviews, interviewers practiced and PSs were pre-tested for length, time and clarity. No changes were made to the survey based on the mock interviews. Rural counties were disproportionately oversampled to assure sufficient responses.

2.5. Data Analysis

Analysis of FGs was iterative and occurred at several levels by the same four trained researchers who attended all FGs. The research team debriefed immediately following each FG, identifying key insights, themes, and unusual findings. Next the FGs were transcribed and transcripts were read individually by each of the researchers who coded and identified emerging themes. Researchers then met as a group to agree upon and define themes. Once themes were identified, researchers identified quotes and organized them according to thematic content. The focus groups were "exploratory" in nature and the insights gained from the groups informed the construction of the PS questionnaires.

For the PSs, summary statistics were generated for demographic data. ANOVA was used to determine if differences existed between PS-1 and PS-2 and PS-2 and control PS-2. Results showed no differences between surveys based on demographic data (county of residence, single/dual parent household, household size); thus, data from the intervention counties were combined for further analysis. Independent *t*-tests were then used to compare changes in variables/belief statements pre/post campaign using predetermined hypotheses based on campaign expectations.

3. Results

Demographic data for FG and PS participants are given in Table 3.

Table 3. Food Hero Formative Evaluation: Focus Group (FG) and Phone Survey (PS) Demographics.

	Focus Groups 1 (FG-1)	Phone Survey 1 (PS-1)	Focus Groups 2 (FG-2)	Phone Survey 2 (PS-2)
Subjects (*n*)	*n* = 25, 4 FG	*n* = 1244	*n* = 11, 2 FG	*n* = 802
Female (%)	92	86	100	84 (Control) 86 (Intervention)
Mean age (year)	36.7	34.5	42.9	33.2 (Control) 34.7 (Intervention)
Household size (3–4 people) (%)	65	55	36	55 (Control) 54 (Intervention)
Household size (1–2 children) (%)	76	71	64	77 (Control) 71 (Intervention)
Single parent households (%)	52	39	45	45 (Control) 43 (Intervention)

3.1. Focus Groups and Phone Survey 1

Step two of the SM benchmark criteria states that a strong understanding of the audience should be developed by combining data from different sources; thus, results from FGs and PS-1 were combined into themes and discussed below. FG and PS-1 results were grouped into five themes/outcomes: (1) audience demographics and characteristics; (2) self-reported FV intake and consumption; (3) grocery shopping and meal preparation habits; (4) preferred communication channels; and (5) responses to previously developed campaigns and messages.

Main Themes

Theme 1: Audience demographics and characteristics.

Overall, the participants were female (86%–100%), mean age range 34–43 years, single parents (39%), working outside the home at least half-time (33%–36%) and had 3–4 people in the household (36%–65%), including 1–2 children (64%–76%). PS-1 results showed that single adult households faced additional time and money constraints compared to two adult households. One FG participant said, "Money, I worry about money, I worry about it all the time, it's a big concern so I try to keep it from my kid so she doesn't see it." Working and stay-at-home parents also expressed time constraints.

Theme 2: Self-reported fruit and vegetable intake and consumption.

Based on PS-1, the mean servings/day of vegetables was 1.7, while the mean serving/day for fruit was 3.1 with juice and 1.4 serving/day without juice. Most PS-1 participants (70%) self-reported being knowledgeable about preparing vegetables and found it easy for their families to eat enough vegetables (60%) and fruit (80%). FG results were similar and responses from the FGs are included below:

- "Potatoes are not just for dinner, we can have them for breakfast and lunch."
- "Carrots are great. I have them as a snack."
- "They are a good snack."
- "My kids like the baby carrots so instead of buying the big long bugs bunny carrots they'll eat the baby carrots."
- "I always have them [bananas] in my house. They are a year round fruit for the most part. When they get home from school they have one."

When shopping for groceries, PS-1 participates reported that "low price" was "very important" (67%), while "fast to prepare" (14%) and "easy to prepare" (15%) were less important. Over half (51%) of the PS-1 participants agreed that a diet rich in FVs was expensive. FGs participants often mentioned price as being important when shopping, "I only buy cereal when it is on sale or with a coupon." Being fast to prepare was also mentioned, but less often, "We eat pasta 'cause it's fast."

Participants from PS-1 and FGs reported that fresh produce was the preferred choice for being most nutritious (i.e., not containing extra sugar/salt or losing nutritional value from canning or freezing), while frozen foods were a good second choice, and canned were less preferred. In PS-1, 39.8% of participants disagreed with the statement "frozen vegetables are just as healthy as fresh," and 63% disagreed with the statement "canned fruit is just as healthy as fresh". Some FG participants said canned was "ok" if nothing else was available, while others said they do not buy canned FV because they thought canned FVs had lower quality and less nutritious, especially if they are "cheap" or on sale. The FG participants also perceived fresh as being costly, since fresh FV are perishable and seasonal.

FG participants could name a wide variety of FVs, yet PS-1 participants reported consistently purchasing the same FVs (e.g., apples, bananas, corn, beans and broccoli). Barriers to eating a larger variety of FVs, reported by FG participants, included inexperience in planning and preparing meals, cost and time commitment, seasonality, and coping strategies to get children to eat them. Some responses are included below:

- "I make stir fry because my son's not a big vegetable eater but he will eat it (stir fry). Now he likes broccoli, caluliflower, stuff like that."
- "I buy fruits and vegetables in season . . . but I buy broccoli year round."

Theme 3: Grocery shopping and meal preparation habits.

Overall, FG participants presented themselves as savvy shoppers, yet found it difficult to provide nutritious meals for their families even with the additional SNAP benefits. Participants indicated they knew how to eat healthfully, wanted their families to have nutritious food, and reported they read product packaging and nutrition labels. One FG participant stated, "I only buy things for her that are good for her. If she wants sweets we make our own and use less sugar."

When asked about preparing dinner, PS-1 participants (46%) reported they 'rarely' had help. Overall, 80% agreed with the statement, "I would like to serve more balanced meals to my family", while 54% disagreed with the statement "healthy food is time consuming to prepare." Some FG participants acknowledged they have little experience with, or knowledge of planning and preparing healthy meals. For example one participant said, "I think I wish that one of them things I could do is to make a more balanced meals, I try really hard but I don't have all the knowledge that I need to make the balanced meals."

Theme 4: Preferred communication channels.

Half of PS-1 participants indicated that the Internet was the preferred method for finding information on healthful food choices, followed by grocery stores (16%), and magazines (12%). The Internet was the preferred method for participants living in both single adult (51%) and multiple adult households (56%). Those individuals between the ages of 25–34 years reported the Internet as the preferred option (58%) versus those 45–54 years (40%) or 55–64 years (30%). PS-1 participants reported using the following sources for cooking tips and ideas: Internet (~28%) friends and family (~25%), cookbooks (~12%) and television (~12%).

FG-1 and FG-2 participants were asked different questions related to communication channels. When FG-1 participants were asked about US Department of Agriculture (USDA), Food and Nutrition Service materials (e.g., SNAP, The Special Supplemental Nutrition Program for Women, Infants, and Children (WIC), and school materials) as healthful eating resources they reported these resources were not motivating and perceived them as having a "government look". FG-2 participants were asked about Internet usage and on-line social networking opportunities. They reported wanting healthful eating websites to provide actionable information, including food advice, healthful recipes, and preparation shortcuts. Specific suggestions included "fast and easy recipes that kids will eat", "recipes with 5 ingredients or less", "gardening tips (when to plant)", and "age appropriate sections so their children could look for items they could cook." Facebook was the participant's main social media site, more "content" and "more of a network" compared to other sites, and Google their main search site. Finally, the majority of participants stated they like to watch cooking shows (i.e., on the Food Network) to learn about new recipes and preparation tips; however, many felt these recipes were too difficult to replicate. For example, one participant said, "sometimes ingredients are too complicated … ".

Theme 5: Responses to previously developed campaigns and messages.

Materials and messages from out-of-state SNAP-Ed funded SM campaigns were tested in FG-1 to determine if they were a "good fit" for our campaign and if the materials could be used "as is" or in a "modified format". Participants were asked to review two campaigns: Iowa's "Pick a Better Snack" and California's "Champions for Change". They preferred Iowa's campaign and indicated that it featured produce items they would buy/eat and responded positively to its message "Ready-to-Serve." For example, one mom expressed, "If you think about a snack versus a candy bar or bag of chips … get some grapes, you don't have to unwrap them, its easy, it's not that hard to eat healthy."

However, Iowa's "Pick a Better Snack" message "It's That Easy" evoked some negative responses indicating it is not always easy to eat healthfully. One comment was, "It's condescending! It's not that easy! Fruits and veggies are expensive, so it's not easy to buy them."

Reponses to the "Champions for Change" campaign were less favorable. Participants felt that this campaign placed primary responsibility for family food choices on mothers, and that it featured overbearing mothers, with such messages as "My Kitchen, My Rules". They also commented that the kitchen is a family space and not solely mom's space. Participants expected to see media ads for these two campaigns at WIC clinics; however, earlier they indicated that nutrition materials at these clinics did not change their eating behavior. Finally, they reported that both campaigns would have a greater likelihood of changing their FV purchasing behaviors if delivered in a grocery store. Although some FG participants mentioned they would like these messages to come home from school in their children's backpacks, earlier in the FGs they said these materials were treated as junk mail.

After reviewing FG-1 and PS-1 results, it was determined that a new SM campaign should be designed. Components of a new campaign were created including two mock-up campaign names, three logos, and seven messages (Figure 2, Table 1). FG-2 was used to test these components. Of the name/logo combinations tested, Food Hero name/logo number 1 tested best (Figure 2). Participants saw themselves as being "Food Heroes" and talked about making their children and others "Food Heroes." They gave feedback on colors and logo use. Participants were asked to rate FV messages (Table 1) on a scale of 1–10 (1 = very bad; 10 = very good). They preferred positive messages that promoted good role modeling within the family, and did not like negative messages or messages that emphasized their financial struggles. They readily accepted messages that were perceived as genuine, and quickly rejected messages they considered disingenuous regardless if they were true or not. The highest rated message was "canned, frozen, or fresh they all start out the same." The other messages are presented in rank order in Table 1.

3.2. Phone Survey 2

The following two key themes/outcomes emerged from PS-2: 1) participant recall and awareness of the Food Hero campaign and 2) beliefs about FVs.

Main Themes

Theme 1: Participant recall and awareness of the Food Hero campaign.

Within the intervention counties, 12% of participants recalled the Food Hero name vs. 3% of participants from the control county. When participants were asked the question, "When you hear the phrase "Food Hero" what is the first word or phrase that you think of?", 60% in the intervention counties correctly interpreted the intended meaning of Food Hero vs. only 23% in the control county. Participants associated Food Hero with eating nutritiously, being a good role model, and eating FVs. For the intervention counties, 68% recalled hearing or seeing at least one of the campaign messages (Table 1). The message with the greatest recall (58%) was "Give them more of the good stuff". SNAP households in intervention counties received this message via direct mail, and on billboards in all counties except Josephine County due to a lack of SNAP-Ed approved billboard locations.

Theme 2: Beliefs about fruits and vegetables.

Campaign participants were asked to respond to a series of eight belief statements regarding FV use (Table 2). With data combined for all intervention counties, three of these belief statements showed significant change from PS-1 to PS-2 ($p < 0.05$). First, participants reported it was easier to get their family to eat fruit. Second, they were less likely to report that it was time consuming to prepare healthful food. Third, they were less likely to report that it was expensive to eat a diet that included "a lot of" FVs.

When comparing PS-2 for the intervention versus the control county for the same eight belief statements (Table 2) the results were similar except for two belief statements ($p < 0.05$). First, the control county had significantly lower confidence in serving balanced meals for their family. Second, they were less likely to report that canned fruit was just as healthy as fresh fruit.

4. Discussion

This study describes the development, implementation and testing of a SM campaign that targets low-income mothers with the goal of increasing child/family FV intake. Three key outcomes resulted from the campaign development: (1) segmentation of the target audience into online and non-online groups, and the inclusion of a secondary target audience (e.g., children); (2) showcasing all forms of FVs (i.e., fresh, frozen, canned, dried and juice); and (3) focusing on positive, actionable messages.

The campaign audience was determined to be SNAP-eligible mothers with children, as they were most often the food buyer/meal preparer in the household. This decision supports data showing that in the US, women do the bulk of these household activities [24,25]. More than 50% of PS-1 participants (86% female) reported wanting to obtain healthful eating information from the Internet, including both single/multi adult households and those age 25–34 years, while the other half did not mention the Internet. Thus, the campaign audience was divided into two segments to address their different communication needs (internet users and non-internet users). The primary segment (53.3%) was mothers who mentioned going online for healthy eating information (i.e., FoodHero.org web site and a campaign social media platform). A secondary segment was for mothers who did not mention going online for healthy eating information (46.7%) (i.e., contents of the community kit such as the printed Food Hero monthly magazine and media buys in grocery stores). It is likely that the segment of mothers who go online for healthy eating information has grown as current Internet usage by US adults with a household income <$30,000/year is 77%; 17% higher than in 2009 [26,27]. Social networking site usage of online adults US adults with a household income <$30,000/year is 79% [28].

The secondary campaign audience was determined to be children of the target mothers who live with their mothers and ≤18 years. In the FGs and PSs mothers talked about engaging and empowering their children with regard to cooking and eating healthy foods. For example, mothers talked about wanting to be healthy eating role models for their children and including children in cooking and increasing children's acceptance of healthy foods. Similar to our results, Treiman et al. [29] found that Maryland WIC participants taking part in FG interviews ($n = 239$) were highly motivated to be good role models for their children, as were mothers ($n = 140$) who participated in the USDA Maximizing the Message FG project [30]. Campaign components developed for the secondary campaign audience were designed to empower children to be positively involved in healthful food shopping and meal preparation (i.e., inclusion of "kids can" tips in the Food Hero Monthly magazine, a statewide search for children's artwork to feature in the annual recipe focused calendar, a large segment of Food Hero on the ground cooking/tasting events occurring in schools).

Recipes became the primary product of the campaign since the FG results indicated mothers wanted quick and healthy recipes their children would enjoy. Research shows that as in-home food preparation increases (including within food insecure households) FV intake also increases [31,32]. A major campaign strategy was to include multiple forms of FVs in Food Hero recipes, thus, promoting different types of affordable FVs. This strategy was adopted to lower the consistently reported time/financial burdens and low household variety of FV types used in the home. Incorporating a greater variety of vegetables into the diet has been shown to increase vegetable intake and overall diet quality, including the diets of low-income women [33,34].

FG-2 participants responded well to messages promoting frozen/canned FV. Research shows that frozen/canned FV are cost effective and healthy, and in most cases only take minutes to heat up and serve [35–39]. However, our participants, in alignment with the USDA Maximizing the Message project participants, felt frozen/canned FV were less healthful and desirable than fresh despite the majority of them reporting "low-price" as a shopping priority and 46% reporting "healthy food is time consuming to prepare" [30]. "Low-price" and "time" have been reported by others as food buying influencers and 'cost' a barrier to FV consumption; yet, canned FV intake continues to decline in the US [40–45]. Canned FV purchases are highest for high-income households, and decline with children in the home [43]. Our results are important since little research exists to describe why mothers prefer fresh FV to canned or frozen. Similar to our results, Black et al., [46] found that Maryland WIC participants (*n* = 223) preferred fresh FV vs. canned due to taste (e.g., disliked the "canned taste") and did not feel comfortable feeding canned to their children. For a low-income audience, actionable strategies to increase intake of healthy, low cost canned and frozen FV along with fresh FV might increase FV consumption, including variety of FV.

Based on the pre-campaign research, campaign development focused on actionable, positive and empowering messages and materials that were genuine, non-governmental looking, and appeared to be delivered by a trusted friend or family member. Participants clearly indicated they understood the importance of healthful eating and were willing to include more FVs in their diets yet, like most US adults, they were not meeting the current FV recommendations (≥ 5 cups FV/day) [11]. Thus, the SM campaign focused on actionable messages that would help mothers increase FV intake amidst their time/financial limited resources and desire to be healthy role models, versus a focus on the importance of FV. Similarly, the USDA Maximizing the Message project also found that moms responded well to actionable, genuine messages, that would fit into their busy lives [30]. Campaign messages were structured to be applicable to the target population's situation, aiming to limit/lower their household burdens, and not emphasizing their financial struggles (i.e., those rated higher in Table 1). Our use of positive (gain-framed) vs. negative (loss-framed) messaging is an effective way to promote health behaviors especially for adherence to preventative behaviors like healthful eating [47–50].

Results showed that participants in the intervention counties recalled awareness of the campaign. When comparing PS-1 to PS-2 questions examining beliefs about FV (Table 2), results were either positive or neutral, providing some feedback on the potential impact of the campaign. We do not know if the Food Hero campaign was responsible for the positive pre/post changes as other factors may have influenced participants' FV beliefs (e.g., other campaigns, changes in the economy, or seasonality). However, the results are useful for future comparisons and have aided in the refinement of the campaign.

4.1. Study Strengths

Overall, this research has four key strengths. First, to our knowledge this is the first SM campaign, aimed at FV intake for SNAP-eligible families by targeting mothers, that has outlined the formative steps used for campaign development, including implementation and testing of a pilot campaign. Research on formative assessment of FV SM campaigns differed from ours in their breath (national campaigns with broad audiences), focus (local campaigns and audiences), audience (focused on low-income parents not mothers), or provided no assessments (focused on mothers but no assessments reported) [15,51–57]

Second, only SNAP participants were recruited using a random sample provided by Oregon's DHS. Third, mixed methods were used to gain in-depth understanding of our target mothers. Fourth, rural and urban counties were included to determine if the same campaign worked for these different populations.

4.2. Limitations

Study limitations are primarily related to funder guidelines: (1) The project needed to be completed within 1-year, which limited key development factors (e.g., in-depth message testing, cognitive testing of the belief questions, comprehensive website development, pilot campaign length); and (2) Only direct education and SM were allowed with SNAP-Ed funds, thus, at the time of development we could not fully engage in PSE change strategies. Consequently, we could only pilot test the Food Hero SM campaign for 2 months, with plans for later assessments that would measure change in FV behavior. Finally, the outcomes from the Food Hero SM campaign may not be generalizable to other population groups, since we had a specific target group of low-income mothers with children in the home and who spoke English.

4.3. Implications for Research and Practice

As a result of this research, the Food Hero SM campaign has evolved and is now a statewide campaign. Currently over 125,000 unique users visit FoodHero.org each month, with over 2.2 million page views in 2015. Since the research described in this paper was conducted, ongoing FGs and PSs with the Food Hero primary and secondary audiences have helped to further refine our campaign components. Behavior change assessments are being done to determine changes in FV intake, PSE strategies incorporated, and both English and Spanish language versions of the campaign are available.

Others working to increase FV intake with low-income mothers can use the insights learned from our target population for their own research/programs. Additionally, we provide an example of potential steps to take to create a new campaign and/or test existing campaigns. Finally, perceptions of different forms of FVs gained from this research can be used to frame FV messaging in health promotion.

5. Conclusions

For SM to demonstrate positive behavior change outcomes, campaigns must follow evidence-based practices, such as being designed and tested for a specific audience. Following such processes will allow research to be compared and aggregated. To use an existing SM campaign, it is imperative that the intended audience is a close match to the audience for which the SM campaign was designed.

Acknowledgments: Oregon SNAP-Ed funding supported the research, but no SNAP-Ed funds were used for publication costs.

Author Contributions: L.N.T. and M.M.M. conceived and designed the experiments; K.H. and N.B collected and analyzed the data; L.N.T. and M.M.M. wrote the paper.

Conflicts of Interest: The authors declare no conflict of interest. The research protocol followed funder guidelines, but the funding sponsors were not involved in the collection, analyses, or interpretation of data, in the writing of the manuscript, and in the decision to publish the results.

Abbreviations

The following abbreviations are used in this manuscript:

FV	Fruits and Vegetables
SNAP	Supplemental Nutrition Assistance Program
BRFSS	Behavioral Risk Factor Surveillance System
SNAP-Ed	Supplemental Nutrition Assistance Program—Education
DHS	The Oregon Department of Human Services
PSE	Policy Systems and Environmental change efforts
FG	Focus Group
PS	Phone Survey
SM	Social Marketing
SCT	Social Cognitive Theory
USDA	United States Department of Agriculture

References

1. Association of Arizona Food Banks. Feeding America. Map the Meal Gap. Available online: http://www.azfoodbanks.org/index.php/hunger/ (accessed on 7 September 2016).
2. Oregon Department of Human Services. July snap caseloads, 2000 through 2013. Unpublished work, 2015.

3. Oregon Department of Human Services, Oregon Public Health. Oregon Overweight, Obesity, Physical Activity and Nutrition Facts. Available online: http://library.state.or.us/blogs/ReadAllAboutItOregon/wordpress/2012/05/oregon-overweight-obesity-physical-activity-and-nutrition-facts/ (accessed on 7 September 2016).

4. Centers for Disease Control and Prevention (CDC). Nutrition, Physical Activity and Obesity Data, Trends and Maps. Available online: https://nccd.cdc.gov/NPAO_DTM/ (accessed on 7 September 2016).

5. Darmon, N.; Drewnowski, A. Does social class predict diet quality? *Am. J. Clin. Nutr.* **2008**, *87*, 1107–1117. [PubMed]

6. Drewnowski, A.; Darmon, N. The economics of obesity: Dietary energy density and energy cost. *Am. J. Clin. Nutr.* **2005**, *82*, 265S–273S. [PubMed]

7. 2015 Dietary Guidelines Advisory Committee. Scientific Report of the 2015 Dietary Guidelines Advisory Committee. Available online: https://health.gov/dietaryguidelines/2015/guidelines/ (accessed on 7 September 2016).

8. Haynes-Maslow, L.; Parsons, S.E.; Wheeler, S.B.; Leone, L.A. A qualitative study of perceived barriers to fruit and vegetable consumption among low-income populations, North Carolina, 2011. *Prev. Chronic Dis.* **2013**. [CrossRef] [PubMed]

9. Mcgurie, S. State Indicator Report on Fruits and Vegetables, 2013, Centers for Disease Control and Prevention, Atlanta, GA. *Adv. Nutr.* **2013**, *4*, 665–666. [CrossRef] [PubMed]

10. U.S. Department of Agriculture; U.S. Department of Health and Human Services. *Dietary Guidelines for Americans, 2015*; U.S. Government Printing Office: Washington, DC, USA, 2015.

11. Centers for Disease Control and Prevention (CDC). *Behavioral Risk Factor Surveillance System Data*; U.S. Department of Health and Human Services: Atlanta, GA, USA.

12. Moser, R.; Clayton, P.F. Obesity, Physical Activity And Nutrition In Kansas. Available online: http://www.kdheks.gov/brfss/PDF/2013_Kansas_Obesity_Burden_Document.pdf (accessed on 7 September 2016).

13. Carins, J.E.; Rundle-Thiele, S.R. Eating for the better: A social marketing review (2000–2012). *Public Health Nutr.* **2014**, *17*, 1628–1639. [CrossRef] [PubMed]

14. Gordon, R.; McDermott, L.; Stead, M.; Angus, K. The effectiveness of social marketing interventions for health improvement: What's the evidence? *Public Health* **2006**, *120*, 1133–1139. [CrossRef] [PubMed]

15. Pollard, C.M.; Miller, M.R.; Daly, A.M.; Crouchley, K.E.; O'Donoghue, K.J.; Lang, A.J.; Binns, C.W. Increasing fruit and vegetable consumption: Success of the Western Australian go for 2 & 5 campaign. *Public Health Nutr.* **2008**, *11*, 314–320. [PubMed]

16. Kotler, P.; Lee, N.; Rothschild, M. *Social Marketing: Influencing Behaviors for Good*; Sage Publications: Thousand Oaks, CA, USA, 2006.

17. Hopwood, T.; Merritt, R. Big pocket guide. In *Social Marketing National Benchmark Criteria*, 3rd ed.; UK National Social Marketing Centre: London, UK, 2011.

18. Thomson, C.A.; Ravia, J. A systematic review of behavioral interventions to promote intake of fruit and vegetables. *J. Am. Diet. Assoc.* **2011**, *111*, 1523–1535. [CrossRef] [PubMed]

19. Truong, V.D. Social marketing: A systematic review of research 1998–2012. *Soc. Mark. Q.* **2014**, *20*, 15–34. [CrossRef]

20. Lefebvre, R.C. Theories and models in social marketing. In *Handbook of Marketing and Society*; Bloom, P.N., Gundlach, G.T., Eds.; Sage Publications: Newbury Park, CA, USA, 2000.

21. Serdula, M.; Coates, R.; Byers, T.; Mokdad, A.; Jewell, S.; Chavez, N.; Maresperlman, J.; Newcomb, P.; Ritenbaugh, C.; Treiber, F.; et al. Evaluation of a brief telephone questionnaire to estimate fruit and vegetable consumption in diverse study populations. *Epidemiology* **1993**, *4*, 455–463. [CrossRef] [PubMed]

22. Oregon State University. Food Hero Website. Available online: http://www.foodhero.org/ (accessed on 7 September 2016).

23. Tobey, L.N.; Manore, M.M. Social media and nutrition education: The food hero experience. *J. Nutr. Educ. Behav.* **2014**, *46*, 128–133. [CrossRef] [PubMed]

24. US Department of Labor. Household Activities. Available online: http://www.bls.gov/tus/charts/household.htm (accessed on 7 September 2016).

25. US Department of Labor. Purchasing Goods and Services. Available online: http://www.bls.gov/tus/current/purchasing.htm (accessed on 7 September 2016).

26. Pew Research Center. Internet, Broadband and Cell Phone Statistics. Available online: http://www.pewinternet.org/2010/01/05/internet-broadband-and-cell-phone-statistics/ (accessed on 7 September 2016).
27. Pew Research Center. Internet User Demographics. Available online: http://www.pewinternet.org/data-trend/teens/internet-user-demographics/ (accessed on 7 September 2016).
28. Pew Research Center. Social Media User Demographics. Available online: http://www.pewinternet.org/data-trend/social-media/social-media-user-demographics/ (accessed on 7 September 2016).
29. Treiman, K.; Freimuth, V.; Damron, D.; Lasswell, A.; Anliker, J.; Havas, S.; Langenberg, P.; Feldman, R. Attitudes and behaviors related to fruits and vegetables among low-income women in the WIC program. *J. Nutr. Educ.* **1996**, *28*, 149–156. [CrossRef]
30. United States Department of Agriculture. Maximizing the Message: Helping Moms and Kids Make Healthier Food Choices. Available online: https://snaped.fns.usda.gov/materials/maximizing-message-helping-moms-and-kids-make-healthier-food-choices (accessed on 7 September 2016).
31. McLaughlin, C.; Tarasuk, V.; Kreiger, N. An examination of at-home food preparation activity among low-income, food-insecure women. *J. Am. Diet. Assoc.* **2003**, *103*, 1506–1512. [CrossRef] [PubMed]
32. Monsivais, P.; Aggarwal, A.; Drewnowski, A. Time spent on home food preparation and indicators of healthy eating. *Am. J. Prev. Med.* **2014**, *47*, 796–802. [CrossRef] [PubMed]
33. Keim, N.L.; Forester, S.M.; Lyly, M.; Aaron, G.J.; Townsend, M.S. Vegetable variety is a key to improved diet quality in low-income women in California. *J. Acad. Nutr. Diet.* **2014**, *114*, 430–435. [CrossRef] [PubMed]
34. Meengs, J.S.; Roe, L.S.; Rolls, B.J. Vegetable variety: An effective strategy to increase vegetable intake in adults. *J. Acad. Nutr. Diet.* **2012**, *112*, 1211–1215. [CrossRef] [PubMed]
35. Rickman, J.C.; Barret, D.M.; Bruhn, C.M. Nutritional comparison of fresh, frozen and canned fruits and vegetables. Part 1. Vitamins C and B and phenolic compounds. *J. Sci. Food Agric.* **2007**, *87*, 930–944. [CrossRef]
36. Rickman, J.C.; Bruhn, C.M.; Barrett, D.M. Nutritional comparison of fresh, frozen, and canned fruits and vegetables II. Vitamin A and carotenoids, vitamin E, minerals and fiber. *J. Sci. Food Agric.* **2007**, *87*, 1185–1196. [CrossRef]
37. Freedman, M.R.; Fulgoni, V.L., III. Canned vegetable and fruit consumption is associated with changes in nutrient intake and higher diet quality in children and adults: National health and nutrition examination survey 2001–2010. *J. Acad. Nutr. Diet.* **2016**, *116*, 940–948. [CrossRef] [PubMed]
38. Comerford, K.B. Frequent canned food use is positively associated with nutrient-dense food group consumption and higher nutrient intakes in us children and adults. *Nutrients* **2015**, *7*, 5586–5600. [CrossRef] [PubMed]
39. Miller, S.R.; Knudson, W.A. Nutrition and cost comparisons of select canned, frozen, and fresh fruits and vegetables. *Am. J. Lifestyle Med.* **2014**, *8*, 430–437. [CrossRef]
40. Hornick, B.A.; Childs, N.M.; Smith Edge, M.; Kapsak, W.R.; Dooher, C.; White, C. Is it time to rethink nutrition communications? A 5-year retrospective of Americans' attitudes toward food, nutrition, and health. *J. Acad. Nutr. Diet.* **2013**, *113*, 14–23. [CrossRef] [PubMed]
41. United States Department of Agriculture. SNAP Households Must Balance Multiple Priorities to Achieve A Healthful Diet. Available online: http://www.ers.usda.gov/amber-waves/2014-november/snap-households-must-balance-multiple-priorities-to-achieve-a-healthful-diet.aspx#.V8kaFjXENOc (accessed on 7 September 2016).
42. Mushi-Brunt, C.; Haire-Joshu, D.; Elliott, M. Food spending behaviors and perceptions are associated with fruit and vegetable intake among parents and their preadolescent children. *J. Nutr. Educ. Behav.* **2007**, *39*, 26–30. [CrossRef] [PubMed]
43. Buzby, J.C.; Wells, H.F.; Kumcu, A.; Lin, B.-H.; Lucier, G.; Perez, A. *Canned Fruit and Vegetable Consumption in the United States, an Updated Report to Congress*; US Department of Agriculture, Economic Research Service: Washington, DC, USA, 2010.
44. Produce for Better Health Foundation. State of the Plate, 2015 Study on America's Consumption of Fruit and Vegetables. Available online: http://www.pbhfoundation.org/pdfs/about/res/pbh_res/State_of_the_Plate_2015_WEB_Bookmarked.pdf (accessed on 7 September 2016).
45. Eikenberry, N.; Smith, C. Healthful eating: Perceptions, motivations, barriers, and promoters in low-income minnesota communities. *J. Am. Diet. Assoc.* **2004**, *104*, 1158–1161. [CrossRef] [PubMed]

46. Black, M.M.; Hurley, K.M.; Oberlander, S.E.; Hager, E.R.; McGill, A.E.; White, N.T.; Quigg, A.M. Participants' comments on changes in the revised special supplemental nutrition program for women, infants, and children food packages: The maryland food preference study. *J. Am. Diet. Assoc.* **2009**, *109*, 116–123. [CrossRef] [PubMed]

47. Wansink, B.; Pope, L. When do gain-framed health messages work better than fear appeals? *Nutr. Rev.* **2015**, *73*, 4–11. [CrossRef] [PubMed]

48. Patterson, R.E.; Satia, J.A.; Kristal, A.R.; Neuhouser, M.L.; Drewnowski, A. Is there a consumer backlash against the diet and health message? *J. Am. Diet. Assoc.* **2001**, *101*, 37–41. [CrossRef]

49. Gallagher, K.M.; Updegraff, J.A. Health message framing effects on attitudes, intentions, and behaviors: A meta-analytic review. *Ann. Behav. Med.* **2013**, *46*, 127. [CrossRef]

50. Rothman, A.J.; Salovey, P. Shaping perceptions to motivate healthy behavior: The role of message framing. *Psychol. Bull.* **1997**, *121*, 3–19. [CrossRef] [PubMed]

51. Pivonka, E.; Seymour, J.; McKenna, J.; Baxter, S.D.; Williams, S. Development of the behaviorally focused fruits & veggies—More matters public health initiative. *J. Am. Diet. Assoc.* **2011**, *111*, 1570–1577. [PubMed]

52. Shive, S.E.; Morris, M.N. Evaluation of the energize your life! Social marketing campaign pilot study to increase fruit intake among community college students. *J. Am. Coll. Health* **2006**, *55*, 33–39. [CrossRef] [PubMed]

53. Glasson, C.; Chapman, K.; Wilson, T.; Gander, K.; Hughes, C.; Hudson, N.; James, E. Increased exposure to community-based education and 'below the line' social marketing results in increased fruit and vegetable consumption. *Public Health Nutr.* **2013**, *16*, 1961–1970. [CrossRef] [PubMed]

54. Woodhouse, L.; Bussell, P.; Jones, S.; Lloyd, H.; Macdowall, W.; Merritt, R. Bostin value: An intervention to increase fruit and vegetable consumption in a deprived neighborhood of dudley, United Kingdom. *Soc. Mark. Q.* **2012**, *18*, 221–233. [CrossRef]

55. Dharod, J.M.; Drewette-Card, R.; Crawford, D. Development of the Oxford Hills Healthy Moms Project using a social marketing process: A community-based physical activity and nutrition intervention for low-socioeconomic-status mothers in a rural area in Maine. *Health Promot. Pract.* **2011**, *12*, 312–321. [CrossRef] [PubMed]

56. Hampson, S.E.; Martin, J.; Jorgensen, J.; Barker, M. A social marketing approach to improving the nutrition of low-income women and children: An initial focus group study. *Public Health Nutr.* **2009**, *12*, 1563–1568. [CrossRef] [PubMed]

57. Sugerman, S.; Backman, D.; Foerster, S.B.; Ghirardelli, A.; Linares, A.; Fong, A. Using an opinion poll to build an obesity-prevention social marketing campaign for low-income asian and hispanic immigrants: Report of findings. *J. Nutr. Educ. Behav.* **2011**, *43*, S53–S66. [CrossRef] [PubMed]

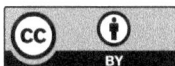

MDPI AG

St. Alban-Anlage 66

4052 Basel, Switzerland

Tel. +41 61 683 77 34

Fax +41 61 302 89 18

http://www.mdpi.com

Nutrients Editorial Office

E-mail: nutrients@mdpi.com

http://www.mdpi.com/journal/nutrients